1985
W. B. SAUNDERS COMPANY
Philadelphia London Toronto
Mexico City Rio de Janeiro
Sydney Tokyo

VETERINARY DENTISTRY

COLIN E. HARVEY, B.V.Sc., M.R.C.V.S.

Professor of Surgery, Department of Clinical Studies,
School of Veterinary Medicine, University of Pennsylvania,
Philadelphia, Pennsylvania

Professor of Surgery, Department of Periodontics,
School of Dental Medicine, University of Pennsylvania,
Philadelphia, Pennsylvania

W. B. Saunders Company: West Washington Square
Philadelphia, PA 19105

1 St. Anne's Road
Eastbourne, East Sussex BN21 3UN, England

1 Goldthorne Avenue
Toronto, Ontario M8Z 5T9, Canada

Apartado 26370—Cedro 512
Mexico 4, D.F., Mexico

Rua Coronel Cabrita, 8
Sao Cristovao Caixa Postal 21176
Rio de Janeiro, Brazil

9 Waltham Street
Artarmon, N.S.W. 2064, Australia

Ichibancho, Central Bldg., 22-1 Ichibancho
Chiyoda-Ku, Tokyo 102, Japan

Library of Congress Cataloging in Publication Data

Harvey, Colin E.
Veterinary dentistry.

1. Veterinary dentistry. I. Title.

SF867.H37 1985 636.089'76 84–13882

ISBN 0-7216-1111-7

Veterinary Dentistry ISBN 0-7216-1111-7

Last digit is the print number: 9 8 7 6 5 4 3 2 1

Contributors

WB Amand, VMD, Director and Chief Veterinarian, Philadelphia Zoological Society

AH Andrews, B Vet Med, PhD, MRCVS, Lecturer in Medicine, Royal Veterinary College, University of London

GJ Baker, BVSc, PhD, MRCVS, Diplomate ACVS, Professor and Head of Equine Medicine and Surgery, College of Veterinary Medicine, University of Illinois

CF Burrows, B Vet Med, PhD, MRCVS, Diplomate ACVIM, Associate Professor of Medicine, College of Veterinary Medicine, University of Florida

AS Dorn, MS, DVM, Diplomate ACVS, Professor of Surgery, College of Veterinary Medicine, University of Tennessee

RR Dubielzig, DVM, DipACVP, Assistant Professor of Pathology, School of Veterinary Medicine, University of Wisconsin, Madison, Wisconsin

DA Garber, BDS, DMD, Dental Practitioner, Atlanta, Georgia; Philadelphia, Pennsylvania

TK Grove, DDS, MS, VMD, Periodontal and Veterinary Dental Practice, Vero Beach, Florida

CE Harvey, BVSc, MRCVS, Diplomate ACVS, Professor of Surgery, School of Veterinary Medicine and School of Dental Medicine, University of Pennsylvania

W Miller, VMD, Assistant Professor of Dermatology, School of Veterinary Medicine, University of Pennsylvania

AM Norris, DVM, Diplomate ACVIM, Assistant Professor of Medicine, Ontario Veterinary College, University of Guelph

RHC Penny, PhD, DVSc, DPM, FRCVS, Professor of Clinical Veterinary Medicine, Royal Veterinary College, University of London

LE Rossman, DMD, Clinical Assistant Professor of Endodontics, School of Dental Medicine, and Adjunct Assistant Professor of Endodontics, School of Veterinary Medicine, University of Pennsylvania

CL Tinkelman, DMD, Clinical Assistant Professor of Endodontics, School of Dental Medicine, University of Pennsylvania, and Dental Consultant, Philadelphia Zoological Society

JP Weigel, DVM, Diplomate ACVS, Associate Professor of Surgery, College of Veterinary Medicine, University of Tennessee

SJ Withrow, DVM, Diplomate ACVS, Associate Professor of Oncology, College of Veterinary Medicine, Colorado State University

SL Yankell, PhD, RDH, Research Associate Professor, School of Dental Medicine, University of Pennsylvania

Preface

This book was written with several purposes in mind. The major purpose is to provide a comprehensive yet concise account of the anatomy, pathogenesis, diagnosis, and management of oral diseases to serve as a textbook for veterinary students.

It should also serve as a reference text for veterinarians in practice, with helpful information for immediate and everyday use in their work. A third purpose is to provide a source of information for dentists interested in collaborating with their veterinary colleagues; much frustration can be avoided by being aware of "what works and what does not" when a health professional with specialized training crosses species lines to treat a superficially familiar problem.

In deciding what information to include in this book, the other contributors and I have used the word "dentistry" in its wider sense of oral disease management, rather than of treatment of diseases affecting the teeth. The technical aspects of repairing dental and gingival diseases continue to be a challenge at times, though much progress has been made. Diagnosis and management of chronic oral inflammatory and ulcerative diseases require much more observation and investigation before we can claim to have a full grasp of the subject; it is no surprise that Oral Medicine is one of the longest chapters in the book.

I would like to thank my coauthors and the editorial and production staff at W. B. Saunders Co. for their expertise and cooperation in producing this book, and Mr. Ray Sze for preparing the line drawings in Chapters 4, 6, 10, 11, and 12.

I welcome comments and constructive criticism of this volume.

COLIN E HARVEY

Contents

Introduction

Diseases of the oral cavity of domesticated animals are common and often severe. They may interfere with function in the animal by preventing eating, and thus lead to economic loss. They may also cause circumstances, such as halitosis, that prevent the normal interaction of companionship with the owner of the animal. The economic consequences have been well known for many years. The consequences of the loss of companionship are only now beginning to be understood.

As advances are made in treatment and control of other major abnormalities affecting companion animals, such as infectious diseases and neoplasia, gradually progressive diseases such as periodontal disease are going to demand more attention and expertise from the health professionals attending these patients. Management of geriatric diseases, including dental disease, is an expanding field; appreciation of efforts expended here is obvious from both the patient and the client who values the longstanding and undemanding friendship of his or her pet.

The range of species that are usually considered to be domesticated is wide. It includes herbivores, omnivores, and carnivores. These three major groups have different needs that must be met by their oral structures; the functional adaptations are described briefly in Chapter 1 and in detail for each species in subsequent chapters. These different needs are reflected in the dissimilarity in the incidence and severity of diseases of the oral cavity of our species, with one exception. Periodontal disease is a common and sometimes severe disease in humans and in all domesticated mammals that are permitted to live their natural lifespan. Effective management and control of this disease in companion animals is the area that most requires investigation in veterinary dentistry.

The study of diseases of the oral cavity in veterinary species has a long history. During the heyday of the horse as a means of transportation, particular attention was paid to the teeth as a means of determining age. After all, a horse 10 years of age was worth a lot more than one 25 years old as a potential source of transportation or energy. Many books devoted to or including sections on the teeth of horses have been written over the centuries, though the medical and surgical management of dental diseases described in most of them seems uninformed and even barbaric. Doctoring horses' teeth to hide their true age is an ancient art, no doubt still practiced by those who think they can get away with it.

Scientific contributions to the understanding of dental diseases in animals did not appear until about the end of the 19th century. Studies were reported but were mostly limited to observations made on dead material because of the difficulties of restraint and examination of live subjects; further progress did not occur until reliable, safe drugs for chemical restraint were available. Often the most available material for study was dried skulls. Soft tissue lesions could only be inferred. The apogee of this era was reached with the publication in 1936 of the monumental book by Sir Frank Colyer on *Variations and Diseases of the Teeth of Animals*. He detailed the results of examining almost 30,000 skulls from numerous species—both domesticated and wild—in 750 pages.

Since that time, there has been a mushrooming of both interest in and reported studies on dental and oral diseases of animals. Austrian and German veterinarians, particularly Joseph Bodingbauer, made many significant contributions, culminating in the publication of a detailed and beautifully illustrated veterinary text in German (*Tierarztliche Zahnheilkunde*) on diseases of teeth by Erich Eisenmenger and Karl Zetner in 1982.

On the other side of the Atlantic, the prime mover for increasing interest in and knowledge of veterinary dentistry has been Donald Ross, who established the first veterinary dental specialist practice. An American Veterinary Dental Society has been growing in membership and activities under the leadership of Dr. Ben Colmery. Veterinarians, dentists, and others interested in veterinary dentistry are invited to join the Society. I will be happy to forward correspondence to the Society Secretary.

There is a long history of cooperation, and sometimes confusion, among human dentists and veterinarians regarding the dental care of animals. Techniques that are routinely successful in humans often are not applicable to veterinary patients because of differences in anatomy, lack of convenient access to the oral cavity, poor home care, and expense. The last several years have seen the gradual development of techniques adapted to veterinary patients, so that a project such as this textbook can reasonably claim to cover veterinary dentistry in an objective and scientific way.

There has been considerable interest among dentists in recent years regarding the establishment of veterinary dental clinics. The regulations covering medical and dental care of animals differ from country to country and from state to state or province to province in North America. Generally, the rules can be summarized as stating that veterinarians are the only professionals permitted to diagnose and treat an animal belonging to a third party. Most states permit other professionals such as dentists to consult with or perform procedures on client-owned animals under the direct supervision of a veterinarian. Because of the diversity of rulings in different administrative areas evident from results of a recent survey of the Veterinary Medical Examining Boards, veterinarians and dentists wishing to collaborate with each other are urged to check with their local practice regulating authorities.

Dental anatomical terms are often confusing and incorrect when applied to veterinary species. The teeth of species of major veterinary interest do not have rather uniform rows of teeth forming a continuous curve in both jaws. Mesial and distal do not apply and are terms that are not in general use in this context by veterinarians. In this book, uniformity of terminology has been attempted. All teeth on the maxilla and premaxilla (incisive) bones are referred to as upper teeth; teeth in the mandible are referred to as lower teeth. The side of the tooth facing inward is called the lingual or palatal surface; the outward-facing surface is the labial or buccal surface. Interdental surface applies only if the tooth is in contact with another on that jaw; otherwise, rostral and caudal are used for surfaces of the teeth on the long axis of the dental arcade. Jaw length abnormalities are a particular source of confusion. When the lower jaw extends abnormally beyond the upper jaw, the condition is usually referred to as prognathia; most animals affected in fact have a mandible of normal length, but the maxilla is pathologically short. This condition is referred to in this book as brachycephalism. The usual name for the opposite condition, brachygnathia, is probably correct for most animals affected, and is used here.

Equipment and supplies for dental procedures are unknown territory for most veterinarians. Not all veterinary schools have a dental engine of any sort; exposure to the terminology of and sources for instruments and supplies is lacking in the veterinary curriculum. Some instruments and supplies are shown in the appropriate sections of this book. Dental practitioners often are willing to discuss options and sources, and may enjoy "hands-on" collaboration. The market for veterinary dental supplies is now being recognized. Companies such as Henry Schein Inc., (5 Harbor Park Drive, Port Washington, New York 11050) provide catalogs and can supply instrument and supplies sets specifically designed for small animal dental practice.

COLIN E HARVEY

Chapter One

Function and Formation of the Oral Cavity

CE Harvey

FUNCTION

The major function of the oral structures can be summarized as the introduction of food and fluids into the alimentary canal. This is true of all animals, but it is met in different ways by different species. Other functions include protection (against external forces such as predators or societal rivals by biting and against microbial invaders) and grooming. In some species, additional functions include heat loss, sexual enhancement by licking and taste stimulation, and communication (both vocal and visual, as in lip raising or teeth baring, which can be either a welcome or a warning).

Food must first be identified, usually by olfactory or visual stimulation. Herbivorous species use their incisor teeth to cut or tear vegetation free. They do not need a mouth with a large opening, but they require long arcades of grinding teeth; a large lip opening would allow ingesta undergoing mastication to fall out of the mouth. Herbivores have little functional use for well-developed canine teeth.

Carnivorous species often must first subdue their food source. They usually do this with their canine teeth, and an opening is needed that is large enough for the sectorial (carnassial) teeth to engage part of the prey so that it can be cut into pieces small enough to swallow.

Omnivorous species, of which the most obvious is the pig, have an oral structure with attributes of both herbivores and carnivores, though the diet of the domesticated pig leaves little need for dental function.

The extent of teeth wear also varies. Herbivores undergo rapid, constant attrition from grinding vegetation. In contrast, carnivores do not grind their food and thus do not have extensive tooth wear. This difference is reflected functionally in the continuous eruption of the teeth in herbivores and the defined eruption of carnivore teeth. This may allow the teeth of carnivores, which are more likely to be subjected to severe lateral stress during the tearing of flesh, to be held more securely by the attachment apparatus.

The ability to move the jaw varies considerably. Carnivores have a much greater angle of maximum oral opening than do herbivores, but they have a very limited ability to move the jaws in other than an open-close maneuver. This allows the temporomandibular joint to be surrounded by ligaments that prevent disruption of the joint when tremendous occlusive forces are applied, for example, during the cracking of bones. Herbivores have a much flatter temporomandibular joint surface, which allows the mandible to slide from side to side and back to front in addition to opening and closing. This movement allows the upper and lower teeth to grind fibrous material between them in several directions.

Once an amount small enough to swallow is separated from the food source, the food is either sent directly to the pharynx, as in cats and dogs, or is directed to the cheek teeth for mastication. Some herbivores, such as ruminants that regurgitate at will, may delay the crushing action of mastication by swallowing the food, which goes into a storage area, while grazing continues. The placement of the food bolus in the mouth, and the entire process of drinking, is accomplished by actions of the tongue, an organ that can move in an almost miraculous fashion, stretching and shortening, tipping up or curling down at will.

A bolus that is ready for passage to the pharynx and beyond is pushed there by the tongue. Deglutition is a complex reflex action that prevents inundation of the airway. The bolus must pass caudally from a ventral position to a dorsal position, crossing the airway between the nasopharynx and the larynx. The process starts by the action of the muscles attached to the hyoid bones, causing the hyoid arch and the root of the tongue and larynx that are attached to it to be pulled rostrally. By a simple hinge mechanism, this causes the epiglottis to cover the laryngeal opening (glottis). The tongue moves, forming the bolus and pumping it caudally. As the bolus reaches the pharynx, the nasopharynx is closed by contraction of muscles in the soft palate and nasopharyngeal wall, which form a sphincteric ring. The bolus is now in the pharynx and cannot escape into the larynx, nasopharynx, or oral cavity (which is closed off by the contracted tongue making contact with the roof of the mouth). The cranial esophageal sphincter (cricopharyngeal muscle) relaxes, opening the passageway into the esophagus, and the pharyngeal muscles contract from a rostral to a caudal position, pushing the bolus ahead of the contraction and into the esophagus. Once the bolus has passed, the cricopharyngeal muscle contracts, preventing regurgitation of material into the pharynx. The nasopharyngeal sphincter muscles and the hyoid muscles relax, allowing the larynx to fall back into its resting position and causing the epiglottis to lift from the glottis. Continuity of the airway is thus restored.

The passage of food material is assisted by the secretions of the salivary glands, which lubricate and macerate the food. Salivary secretion is also controlled by reflex, except for a basal secretion level. Parasympathetic fibers in the trigeminal and facial (chorda tympani) nerves cause secretion in response to olfactory, visual, and glossal stimulation.

Grooming in most veterinary species is accomplished by the tongue, which coats the hair with saliva and then removes it. Grooming is an important method for controlling external parasites.

Heat loss in dogs, which have few sweat glands in their skin, is achieved by evaporation of nasal and salivary secretions during panting. The lateral nasal gland, which has a secretion rate that is proportional to ambient temperature, is the major source of fluid for evaporative loss, though the salivary and scattered mucosal glands in the oral cavity contribute. Panting is an efficient one-way (in through the nose, out through the mouth) system that depends on the muscles in the soft palate and the hyoepiglottic muscle for its function.

The immunological function of the lymphatic tissue ring in the oronasal pharynx is discussed in Chapter 11.

Taste is usually thought of as a way of stimulating appetite. This is of unknown importance in veterinary species; the macrosmatic carnivorous species probably depend more on olfaction than gustation as an appetite stimulant.

FORMATION

The digestive tract consists of a blind-ended tube that is formed by entodermal proliferation very early in embryonic development. Connection to the outside world is made by two depressions that form over the cranial and caudal extensions of the primitive gut. The cranial depression, the stomodeum, sinks in until only a thin layer of tissue, the oral plate, separates the two spaces. The oral plate ruptures to establish continuity; it is located at the equivalent of the tonsillar area in the adult. Thus, the oral cavity and related structures are all formed from stomodeal ectoderm and supporting mesenchymal connective tissue.

At the time that the oral plate ruptures, the stomodeum is still very shallow compared with the complex oral cavity present at birth. Subsequent development occurs by forward growth of the structures forming the jaws and face. The mandible and maxilla both start as paired processes. The mandibular processes grow together and join to form the complete mandibular arch. The upper jaw is somewhat more complicated, because the maxillary processes grow together but do not join; they remain separated but fuse with the premaxilla that forms from paired nasomedial processes. The multiple sites of origin of the upper jaw are a major reason for the several, complex congenital anomalies that can occur in this area.

The area formed by the median nasal process (the premaxilla and the site of origin of the upper incisor teeth) is called the primary palate. It may fail to fuse in the midline or on one or both sides with the structures formed from the maxillary processes (the maxilla, all of the upper teeth other than the incisors, which is called the secondary palate). The palate itself is formed in three parts (Fig. 1–1). One part is formed by a triangular rostral contribution from the conjoined me-

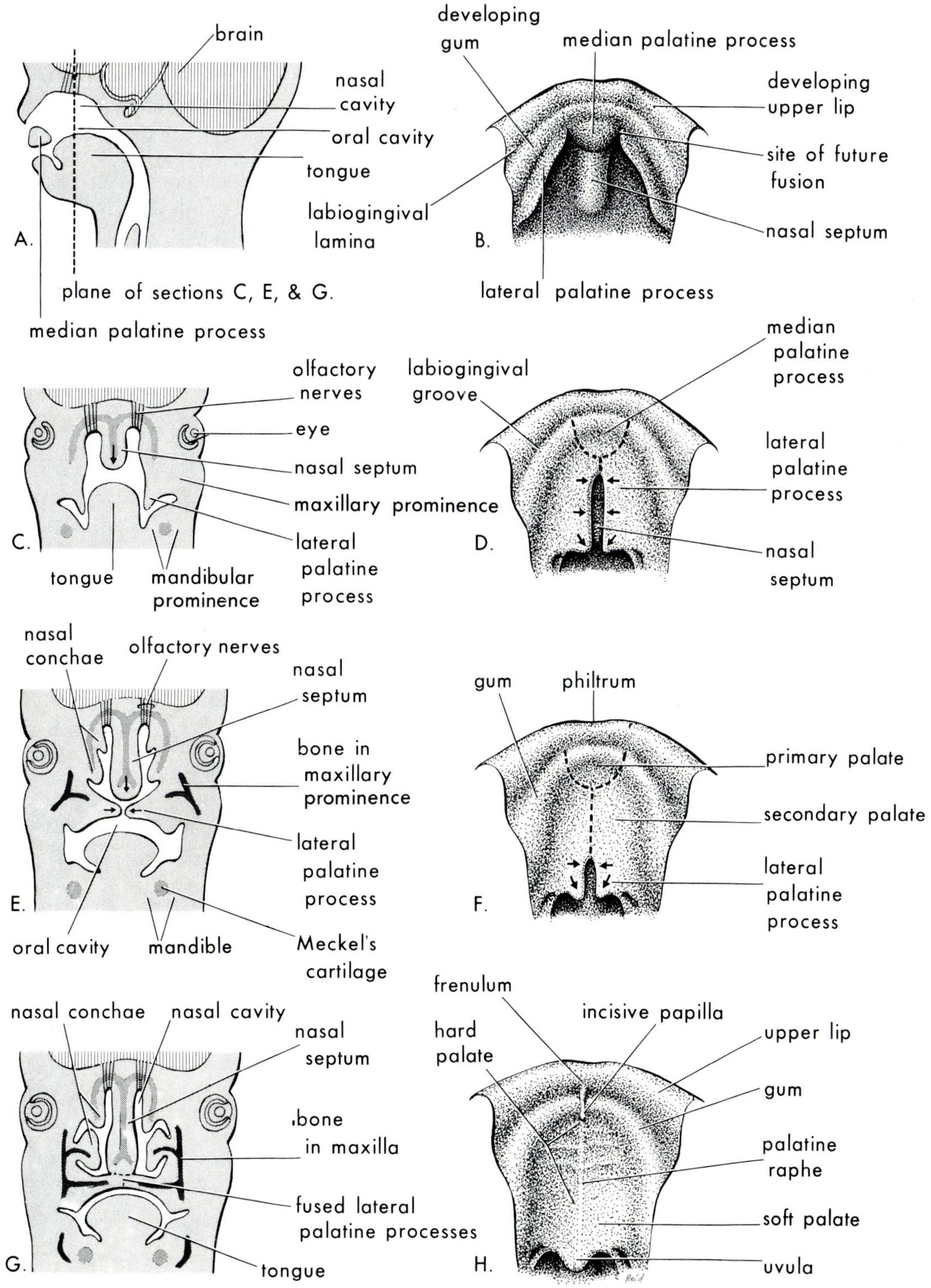

Figure 1–1. Development of the structures forming the roof of the mouth. (From Moore KL: The Developing Human, 3rd ed. Philadelphia, WB Saunders Co., 1982.)

dian nasal processes forming the premaxilla, which becomes the area rostral to and including the incisive papilla. The larger portion of the palate is formed by shelf-like projections that grow in medially from the maxillary processes; these join to separate the nasal cavity from the oral cavity.

The tongue arises from a midline prominence and two lateral swellings that form most of its substance. The origins of the muscles of the tongue are occipital somite myotomes that migrate, carrying with them the hypoglossal nerve, which thus takes a long passage across the lateral tissues of the pharynx. The sensory supply of the tongue is derived from the nerves associated with branchial arches 1 to 4 that form the epithelial surface of the tongue; these nerves are the trigeminal, facial, glossopharyngeal, and vagus nerves.

Teeth arise from a thickening on the jaws called the dental ledge. Epithelial cells push into the underlying mesenchymal tissues to form two structures—a labiogingival lamina that forms the lips, and a dental lamina. The longitudinal dental lamina separates to form buds, the enamel organs (Fig. 1–2). They differentiate into cup-shaped structures with an inner ameloblast layer that surrounds a papilla of mesenchymal cells that proliferate

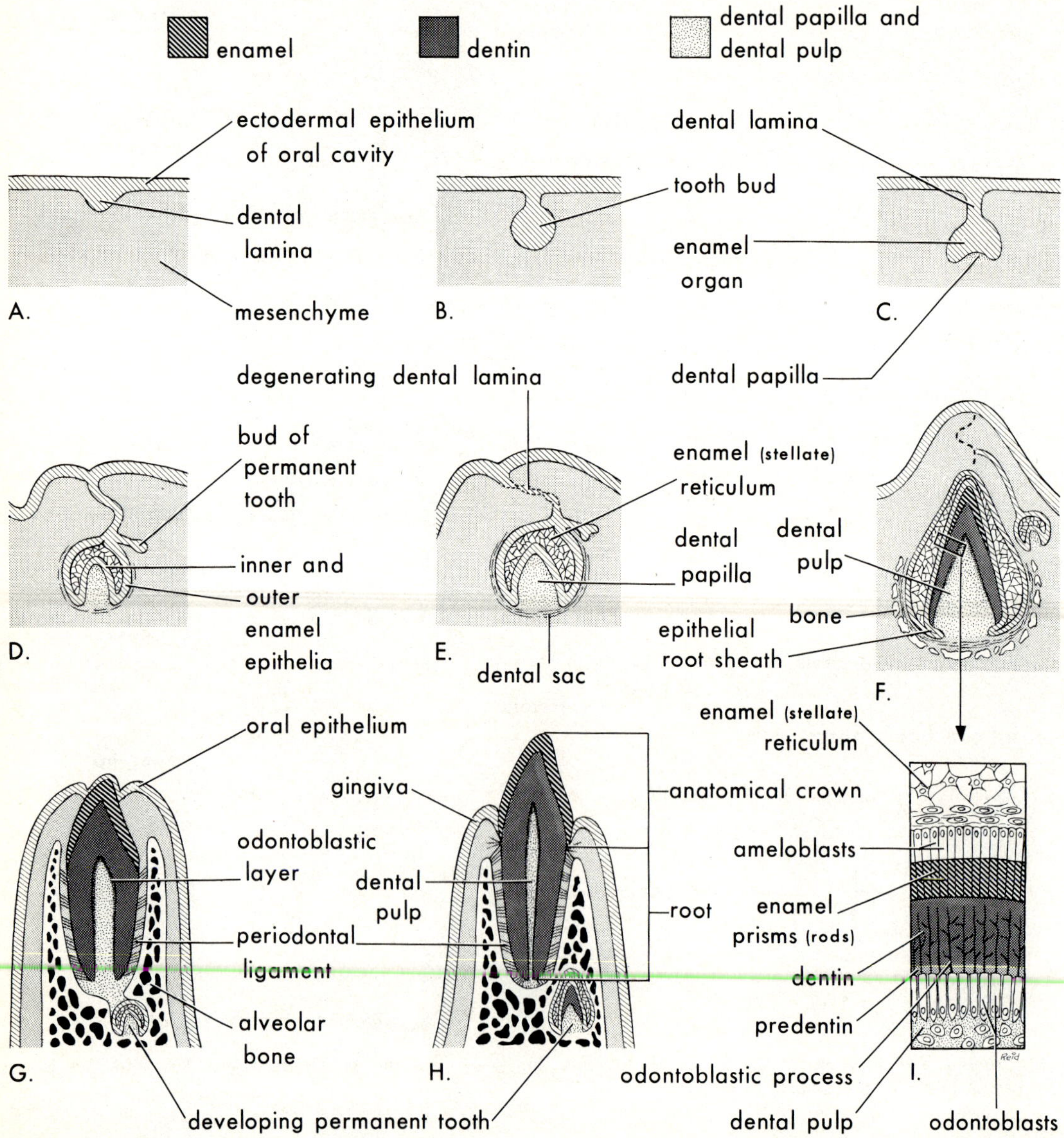

Figure 1–2. Development of a tooth. (From Moore KL: The Developing Human, 3rd ed. Philadelphia, WB Saunders Co., 1982.)

to form the dentin and pulp of the tooth. Nerves and vessels proliferate, sending branches into each papilla, and mandibular or premaxillary-maxillary bone also proliferates so that the calcified structures of the jaws are in place. Both deciduous and permanent teeth buds form within a short time of each other, though the permanent teeth stay dormant for some time, until jaw length has provided space for them.

Dentin is formed by odontoblasts, the outer layer of the mesenchymal dental papilla. Dentin matrix is secreted and later strengthened by deposition of calcium salts. Cytoplasmic strands of the odontoblast cells remain embedded in the dentin. The tissues remaining in the pulp are blood vessels, nerves, and supporting connective tissue.

Enamel is formed by ameloblasts in the inner lining of the enamel organ. A prism of calcified organic matrix forms perpendicular to each ameloblast, providing the strong, rigid surface of the tooth. Crown formation is completed well before root formation. Teeth erupt because of the progressive growth of roots.

Cementum formation does not occur until the tooth is almost full grown and in position. Prior to eruption, the tooth is surrounded by a specialized layer of mesenchymal tissue, the dental sac. Part of this sac is lost during eruption, but the deeper part forms cementum on the dentin surface of the root, much as periosteum forms bone. Between the periosteum of the surrounding bone and the cementoblasts of the dental sac remnant, and embedded in the organic matrix of the two structures, are the periodontal fibers formed from connective tissue in the narrow space.

Formation and mineralization of the calcified structures forming the teeth are described in more detail in Chapter 13.

Permanent teeth erupt at various times in each species. During eruption, the developing permanent tooth enlarges and pushes the deciduous tooth out of position, disrupting its blood supply. The root of the deciduous tooth is resorbed, and the tooth becomes so weakly held in position that occlusal pressure dislodges it from the mouth. Growth of the root of the permanent tooth continues until it is in normal position. Growth of the upper and lower jaws is relatively independent. The succession of deciduous and permanent teeth provides functional dentition of a size suitable for the jaw at the time of eruption and replacement at a later time by a larger set of teeth appropriate for the larger jaws of the mature animal. Jaw growth may be affected by the teeth if the upper and lower teeth lock into position with each other, as is most obviously the case with carnivores. Dental interlock can occur with the deciduous teeth in an abnormal position early in jaw growth, and it can interfere with subsequent normal development of the jaws.

The salivary glands and ducts develop from invaginations of oral epithelium. Myoepithelial cells and autonomic nerves and vessels develop to form the functional unit.

Section One

Oral Disease in the Dog and Cat

Chapter Two

Anatomy of the Oral Cavity in the Dog and Cat

CE Harvey and RR Dubielzig

The oral cavity of the dog and cat differs from other veterinary species in that there is variation in the size and shape of the teeth, and the lips and mouth can be opened to a greater extent.

ANATOMICAL FEATURES

Lips

The opening of the lips is wide, extending to the level of the first molar teeth (Fig. 2–1). The lips themselves are soft and fleshy and are covered by normal hairy skin on the external surface and by non-keratinized squamous epithelium on the inner surface. Between the epithelial surfaces lie the facial muscles, connective tissue and vessels, and the large trigeminal nerve branches serving the vibrissae. As with all oral cavity surfaces, the lips normally are moistened continuously by salivary gland secretions. The upper lip usually overhangs the junction of the lower lip and oral tissues so that the oral epithelium is not normally visible except during eating and drinking or during panting in dogs.

In the dog, the lower lip is rather loosely attached to the mandible and may form a furrow that allows salivary secretions to leak from the mouth. There is a shorter, firmer attachment of the lower lip to the mandible at about the level of the first premolar tooth that causes an indentation of skin; it is this area that forms a valley of skin that becomes diseased in lip-fold dermatitis. The lips, and sometimes the tongue, are often partially pigmented (with the exception of chows, whose tongues are also pigmented).

If the upper lip is lifted and curled out, the openings of two salivary ducts can be seen: the parotid, which appears as a single papilla on the mucosa that normally lies opposite the upper carnassial tooth, and the zygomatic, which appears as a line of several papillae on a ridge of mucosa caudal and medial to the parotid papilla and opposite the last molar tooth.

Teeth[1]

When the lips are raised or the mouth is opened, the most obvious visible structures are the teeth. The surface of normal teeth of dogs is dense white and smooth; the teeth of cats are often slightly yellow compared with those of dogs.

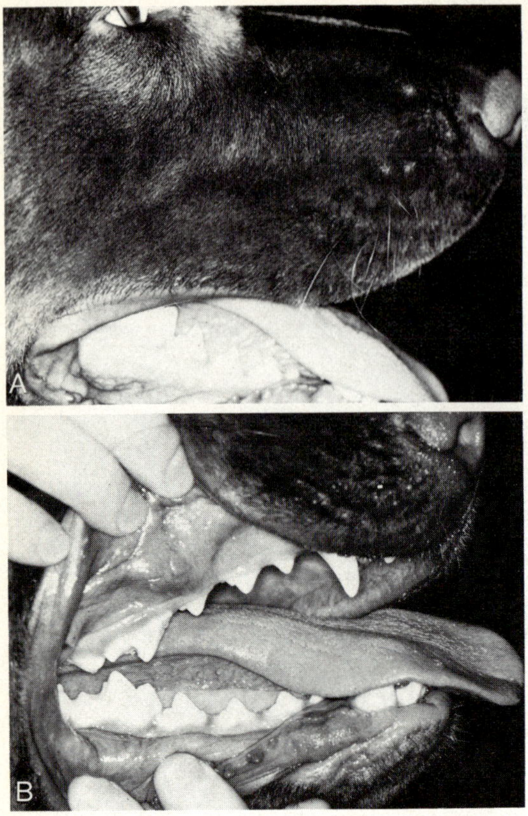

Figure 2–1. Lateral view of the mouth of a dog. *A,* The lip in normal position. *B,* The lip raised to show the teeth, gingivae, and tongue.

Table 2–1. Teeth Eruption Schedules for the Dog and Cat*

	Deciduous Teeth (weeks)		**Permanent Teeth (months)**	
	Dog	***Cat***	***Dog***	***Cat***
Incisors	3–4	2–3	3–5	3–4
Canines	3	3–4	4–6	4–5
Premolars	4–12	3–6	4–6	4–6
Molars	—	—	5–7	4–5

*Variations occur with breed and size of animal. Gingival eruption is followed by extrusion to full crown height over a period of several weeks (or in the case of the canine tooth, several months).

The dental formula of the dog[2] is:

Deciduous: $2\,(I\frac{3}{3}, C\frac{1}{1}, P\frac{3}{3}) = 28$

Permanent: $2\,(I\frac{3}{3}, C\frac{1}{1}, P\frac{4}{4}, M\frac{2}{3}) = 42$

The dental formula of the cat[3] is:

Deciduous: $2\,(I\frac{3}{3}, C\frac{1}{1}, P\frac{3}{2}) = 26$

Permanent: $2\,(I\frac{3}{3}, C\frac{1}{1}, P\frac{3}{2}, M\frac{1}{1}) = 30$

Eruption times are variable;[4–6] eruption schedules and the number of roots of each tooth are shown in Table 2–1 and Figure 2–2. Factors affecting the time of eruption include general health and nutritional state, sex (teeth of females erupt earlier than those of males), body size (teeth of larger breed dogs erupt earlier), and season of birth (teeth of dogs born in the summer erupt earlier).[7] Once the teeth are fully erupted, tooth development ceases except for the laying down of dentin on the inside pulpal surface.

The four canine teeth are the largest teeth and are situated at the rostral corners of the jaws. The single, slightly curved crown tapers smoothly to a rounded tip in the dog and is more pointed in the cat. The canine teeth crowns often have linear grooves in their surface, particularly in cats. In normal occlusion (the so-called scissors bite), the lower canine tooth sits between the upper canine tooth and the upper third incisor tooth. The roots of the canine teeth are single but very large and long—often up to twice as long as the crown and wider than the crown in the midsection. They curve caudally, lying beneath the first and sometimes the second premolar teeth. The upper canine tooth root is indicated by a palpable smooth protuberance on the surface of the maxilla. There is usually a space (diastema) between the canine teeth and the incisor and first premolar tooth. The root apex of the mature tooth contains several small openings (apical delta) for passage of blood vessels and nerves into the pulp cavity.[1] The pulp cavity is much larger and the dentin is thinner in growing dogs; however, by the time the animal has matured, the dentin has thickened so that the adult tooth has a pulp cavity of about one quarter or less of the diameter of the tooth.[8]

The six upper and lower incisor teeth sit in curved lines between the canine teeth; they are usually even in size and, at least early in life, have three cusps at the tip of the crown. Attempts to age dogs by the wear on the cusps of the incisor teeth are not satisfactory because of the variable wear caused by dietary differences. The incisors of cats have a large central cusp and two small lateral protuberances. The roots of the incisor teeth are single and narrower but usually longer than the crowns. The crowns of the incisor teeth usually contact those of adjacent incisor teeth, though in large dogs with dolichocephalic skulls there may be an obvious interdental

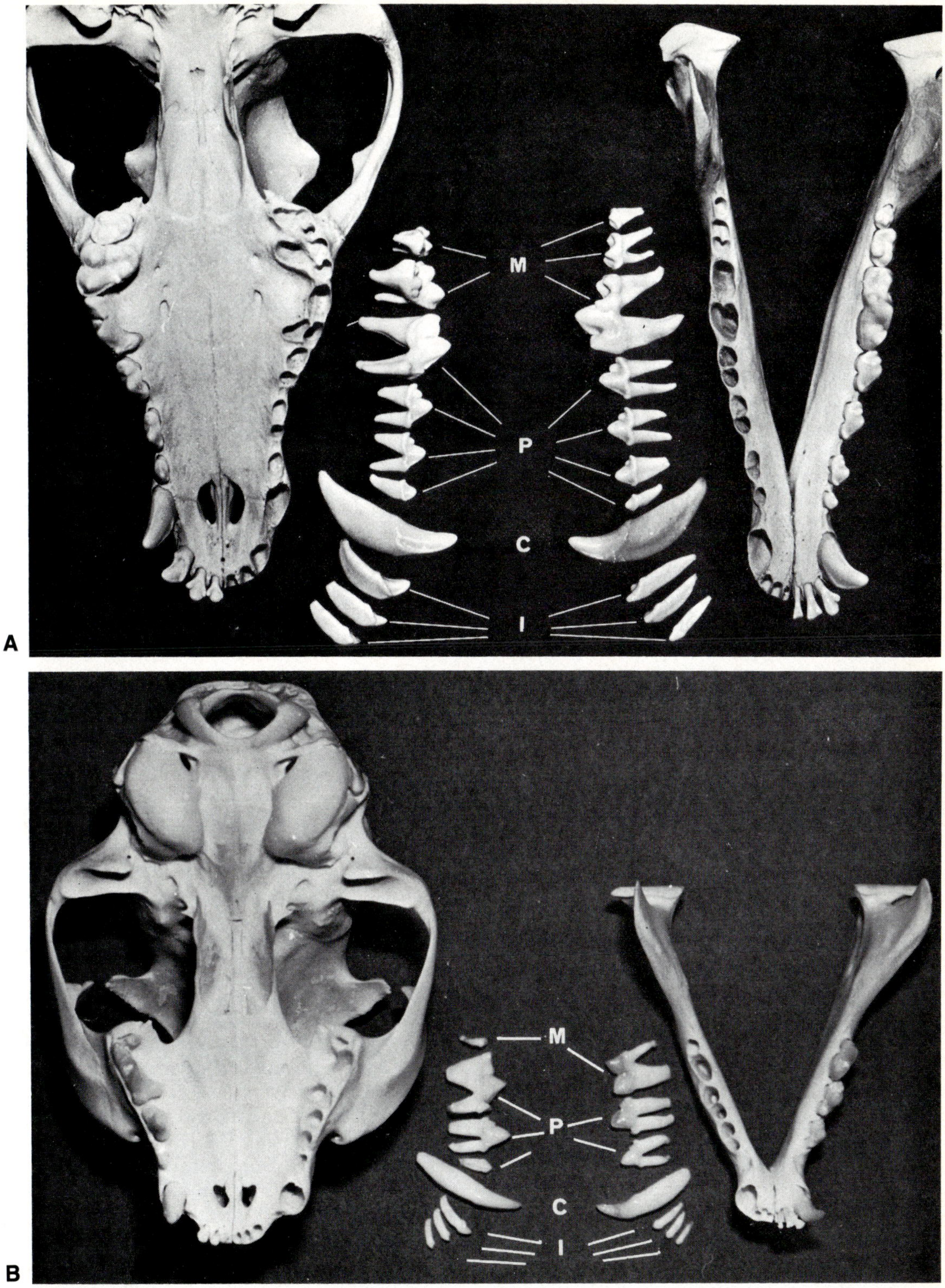

Figure 2–2. *A*, Skull and mandible with the teeth in place on one side and removed and displayed on the other side. *A*, A dog. *B*, A cat. The incisive foramina lie close to the midline between the canine teeth. (C = canine; I = incisor; M = molar; P = premolar teeth.) (From Getty R: Sisson and Grossman's Anatomy of the Domestic Animals, 5th ed. Philadelphia, WB Saunders Co., 1975.)

space. In a dog or cat with normal occlusion, the upper incisor teeth crown tips lie just rostral to and slightly overlap the tips of the lower incisor teeth when the jaws are closed. There is widespread variation in incisor occlusion among dogs; lower incisor placement well rostral to the upper incisors is considered normal in brachycephalic breeds.

The largest and most obvious of the cheek (premolar and molar) teeth are the carnassial teeth, which provide a shearing or scissors action for reducing large sections of meat to a size suitable for swallowing. These teeth are the upper fourth premolar and lower first molar teeth in dogs, and the upper third premolar and lower first molar teeth in cats. The crown of the upper carnassial tooth occludes against the crown of the lower carnassial tooth, which normally lies slightly medial to the upper crown in resting occlusion. The crowns are large and multicusped. The other cheek teeth are usually pointed and, except for the first premolar, are usually multicusped. The upper first molar tooth has three cusps of almost equal size, forming an occlusal surface for crushing. Although caries formation is rare in dogs, the shape of the crown of this tooth makes it the one most likely to be affected. The larger cheek teeth are multirooted (Fig. 2–2), the upper fourth premolar and first molar in dogs and the upper third premolar in cats having three roots. The traditional division into premolar and molar teeth in dogs has been questioned recently. From examination of the anatomy and eruption sequence, it has been suggested that the first upper premolar, fourth upper premolar, and first lower premolar of dogs should be renamed the postcanine, canine premolar, and canine molar, respectively.[9]

Deciduous teeth are smaller and slimmer than permanent teeth. Occlusal contact of deciduous teeth is minimal in dogs.[10]

On microscopic examination, the teeth are seen to be composed of three mineralized matrices (Fig. 2–3). Dentin is the inner layer, which forms the main supporting structure of the tooth apparatus. Both the enamel and the cementum are adherent to the outside surface of the dentin. The enamel makes up the exterior surface of the crown, which is the exposed portion of the tooth. Enamel is approximately 98 percent inorganic, making histological examination difficult because the enamel substance is dissolved during routine decalcification. The gingival epithelium attaches to the tooth at the cemento-enamel

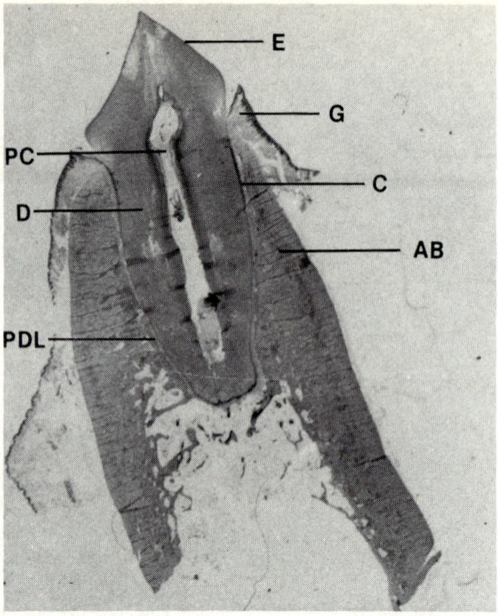

Figure 2–3. Histological section through a tooth in the mandible. (AB = alveolar bone; C = cementum; D = dentin; E = enamel [removed in processing]; G = gingiva; PC = pulp cavity of tooth; PDL = periodontal ligament.)

junction at the bottom of the gingival crevice. The cementum lines the outside portion of the tooth root and provides a point of attachment for the periodontal ligament. Cementum is similar in composition to woven bone; cementocytes can be seen in lacunar spaces in much the same manner as osteocytes occur in bone. Dentin is acellular and approximately 70 percent mineral, making it the second hardest tissue, after enamel, in the body. The dentin matrix is made up of collagen, as is the cementum and bone matrix. Dentin, unlike enamel, is viable tissue capable of reacting to injury and undergoing change. It is formed and maintained throughout life by the odontocytes that line the dental pulp cavity and send apical processes into the dentin matrix. Each apical process is responsible for the formation and maintenance of the dentin matrix immediately around it. The tunnels in which the odontoblastic processes lie are known as the dental tubules. Nerve endings also extend into the dentin through these tubules, making the dentin a sensitive layer in the tooth. The formation and crystal structure of the hard tissues of the teeth are described in more detail in Chapter 13.

The pulp cavity is filled with loosely arranged primitive mesenchymal tissue. Spindle and stellate cells are widely separated by gelatinous ground substance, and the cavity is well vascularized and innervated. The periodontal ligament consists of Sharpey's fibers, which are anchored on the tooth side in the cementum and on the jaw side in the alveolar bone. The ligament is made up of dense connective tissue with abundant collagen bundles. The collagen bundles are less tightly packed and more fibrillar than in the subgingival stroma. Blood vessels generally are widely dilated and evenly distributed in the periodontal ligament.

Jaws

The teeth sit in sockets within the mandible, maxilla, or incisive bone (Fig. 2–4) and are held in place by the periodontal fibers that penetrate both tooth and bone.

The mandible consists of two bones joined rostrally by a fibrous joint. The teeth are contained in the horizontal ramus, a slightly curved section of bone with an obvious medullary cavity and one or more mental foramina piercing the cortex just caudal to the canine tooth. The medullary cavity carries the sensory mental nerves and vessels supplying the teeth. The vertical ramus at the caudal end of the horizontal ramus has three main parts. The most dorsal is the coronoid process, a broad but thin and flat area of bone for attachment of the temporal muscle. Projecting caudally is the articular process; the transversely oriented condyle at its caudal end articulates with the temporal bone. The angular process extends caudoventrally, forming the site of insertion of the pterygoid and masseter muscles. The muscles of mastication (temporal, medial and lateral pterygoid, and masseter) close the jaws, with great force when necessary. The digastricus, a smaller muscle originating on the jugular process of the skull and inserting on the ventral surface of the mandible, causes the jaws to open. The muscles of mastication, and the rostral part of the digastricus muscle, are supplied by the mandibular branch of the trigeminal nerve. The caudal part of the digastricus muscle is supplied by the facial nerve.

The temporomandibular joint is formed between the articular process of the mandible and the mandibular fossa of the temporal bone (Fig. 2–5). The joint surface is separated into a dorsal (temporal) and a ventral (mandibular) compartment by an articular disc. The shapes of the mandibular process and the temporal facet do not match exactly, allowing some sliding as well as hinge movements, though the sliding movement option is less available in the dog and cat than in most other veterinary species. The joint capsule is surrounded by fibrous tissue, which is formed into an obvious ligament laterally.

The incisive, maxillary, and palatine bones form the roof of the mouth and support the

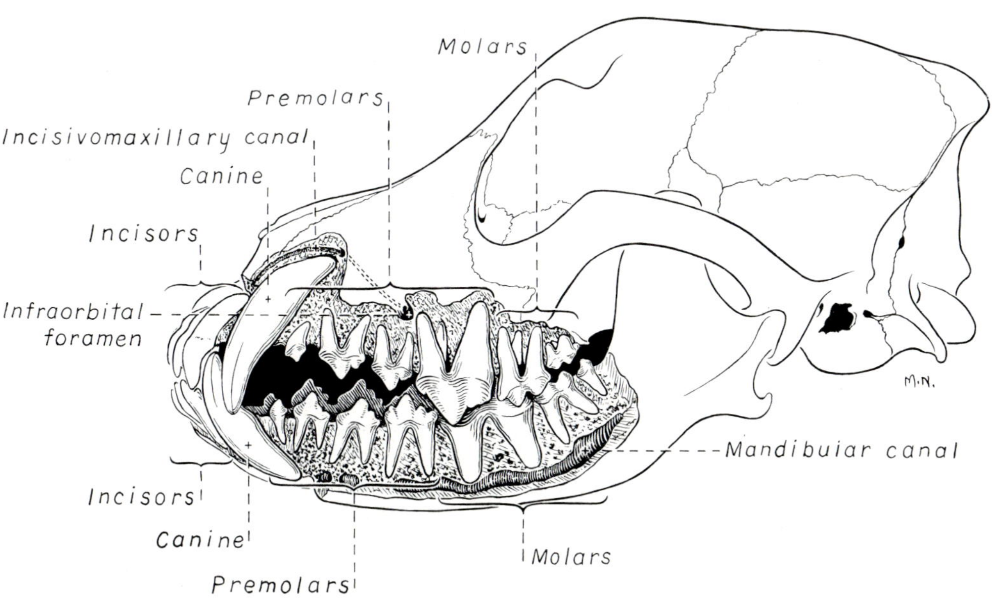

Figure 2–4. Jaws of a dog dissected to show the position of the roots of the teeth. (From Evans HE, Christiansen GC: Miller's Anatomy of the Dog, 2nd ed. Philadelphia, WB Saunders Co., 1979.)

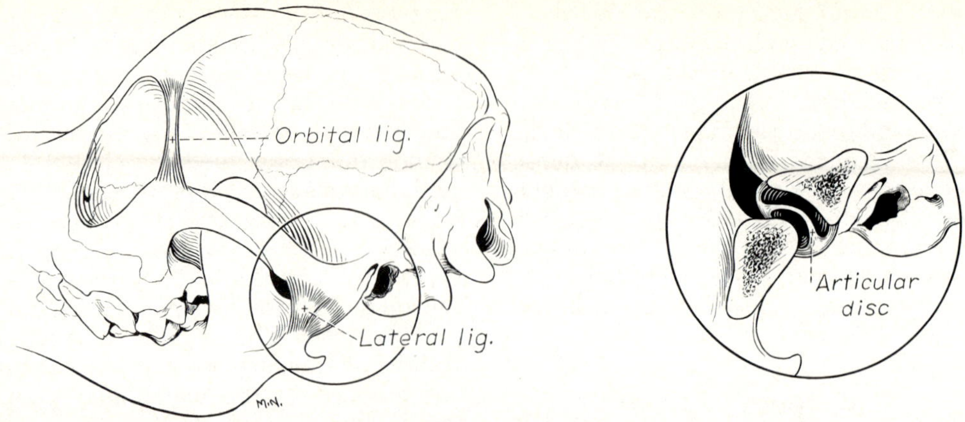

Figure 2–5. Temporomandibular joint of the dog. Lateral aspect and section. (From Evans HE, Christiansen GC: Miller's Anatomy of the Dog, 2nd ed. Philadelphia, WB Saunders Co., 1979.)

upper teeth. Incisor teeth are carried on the incisive bone; "primary" palate abnormalities are restricted to the structures supported by this bone and consist of harelip and asymmetrical rostral cleft palate. There are two large openings in the incisive bones, the palatine fissures (see Fig. 2–2); these openings can often be palpated as soft areas at the rostral end of the palate.

The maxilla carries the canine and cheek teeth. There is a slight alveolar process (dental ridge); however, the cemento-enamel junction of the teeth is generally level with the surface of the mucoperiosteum of the palate. The roots of the teeth thus extend into the maxilla proper, and bony prominences can be seen or felt on the external surface of the maxilla, or they may extend into the nasal spaces. The infraorbital canal, carrying the infraorbital nerves and vessels, is present just dorsal to the roots of the cheek teeth on the lateral aspect of the maxilla.

The upper and lower jaws grow independently of each other. Upper and lower jaw length is also inherited independently.[11] Jaw growth that occurs after eruption of the canine teeth is modified by the interlocking of the canine and corner incisor teeth.

The palatine bones do not contain teeth. They separate the oral and nasal cavities. "Secondary" palate abnormalities affect this area and are seen as a failure to fuse in the midline, usually extending into the soft palate. The soft palate is attached to the caudal end of the palatine bones.

Oral Soft Tissues

The gingivae surrounding the teeth are normally tightly adherent and should not admit a periodontal probe more than 2 mm to 3 mm into the potential space between the gingiva and the tooth. Histologically, the gingivae are composed of epithelium and stroma. The epithelium is tightly attached to the relatively non-elastic stroma and through that to the underlying bone. The epithelium is a multilayered stratified squamous epithelium that is generally considered to be non-keratinizing; however, a thin layer of keratinocytes may occasionally be seen. There are no adnexal or glandular structures in the gingivae, and the epithelium and stroma interdigitate in a series of stromal papillae and epithelial rete pegs. The stroma consists of a rather haphazardly arranged network of dense collagen fibers and blood vessels. The gingivae and periodontal tissues are described in more detail in Chapter 5.

Laterally, the gingivae are continuous with the mucosa of the lips at the mucogingival junction. Medially, on the upper jaw, the gingivae are continuous without obvious demarcation with the mucoperiosteum of the palate; on the lower jaw, the sublingual mucosa attaches to the gingivae at the mucogingival junction, forming a trough between the mandible and the tongue. The mandibular and sublingual salivary gland ducts run submucosally in this tissue before opening onto the lingual caruncle lateral to the frenulum of the tongue. Large sublingual veins are often visible through the mucosa in this area. The palatal mucosa is thrown into obvious folds that lie perpendicular to the long axis of the palate; in the cat, these folds often have a line of small projections. At the rostral end of the palate lies a midline protuberance, the incisive papilla (Fig. 2–6). The nasopalatine ducts open just lateral to this papilla;

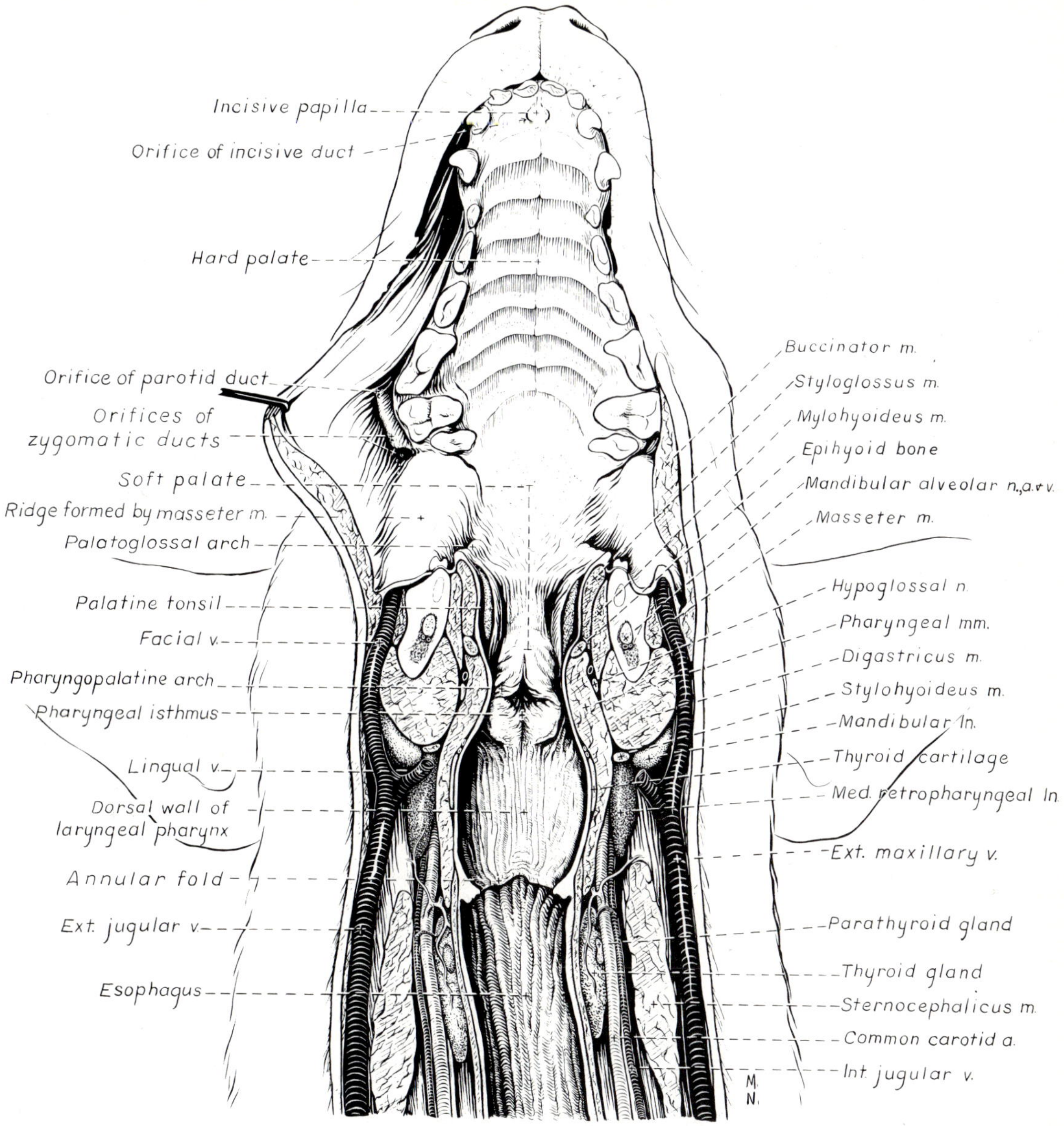

Figure 2–6. Frontal section of head and neck of a dog showing the palate and pharynx. (From Evans HE, Christiansen GC: Miller's Anatomy of the Dog, 2nd ed. Philadelphia, WB Saunders Co., 1979.)

fluid may squirt out of these ducts during nasal flushing.

The tongue, though very long, is usually retained in the mouth except when the animal is sleeping or panting; brachycephalic dogs may carry their tongues in an extruded position at other times. Its dorsal surface is covered by a thick mucosa that is thrown into papillae. Specialized areas of mucosa form the taste buds. Taste sensation is of little clinical significance in companion animals and has been described in detail elsewhere.[2] In the dog, the surface of the tongue is soft, compared with the rather stiff, rough surface of the tongue of the cat. A dorsal midline groove extends along the rostral surface of the tongue. Hairs arranged in a midline row or in two symmetrical rows parallel to the midline are seen in occasional dogs. In newborn animals, the lateral surfaces of the tongue are fimbriated. The rostral end of the tongue is free, and the lingual frenulum ventrally is loose, allowing the tongue to extend a considerable distance.

The major function of the tongue is to form food boluses and to lap fluids. Its muscular structure is complex. The free rostral end contains a stiffening rod, the lyssa (septum linguae), which is formed of fat and muscle in a fibrous sheath; the ancients believed that this structure was the source of rabies and attempted to prevent or treat the disease by excising the lyssa. The motor nerve supply is the hypoglossal (XII) nerve. The sensory supply is a combination of trigeminal (V), facial (VII), glossopharyngeal (IX), and vagus (X) nerves, combining special sensory responses from the taste buds with normal sensory function.

The principal blood supply to the oral region is via the maxillary, facial, and lingual arteries, which are branches of the external carotid arteries. The maxillary artery supplies the palate, mandible, and associated muscles and gives off the infraorbital artery supplying the maxilla. The facial artery, together with branches from the infraorbital artery, supplies the lips and superficial facial muscles. The lingual artery supplies the tongue. The collateral circulation system in the dog and cat is very well organized; both common carotid arteries can be ligated in dogs with no clinically obvious effects.[12] Venous drainage is via the linguofacial vein and branches of the maxillary vein; these two systems join to form the external jugular vein. A major branch of the lingual vein, the hyoid venous arch, crosses the ventral midline in a superficial position rostral to the larynx. Lymphatic channels are plentiful in the head and neck. The major lymph nodes draining oral and pharyngeal structures are the facial, parotid, mandibular and, of major importance, the retropharyngeal nodes; lymphatic drainage caudally is via the cervical lymph nodes and tracheal trunks, which terminate either in the thoracic duct or directly into a venous structure at the thoracic inlet.[2]

Pharynx

The pharynx is a muscular tube that is lined by stratified squamous epithelium (Figs. 2–6 and Fig. 2–7). It connects the oral cavity, the nasal meatus at the caudal end of the nasal cavities, and the esophagus and larynx caudally. The airway spaces are supported by the hyoid bony arch, which also provides a point of insertion for many of the muscles that cause closure of the nasopharynx as well as contraction of the pharynx itself during deglutition. Motor nerve supply is via the glossopharyngeal and vagus nerves. The pharynx contains a prominent ring of lymphatic tissue, the most obvious part being the paired palatine tonsils that lie in folds of the

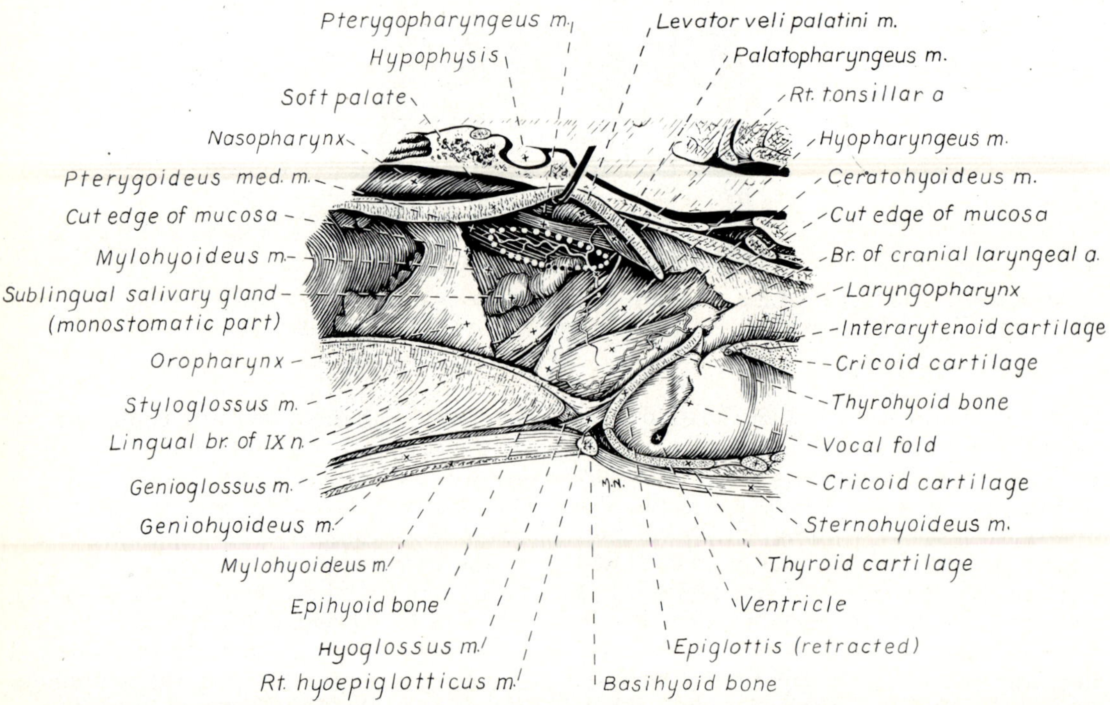

Figure 2–7. Median section through the pharynx of a dog. Location of tonsil indicated by dotted oval. Mucosa has been partly removed, and the soft palate is elevated. (From Evans HE, Christiansen GC: Miller's Anatomy of the Dog, 2nd ed. Philadelphia, WB Saunders Co., 1979.)

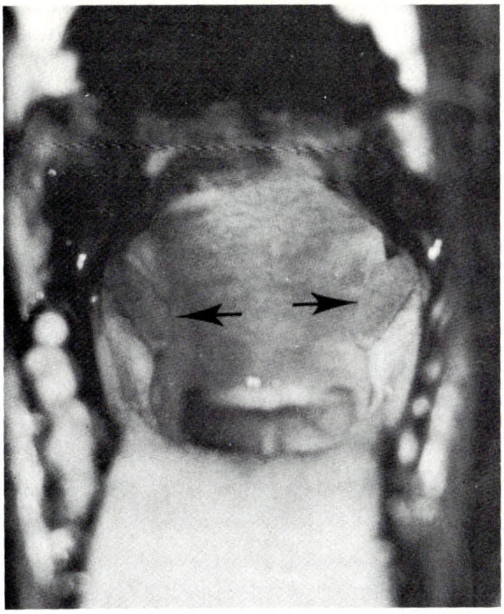

Figure 2–8. View of the dog's pharynx from the mouth. The tonsils are indicated (*arrows*). (From Ettinger SJ (ed): Textbook of Veterinary Internal Medicine, 2nd ed. Philadelphia, WB Saunders Co., 1983.)

pharyngeal mucosa on the lateral surface of the oropharynx (Figs. 2–7 and 2–8).[13] The soft palate, a caudal extension of the hard palate separating the nasal and oral cavities, forms the dorsal margin of the oropharynx. The soft palate contains muscles, which contract to close off the nasal cavity during swallowing; glandular tissue and supporting connective tissue; and nerves and vessels between the nasal and oral epithelia. The parallel hamular processes projecting ventrally from the base of the skull can be palpated through the soft palate. The caudal edge of the soft palate is at approximately the level of the cranial tip of the epiglottis, though there is considerable variation, particularly in brachycephalic dogs. The close appositional relationship between the soft palate and the epiglottis in horses is not essential in dogs and cats. The uvula, which is the midline soft fleshy protuberance found on the free edge of the soft palate in some other species, is not present in the dog and cat.

Salivary Glands

The mouth is richly endowed with serous and seromucous glands and mucus-secreting cells on the epithelial surface. Scattered areas of glandular tissue are present submucosally in the lips and are sometimes identified as the dorsal and ventral buccal glands. The tongue, soft palate, and pharyngeal wall also contain acinar groups. The major salivary glands of the dog and cat are the paired parotid, mandibular, sublingual, and zygomatic glands (Fig. 2–9).

The triangular parotid gland is a serous gland located on the side of the face, surrounding the horizontal ear canal. Compared with the other major glands, its margins are indistinct because the lobules at the periphery of the gland are held together loosely by connective tissue and blend with the subcutaneous fat and connective tissue of the muscles of the external ear. The duct of the parotid gland lies in an exposed position on the side of the face. It forms from a branched collecting system within the gland that leaves the gland on the rostral edge and runs over the aponeurosis of the masseter muscle. It bends medially and opens into the mouth on a prominent papilla at the level of the upper fourth premolar (carnassial) tooth. The secretory nerve supply is carried in the glossopharyngeal nerve and auriculotemporal branch of the trigeminal nerve.

The mandibular gland is a large, ovoid structure lying within a strong fibrous capsule caudal and ventral to the parotid gland. The maxillary vein covers the caudodorsal aspect of the gland, and the mandibular lymph nodes lie on the dorsal and ventral surfaces of the linguofacial vein, which runs along the ventral aspect of the mandibular gland. The mandibular duct runs rostrally between the mandible and the root of the tongue, and it opens into the mouth on the lateral surface of the lingual caruncle at the base of the frenulum of the tongue.

The sublingual gland is a longer, less compact gland. The caudal lobe of the gland is intimately attached to the cranial surface of the mandibular gland. The sublingual gland and duct accompany the mandibular duct, running deep to the digastricus muscle. The gland is formed into caudal and rostral lobes, though there is considerable variation in the shape and location of the lobules. The sublingual duct either opens as a separate passage on the lingual caruncle or joins with the mandibular duct, in which case there is only one opening. The mandibular and sublingual glands are both mixed glands.

The zygomatic gland is a mixed gland with an irregular ovoid shape that lies on the floor of the orbit ventrocaudal to the eye. The gland lies immediately medial to the zygomatic arch and on top of the infraorbital nerve and vessels. Several ducts, of which the

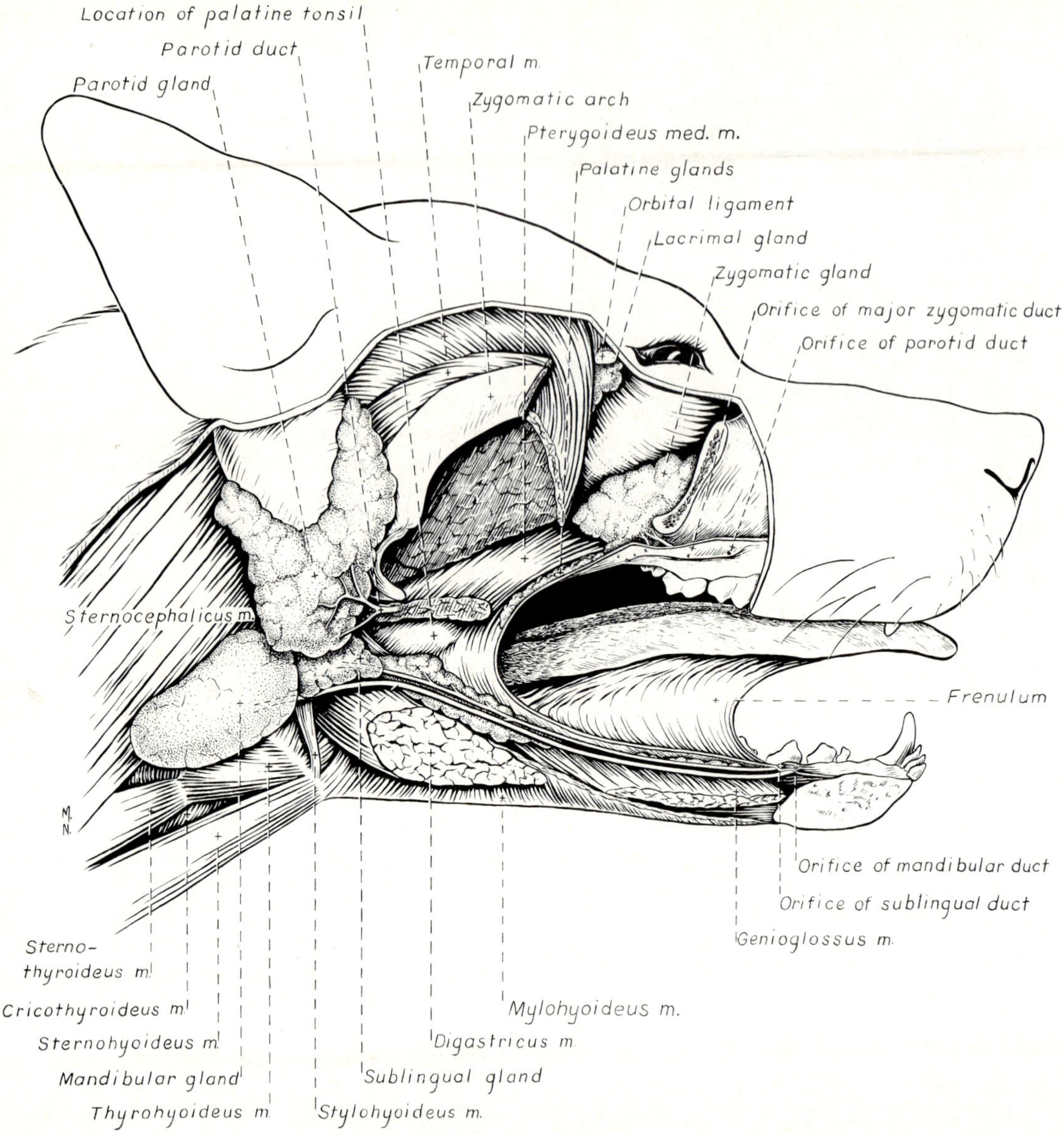

Figure 2–9. Lateral view of a partially dissected head of a dog showing the major salivary glands and ducts (parotid duct partially removed). (From Evans HE, Christiansen GC: Miller's Anatomy of the Dog, 2nd ed. Philadelphia, WB Saunders Co., 1979.)

most rostral is the largest, run ventrally and open on a fold of mucosa lateral to the maxillary second molar tooth.

The radiographic anatomy of the salivary glands as demonstrated by sialography is shown in Chapter 12.

RADIOGRAPHIC APPEARANCE OF NORMAL ORAL STRUCTURES

The dental structures are generally more dense than surrounding bone, and the enamel surrounding the crown is particularly dense. Between the root of the tooth and the adjacent alveolar bone is the periodontal ligament, seen radiographically as a radiolucent line. The cortex of the alveolar bone is more compact than the bone forming the rest of the maxilla and mandible; this layer of dense bone between the radiolucent periodontal ligament space and the surrounding bone is known as the lamina dura.[14] On detailed radiographs of normal teeth and jaws, the pattern formed by the varying densities of structures forming the jaws is very obvious (Fig. 2–10). Variations in pattern, number of

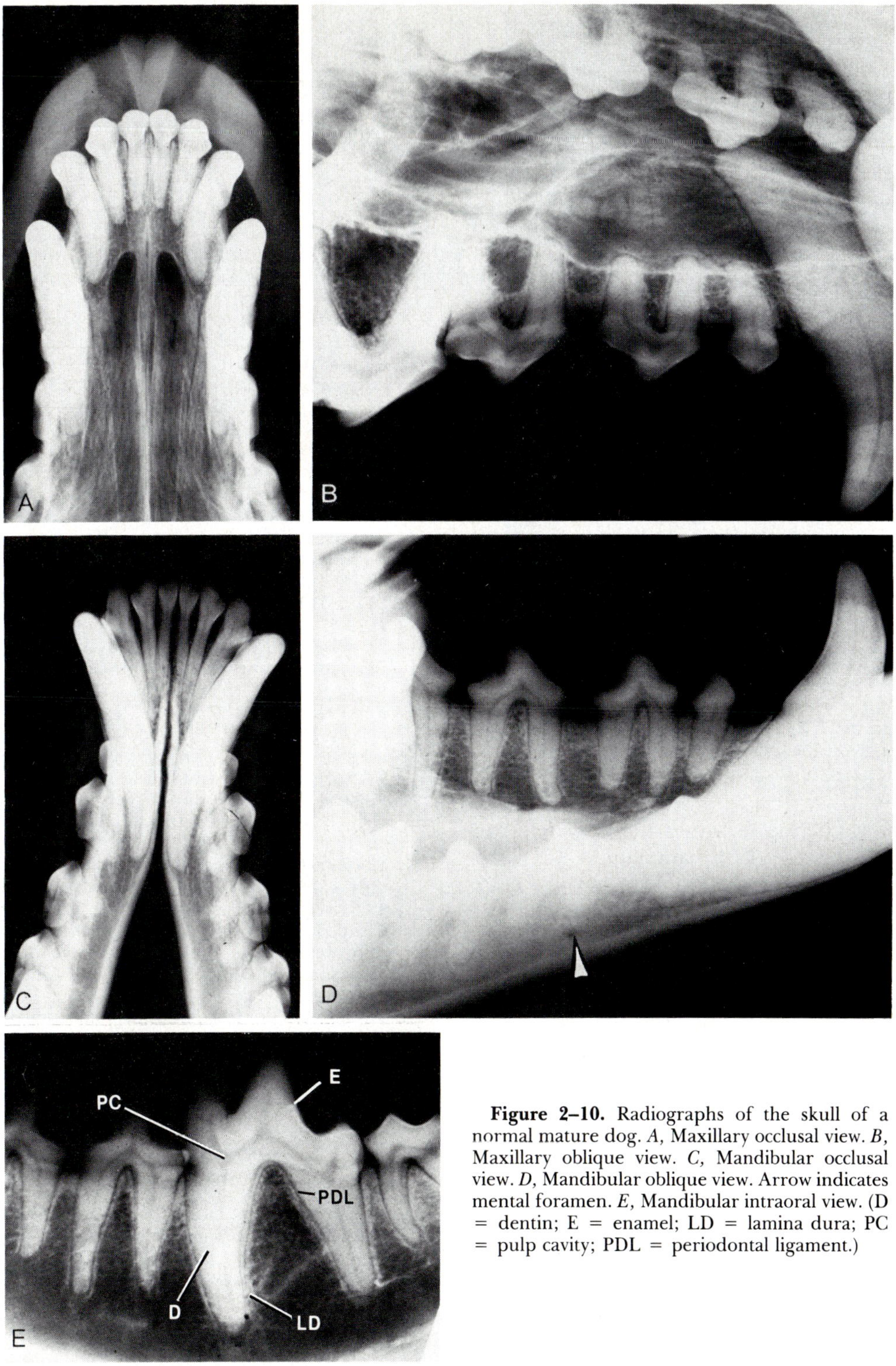

Figure 2–10. Radiographs of the skull of a normal mature dog. *A,* Maxillary occlusal view. *B,* Maxillary oblique view. *C,* Mandibular occlusal view. *D,* Mandibular oblique view. Arrow indicates mental foramen. *E,* Mandibular intraoral view. (D = dentin; E = enamel; LD = lamina dura; PC = pulp cavity; PDL = periodontal ligament.)

teeth, smoothness of the enamel, cementum and dentin of the teeth, height of alveolar bone, and density of bone are indicative of disease. Normal anatomical features include the mental foramina (Fig. 2–10), which can be confused with apical abscesses or cysts. There is a tremendous variation in the position, and less often the number, of teeth in the jaws of dogs. There is less variation in cats.

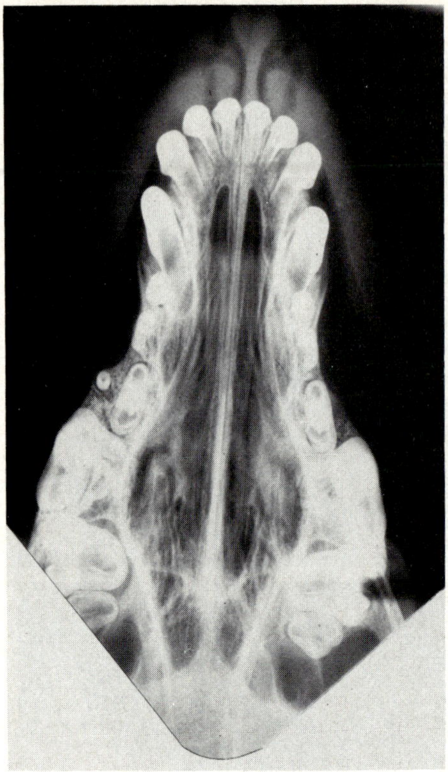

Figure 2–11. Radiographs of the maxilla of a 5 month old dog. Note the wide, open ended pulp cavities in this figure compared with Figure 2–7.

The radiographic appearance of teeth varies with the age of the animal. At birth, the crowns of all the deciduous teeth are calcified; the roots begin to become calcified at 5 to 10 days of age and are completely calcified at 30 to 40 days of age. The permanent crown of the lower carnassial tooth is calcified at birth. Calcification of the other permanent crowns starts at 5 to 10 days for the incisors and canines; at 20 to 30 days for the premolars, first upper molar, and second lower molar; and at about 70 days for the second upper molar and the third lower molar in dogs.[15–17] The deciduous teeth are usually exfoliated by 6 months of age (see Table 2–1).

The pulp cavity of the permanent teeth in immature animals is wide, and is surrounded by a narrow rim of enamel, cementum, and dentin (Fig. 2–11). As the animal ages, the width of the radiodense tissue increases so that at maturity there is only a narrow pulp cavity present (see Fig. 2–10),[14] unless development of the dentin is interfered with by a traumatic insult.[18] Immature teeth have an open root apex; the root appears closed on radiographs of mature dogs, because the channels in the apical delta are too fine to be seen.

References

1. Lawson DD, Nixon GS, Noble HW, Weipers WL: Dental anatomy and histology of the dog. *Res Vet Sci* 1:201–204, 1960.
2. Evans HE, Christensen GC: Miller's Anatomy of the Dog, 2nd ed. Philadelphia, WB Saunders Co., 1979.
3. Berman E, Davis J, Stara JF: Dental chart of the domestic cat. *Lab Anim Care* 17:511–513, 1967.
4. Arnall L: Some aspects of dental development in the dog: Eruption and extrusion. *J Small Anim Pract* 1:259–267, 1961.
5. Berman E: The time and pattern of eruption of the permanent teeth of the cat. *Lab Anim Sci* 24:929–931, 1974.
6. Kremenak CR: Dental eruption chronology in dogs: Deciduous teeth gingival emergence. *J Dent Res* 48:1177–1184, 1969.
7. Lawer DR: Canine tooth eruption. *Calif Vet* 33:6, 1979.
8. Lawson DD, Nixon GS, Noble HW, Weipers WL: Development and eruption of the canine dentition. *Br Vet J* 123:26–30, 1967.
9. Ross DMJ, Neuhaus RG, de Neuhaus IP, Pagliari de Ross MC, Marx G: Chronologie der zahnentwicklung des hundes. *Tierarztl Umschau* 34:418–430, 1979.
10. McKeown M: The deciduous dentition of the dog—Its form and function. *Irish Vet J* 25:169–173, 1971.
11. Stockard CR: The genetic and endocrinic basis for differences in form and behavior. *Am Anat Memoir* 19, Wistar Inst, Philadelphia, 1941.
12. Clendenin MA, Conrad MC: Collateral vessel development after chronic bilateral common carotid artery occlusion in the dog. *Am J Vet Res* 40:1244–1246, 1979.
13. Frewein J: Zur topographischen anatomie der tonsilla palatina des hundes. *Schweiz Arch Teirheil* 118:265–270, 1976.
14. Zontine WJ: Dental radiographic technique and interpretation. *Vet Clin North Am* 4:741–762, 1974.
15. Arnall L: Some aspects of dental development in the dog: Calcification of crown and root of the deciduous dentitions. *J Small Anim Pract* 1:169–173, 1961.
16. McKeown M: Calcification of the dentition of the domestic dog: Longitudinal radiographic study. *Irish Vet J* 26:221–224, 1972.
17. Hooft J, Mattheeuws D, Van Bree P: Radiology of deciduous teeth resorption and definitive teeth eruption in the dog. *J Small Anim Pract*, 20:175–180, 1979.
18. Gibbs C: Radiological refresher: Dental disease. *J Small Anim Pract* 19:701–707, 1978.

Chapter Three

Oral Examination and Diagnostic Techniques

CF Burrows and CE Harvey

Oropharyngeal disorders are common in the dog and cat; however, signs of disease may not always be apparent to the client until the process is well advanced. In some patients the presenting signs may suggest either primary or secondary oral disease, whereas in others oropharyngeal disease may be detected only during detailed clinical examination. Although diagnosis is sometimes evident from the history and the results of clinical examination, diagnostic studies such as culture for infectious organisms, radiographs, biopsy, specific functional tests and possibly tests of immune function are often required. A hemogram and serum biochemistry tests are also indicated in many patients, not so much to facilitate a specific diagnosis but more as a guide to the severity of any local or systemic disease process. The history and physical examination findings are the key to diagnosis, providing essential information about the nature and severity of the disease process.

HISTORY

Age, breed, and occasionally the sex of an affected animal are often useful guides to a diagnosis. Information about the health of siblings, other animals in the house, vaccination history, and history of any previous illnesses should be obtained and recorded, particularly for animals in whom inherited disease is a possibility.

Signs of oropharyngeal disease include inappetence or anorexia, halitosis, dysphagia, pawing at the mouth or face, ptyalism, retching or vomiting, rapid "chattering" jaw movements, inability to open or close the jaws, and facial swelling or disfigurement.

Inappetence and anorexia are frequently associated with oropharyngeal disease, though these signs may also reflect the fever and malaise associated with severe disease of any organ system. Inappetence without additional signs is usually attributed to the pain associated with inflammation and ulceration of the oral cavity. Anorexia (total lack of interest in or unwillingness to eat food) occurs if oral pain is severe; with less severe oral disease, inappetence or a willingness to eat soft food in preference to other foods is more common.

Halitosis is a frequent presenting complaint and can be associated with either systemic or oral disease. An unpleasant necrotic odor can result from local necrotizing conditions such as stomatitis or periodontal or neoplastic disease, or from systemic diseases such as uremia, necrotic respiratory disease, or gastrointestinal disturbances. Extensive subgingival periodontal disease can cause severe halitosis in an animal with an apparently normal mouth, particularly if mild gingival hyperplasia is present. If systemic causes of halitosis have been eliminated, a detailed dental examination under sedation or anesthesia is indicated. Some dogs exhibit halitosis in the absence of obvious oral or systemic disease. Gastrointestinal disturbances have been most frequently incriminated as the cause of this problem in human patients, with the suggestion that enteric microbial degradation of nutrients, particularly of proteins, produces gases that are absorbed and excreted via the respiratory tract.[1] A similar process probably occurs in the dog, since the complaint can sometimes be ameliorated by a change in diet.

Dysphagia shown with either solids or liquids suggests inflammatory, proliferative, neoplastic, necrotic, or neuromuscular disorders of the tongue, pharynx, or proximal esophagus. It may also cause aspiration pneumonia with subsequent fever, cough, or dyspnea. Dysphagia noticed at or before weaning usually suggests a congenital oral, pharyngeal, or esophageal abnormality, though severe pharyngeal ulceration in puppies or kittens may cause similar signs. Dysphagia of sudden onset suggests an acute or traumatic process, whereas an insidious onset is more suggestive of a neoplastic, chronic inflammatory, or degenerative neurological condition. Congenital or neuromuscular abnormalities can often be differentiated from painful ulcerative disease by the way in which the patient eats, inasmuch as animals with congenital or neuromuscular disorders frequently make multiple unsuccessful attempts to swallow, whereas animals with painful ulcerative diseases make only infrequent, short-lived attempts.

Pawing at the face or mouth in the absence of any obvious external lesion or ear disease is a reliable sign of oral pain in the dog and cat. It always indicates the need for a thorough oral examination, especially since uncommon causes of pain, such as caries, may not be apparent on routine examination. Other signs of oral pain or discomfort include rubbing the face on the floor or furniture as well as excessive or inappropriate chewing or swallowing movements. Clients commonly present a pet with disease of the caudal oropharynx complaining that "there is something stuck in the throat," a condition usually manifested by excessive and apparently unsuccessful swallowing movements. Although pharyngeal foreign bodies are a possible cause of this behavior, it is more frequently associated with inflammatory disease such as pharyngitis or tonsillitis. Rapid jaw movements, resulting in "chattering" of the teeth, are caused by localized dental disease that has penetrated to the sensitive tooth dentin, such as dental caries or osteoclastic activity in the root cementum associated with periodontal disease. A similar abnormality results from the neurological damage caused by distemper virus infection.

Ptyalism, manifested by drooling of saliva from the mouth, is a feature of many oropharyngeal diseases and is seen, for example, in organophosphate intoxication or systemic diseases that cause nausea and vomiting. Periodic drooling is normal in some dogs, particularly the larger floppy lipped breeds such as the Newfoundland, Saint Bernard, and Great Dane. Drooling in most patients is due to a reluctance or inability to swallow, rather than to the increased production or flow of saliva. However, reflex stimulation of the salivary glands may occasionally result from oropharyngeal disease and is relieved by treatment of the underlying primary disease.

Normal saliva is either clear and watery or somewhat mucoid depending on the source of the sample; clear, viscid saliva suggests dehydration. Blood-tinged saliva suggests damage to the oral epithelium and is associated with oral or facial trauma, inflammation, tumors, or bleeding disorders. Brown or green-tinged, foul-smelling saliva suggests necrosis of oral tissues. Abnormal dryness of the mouth (xerostomia) is rare in the dog and cat; it may be seen in dogs with immune-mediated disease or in association with keratoconjunctivitis sicca.[2]

Severe inflammation of the oropharyngeal mucosa directly stimulates the emetic center via vagal afferent nerves to result in retching or vomiting. Accumulation of mucus in the oropharynx in an animal unwilling to swallow is a more common cause of retching. Retching is also one of the major signs of tonsillitis, and afflicted animals are frequently presented with the spurious history of "vomiting." A description of white frothy "vomitus" should be cause for a detailed examination of the oropharynx, rather than the rote prescribing of an antiemetic.

Facial swelling and edema are associated with a variety of inflammatory, traumatic, and neoplastic diseases. An acute, bilaterally symmetrical lesion is most likely due to anaphylaxis, whereas an acute unilateral lesion is most likely caused by trauma. Snake bites can cause rapidly progressive and severe facial edema with subcutaneous ecchymotic hemorrhage. Insidious, unilateral swellings over the maxilla, ventral and rostral to the eye, are usually associated with carnassial abscess, whereas unilateral swelling in other locations can be associated with tumors or chronic abscesses.

Loss of tissue is uncommon in oral disease. The most frequently observed causes are loss of teeth from periodontal disease and atrophy of the temporal and masseter muscles in association with either neuromuscular abnormalities or nasal disease.

Gradually increasing inability to open the jaws is a feature of inflammatory or degenerative disease of the muscles of mastication or of a developing mass lesion arising from or impinging on the vertical ramus of the mandible. Craniomandibular osteopathy is one of the few causes of this problem in young dogs.

An acute inability to open the jaws is usually caused by trauma; temporomandibular joint dislocation and mandibular fractures are typical causes, but protrusion of the jaw to one side or dropping of the jaw on one or both sides are more common presenting signs.

Inability to close the mouth ("dropped jaw") usually results from trauma. Symmetrical, non-painful dropped jaw ("mandibular neuropraxia") is seen occasionally in dogs and is believed to be due to stretching of trigeminal nerve branches that supply the muscles of mastication.[3]

Signs relating to the oral cavity seldom occur in isolation. Their rate of onset, severity, and specific characteristics should be evaluated against the history, clinical background, and the results of physical examination. Although the preceding features alone might suggest a specific disease, the need for more specific diagnostic studies should never be discounted.

PHYSICAL EXAMINATION

A thorough oral examination is an essential part of the routine physical examination. It is, however, unfortunately too often neglected because of the sometimes very real risk of being bitten. Although the teeth and the lateral gingival margins can usually be examined with the patient muzzled, the limited usefulness of this examination or the lack of cooperation by the patient may necessitate a more detailed oral examination under sedation or anesthesia.

Examination of the oral cavity is preceded by visual inspection of the head, noting any swelling, facial asymmetry, or abnormal posturing or movements. The examination is carried out in a systematic and routine fashion. Both sides of the mouth should always be examined. First, the outer surfaces of the lips and muzzle are viewed and palpated. Gentle retraction allows examination of the inner surfaces of the lips, the labial mucosa, and the rostral or lateral surfaces of the incisor, canine, and premolar teeth. Most patients do not resent this procedure if it is carried out quietly and gently.

The mouth may be opened by grasping the upper jaw with a hand placed over the nose so that the thumb lies on one side and the fingers lie on the other side (Fig. 3–1). The thumb is then slipped behind the canine teeth to exert upward and backward pressure on the hard palate. This forces the head back while at the same time partly opening the mouth. The lower jaw can be depressed by placing the index finger over the dorsal surface of the tongue between the lower canine teeth (Fig. 3–2). A gauze sponge may assist in grasping and manipulating the tongue. Downward and backward pressure on the tongue pulls it forward to permit examination of the oropharynx. The mouth should never be forced open by pressing the lips onto the teeth (Fig. 3–3); this maneuver is painful, causes struggling, and increases the risk of being bitten.

In dogs that resent being handled, the mouth may be opened by lengths of tape or gauze placed over the upper and lower jaws behind the canine teeth (Fig. 3–4). Chemical restraint, however, is usually necessary in

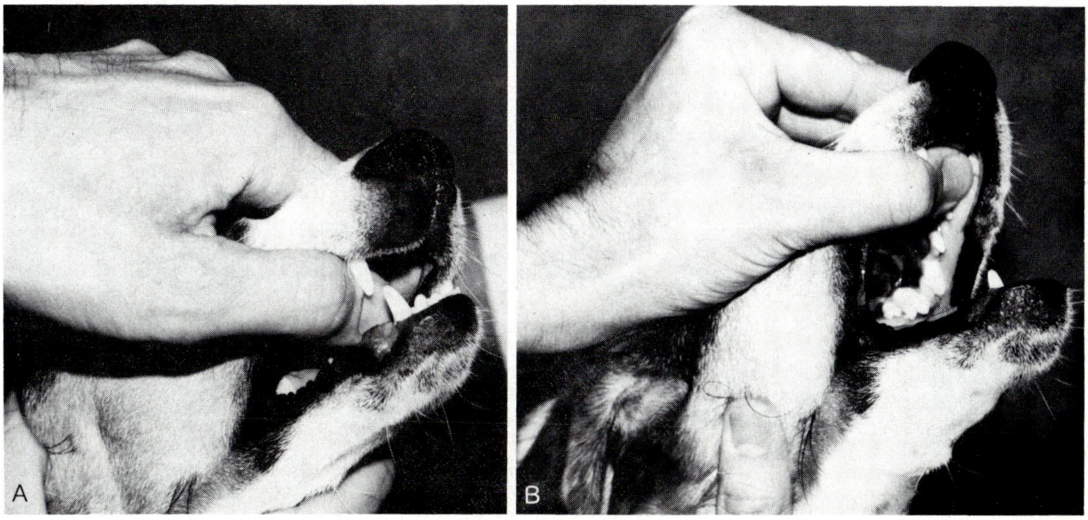

Figure 3–1. *A* and *B*, Correct technique for opening the mouth of a dog.

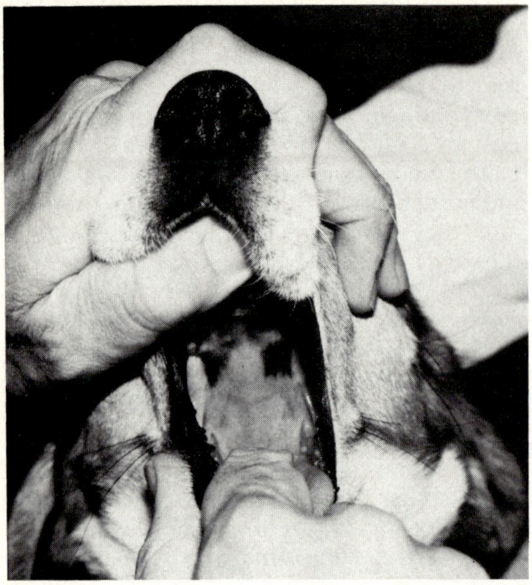

Figure 3–2. Examination of the oropharynx. The head is tilted back in order to force the mouth open.

such patients to permit a thorough examination. Sedation or anesthesia is essential in brachycephalic breeds because the relatively large size of the tongue and soft palate in relation to the rest of the oral cavity precludes examination of the pharynx, tonsils, and larynx.

In cats the mouth may be opened by grasping the head firmly with one hand placed so

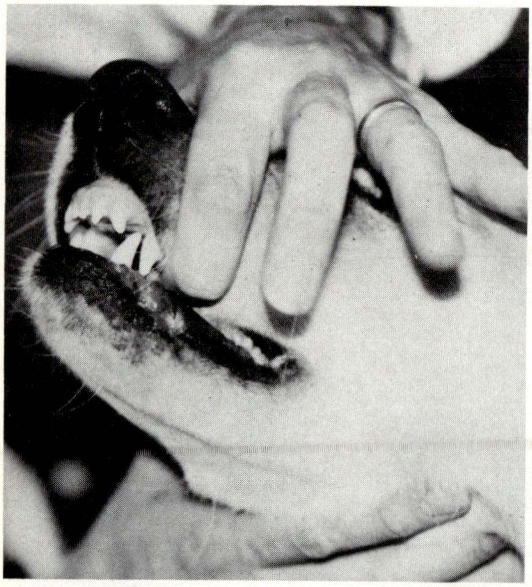

Figure 3–3. Incorrect method for opening the mouth of a dog. The lips may be injured if pressed between the teeth.

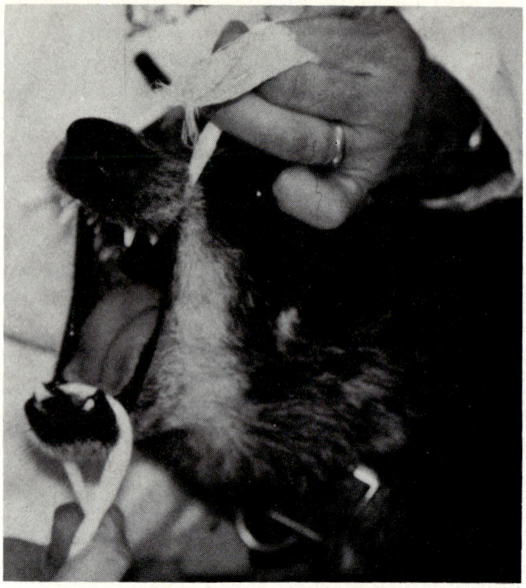

Figure 3–4. Technique for examining the oral cavity of a dog that may bite. Pieces of tape or gauze are placed behind the canine teeth, and the jaws are pulled open.

that the thumb and fingers lie in front of the ears. Tilting the head backward and upward forces the mouth open. The tongue can be depressed and pulled forward with the index finger of the opposite hand to allow examination of the caudal pharynx (Fig. 3–5). The ventral portion of the tongue can be examined by upward pressure exerted with the tip of the thumb between the rami of the mandibles (Fig. 3–6). This is an important maneuver, since string foreign bodies frequently

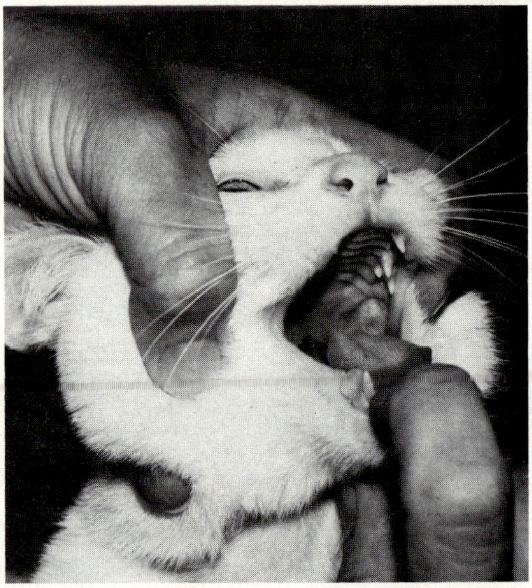

Figure 3–5. Opening the mouth of a cat.

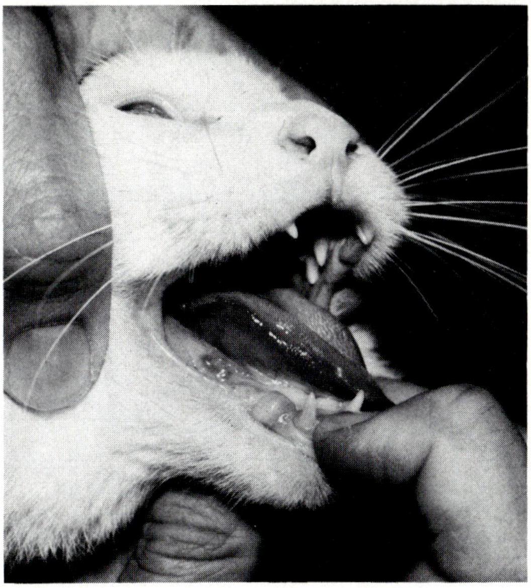

Figure 3–6. Lifting the tongue of a cat with a finger between the rami of the mandibles in order to examine the base for linear foreign bodies.

lodge under the tongue in cats. Chemical restraint may be required to permit a detailed examination.

Examination should include a detailed inspection of the mucous membranes of the tongue, gums, and cheeks, which are normally reddish pink and appear moist. Dry, tacky gums suggest dehydration. Pale mucous membranes suggest either anemia or perhaps shock if refill time is more than 2 seconds. Other common mucosal abnormalities include inflammation, ulceration, petechial hemorrhage, vesicles, tumors, and foreign bodies.

Examination of the teeth may reveal malocclusion, retained deciduous teeth, attrition or other enamel abnormalities, fractures, root exposure, or absence of teeth. Any asymmetry in the placement or shape of the teeth may be helpful in assessing whether the jaw is normal.

Following inspection of the oropharyngeal cavity, the external surfaces of the head, face, and neck should be palpated for areas of pain, heat, or swelling. Associated lymph nodes should be palpated, and any asymmetry, abnormal firmness, or enlargement should be noted and scheduled for further investigation.

A form suitable for recording results of a detailed oral and periodontal examination is shown in Figure 3–7.

FUNCTIONAL STUDIES

Much can be learned by offering the patient food if there is either a history of dysphagia or coughing when swallowing, or signs of pain on eating. Some animals may be too distracted to eat in the examination room, but small quantities of a palatable food should be offered nonetheless and the reaction observed. Observation by the veterinarian should allow differentiation of vomiting from coughing and gagging, the detection of pain on eating, and the inability to swallow. Observation of eating can be delayed if the patient is to be hospitalized, but it is essential that the veterinarian observe the reaction and not rely on anecdotal reports.

Repeated unsuccessful attempts to swallow suggest either a painful lesion or a functional disorder. In a young dog, immediate regurgitation suggests pharyngeal dysphagia, cricopharyngeal achalasia, or esophageal disease. Coughing associated with the swallowing of liquids may be associated with neuromuscular disorders or aspiration pneumonia, or both.

DIAGNOSTIC TECHNIQUES

Culture for Infectious Organisms

The oral cavity and pharynx of the dog and cat contain a vast and varied flora.[4–11] In early life most bacteria are found on the dorsum of the tongue; with eruption of the teeth, however, colonization of the tooth surfaces begins. Most bacteria are found at the gingival sulcus, but others colonize the surfaces of the teeth to form bacterial plaque (see Chapter 5).

Within the first days of life a predominantly streptococcal flora is established; other bacteria are isolated only after eruption of the teeth, and they predominate in the gingival sulcus. Bacteria routinely isolated from the oral cavity or pharynx of normal dogs are shown in Table 3–1. There are no discernible differences in bacterial isolates among breeds.[5] Cats probably have a similar flora but *Pasteurella* spp. predominate; the incidence of *Pasteurella* isolation in both species increases concomitantly with the severity of periodontal disease.[10]

Almost any organism might conceivably be found in the mouth at one time or another; those that may be of pathogenic significance

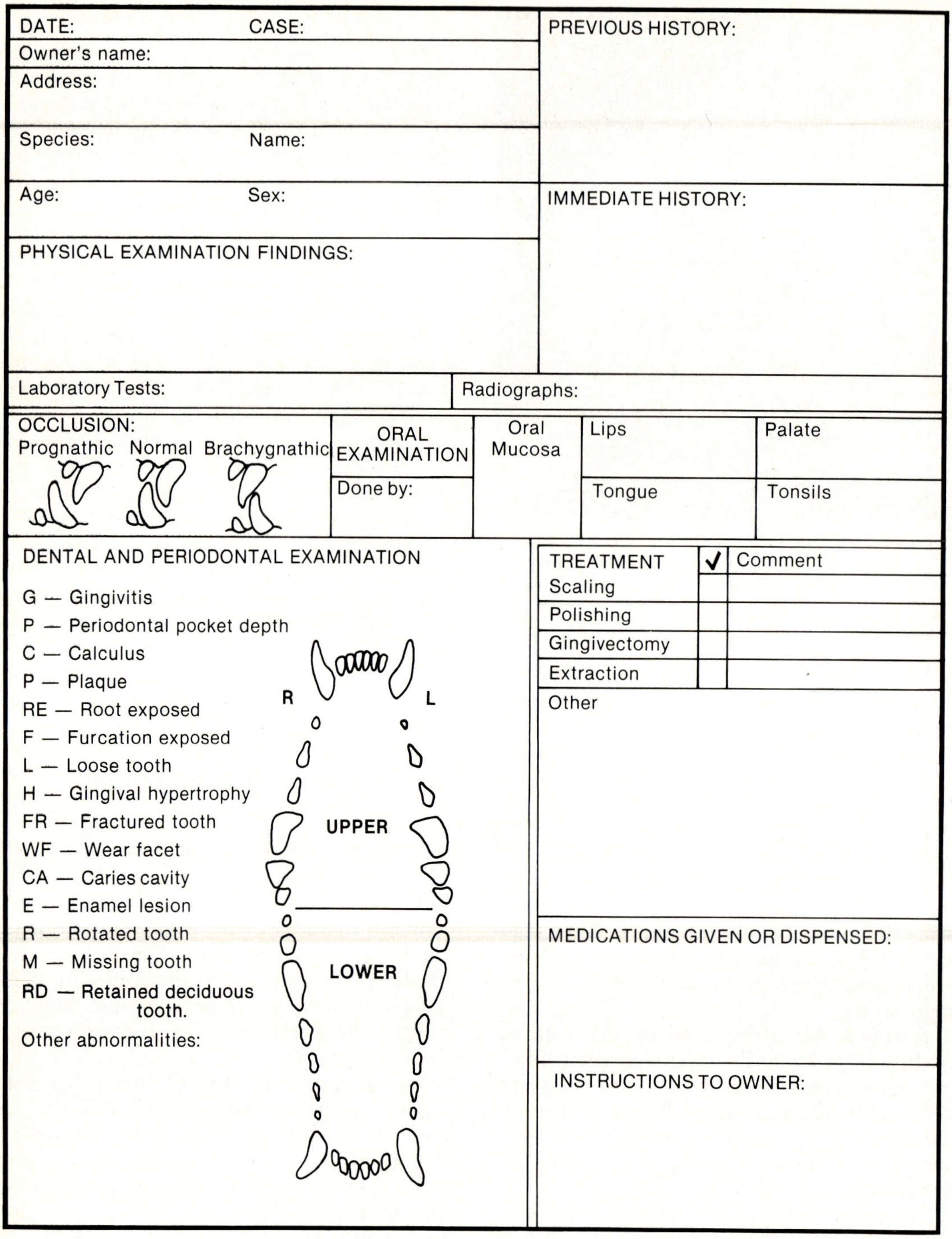
DATE: CASE:
Owner's name:
Address:
Species: Name:
Age: Sex:
PHYSICAL EXAMINATION FINDINGS:
PREVIOUS HISTORY:
IMMEDIATE HISTORY:
Laboratory Tests:
Radiographs:
OCCLUSION:
Prognathic Normal Brachygnathic
ORAL EXAMINATION
Done by:
Oral Mucosa
Lips
Palate
Tongue
Tonsils
DENTAL AND PERIODONTAL EXAMINATION
G — Gingivitis
P — Periodontal pocket depth
C — Calculus
P — Plaque
RE — Root exposed
F — Furcation exposed
L — Loose tooth
H — Gingival hypertrophy
FR — Fractured tooth
WF — Wear facet
CA — Caries cavity
E — Enamel lesion
R — Rotated tooth
M — Missing tooth
RD — Retained deciduous tooth.
Other abnormalities:
R
L
UPPER
LOWER

TREATMENT	✓	Comment
Scaling		
Polishing		
Gingivectomy		
Extraction		

Other
MEDICATIONS GIVEN OR DISPENSED:
INSTRUCTIONS TO OWNER:

Figure 3–7. Oral and periodontal examination record.

include spirochetes, anaerobic *Streptococcus, Staphylococcus, Pasteurella, Candida,* and perhaps some viruses.

Although bacteria may occasionally invade oral soft tissues, local resistance usually precludes overt infection. Exogenous oral infections that are not the result of trauma or foreign body penetration are extremely rare, and infection by endogenous organisms becomes evident only after one group becomes dominant. In some instances, culture may reveal heavy bacterial or fungal contamination, but the infection need not necessarily be primary. Excessive numbers of microbial

Table 3–1. Bacteria Isolated from the Oropharynx in Normal Dogs[4–11]

Genus of Bacterium	Incidence in Gingivae (%)	Incidence in Throat (%)
Streptococcus	82–85	35–100
Staphylococcus	50	24–65
Pasteurella	25–75	10–65
Micrococcus	5–60	30–65
Escherichia	20	15–75
Neisseria	20	20–100
Proteus	15	15–40
Pseudomonas	30	5–20
Enterobacter	2–5	40
Corynebacterium	25	1–15
Bacillus	10–15	5–40
Moraxella	5–40	
Diphtheroids		10–35
Alcaligenes		25–40

agents might well be secondary to other processes (see Chapter 4).

Ulceromembranous stomatitis (Vincent's stomatitis, see page 36) and candidiasis (see page 37) are conditions in which microbial agents are of primary importance.

Specimens for bacteriological culture should be taken from obviously diseased areas using sterile culture swabs; material for smears should be taken using clean swabs and transferred by rolling onto a clean glass slide. Once specimens have been collected, they should be sent to the laboratory as soon as possible. Delay in transmission may severely diminish the success of a diagnostic investigation. Specimens should be placed in suitable transport media if they are to be sent to an outside laboratory.

Clinicians sometimes tend to rely too heavily on the results of oral microbial cultures and antibiotic sensitivity testing. The question of which microbes are present and which drugs should be used to eliminate them should never displace the more rational question of *why* the microbes are present and what can be done to render conditions less favorable for colonization.

Little detailed information is available regarding the normal viral oral flora in dogs. Viruses in the oral cavity and pharynx of the cat have been studied extensively because of the association of feline viral rhinotracheitis and feline calicivirus infection with oropharyngeal ulceration.[13–15] Viral culture is indicated in cats with chronic non-responsive oral lesions, particularly in catteries in which the results may be of epizootiological significance. A sample of tissue or oral fluid is obtained under sterile conditions and is sent to the virus diagnostic laboratory in virus transport medium.

Hematology, Serum Chemistry, and Immune System Tests (Table 3–2)

Oral disease is not associated with any *specific* hematological or blood chemical abnormality, but routine studies are useful nevertheless because they may eliminate some diseases from consideration and indicate the severity of the disease process. In severe oral inflammatory disease, for example, the hemogram may reveal a leukocytosis, which is most frequently manifested as a neutrophilia, but an eosinophilia may be present in eosinophilic granuloma. Anemia may be present in patients with subacute or chronic bleeding oral lesions.

Blood chemical analysis may reveal increases in serum creatinine, phosphorus, and urea nitrogen concentration, suggesting renal disease. Since oral ulceration is common in this disorder, these tests become important in its differentiation. An increase in blood glucose concentration may suggest diabetes, and this is also important in oral disease, inasmuch as periodontal disease is believed to be more severe in this disorder.

A variety of tests are available to evaluate an animal's immune system. Unfortunately, many of these tests require viable cells, so blood samples cannot be sent in the mail. A practical approach for diagnosis of an immunodeficiency is to perform a hemogram, a protein electrophoresis, and an immunoelectrophoresis or radial immunodiffusion.[16] These tests are readily available, and samples can be sent by mail. The hemogram indicates whether or not the animal has sufficient numbers of neutrophils and lymphocytes to mount an immune response. However, the animal may have a functional neutrophil or lymphocyte defect with a normal number of cells. Serum electrophoresis has limited use in the documentation of these conditions, since immunoglobulin deficiencies are difficult to recognize. The immunoelectrophoresis or radial immunodiffusion give qualitative and quantitative measures, respectively, of the animal's immunoglobulins. Since the radial immunodiffusion test gives a quantitation of the immunoglobulins, it is a much more useful test. If these tests are normal or are suggestive of an immunodeficiency state, the animal should be re-

Table 3–2. Laboratory Studies in Oral Disease

Study	Abnormality	Disease
Hemogram	Packed cell volume, hemoglobin, red blood cell count decreased	Subacute and chronic bleeding lesions, clotting defects.
White blood cell count	Increased	Neutrophilia in chronic inflammatory diseases. Eosinophilia in eosinophilic granuloma.
	Decreased	Lymphopenia may be associated with immunodeficiency.
Creatinine, phosphorus, BUN	Increased	Renal disease (oral ulceration, necrosis).
Blood glucose	Increased	Diabetes. Increased severity of periodontal disease.
T_3, T_4, TSH stimulation	Decreased	Hypothyroidism. Increased severity of periodontal disease.
Test for feline leukemia virus (FeLV)	Positive	Possible association with immunosuppression and chronic ulcerative glossopharyngitis in cats. Increased severity of periodontal disease.
Antinuclear antibody (ANA)		
Lupus erythematosus preparation (LE Prep)		
Immunoelectrophoresis		Immune-mediated diseases with oral manifestations.
Bactericidal assay		
Lymphocyte transformation		
Serum electrophoresis		

ferred to an institution with an immunology laboratory for cellular studies such as bactericidal assay and in vitro lymphocyte transformation.[16]

Oral Radiography

Oral radiographs require correct positioning and use of appropriate films and techniques to be of value because the radiographic appearance of normal oral structures is complex, and radiographically demonstrable changes resulting from disease are often minor. There are no special requirements for the x-ray machine itself, though a tilting or rotating x-ray head is very helpful. Good quality films can be obtained with machines of low power if the exposure factors are set correctly.

Film Type. Non-screen film is by far the most satisfactory because it provides the most detail. This film is available for both manual and automatic processing. In the darkroom, large-sized paper-covered non-screen film can be cut to fit the oral cavity; the cut edges must be taped with light-proof tape.[17] Custom-made packets of this sort or commercially available oral occlusal (8 cm × 6 cm) or bite wing (4 cm × 3 cm) films available for human patients can be made to conform to the shape of the canine or feline jaw. Normal veterinary cassettes are too large or unwieldy for intraoral use in cats and in many small- or medium-sized dogs, and they provide poorer radiographic detail.

Control of the Animal. Reliable interpretation of oral radiographs requires comparison of the two sides of the head or mouth. Symmetrical positioning is essential. This mandates a well-controlled and immobile patient, and results are usually best when radiographs are made with the animal under deep sedation or anesthesia. An anesthetized patient can be positioned so as to avoid the overlying jaw, or obtain exact symmetry. Oral films made without using chemical restraint of some kind are generally useful only for confirming the existence of gross lesions such as large tumors that are clinically evident, and these films rarely allow evaluation of the margins of such lesions.

Positioning. Positioning of the animal and film depends on the reason for the examination. Lateral and ventrodorsal views of the entire head are rarely useful because of the superimposition of the jaws. Simple occlusal films are excellent for obtaining a symmetrical view of the maxilla or mandible, as well as for assessing bone erosion or the extent of general bone calcification. For these views the animal is placed in either dorsal (for mandibular radiographs) or ventral (for maxillary radiographs) recumbency, with the film in the animal's mouth.

Examination of specific sections of the jaw or teeth requires more careful positioning because the most diagnostically useful information is obtained when the long axis of both the film and the tooth are as close to perpendicular to the x-ray beam as possible. This position is best obtained for the incisor and canine teeth by an angled beam with the x-ray film flat in the mouth. An oblique view is required for the premolar and molar teeth, since the crown and roots are superimposed when the x-ray beam is directed laterally. An angle of approximately 30° rotation of the head compared with the beam gives best results. This can be achieved by placing a radiolucent foam block beneath one side of the head or by tilting the x-ray beam (Fig. 3–8). Radiographs should always include a

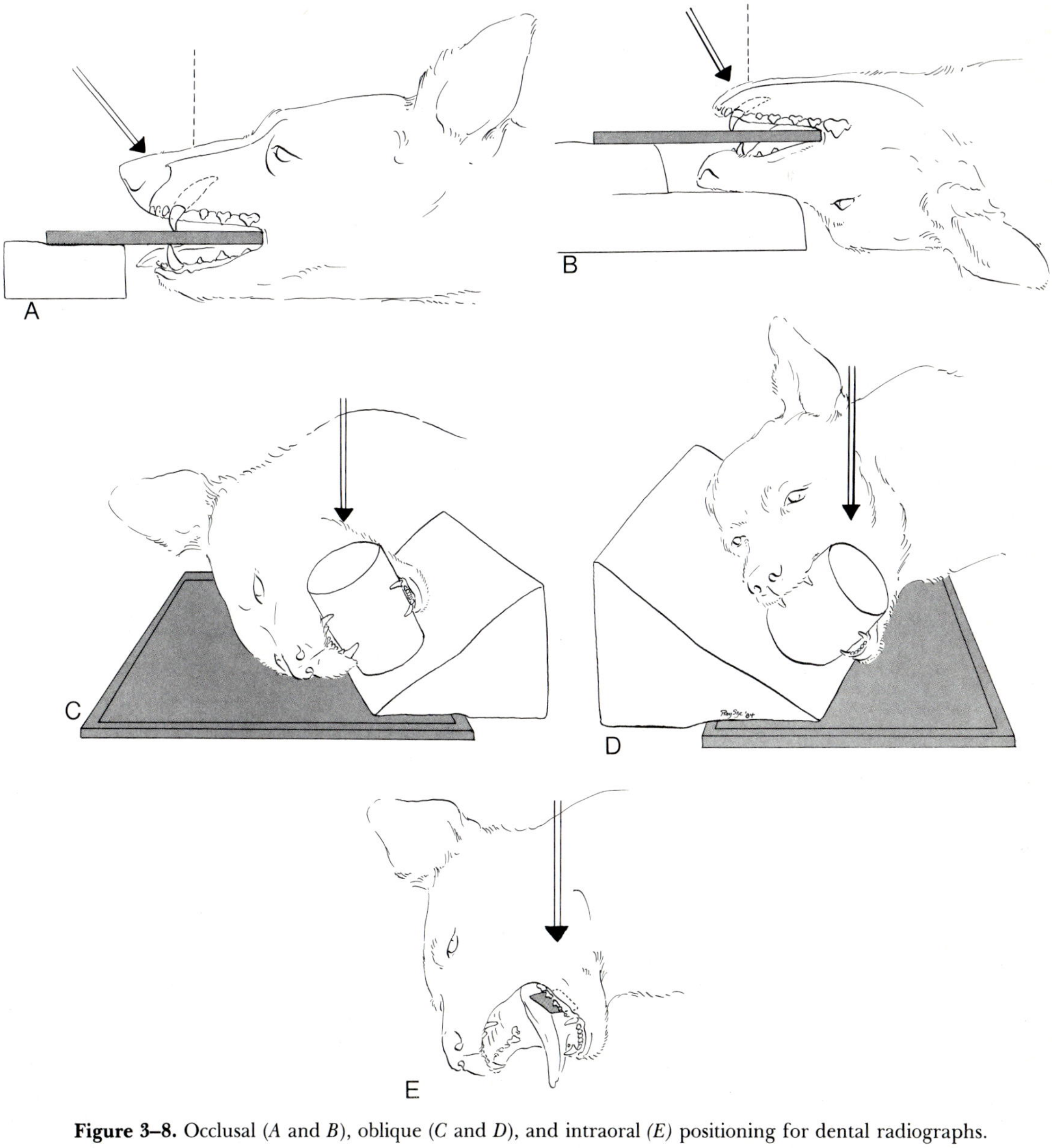

Figure 3–8. Occlusal (*A* and *B*), oblique (*C* and *D*), and intraoral *(E)* positioning for dental radiographs.

side marker. When using non-screen films, a shorter distance (40 cm) than normal from the machine to the film is recommended.

The following machine settings have been recommended[18] for intraoral technique:

Cats, small dogs, and puppies: 7.5 milli ampere seconds (mAs) to 10 (mAs), 60 kilovolt peak (kVp)
Medium-sized dogs: 12.5 mAs, 60 kVp
Large-sized dogs: 12.5 mAs, 65 kVp to 80 kVp

Radiographs should be mounted in black opaque film mounts to exclude stray light when viewed in a darkroom. The stray light produced when dental radiographs are viewed unmounted on a viewbox can be enough to cause missed carious lesions, calculus, and incipient bone resorption.

Interpretation of Oral Radiographs. The most common reasons for radiographic examination are to assess (1) the nature of mass lesions, (2) the extent of disease associated with periodontal disease, and (3) the extent and nature of trauma to teeth. The examination of an oral radiograph should proceed logically, answering the following questions:

1. General features: Is the positioning adequate for viewing the area of interest? Are both sides of the jaw visible so that comparisons can be made? Is the technique (exposure factors) adequate? Is the extent of calcification of the bone compatible with the radiographic technique used? Osteoporosis associated with primary or secondary hyperparathyroidism is easy to "diagnose" on an underexposed radiograph. Is the general shape of the skull and mandible normal? There is a wide variation in the skull shape of dogs. A certain position and number of teeth is accepted as normal in some breeds (particularly brachycephalic dogs), whereas the same conditions would be regarded as grossly abnormal in others.

2. Specific examination of the area of interest: Can the expected normal tissue margins be followed? Is the ratio of soft tissue to bone normal? Are the teeth normal in number and position (or is there a history of tooth loss unrelated to the present reason for examination)? Is the appearance of the teeth normal for an animal of this age?

The radiographic appearance of oral structures in normal dogs and cats is described on page 20. The radiographic findings in animals with specific diseases are discussed in the appropriate disease sections.

Mass Lesions. Radiographic examination cannot discriminate between malignant and benign disease. Severe gingival hyperplasia associated with longstanding periodontal disease that has progressed to loss of alveolar bone will show a radiographic pattern that is similar to an early infiltrating gingival or subgingival tumor. One differentiating feature, however, is that tumors will often push a tooth out of its normal position. These displaced teeth may be visible on inspection of the mouth, but some may be hidden in the soft tissue mass and may only be visible radiographically. Differentiation is easier with more deeply infiltrating tumors, since the associated irregular pattern of bone loss is unlikely to be due to benign disease. The extent of tissue infiltration by oral tumors cannot be accurately assessed from radiographs, since the common oral malignancies are notorious for extending well beyond the grossly or radiographically visible margins. Benign tumors or cysts of the jaw can usually be differentiated from malignant lesions by examining the radiographic margins, since a slow-growing benign lesion is surrounded by a clearly visible margin of sclerotic bone.

Periodontal, Dental, and Periapical Disease. Radiographic changes associated with periodontal disease are discussed in Chapter 5. Common abnormalities include loss of alveolar bone starting at the crest, widening of the radiolucent space formed by the periodontal ligament, and extension of the crevicular groove as periodontal attachment is lost. Loss of periapical bone occurs when a disease process extends into the pulp cavity or deeply into the periodontal ligament. This process is usually referred to as a root abscess, though the root is not necessarily infected. The structure of the involved tooth should be examined carefully for gross and radiographic signs of fracture. Confusion of bone resorption around a root with the normal mandibular mental foramina is a common mistake (see Fig. 8–2).

Radiographic examination of the temporomandibular joints is described on page 111. Radiographic examination of salivary glands is described on page 190.

Biopsy Techniques

Biopsy of an oral lesion is usually simple compared with biopsy of lesions in some other areas of the body. Some lesions, such as protuberant hyperplastic or neoplastic lesions, require no anesthesia or analgesia for biopsy in a cooperative animal; a biopsy punch or even a pair of scissors can be used to remove a portion of the mass. Necrotic debris should be avoided so that a representative piece of viable tissue is obtained. The site sometimes bleeds for some time after the biopsy has been taken, but firm pressure with a gauze sponge is usually sufficient for hemostasis. This approach will allow a definitive diagnosis of protuberant epithelial lesions to be obtained at the first visit, without the expense or risk of anesthesia.

Sedation or anesthesia is usually necessary in small animals in whom the lesion is attached to the mucosal surface and is likely to contain pain receptors or is covered by normal gingiva. Biopsies can be obtained by wedge incision using a scalpel or by means of a skin biopsy instrument. The area to be biopsied should be chosen with care. If the condition has a number of separate lesions of varying maturity on the mucosal surface, it is advisable to include a section that has normal tissue adjacent to a newly formed lesion, because mature lesions may not possess a characteristic microscopic appearance. This is especially true with some of the autoimmune conditions. Representative lesions from the skin or from other mucocutaneous junction areas should also be biopsied. Some gingival lesions will tend to shed and may lose their identity or even be lost before or during processing. A piece of tissue at least 5 × 10 mm in diameter should be submitted whenever possible. It is always best to take more specimens and submit an unnecessary volume of material than to make do with a small piece of tissue that may not be diagnostic. A piece of tissue large enough for normal histopathological processing is much more likely to provide a diagnosis than is a smear submitted for cytological examination.

Tumors arising from the oral connective tissues or tooth-forming structures require a deeper biopsy. If a mass lesion is covered by normal epithelium, the biopsy should be made by a deep incision down to underlying bone with the patient either sedated or under general anesthesia. Skin biopsy instruments that core out a circular piece of tissue are ideal for this purpose. Hemorrhage can be controlled by deep sutures of absorbable material placed to forcefully appose the edges of the biopsy incision.

Cytological examination is a useful diagnostic technique and may provide a rapid means of diagnosing lesions such as squamous cell carcinoma or eosinophilic granuloma. Samples are obtained by scraping the lesion vigorously after any superficial necrotic debris has been removed. A smear is made on a microscope slide, is sprayed with one of the commercially available cytological fixation agents, and is stained. Since some lesions cannot be diagnosed from superficial smears, a biopsy specimen suitable for normal microscopic fixation and sectioning should be obtained at the same time.

Electromyographic examination and muscle biopsy are useful for diagnosing myositis of masticatory muscles, or differentiating the causes of abnormalities in the pharyngoesophageal phase of swallowing; they are rarely useful or necessary for oral or oropharyngeal disorders.

References

1. Levitt MD: Intestinal gas production—recent advances in flatology. *N Engl J Med* 302:1474–1475, 1980.
2. Kaswan RL, Martin CL, Dawe DL: Rheumatoid factor determination in 50 dogs with keratoconjunctivitis sicca. *J Am Vet Med Assoc* 183:1073–1075, 1983.
3. Robins GM: Dropped jaw—mandibular neuropraxia in the dog. *J Small Anim Pract* 17:753–758, 1976.
4. Saphir DA, Carter CR: Gingival flora of the dog with special reference to bacteria associated with bites. *J Clin Microbiol* 3:344–349, 1976.
5. Snow HD, Donovan ML, Washington JO, Fonkalsrud EW: Canine respiratory disease in an animal facility. *Arch Surg* 99:126–128, 1969.
6. Clapper WE, Meade GH: Normal flora of the nose, throat, and lower intestine of dogs. *J Bacteriol* 85:643–648, 1963.
7. Clapper WE, Rypka EW: *Brucellaceae* in noses and throats of dogs and a method for their identification. *Bacteriol Proc* M41:67, 1967.
8. Smith JE: The aerobic flora of the nose and tonsils of healthy dogs. *J Comp Pathol* 71:428–433, 1961.
9. Keyhani M: Characteristics of coagulase-positive staphylococci from the nose and tonsils of apparently healthy dogs. *J Comp Pathol* 87:(2)311–314, 1977.
10. Singh G, Parniak DT: Observations on bacterial flora of nose and throat of sick dogs with clinically non-respiratory affections. *Ind Vet J* 42:159–168, 1965.
11. Esterre P: Flore buccale des carnivores domestiques et pathologie de la muqueuse associee. *Le Point Vet* 12:73–79, 1981.
12. Arnjberg J: Pasteurella multocida from canine and feline teeth, with a case report of glossitis calcinosa in a dog caused by P. multocida. Nord Med Vet 30:324–332, 1978.
13. Gaskell RM, Wardley RC: Feline viral respiratory disease: a review with particular references to its epizootiology and control. *J Small Anim Pract* 19:1–16, 1978.
14. Johnson RP, Povey RC: Effect of diet on oral lesions of feline calicivirus infection. *Vet Rec* 110:106–107, 1982.
15. Thompson RR, Wilcox GE, Clark WT, Jansen KL: Association of calicivirus infection with chronic gingivitis and pharyngitis in cats. *J Small Anim Pract* 25:207–210, 1984.
16. Schultz RD, Adams LS: Immunologic methods for the detection of humoral and cellular immunity. *Vet Clin North Am* 181:1134–1141, 1982.
17. Zontine WJ: Canine dental radiology: radiographic technique, development and anatomy of the teeth. *Vet Radiol* 16:75–83, 1975.
18. Zontine WJ: Dental radiographic technique and interpretation. *Vet Clin North Am* 4:741–762, 1974.

Chapter Four

Oral Medicine

CF Burrows, WH Miller, and CE Harvey

Lesions in the oral cavity are common in the dog and cat. They may be the result of either local or systemic disease. Diagnosis of the causes of these lesions is sometimes simple, but in other instances it is time-consuming, expensive, and frustrating. In some cases, a definitive diagnosis cannot be made. Treatment of oral lesions, by contrast, is often simple and successful if a definitive diagnosis can be reached.

A major reason for the difficulty in diagnosing oral diseases is that the epithelial surfaces of the oral cavity are subject to constant contact with a wide variety of microorganisms under differing conditions of temperature and humidity, as well as the effects of abrasion by ingesta. Thus, any factor that causes a change in the efficiency of local defense mechanisms is likely to result in similar pathological effects. Many disease processes present with a similar history and clinical findings. In some patients, symptomatic and supportive therapy is curative, whereas in others specific diagnosis and treatment are necessary to obtain a satisfactory clinical response.

Diagnosis of oral diseases is most often made by elimination. Periodontal disease is by far the most common oral disease in dogs and cats (Fig. 4–1). Most lesions affecting the gingival margin should, at least initially, be presumed to be due to periodontal disease and should be treated as such (see Chapter 5). Ulcers may develop on the mucosal surfaces of the cheek or tongue from contact with severe gingival disease; treatment directed at the gingival or periodontal disease results in rapid healing of these contact ulcers. Additional diagnostic studies are indicated if the response to periodontal therapy is poor.

The oral mucosal protective barrier is strengthened by abundant vascular and lymphoreticular tissue. Oral stratified squamous epithelial cells have a high turnover rate and are shed in large quantities. The cell turnover rate is decreased in many chronic diseases, but when traumatized, oral mucosa heals more rapidly than skin.

Inflammation of oral structures (stomatitis, glossitis, gingivitis, pharyngitis) indicates that the oral environment is disturbed. Causes can be either internal (genetic, immunological, nutritional, neoplastic, or metabolic) or external (traumatic, toxic, bacterial, viral, or fungal).

In some diseases, such as the feline viral respiratory disease complex, the lesions are obvious and are an important diagnostic feature, whereas in others, such as gingivitis

---

Figure 4–1. Periodontal disease. *A,* Acute gingivitis. *B,* Gingival hyperplasia. *C,* Gingival recession and root exposure.

Figure 4–2. A 4 year old dog with severe ulcerative stomatitis. Note the gingival hyperemia, cheilitis, salivation, and severe periodontal disease. The patient responded to teeth cleaning, metronidazole therapy, and improved nutrition.

Figure 4–3. *A* and *B,* A 1 year old dog with suspected immunodeficiency and candidiasis involving the mucocutaneous junctions and gingivae. *Candida* was cultured from the oral lesions, the nailbeds, the ear, and the vulva.

Figure 4–4. A 6 year old dog that has recovered from uremia caused by infection with *Leptospira canicola.* The rostral one third of the tongue has sloughed. Food prehension is unimpaired.

Figure 4–5. Lesions on the tongue of a cat caused by infection with calicivirus.

Figure 4–6. Herpesvirus (rhinotracheitis) lesions on the tongue of a cat.

For comparison, see Color Plates on pages 40, 44, and 50.

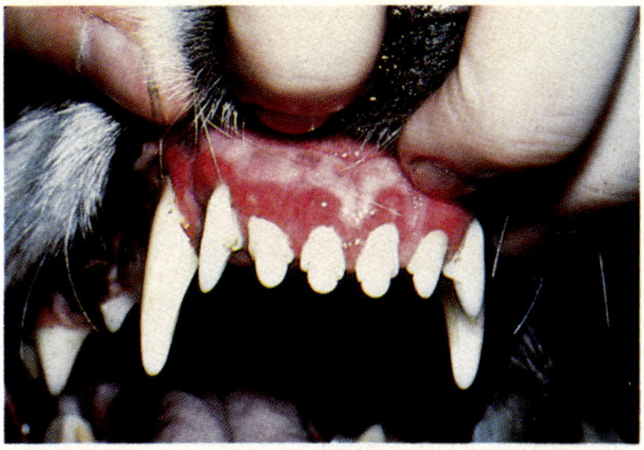

Figure 4–1A

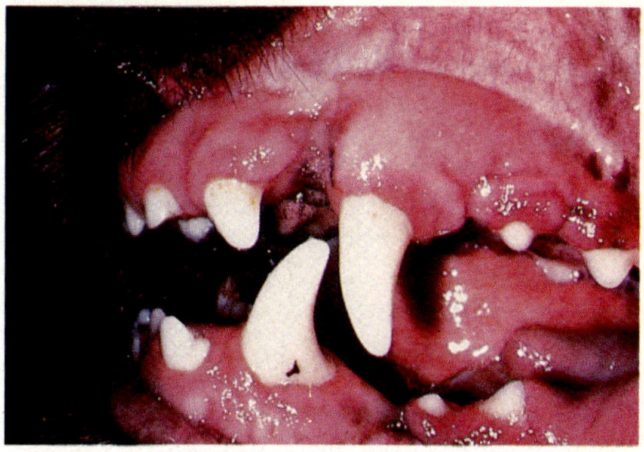

Figure 4–1B

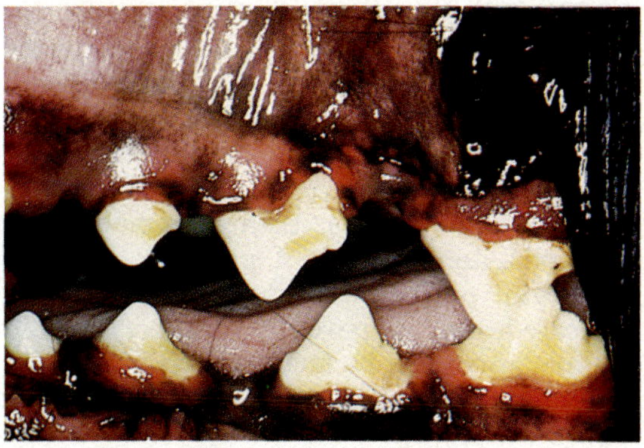

Figure 4–1C

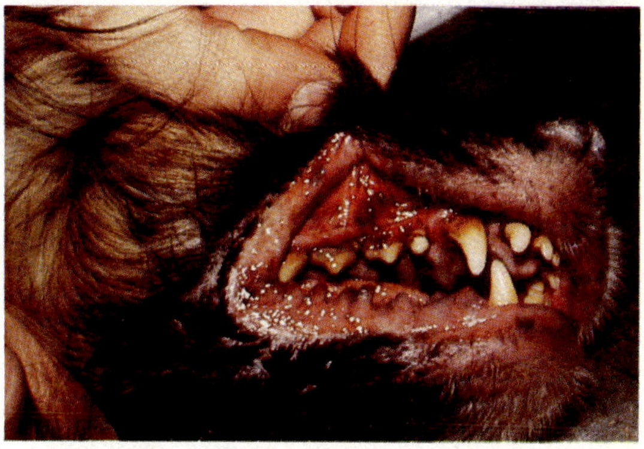

Figure 4–2

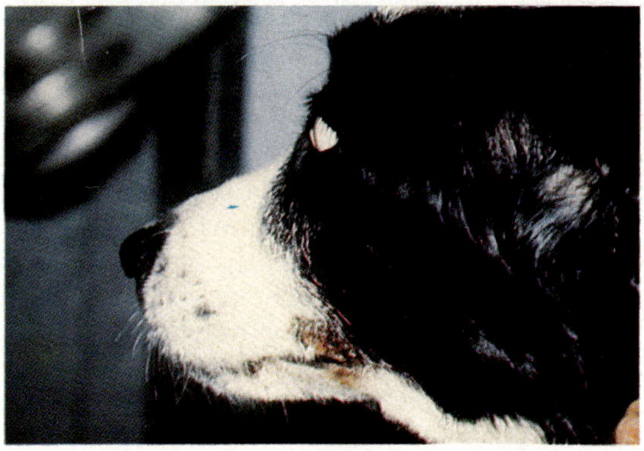

Figure 4–3A

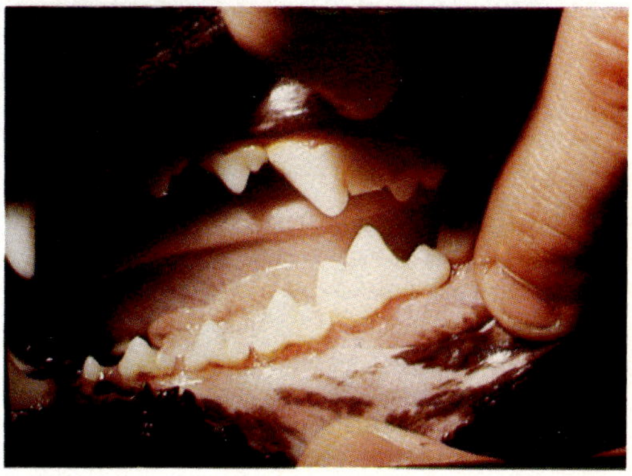

Figure 4–3B

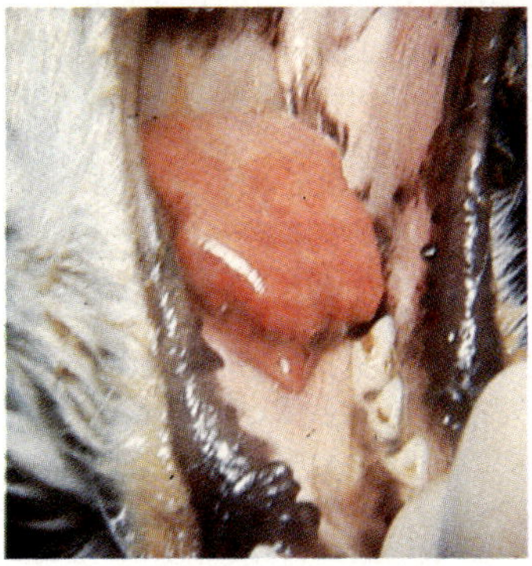

Figure 4–4

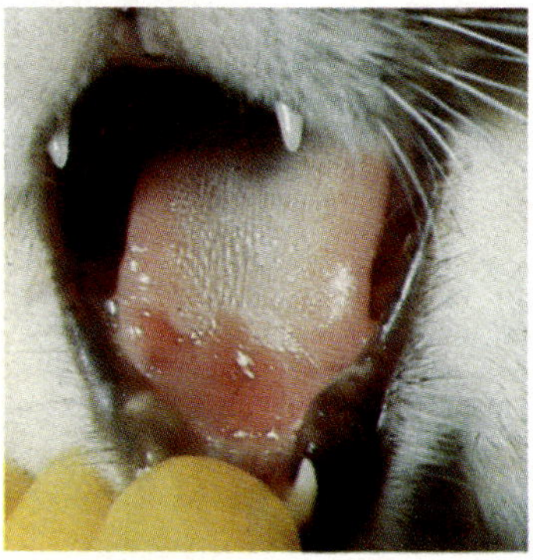

Figure 4–5

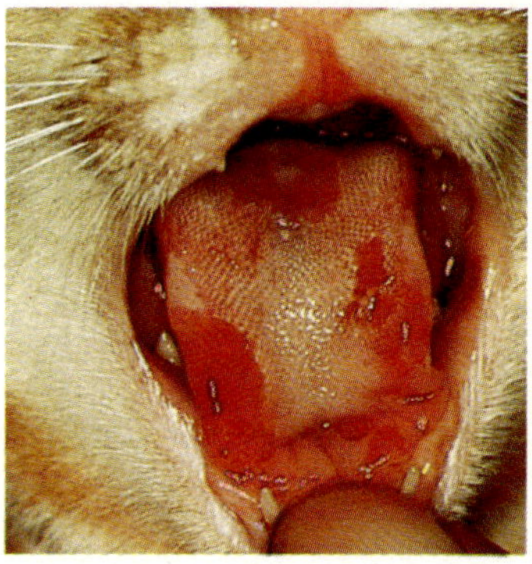

Figure 4–6

Figures 4–1 to 4–6. *See legends on opposite page.*

associated with hypothyroidism, the relationship between the systemic disease and the oral lesions is more subtle. Primary and secondary oral diseases are listed in Table 4–1.

This chapter describes those non-neoplastic conditions affecting the mucosal surface of the oral cavity and adjacent skin. Conditions affecting the oral hard tissues are described in Chapters 6 and 7. Oral neoplasms are described in Chapter 8.

Table 4–1. Primary and Secondary Diseases of the Oral Cavity of the Dog and Cat

Periodontal Disease (See Chapter 5)
Diseases Associated with Infectious Organisms
Ulcerative stomatitis
Mycotic stomatitis
Leptospirosis
Feline influenza
Feline leukemia virus infection
Canine distemper
Infectious canine hepatitis
Blastomycosis
Aspergillosis-penicillosis
Endocrine Metabolic and Toxic Diseases
Hypothyroidism
Diabetes mellitis
Hypoparathyroidism
Bleeding disorders
Uremia
Poisons
Genetic and Congenital Diseases (See Table 4–3)
Traumatic Disease
Snakebite
Lacerations
Electric cord injury
Phytogranulomatosis
Foreign bodies
Caustic agents
Immune-mediated Disorders
Contact dermatitis
Bullous autoimmune skin diseases
Systemic lupus erythematosus
Discoid lupus erythematosus
Secondary immune complex diseases
Drug eruptions
Immunodeficiency diseases
Neoplastic Diseases (See Chapter 8)
Non-specific Oral Diseases
Tonsillitis (See Chapter 11)
Pharyngitis (See Chapter 11)
Chronic feline gingivitis-stomatitis
Ulceration following protein-calorie malnutrition
Lingual calcinosis
Glossitis of military working dogs
Idiopathic stomatitis
Skin Diseases Affecting the Face and Mouth
Lip-fold pyoderma
Ectodermal defects
Depigmentation disorders
Cutaneous lymphosarcoma
Erythema multiforme

DISEASES ASSOCIATED WITH INFECTIOUS ORGANISMS AS A PRIMARY OR SECONDARY CAUSE

Ulcerative Stomatitis

This relatively uncommon canine disease (also known as Vincent's stomatitis or trench mouth) is manifested by severe gingivitis, ulceration, and necrosis of the oral mucous membranes (Fig. 4–2).

The cause is unknown, but it is believed to be associated with the fusiform bacilli and spirochetes that constitute part of the normal canine oral flora. The disease may result from an acquired immunodeficiency, allowing proliferation of normal oral flora.

Afflicted animals are presented with a history of halitosis, oral pain, inappetence or anorexia, and ptyalism. There may be a long history of periodontal disease, together with repeated and apparently unsuccessful attempts at control by teeth scaling.

Examination reveals cheilitis (inflammation of the lips), generalized hyperemia of the oral mucous membranes, and severe gingivitis with gingival recession. The mucous membranes are frequently ulcerated and necrotic. The gums denude and bleed when touched, and bone may be exposed if ulceration is severe. The mouth is extremely painful, and general anesthesia is often required to permit a thorough examination.

The patient is frequently depressed and febrile and may be cachexic as a result of severe and prolonged malnutrition. Culture and impression smears of the oral mucosa reveal a variety of organisms. Spirochetes predominate, but *Staphylococcus* and *Candida* spp. may also be identified.

The differential diagnosis includes severe periodontal disease, bullous autoimmune skin disease, uremia, thallium poisoning, and leptospirosis.

Treatment is symptomatic and consists of teeth cleaning or extraction as appropriate, debridement of necrotic areas and broad-spectrum antibiotic therapy (e.g., lincomycin, cephalosporins, tetracycline, or metronidazole) (Table 4–3, page 54). Long-term therapy (6 to 8 weeks) is frequently necessary. Oxygenated mouth rinses (e.g., 3 per cent hydrogen peroxide diluted 1:1 with water) are often helpful.[1]

In many patients, oral pain may prevent

eating, yet continued food intake is essential, since malnutrition may exacerbate the disease process and delay healing. Soft, highly palatable food may be accepted by some patients, whereas liquid diets or dog food blended with water may be accepted by others. Some patients may eat if hand-fed, but feeding via pharyngostomy tube (page 54) may be necessary in advanced cases. Multivitamin supplementation is advisable.

Mycotic Stomatitis

Mycotic stomatitis is a rare condition caused by an overgrowth of *Candida albicans* in the oral cavity. It is usually associated with long-term antibiotic therapy, with an underlying immunodeficiency disease, or is a complication of other oral diseases.

The disease is characterized by diffuse creamy white plaque-like lesions on the tongue and oral mucosa or by inflammation at the mucocutaneous junctions (Fig. 4–2). The adjacent mucosa is usually erythematous; scraping the lesions usually reveals a raw, bleeding surface.

Afflicted animals are presented with a history of chronic dysphagia, inappetence or anorexia, ptyalism, halitosis, and sometimes obvious lesions at the mucocutaneous junctions. Examination may reveal ulcerating, crusting lesions at the commissures of the lips, chronic gingivitis, gingival recession, or in some patients glossitis characterized by white plaque-like friable lesions on the surface of the tongue. Other mucocutaneous junctions may also be involved in immunosuppressed patients. Otitis, vulvovaginitis, and paronychia of varying severity are common, but concomitant gastrointestinal candidiasis is rare.

The differential diagnosis includes ulcerative stomatitis, bullous autoimmune skin disease, and extension of nasal aspergillosis into the oral cavity. Diagnosis is by culture of *Candida albicans* from the lesions or by identification of yeast hyphae in periodic acid-Schiff (PAS)-stained biopsies, or by a combination of both. Tests of immune function may show abnormal results.

Treatment is directed at the elimination of any underlying cause, the discontinuation of antibiotic therapy, the performance of teeth cleaning, and the administration of oral ketoconazole (10 mg/kg BID) until lesions regress.[2] Nystatin was the recommended treatment at one time but is less effective than ketoconazole. Immunotherapy is not generally successful. The prognosis is guarded, since the lesions may recur if the underlying disorder cannot be treated.

Leptospirosis

Canine leptospirosis is an acute infectious disease caused by *Leptospira canicola, L. icterohaemorrhagiae*, or, rarely, by *L. pomona*. Infection results in systemic disease with a spectrum of organ involvement. *L. canicola* primarily affects the kidney, and *L. icterohaemorrhagiae* affects the liver and blood; overt infection with any organism, however, is now rare.

The usual source of infection is believed to be the urine of convalescent dogs *(L. canicola)* and rats *(L. icterohaemorrhagiae)*. The organisms enter through cutaneous or mucosal abrasions.

Fever, depression, anorexia, and mucous membrane congestion characterize the bacteremic stage of the disease. Both *L. canicola* and *L. icterohaemorrhagiae* can cause severe congestion of the oral mucous membranes. Oral manifestations then differ; infection with *L. icterohaemorrhagiae* is associated with thrombocytopenia that may lead to gingival petechiation or oral hemorrhage, whereas *L. canicola* causes acute uremia with oral ulceration, oral hemorrhage, glossitis, and necrosis. The tip of the tongue may slough in severely afflicted animals (Fig. 4–4).

Treatment is based on attempts to eliminate the organism with penicillin and streptomycin or with tetracycline, in conjunction with appropriate nutritional and fluid support.[3] Necrotic areas may be left to slough spontaneously or may be cautiously debrided after they become defined.

Feline Viral Respiratory Disease

Two viruses, feline herpesvirus and feline calicivirus, have been implicated as the major cause of respiratory infection in cats. These viruses have been isolated with approximately equal incidence and are responsible for the majority of feline respiratory disease.[3, 4]

Both of these now relatively uncommon diseases can cause ulcerative stomatitis. Ulceration is more common in calicivirus infection but is more extensive and severe in herpesvirus infection. It is not possible, however, to distinguish between the two diseases from the clinical signs or from the extent of the ulceration alone.[4] Calicivirus has been isolated from gingival tissue of cats with chronic periodontal disease.[111]

Depending on the stage of the disease at presentation, afflicted cats may be febrile, depressed, and sneezing, and may have serous, mucopurulent, or purulent ocular and nasal discharges. Painful oral lesions prevent normal grooming, and the coat has an unkempt appearance. Ptyalism is common. Examination of the mouth frequently reveals ulcers on the tongue and hard palate (Figs. 4–5 and 4–6). Dry cat food has been shown to increase the severity of oral ulcers, but it is unclear whether dry food first abrades the epithelium, thereby making it more susceptible to virus, or whether virus-infected epithelium is more susceptible to abrasion.[5]

Treatment is symptomatic and supportive; broad-spectrum antibiotics, such as ampicillin or chloramphenicol, should be administered in conjunction with parenteral fluids if dehydration is present. Adequate nutrition is a prerequisite for proper therapy. Since painful oral lesions and loss of the sense of smell frequently combine to cause total anorexia, feeding via a pharyngostomy tube (page 54) can benefit severely ill cats. Normal feeding can be reintroduced as recovery begins, but dry food is best avoided and the cat should be offered soft food only. Recurrent episodes are common, particularly when cats are subjected to stressful situations such as those induced by intercurrent disease, hospitalization, or steroid therapy. Oral ulceration is less common in subsequent episodes.[6]

Feline Leukemia Virus Infection

One of the many manifestations of feline leukemia virus (FeLV) infection is suppression of the immune system, which can lead to chronic gingivitis and stomatitis, with ulceration of the tongue and oral mucous membranes.[7] An association between FeLV infection and oral lesions is controversial, since not all cats with oral ulceration, chronic gingivitis, and stomatitis can be shown to be infected with FeLV. Oral lesions are common in cats shown to be positive on the FeLV immunofluorescence test;[7,8] however, cats presented because of oral disease often do not show positive results on this test, even in the presence of severe chronic granulomatous gingivitis.

Canine Distemper

Hyperemia and ulceration of the oral mucous membranes are occasionally observed in dogs infected with canine distemper. The membranes may also appear dry as a result of dehydration, but ptyalism is a more common sign.[3]

Infectious Canine Hepatitis

Infection with canine adenovirus type 1 (CAV 1), the virus responsible for infectious canine hepatitis, is now rare. The virus causes a systemic disease characterized by damage to the liver, lymphatic tissues, and vascular endothelium. Afflicted animals are depressed, febrile, and anorexic. Vomiting and abdominal pain are other common signs. Oral lesions consist of tonsillar enlargement, injected or hyperemic mucous membranes, and occasional oral hemorrhage or petechiation.[3]

Blastomycosis

Blastomycosis is a suppurative granulomatous disease caused by the yeast-like fungus *Blastomyces dermatitidis*. The disease occurs primarily in 2 to 5 year old dogs and is endemic in the midwestern states, along the eastern seaboard, and in southern Canada. Infection causes a systemic chronic wasting disease, which most frequently involves the lungs and the bronchial and mediastinal lymph nodes.[9] Granulomatous yellow or white oral lesions, up to 1.5 cm in diameter, are occasionally observed on the tongue or oral mucous membranes (Fig. 4–7).

Clinical signs include weight loss, inappetence, emaciation, dyspnea, fever, and lymphadenopathy; signs of other organ involvement may also be present.[9]

The differential diagnosis includes other systemic fungal diseases such as sporotrichosis, histoplasmosis, cryptococcosis, and coccidioidomycosis, but oral lesions are uncommon in all systemic fungal infections. Diagnosis is made by identification of the organism in aspirates or culture.[9] No specific treatment of the oral lesions is required, since they usually resolve rapidly when the patient is treated with ketoconazole (10 mg/kg SID or BID for 6 to 8 weeks).[2]

Aspergillosis-Penicillosis

Nasal lesions caused by infection with *Aspergillus fumigatus* may occasionally extend through the nasopalatine duct onto the palatal surface causing a lesion similar in appearance to oral candidiasis (Fig. 4–8). Signs of upper airway involvement, such as nasal discharge, sneezing, and snuffling are obvious. Diagnosis is by smear or culture of the nasal discharge or by serological examination.[10]

Treatment is with oral ketoconazole (10 mg/kg SID or BID daily for 6 weeks), though not all dogs respond to therapy. Turbinectomy is necessary in some dogs. Specific treatment of the oral lesions is usually unnecessary.

ENDOCRINE, METABOLIC, AND TOXIC DISEASES

Hypothyroidism

Hypothyroid dogs and cats do not appear to be more susceptible to periodontal disease than are normal animals; however, periodontal disease is often wide-spread and more severe when present. For example, Doberman pinschers, as a breed, have a high incidence of hypothyroidism, and periodontal disease tends to be extensive[11] (Fig. 4–9). Afflicted animals have severe gingivitis with less calculus accumulation than might be expected, and are reluctant to eat hard food. The tests most useful in confirming hypothyroidism are the thyroid-stimulating hormone (TSH) response test in conjunction with measurement of serum T_3 and T_4 concentrations.[11] Afflicted animals respond to dental prophylaxis, broad-spectrum antibiotic therapy and thyroid hormone supplementation.

Cats with chronic oral ulceration may occasionally respond to thyroid hormone supplementation even if thyroid function tests are normal.

Diabetes Mellitus

Periodontal disease may be more severe in diabetics, possibly because of the xerostomia that occurs in this disease.[12] Urinalysis or serum glucose determination is indicated in animals with chronic recurrent or non-responsive stomatitis and in those with severe periodontal disease.

Hypoparathyroidism

One of the less common manifestations of hypoparathyroidism and hypocalcemia is the development of oral ulcers.[13] These are usually found at the margins of the tongue or on the mucocutaneous junctions and are manifested by necrosis, halitosis, and ptyalism. The mouth is extremely painful, but lesions regress and heal spontaneously following treatment of the underlying disorder. The pathogenesis of ulcer formation is unclear.

Bleeding Disorders

Oral hemorrhage or petechiation is common in bleeding disorders, presumably because of the constant trauma to the oral tissues and the failure of one or more steps in the clotting process.[14] Although any of the disorders that cause bleeding can be associated with oral hemorrhage, thrombocytopenia and ingestion of the anticoagulant rodenticides are most frequently implicated. Thrombocytopenia is manifested by petechiation of the oral mucous membranes or gingival bleeding, or a combination of both, whereas warfarin poisoning is more often associated with overt oral hemorrhage.[14] In many of the hereditary bleeding disorders, bleeding is frequently initiated by minor trauma such as tooth extraction.[14]

Petechiation and hemorrhage are seldom restricted to the oral cavity. Diagnosis of a bleeding disorder and differentiation of the cause can be made by standard laboratory tests (platelet count, prothrombin time, partial thromboplastin time, and activated clotting time).[14] Treatment is directed at correction of the underlying disease if possible, or with hereditary bleeding disorders, by minimizing the possibility of trauma. Bleeding after tooth extraction is common but can be prevented by filling the socket with gauze sponge or bone wax.

Bleeding restricted to the oral cavity is more often associated with oral trauma or with an underlying primary oral disease process.

Uremia

Uremia is frequently associated with stomatitis and oral ulcers.[15] Such lesions can occur in both acute and chronic uremia, but they are more severe in acute disease. Oral

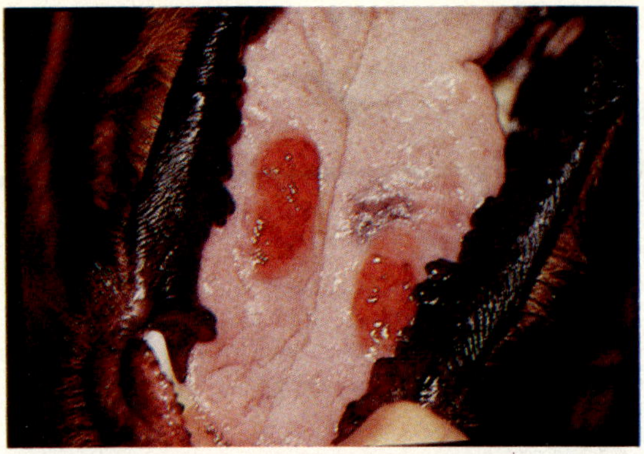

Figure 4–7

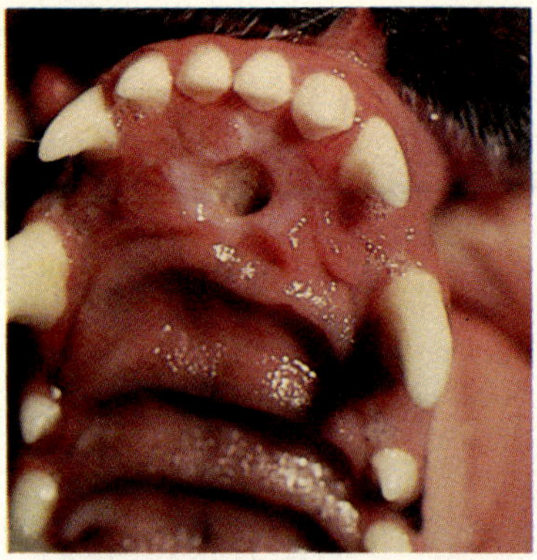

Figure 4–8

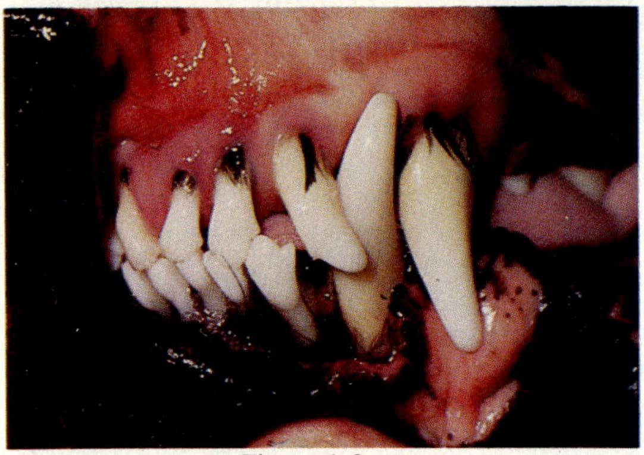

Figure 4–9

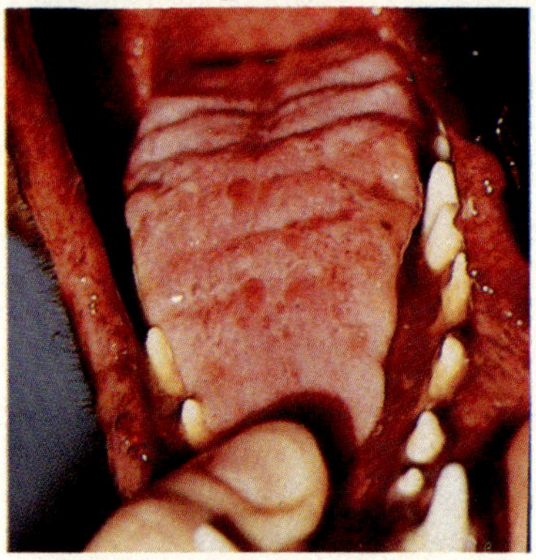

Figure 4–10

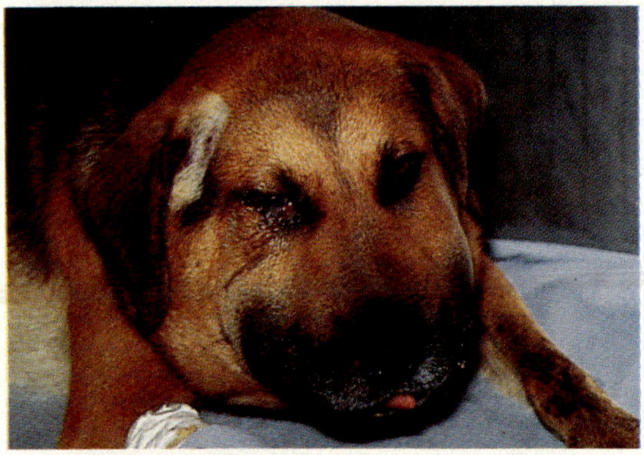

Figure 4–11

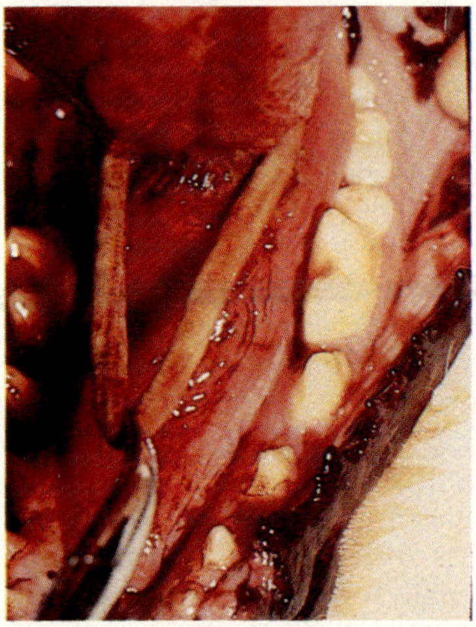

Figure 4–12

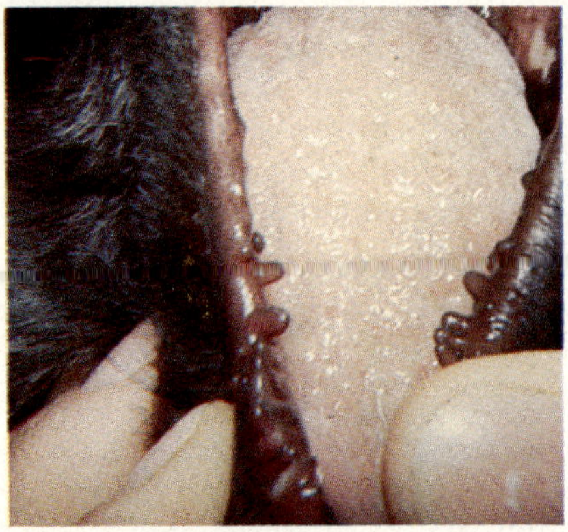

Figure 4–13

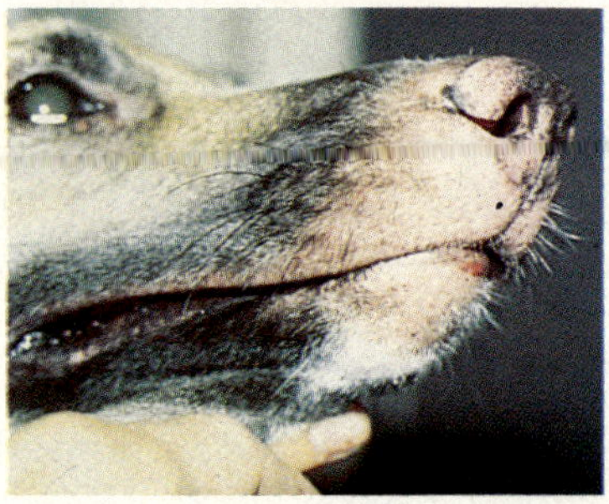

Figure 4–14

Figures 4–7 to 4–14. *See legends on opposite page.*

hemorrhage may also be reported in some uremic patients. Most ulcers are located over contact points such as the labial mucosa overlying the carnassial and canine teeth (Fig. 4–10). In severe uremia the rostral portion of the tongue may necrose and slough (Fig. 4–11).

The causes of oral ulceration are multifactorial, but the major cause is believed to be the cytotoxic effect of ammonia produced by the bacterial degradation of urea. Uremia also impairs platelet function, with subsequent bleeding from traumatized or ulcerated tissue. Immunodeficiency and the decreased rate of tissue repair in uremia exacerbate the condition.[15]

Treatment is directed at restoration of fluid and electrolyte balance and correction of the uremic state by dietary manipulation and appropriate drug therapy. Dogs that lose the tip of their tongue through necrosis adapt quickly and are able to prehend and swallow food and water with little problem.

Poisons

Anticoagulant Rodenticides. Warfarin and the indanedione compounds inhibit the hepatic synthesis and function of clotting factors II, VII, IX, and X.[14] This results in bleeding abnormalities that range from mild petechiation to severe bleeding into the gut, skin, muscle, and thoracic or abdominal cavities. One of the most common sites for bleeding abnormalities is the mouth, in which they are manifested as gingival hemorrhage or petechiation of the oral mucosa, or a combination of both.[14]

Heavy Metals. The incidence of heavy metal poisoning and the associated oral inflammation and ulceration has decreased in the past few years. When ingested, all heavy metals cause oral inflammation to a varying degree, but thallium produces the most severe and dramatic clinical signs. After ingestion, thallium becomes bound intracellularly and substitutes for potassium, inhibiting mitochondrial function. This results in a variety of signs, such as ulceration and necrosis of skin, muscle, gastrointestinal mucosa, kidney, and nerves. The mucocutaneous junctions are frequently involved.[16] Early signs of intoxication are non-specific, often presenting merely as malaise. A pronounced and generalized erythema soon develops, however, and progresses into exudative inflammation of the feet, oral mucous membranes, lips, and conjunctiva.[16] These signs, along with the generalized severe pain and metabolic acidosis, are virtually diagnostic. The differential diagnosis, however, includes lead poisoning, immune-mediated diseases such as pemphigus, and, in the early stages before ulcers become apparent, acute gastroenteritis, intestinal foreign body, and canine distemper.[16]

GENETIC AND CONGENITAL DISEASES

A variety of hereditary and congenital diseases can be associated with oral lesions (Table 4–2); the pattern of inheritance of many of them has not been studied in detail. Stomatitis is a severe recurrent problem in silver-gray collies afflicted with the recessive autosomal disease that causes cyclic neutropenia (gray collie syndrome).[17]

The hereditary clotting factor deficiencies associated with bleeding disorders can also be associated with oral hemorrhage[14] (see page 39). Other genetic diseases affecting the

---

Figure 4–7. Oral lesions in a 3 year old dog with systemic blastomycosis. The granulomata disappeared within 5 days of the commencement of therapy with ketoconazole; treatment for 60 days resulted in a complete cure.

Figure 4–8. Oral aspergillosis spreading from the nasal cavity. The incisive papilla has been eroded away.

Figure 4–9. Periodontal disease and gingival recession in a 4 year old Doberman pinscher with severe hypothyroidism. Note the hairs impacted in the gingival sulcus.

Figure 4–10. Oral ulcers in a dog with chronic uremia. Small ulcers can be seen on the dorsal surface of the tongue. Extensive ulcers were present on the labial mucous membranes over the upper incisors and canine teeth.

Figure 4–11. Facial edema in a dog some 4 hours after being bitten on the muzzle by an Eastern diamondback rattlesnake.

Figure 4–12. Lingual lesion in a dog caused by a linear foreign body.

Figure 4–13. Cockleburs embedded in the tongue of a dog.

Figure 4–14. Contact dermatitis caused by hypersensitivity to plastic.

For comparison, see Color Plates on pages 35, 44, and 50.

Table 4–2. Genetic and Congenital Diseases Affecting Oral Structures in Dogs and Cats[109, 110]

Dog
Bleeding disorders[14]
Craniomandibular osteopathy[78]
Otocephaly[79, 80]
Brachygnathism and prognathism[81–84]
Cleft lip and palate[85–90]
Dental abnormalities[91–96]
Gingival hyperplasia[97]
Misshapen tongue[98]
Ectodermal defects[63]
Depigmentation disorders[64]
Stomatitis in gray collie syndrome[17]
Cat
Micrognathia[99]
Dental abnormalities[100, 101]
Cleft palate[102, 103]
Harelip[104, 105]
Porphyria (teeth discoloration)[106–108]

oral cavity are usually specific and apparent on routine inspection. They include macroglossia and other rare anomalies of the tongue, and failure of the palatal ledges to fuse, with subsequent harelip, and hard or soft cleft palate (see Chapter 10).

TRAUMATIC DISEASES

Snakebite

Lesions of the face and lips following a rattlesnake bite are relatively common in the dog, particularly in the southern United States. Snake venom contains proteinases and enzymatic toxins such as phospholipase A, L-amino-oxidase, and hyaluronidase that cause a variety of local and systemic effects.

A history of snakebite is usually available; however, the bite wound may not always be obvious, and diagnosis may be delayed if no history is available. Edema is the most obvious local sign (see Fig. 4–11).[18] This becomes progressively more severe and may later be accompanied by petechiation, echymotic hemorrhage, or hematoma formation. Edema may impair respiration, and shock may develop; local tissue necrosis, cardiac arrythmias, hemolysis, and hemoglobinuria may complicate recovery.[19]

The differential diagnosis includes other causes of facial edema, particularly electric cord injury and anaphylaxis.

Initial treatment consists of antivenin, fluids, anti-inflammatory steroids, and antibiotics.[18, 19] Blood transfusion and local debridement of necrotic tissue are sometimes required. The prognosis is usually good provided that enough antivenin is administered early in the disease process and oral necrosis is not sufficiently severe to impair swallowing.

Oral Trauma

Trauma to the oral cavity, particularly to the tongue, can result from licking sharp objects, ingesting caustic materials, or biting on an electric cord (page 157, Chapter 10). Another cause of injury is a linear foreign body such as string or fishing line that becomes caught around the base of the tongue (Fig. 4–12). The animal moves the tongue constantly, and the string saws into the frenulum. Embedded foreign material occasionally causes chronic inflammation of the deeper tissues of the tongue; cockleburs and other seeds equipped with hooks are the best known cause (Fig. 4–13). Licking at plant material caught in the coat results in penetration of the burrs into the tongue, in which they cause a chronic inflammatory process called phytogranulomatosis.

Signs of oral trauma include ptyalism (the saliva may be blood-tinged), pawing at the mouth, ineffectual swallowing movements, inappetence, anorexia, or dysphagia.

Treatment is based on identification and elimination of the underlying cause, when possible, in conjunction with appropriate supportive and symptomatic care.

IMMUNE-MEDIATED DISORDERS

Contact Dermatitis

The most frequently recognized immune-mediated abnormality is allergic contact dermatitis of the lips and oral cavity, which is caused by a sensitivity to plastic food or water dishes and plastic toys.[21] Afflicted dogs show alopecia, depigmentation, and erythema of the muzzle, nose, lips, and gums (Fig. 4–14). The condition results in mild to moderate pruritus.

Diagnosis of plastic hypersensitivity is based on the history. Avoidance of contact with plastic for 5 to 7 days should result in spontaneous resolution of the lesion. If the pruritus is bothersome, a short course of oral prednisolone (0.5 mg/kg/day) can hasten resolution. Since re-exposure is not dangerous, the diagnosis can be confirmed by observing a relapse within 48 hours of re-exposure. Once confirmed, the condition is cured by avoiding contact with plastics.

Bullous Autoimmune Skin Diseases

Bullous autoimmune skin diseases have been documented in companion animals since 1975.[22] To date, pemphigus vulgaris and bullous pemphigoid have been documented to involve the oral cavity of the dog,[23] whereas only pemphigus vulgaris has been documented in the mouth of the cat.[24,25] There is no sex predilection. All breeds are at risk, but there appears to be a high incidence of bullous pemphigoid in the collie dog.[23] No breed predisposition has been recognized in the cat. An animal can be afflicted at any age, but the disease is seen most often in young adult or middle-aged dogs.[23]

In these disorders the animal produces antibodies against a component of the apparently normal epidermis. In the pemphigus group, the intercellular cement substance between the keratinocytes is the target antigen, whereas in bullous pemphigoid, a component of the basement membrane acts as the antigen. After the antibodies bind to the antigen, separation occurs between the keratinocytes or between the epidermis and dermis, and blisters form. Since the epidermis of the dog and cat is thin, blisters are fragile and rupture when small. At presentation the typical lesion is an erosion or an ulcer that may or may not be crusted, rather than an intact vesicle or bulla.

Pemphigus Vulgaris. Typically, an animal with pemphigus vulgaris presents with an erosive or ulcerative disease involving the oral cavity, mucocutaneous junctions, or skin, or any combination. Approximately 90 percent of the reported cases of pemphigus vulgaris in dogs, and 100 percent of cases in cats, have oral involvement at presentation.[23–25] In both the dog and cat, oral disease is the initial site of involvement in approximately 50 percent of afflicted animals.

Clinical signs can be acute or chronic in onset. With widespread involvement, the animal is often depressed, anorexic, and febrile.[26] Halitosis and dysphagia are usually reported if oral disease is the sole complaint or a significant component of generalized disease.

Oral lesions can present as discrete ulcers on the lips, tongue, or palatine mucosa or as diffuse inflammation such as glossitis, cheilitis, or gingivitis (Fig. 4–15). Any of the mucocutaneous junctions can be affected by a non-healing ulcerative process. Skin lesions often occur both in intertriginous areas and over pressure points and are identified as irregular ulcers with a peripheral epidermal collarette. The pinna and nail beds are frequently involved.[26,27]

Bullous Pemphigoid. Bullous pemphigoid and pemphigus vulgaris are often clinically indistinguishable. Approximately 80 percent of reported cases have oral lesions, but these lesions are usually noted concurrently with skin lesions.[23] The oral cavity, mucocutaneous junctions, or skin, or any combination thereof, can be affected by vesicobullous ulcerative lesions. There is a high incidence of bullous pemphigoid in the collie dog.[23]

The onset of bullous pemphigoid is often more acute than that of pemphigus vulgaris, but chronic cases do occur.[25] The oral, mucocutaneous, and cutaneous lesions are indistinguishable from those seen in pemphigus vulgaris. The cutaneous lesions are usually most marked in the inguinal and axillary areas and often assume a serpiginous configuration. Intact lesions are infrequent, and the typical lesion is an ulcer with an epidermal collarette. Although pemphigus vulgaris affects the nail bed, bullous pemphigoid more often affects the interdigital skin, pads, or pad-skin junctions.[28,29]

Routine laboratory evaluations (hemogram, serum chemistry profile, and urinalysis) are usually normal or show non-specific changes;[23] these tests provide a data base for monitoring treatment. Immunoserological tests such as the lupus erythematosus preparation (LE Prep), the antinuclear antibody test, and the direct Coombs' test are usually negative. The indirect immunofluorescence test that detects circulating pemphigus or pemphigoid antibodies is often negative in confirmed cases and is of little value.[23]

Pemphigus vulgaris and bullous pemphigoid are best confirmed by epithelial biopsies. Routine histopathological examination may be sufficient to diagnose either of these conditions, but simultaneous histopathology and direct immunofluorescence testing more completely documents the condition; multiple biopsy samples are often necessary for locating the typical lesions or immunoglobulin deposits. New lesions should be biopsied. Intact vesicles are removed intact. If no intact lesions are present, the freshest ulcers should be biopsied at their leading edge, at which point the epidermal collarette is visible. Crusted lesions should be avoided. For direct immunofluorescence testing, normal peri-

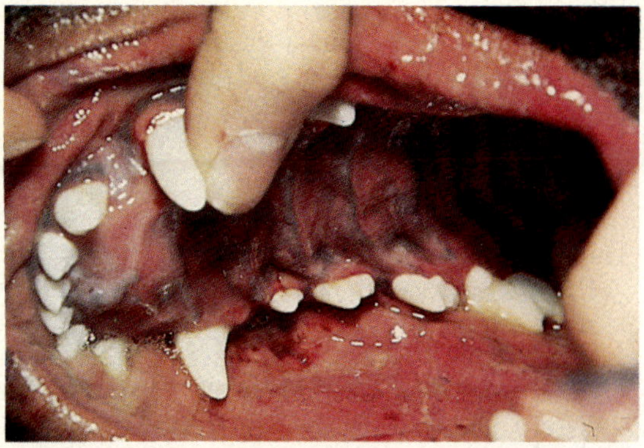

Figure 4–15

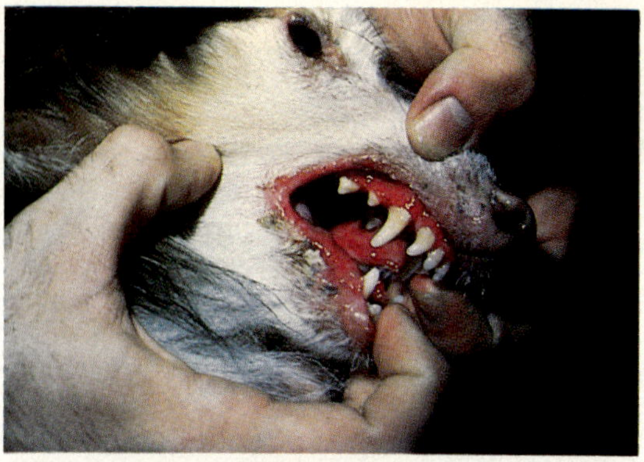

Figure 4–16

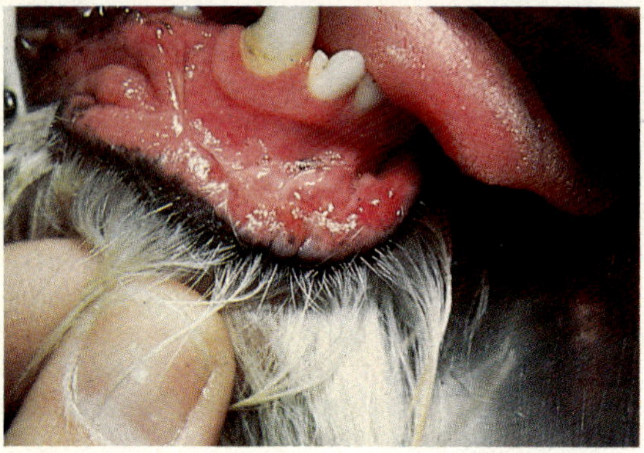

Figure 4–17

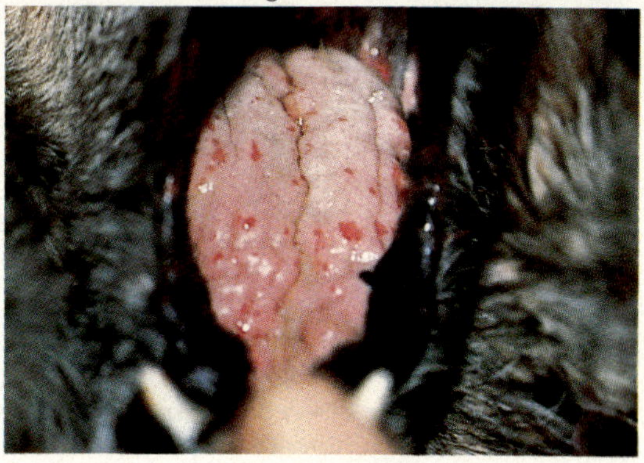

Figure 4–18

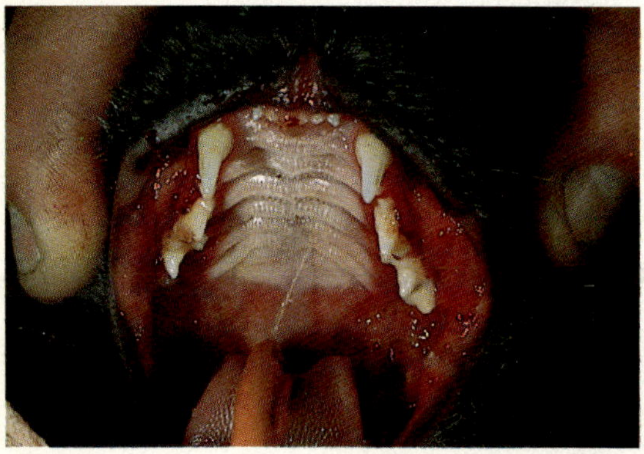

Figure 4–19

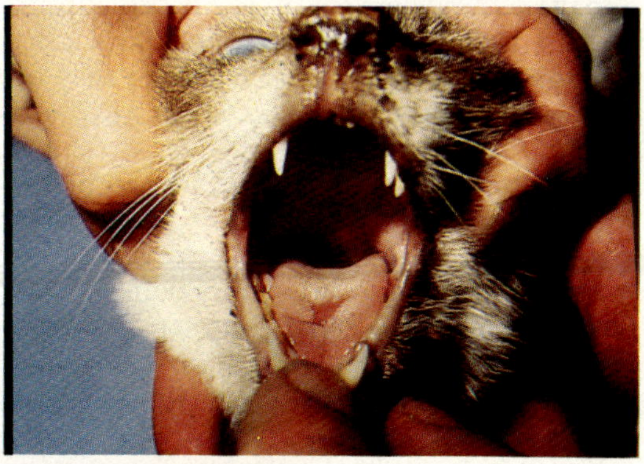

Figure 4–20

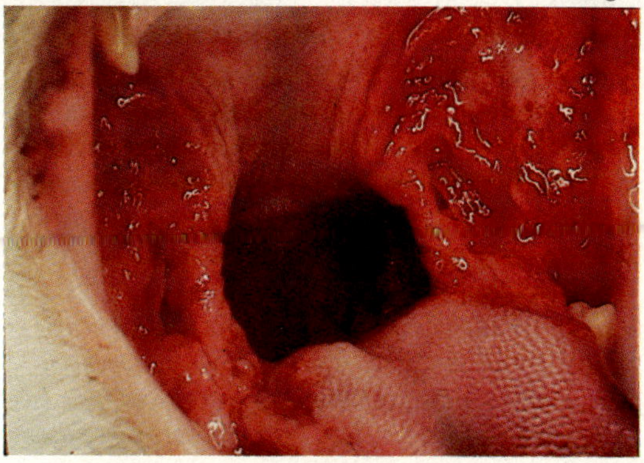

Figure 4–21

Figures 4–15 to 4–21. *See legends on opposite page.*

lesional skin should be sampled. A small portion of lesional skin can be included. Intact lesions, unless they are very small and are surrounded by normal skin, should not be submitted for direct immunofluorescence testing, since the inflammatory response will often destroy the immunoglobulins. Biopsies for immunofluorescence should be stored in Michel's fixative and sent to a laboratory that has feline and canine antisera available.

Pemphigus vulgaris is easily differentiated from bullous pemphigoid by direct immunofluorescence testing. Pemphigus vulgaris shows intercullar fluorescence in the epidermis, whereas bullous pemphigoid shows a linear deposition of immunoglobulin along the basement membrane.

Both pemphigus vulgaris and bullous pemphigoid are serious diseases with relatively poor prognoses and both require aggressive therapy. Apart from symptomatic therapy and antibiotic administration to treat a current or potential pyoderma, the main mode of therapy is immunosuppression.

Originally, only massive doses of corticosteroids (prednisolone: 4 mg to 12 mg/kg daily in two or three divided doses) were used. This therapy is often unsatisfactory because of unacceptable side effects, serious metabolic consequences, or incomplete response.[23] Cytotoxic immunosuppressive drugs were added to the regime to lower the doses of the corticosteroid, and therefore its side effects, and to improve the clinical response.[25] The drugs most frequently used are cyclophosphamide (1.5 mg/kg daily for 4 days each week) or azothioprine (1.5 mg/kg daily). Cyclophosphamide is more potent and has a synergistic immunosuppressive effect with prednisolone so that the dose of prednisolone required can be reduced to 1 mg to 2 mg/kg/day;[30] however, bone marrow suppression and sterile hemorrhagic cystitis can follow its use, and this drug is no longer widely used.[26] Azathioprine is a less potent immunosuppressive agent but has proved very effective in treating autoimmune disorders.[30] Apart from the potential for bone marrow suppression, this drug is relatively safe in the dog; the cat appears to be more sensitive to azothioprine, and hemograms should be monitored weekly. Azothioprine allows the dose of prednisolone to be reduced to 2 mg to 4 mg/kg/day.

Regardless of which agent or agents are used, the full dose should be administered until the lesions are completely healed, then a lifelong maintenance regime should be determined. Typically, the cytotoxic immunosuppressant is maintained at full dose while the prednisolone is switched to an alternate-day regime at the lowest possible dose. If the dose of prednisolone cannot be lowered to less than 1 mg to 2 mg/kg every other day, the cytotoxic drug probably cannot be discontinued.

Recently, chrysotherapy has been used in the treatment of pemphigus in the dog and cat and appears to be effective and safe.[25, 31] Aurothioglucose is administered at a dose of 1 mg/kg intramuscularly once weekly after two test doses have been given. Weekly injections are continued until remission is seen, then the frequency is lowered to semimonthly or monthly. In some dogs the drug can be discontinued.[31] The response time usually is slower than with other forms of therapy and can take at least 6 to 9 weeks. Corticosteroids can be used with chrysotherapy to lessen the animal's discomfort during the lag period. Cytotoxic immunosuppressive agents should not be used with chrysotherapy; recent immunosuppressant therapy may increase the possibility of an adverse reaction.[32] Because

---

Figure 4–15. Bullous autoimmune skin diseases. There are multiple oral ulcers and diffuse inflammation. This could be either pemphigus vulgaris or bullous pemphigoid.

Figure 4–16. Systemic lupus erythematosus. Note the depigmentation of the eyelids, nose, muzzle, and lips, and the gingivitis.

Figure 4–17. Discoid lupus erythematosus. There is depigmentation and focal ulceration of the lower lip, and an ulcer on the tongue.

Figure 4–18. Toxic epidermal necrolysis. Note the multiple ulcers on the tongue.

Figure 4–19. Ulcerative gingivitis in an FeLV positive cat.

Figure 4–20. Oral lesions in a 2 year old Siamese female cat with gingivitis, glossitis, stomatitis, fever, inappetence, and periodic anorexia. No cause was determined. Tests for FeLV and feline infectious peritonitis were negative, and thyroid function, hemograms, and metabolic profiles were normal.

Figure 4–21. Proliferative gingivitis in a cat.

For comparison, see Color Plates on pages 35, 40, and 50.

this drug has the potential to cause bone marrow suppression and renal damage, a weekly hemogram and blood urea nitrogen concentration should be evaluated during the loading period.

Systemic Lupus Erythematosus

Systemic lupus erythematosus is a multisystem disorder of unknown cause. Affected animals develop antibodies to their own nuclear proteins and other tissues, causing a variety of clinical signs.[33]

Cutaneous lesions occur in approximately 50 percent of dogs with systemic lupus erythematosus. They present as areas of depigmentation or leukoderma, with or without ulceration of the nose, lips, and oral cavity, and seborrheic-like skin lesions. Other typical and more striking abnormalities are shifting leg lameness, Coombs' positive anemia, thrombocytopenia, and glomerulonephritis.[33] The simultaneous occurrence of one or more of these disorders in an animal with skin disease should suggest a diagnosis of systemic lupus erythematosus.

Oral involvement other than depigmentation is infrequent, but is manifested as gingivitis or oral ulceration (Fig. 4–16).[34] Oral lesions have not been described in cats with systemic lupus erythematosus.[35]

Diagnosis of systemic lupus erythematosus is made when two major systems are involved and the immunoserological tests are positive. A tentative diagnosis of systemic lupus erythematosus can be offered if only one organ system is involved, and the serological tests are positive, or if two organ systems are affected, but the immunoserological tests are negative. The immunoserological tests include the lupus erythematosus preparation (LE Prep) and the antinuclear antibody test. The LE Prep is fairly specific, but it is of such poor sensitivity that it produces false-negative results in 30 to 80 percent of afflicted animals.[36, 37] False-positive results can occur but are rare. The antinuclear antibody test is not specific for systemic lupus erythematosus but is invariably positive; a positive antinuclear antibody test can occur in other diseases, as well as in normal dogs.[33, 37] To be of value, the results of any immunoserological test must be considered in conjunction with the clinical signs shown by the animal.

The diagnosis of cutaneous or oral lesions associated with systemic lupus erythematosus can be substantiated by biopsies for direct immunofluorescence. One sees either patchy and granular, or linear and continuous deposits of immunoglobulin at the dermoepidermal junction.

Since systemic lupus erythematosus is an immune-mediated disorder, immunosuppressive therapy as described for the bullous autoimmune diseases is appropriate. Because of its potential nephrotoxicity, chrysotherapy should not be used.

Discoid Lupus Erythematosus

Discoid lupus erythematosus is a mild, benign variant of systemic lupus erythematosus that is restricted to the skin and oral cavity. Discoid lupus erythematosus has been documented in the dog but not in the cat.[38, 39]

One of the striking features of discoid lupus erythematosus is the loss of normal pigmentation of the planum nasale and the lips and gums, with or without subsequent ulceration (Fig. 4–17). Additionally, the bridge of the nose is usually afflicted by a seborrheic-like condition with alopecia, erythema, scaling, crusting, hypopigmentation, and ulceration. Oral ulcers can be seen, especially on the tongue.

The tentative diagnosis of discoid lupus erythematosus can be made by the clinical findings and negative immunoserological tests. The diagnosis is confirmed by dermatohistopathological examination and direct immunofluorescence testing; results are similar to those seen in systemic lupus erythematosus.

Because discoid lupus erythematosus is typically a benign disease, intense immunosuppressive therapy is usually not necessary. Prednisolone at a daily dose of 2 mg/kg or less usually results in resolution of the lesions.[38] Oral vitamin E (*dl*-tocopherol acetate, 400 IU BID) has also been shown to be effective, but the response time is slower than that seen with prednisolone.[39] If the animal is pruritic, a combination of prednisolone and oral vitamin E can be useful; corticosteroids are continued until the lesions have healed and are then slowly withdrawn. Vitamin E therapy is continued to maintain the animal in remission.

Secondary or Idiopathic Immune Complex Diseases

Circulating immune complexes form when an antigen is in slight excess of the antibody produced by the host. The most frequently recognized immune complex disease of companion animals is systemic lupus erythematosus, but any chronic viral, bacterial, or neoplastic condition can induce immune complex formation and subsequent skin disease. In these instances, the cutaneous and oral lesions mimic those seen in systemic lupus erythematosus.

When an animal presents with skin lesions typical of systemic lupus erythematosus, but the immunoserological tests are negative, one should search for an antigen source. Skin lesions usually resolve spontaneously if the antigen source (such as a low-grade chronic bacterial infection) can be identified and resolved. If the antigenic source defies detection, the treatment regimen used for systemic lupus erythematosus is usually effective.

Drug Eruptions

A drug eruption is described as a cutaneous or mucocutaneous reaction to the administration of a drug,[36, 40] and is an allergic hypersensitivity reaction. In contrast, a drug reaction is an untoward or unexpected reaction of a non-allergic nature. Drug eruptions, though infrequent in veterinary patients,[26] may result from exposure to sulfa drugs and antibiotics such as the penicillins, chloramphenicol, and tetracycline.[36]

There is no classic presentation for a drug eruption; the same drug can produce a different reaction in different animals. The eruption usually occurs 7 to 14 days after the drug is started or anytime thereafter, but the reaction can occur earlier if the animal has received the drug previously.

The most serious form of a drug eruption is toxic epidermal necrolysis.[41] In this disorder, the epidermis becomes necrotic and sloughs to leave large areas of ulcerated skin. The mucocutaneous junctions are usually involved, and oral lesions are common (Fig. 4–18). Cutaneous lesions can occur anywhere on the body, especially over pressure points or in friction areas. Skin ulcers have a peripheral epidermal collarette. The animal is usually depressed, febrile, and anorectic, and often shows signs of cutaneous pain. It can be difficult if not impossible to differentiate between toxic epidermal necrolysis and pemphigus vulgaris or bullous pemphigoid, but the presence (with epidermal necrolysis) or absence (with bullous autoimmune disease) of cutaneous pain can be a useful diagnostic aid.

Drug eruptions, especially the milder forms, can be difficult to document; toxic epidermal necrolysis is relatively easy to confirm by biopsy. Apart from careful consideration of the history and skin biopsy results, there are no other uniformly valuable diagnostic tests. The diagnosis can be confirmed by readministration of the drug, but this may be dangerous and is not recommended.

Withdrawal of the drug should prove curative within 7 to 14 days, though the reaction can last longer. No additional therapy is necessary if the epithelial lesions are mild. In severe disorders such as toxic epidermal necrolysis, intensive supportive therapy will be necessary.

IMMUNODEFICIENCY DISEASES

Immunodeficiency diseases are those in which one or more components of the animal's immune system fail to function normally. The parts of the immune system that can be affected are non-specific immunity (such as complement pathway, polymorphonuclear leukocyte function), humoral immunity (B cells), and cell-mediated immunity (T cells).[42] The deficiency state can be inherited or acquired. Inherited immunodeficiencies are rare, since afflicted animals usually die when young. Acquired immunodeficiencies now are being recognized more frequently, since tests to document the deficiency state are more available. However, these diseases are rare, especially those involving the oral cavity.

Oral Diseases Associated with Immunodeficiency

If one discounts the immune-mediated diseases and the lymphoreticular neoplasms, which can be immunosuppressive, the primary oral sign of immunodeficiency is infection, either of a recurrent or resistant nature or associated with an organism that is not usually pathogenic. The infectious agent can be bacterial, viral, or fungal. In the dog, mucocutaneous candidiasis (see Fig. 4–3) and ulcerative stomatitis (see Fig. 4–2) are the most frequent diseases associated with immunodeficiency. Chronic, recurrent bacterial stomatitis-gingivitis (Fig. 4–19) is seen in the cat, sometimes secondary to FeLV infection.[7, 8, 43] The diagnosis and treatment of these disorders is described elsewhere in this chapter.

The immune system of any animal that has an unusual or recurrent oral infection should be evaluated (see Chapter 3), and a FeLV test specimen should be submitted from all afflicted cats.

The treatment of immunodeficiency disorders is often unrewarding. Immunopotentiating drugs can be tried (levamisole, 0.5 mg to 1 mg/kg every other day), but treatment achieves variable success.[44] Treatment of secondary infections or symptomatic treatment of oral ulcers is occasionally beneficial.

NON-SPECIFIC ORAL DISEASES

There are a variety of primary and secondary oral lesions that represent distinct clinical entities though no specific cause is recognized. They include tonsillitis, pharyngitis, idiopathic stomatitis, chronic feline gingivitis-stomatitis, and oral ulceration secondary to protein-calorie malnutrition. Tonsillitis and pharyngitis are discussed in Chapter 11.

Chronic Feline Gingivitis-Stomatitis

Chronic gingivitis, often in association with diffuse oral ulceration, stomatitis, glossopharyngitis, and granulation tissue in the caudal oropharynx, is a problem apparently unique to the cat.[20] No single cause is apparent. Although association with a deficient immune system and FeLV infection has been proposed,[7, 8, 42] it remains unproved. A calicivirus, one of the two major causes of upper respiratory viral infections in cats, was isolated from gingival tissue from eight of 10 cats with chronic gingivitis.[111]

The condition affects cats of any age and breed, and though there is no reported age or breed incidence, the Siamese seems especially susceptible. The disease is characterized by chronicity with intermittent exacerbations and a failure to permanently respond to any of a variety of therapeutic regimens.

Presenting signs include ptyalism, halitosis, dysphagia, inappetence or anorexia, and weight loss that can progress to severe emaciation.

Examination of the mouth reveals generalized hyperemia, gingivitis, gingival recession, or less frequently a proliferative gingivitis, periodontal disease, and loss of teeth. The premolar and molar gingivae are usually much more severely afflicted than the incisor and canine gingivae. In more advanced cases, severe lesions are seen at the mucosal commissures or on the palatine arches, soft palate, or oropharynx (Figs. 4–20 and 4–21). Histological examination of biopsy specimens made from the proliferative tissue frequently reveals an ulcerated mucosa with a dense submucosal inflammatory cell infiltrate that is characterized by a preponderance of plasma cells, neutrophils, lymphocytes, and histiocytes. This has led to the designation of the disease as feline plasma cell gingivitis-pharyngitis.[45]

Routine laboratory studies are of no help either in making a diagnosis or in pinpointing the cause. Mild anemia may be present in longstanding cases; some cats have a leukocytosis with a neutrophilia or eosinophilia, whereas others have a lymphopenia. Serum chemistry determinations are normal except for total protein elevation in many patients. Electrophoresis reveals a polyclonal elevation in the gamma globulin region.[45] Tests for feline leukemia virus and infectious peritonitis are usually negative. Similarly, tests of thyroid and adrenal function reveal no abnormality. Culture does not reveal any apparent pathogen.[45]

The differential diagnosis includes severe periodontal disease, feline leukemia virus–associated immunosuppression, eosinophilic granuloma complex, and periodontal disease secondary to hypothyroidism or diabetes mellitus.

Treatment is symptomatic and is seldom totally successful. Teeth cleaning, debridement of necrotic tissue, and extraction of any loose teeth are the first and most important steps. Antibiotics such as metronidazole or ampicillin appear to help, at least on a temporary basis. Multivitamin therapy, megestrol acetate, prednisolone, levamisole, thyroid hormone, and oral mouthwashes have all been used with varying but usually limited success. Many afflicted cats refuse to eat dry cat food, presumably because it causes too much oral pain, but such diets should nevertheless be offered for their benefit on oral health.[46] Maintenance of an adequate plane of nutrition is essential to prevent secondary lesions associated with protein-calorie malnutrition (see page 51), and cats should be coaxed to eat as much high-quality protein as possible, regardless of its consistency. The prognosis is poor with conservative treatment, but the usually excellent response to extraction of all the premolar and molar teeth suggests that the condition may be a variation of periodontal disease.

Feline Eosinophilic Granuloma Complex

The eosinophilic granuloma complex consists of three disorders: eosinophilic ulcer, eosinophilic plaque, and linear granuloma. The etiology of each of these conditions is unknown, and it is unclear whether they are related.[48] Although each disorder has a predilection for certain areas of the body, lesions can occur anywhere on the skin or in the oral cavity, or a combination of the two. When oral lesions are present, the initial complaint usually is dysphagia or ptyalism.[47]

Eosinophilic ulcer occurs primarily in middle-aged cats, with a three-fold higher incidence in females.[48] Lesions can occur anywhere on the skin or oral cavity, but 80 percent involve the upper lip. The lesions vary in size, depending on their chronicity, and are red and painless proliferative ulcers with raised borders (Fig. 4–22). Oral lesions present either as discrete nodules or plaques anywhere in the mouth or as one or more areas of ulcerative proliferative tissue.

Linear granuloma is typically a disease of the young cat, with a twofold higher incidence in females; oral lesions are common and present as single or multiple well-circumscribed, raised, firm, and yellowish-pink nodules in the mouth (Fig. 4–22).[48] Eosinophilic plaque oral lesions are rare.[48]

The clinical presentation usually suggests the tentative diagnosis of the eosinophilic granuloma complex. Because each of the disorders can occur anywhere on the body, lesions should be biopsied to confirm the diagnosis. Skin biopsies are essential to rule out squamous cell carcinoma or other tumors or when the lesion fails to respond to conventional therapy.

A sample for the FeLV test should be submitted from all afflicted cats, especially those with ulcerative oral disease. An absolute peripheral eosinophilia usually is present in animals with eosinophilic plaque or oral linear granuloma.[38] Other diagnostic tests are usually unrewarding.

Many forms of therapy have been used to treat the eosinophilic granuloma complex, but medical management, especially with glucocorticoids, is most rewarding. For small, solitary lesions, surgical excision or cryosurgery may be of benefit, but the success rate is variable.[47] Corticosteroids can be given intralesionally or systemically, or both.[47, 48] For solitary lesions, intralesional injections of 3 mg of triamcinolone are given weekly until the lesion has healed; three or four injections are usually required. High doses of oral prednisolone (1 mg to 2 mg/kg BID) are effective, but may be impractical depending on the nature of the cat and the presence of painful oral lesions. Methylprednisolone acetate injections (20 mg/cat, given subcutaneously every 2 weeks) are effective and avoid the need for oral drug administration. Regardless of the route of administration, the corticosteroid should be continued until the lesion has healed completely. A month or more of therapy is usually required.

Progestational compounds have gained wide acceptance for the treatment of the eosinophilic granuloma complex. Repository progesterone (2 mg to 20 mg/kg) or medroxyprogesterone acetate (50 mg to 175 mg/cat) can be given intramuscularly or subcutaneously every 2 weeks, or oral megestrol acetate can be administered at a dose of 2.5 mg to 5 mg every other day.[48] No matter which route of administration is used, treatment should be continued until the lesions are healed completely. Progestational compounds are not licensed for use in the cat and have a number of side effects, which include adrenocortical suppression, polydipsia, polyuria, polyphagia, obesity, personality changes, reproduction abnormalities, mammary hypertrophy, neoplasia, and diabetes mellitus.[49] Because of the side effects, these drugs should be used only when necessary and not as the first mode of therapy.

Inadequate drug doses or insufficient duration of corticosteroid or progestational therapy are the usual reasons for treatment failure. A staging system has been proposed to evaluate whether a recurrence is likely.[47] Cats with lesions that have never been treated before, cats that have had a previous lesion that has responded to therapy, or cats that have failed to respond to glucocorticoids have a 50 percent recurrence rate within 5 months.

The prognosis is poor in animals in whom the lesions have failed to respond to glucocorticoids and progestational compounds, or when intercurrent diseases, such as diabetes mellitus, negate the use of such drugs. Radiation therapy, cryotherapy, or immunotherapy may be of benefit.[47, 50]

Canine Eosinophilic Granuloma

A pathological process similar to the linear granuloma of the cat has been described in the dog.[51–53] The disorder has been reported

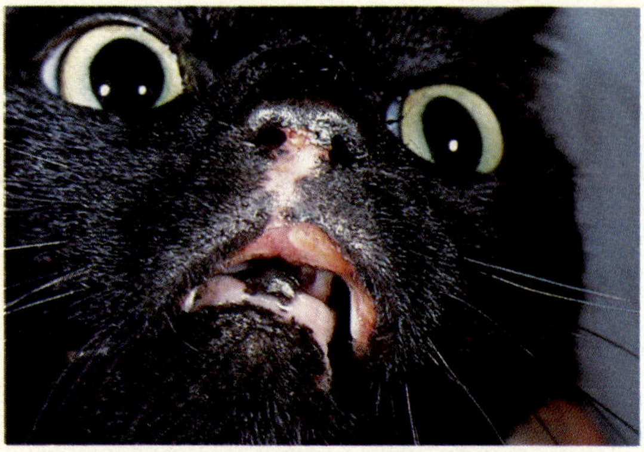

Figure 4–22A

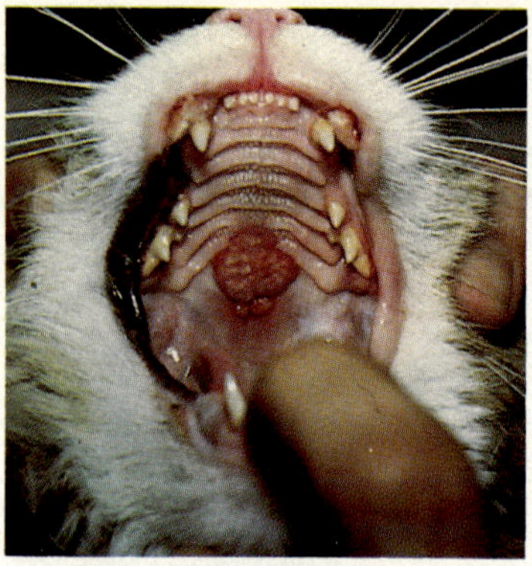

Figure 4–22B

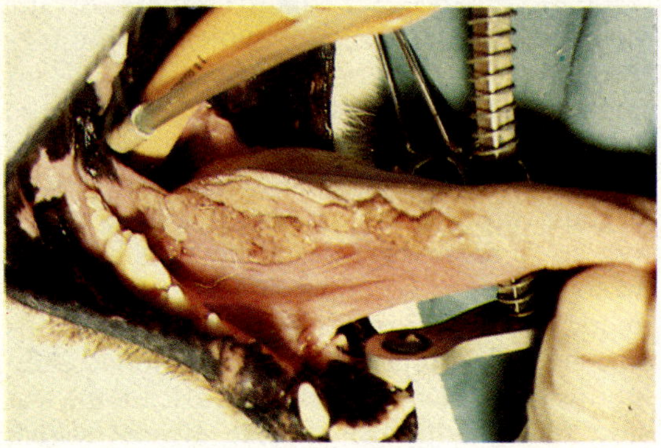

Figure 4–23

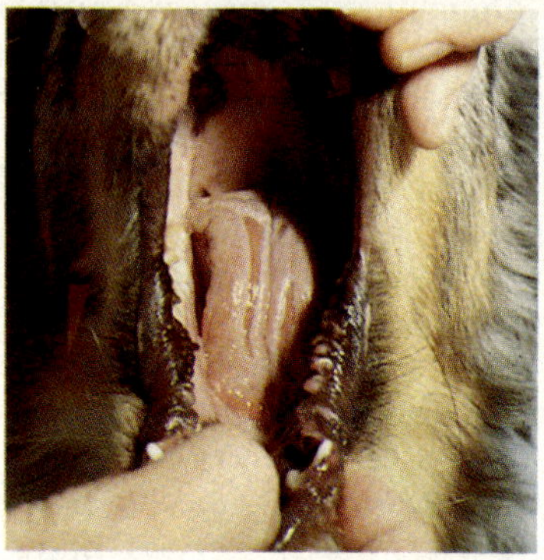

Figure 4–24

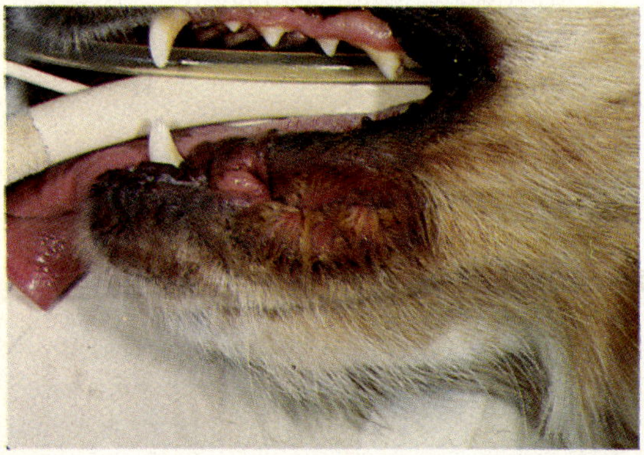

Figure 4–25

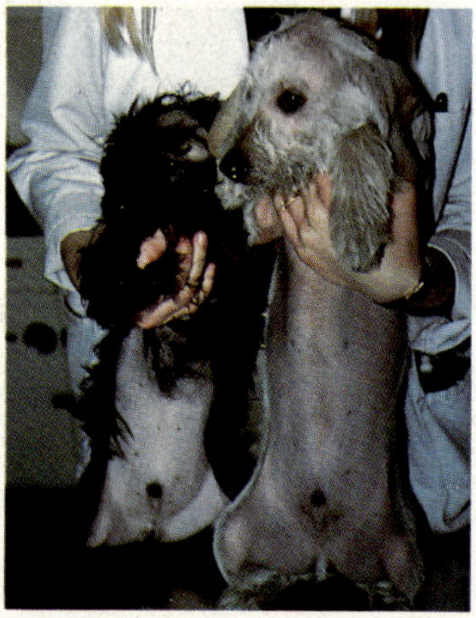

Figure 4–26

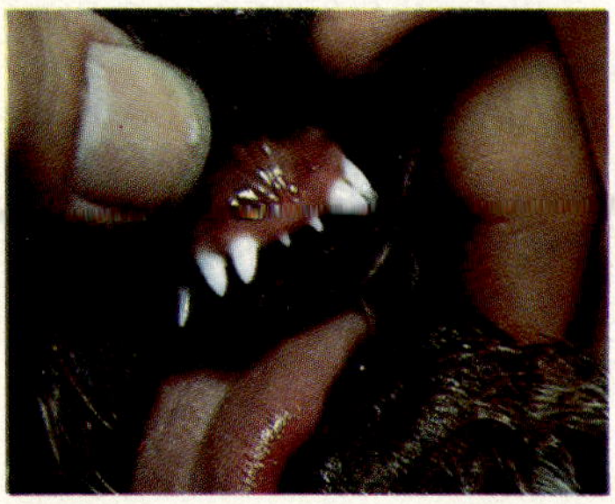

Figure 4–27

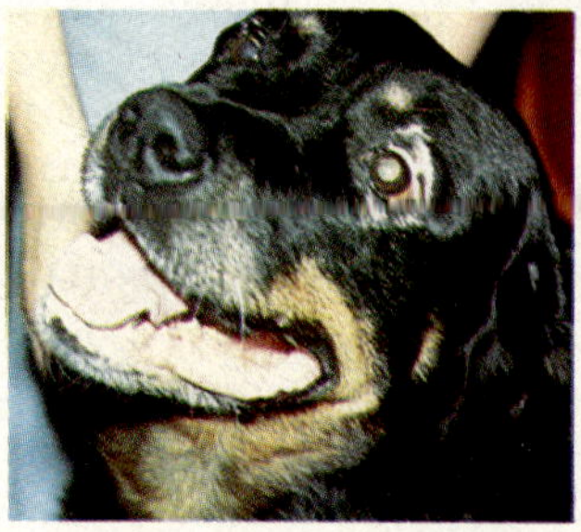

Figure 4–28

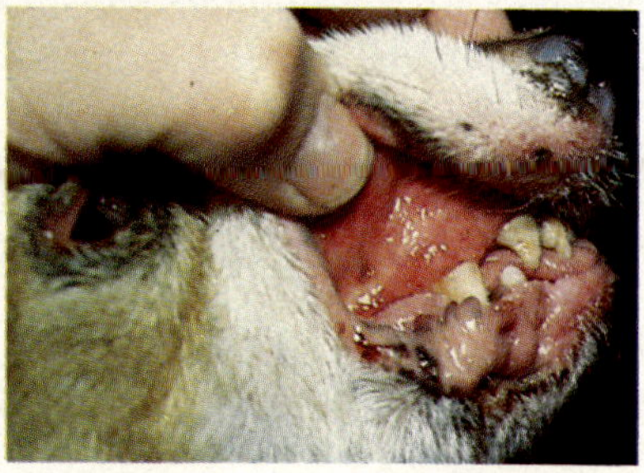

Figure 4–29

Figures 4–22 to 4–29. *See legends on opposite page.*

most frequently in the oral cavity of the Siberian husky, but cutaneous lesions have been recognized in other breeds,[52, 53] and oral lesions have been seen in the Samoyed.[52] Apart from the marked breed predilection, which suggests a hereditary influence, the etiology is unknown.

Approximately 90 per cent of animals with oral lesions are purebred Siberian huskies. There is no sex predilection, but the majority of afflicted animals are less than 3 years old. Lesions tend to occur on the ventral or lateral surface of the tongue or on the palatine mucosa. Animals with lingual lesions are usually presented for halitosis and oral pain, whereas the palatine lesions seem to cause little symptomatology.

Physical examination reveals one or more raised, irregular proliferative masses on or around the tongue (Fig. 4–23) or discrete raised ulcers on the palatine mucosa. A regional lymphadenopathy may be present.

The diagnosis is confirmed by biopsy. A hemogram evaluation yielded an absolute peripheral eosinophilia in approximately 80 percent of afflicted animals. Other diagnostic tests are usually unrewarding.

The condition responds rapidly to the oral administration of prednisolone (0.5 mg to 2 mg/kg daily); palatine ulcers may regress spontaneously.[52] A relapse can be expected in approximately 40 percent of dogs with lingual lesions. Each episode can be treated successfully with prednisolone. If the frequency of recurrence is high, the animal may be maintained with a course of alternate-day prednisolone.

Oral Ulceration Secondary to Protein-Calorie Malnutrition

Oral ulcers are common in dogs and cats with severe malnutrition, especially in animals that have an underlying disease process associated with excess loss of protein, such as protein-losing enteropathy or nephropathy (Fig. 4–24).

Malnutrition consistently and severely depresses the cell-mediated immune response,[54] though all aspects of immunity are depressed. The rate of cell turnover is decreased during protein depletion and this, coupled with a decrease in the immune response, predisposes animals to secondary ulceration. Stress, as an immune suppressant, may also be involved in the development of oral lesions. In humans, stress reduces salivary secretion of immunoglobulin A,[55] and in animals stress has been shown to increase susceptibility to viral, bacterial, and parasitic infections.[56]

When possible, treatment should be directed at correction of the underlying disease process.

Lingual Calcinosis

Heterotopic deposition of calcium salts in the submucosa of the tongue, and less frequently in the gingivae, is seen occasionally as a gritty mass; it occurs particularly in immature dogs of the larger breeds.[57] The pathogenesis is unknown but *Pasteurella multocida* has been isolated in pure culture from such a lesion and has been incriminated as the cause, even though this organism comprises part of the normal canine oral flora.[58] The breed, age, and appearance of the animal are diagnostic. The microscopic appearance is similar to that of subcutaneous calcinosis circumscripta.[59] Treatment is seldom necessary, but lesions may be surgically excised for cosmetic reasons or if dysphagia is evident.

Glossitis of Military Working Dogs

In 1973, an apparently unique pathological lesion affecting the tongues of military work-

Figure 4–22. Feline eosinophilic granuloma complex. *A*, Ulcers on the upper lip. *B*, A plaque-shaped lesion on the palate.

Figure 4–23. Canine eosinophilic granuloma. A proliferative, ulcerated mass can be seen on the ventrum of the tongue.

Figure 4–24. Linear ulcers in a dog with severe diarrhea and protein-losing enteropathy. The ulcers healed when the underlying disease was treated and the caloric intake improved.

Figure 4–25. Lip fold pyoderma, with alopecia, erythema, and exudation in the fold of the lower jaw.

Figure 4–26. Inherited ectodermal dysplasia. Hair loss is obvious on the head and ventrum.

Figure 4–27. Dental abnormality associated with ectodermal dysplasia.

Figure 4–28. Vitiligo. There is a lack of pigment on the lips, gums, and eyelids.

Figure 4–29. Mycosis fungoides causing depigmentation of the muzzle, lips, and eyelids, and proliferative gingivitis.

For comparison, see Color Plates on pages 35, 40, and 44

ing dogs was observed in South Vietnam.[60] The disease was characterized by an erosive glossitis with inflammation and loss of the dorsal lingual epithelium. Clinical signs included ptyalism, inappetence or anorexia, and in some cases the inability to lap water.[60] The tip of the tongue appeared reddened and smooth at physical examination. There were no characteristic hematological or blood chemical abnormalities. The condition is believed to be caused by excessive exposure to sunlight, which produces irreversible changes in lingual epithelial regeneration.[61] Treatment is symptomatic and involves rest and avoidance of sunlight. The disease thus far has not been reported elsewhere.

Idiopathic Stomatitis

Oral lesions in some animals defy diagnosis and do not appear to fall into any of the preceding categories. It is generally neither necessary nor practical to eliminate the likelihood of many of these diseases at the time of initial presentation. If the disease primarily affects the periodontium and the history and clinical signs do not indicate a separate disease, the condition should be treated as periodontal disease. Only when the response is poor are additional diagnostic tests, such as those detailed in Chapter 3 and Table 3–1, indicated.

In some patients, the response to antifungal or immunostimulant therapy may be good, even when diagnostic tests indicate no immunological abnormality. Extraction of some or all of the teeth is a practical and frequently successful last resort in patients with chronic, non-responsive, or undiagnosed gingival disease.

SKIN DISEASES AFFECTING THE MOUTH AND FACE

Lip-fold Pyoderma

Lip-fold pyoderma is a surface bacterial infection of the lip area that is seen in spaniels, setters, and other breeds that have large, pendulous upper lips and pronounced lower lip folds.[20, 62] Because of this anatomical abnormality, saliva and food accumulate in the folds and macerate the tissues. This maceration, combined with the dark, warm, and moist environment of the fold, predisposes the area to surface infection that results in an extremely fetid odor. As a result, the primary complaint is usually halitosis rather than skin disease.

Physical examination reveals red, glistening, and ulcerated skin in the folds along the lower jaw (Fig. 4–25). The area usually stinks and may be tender, depending on the degree of involvement. Afflicted animals often have concurrent dental disease that contributes to the halitosis.

Since lip-fold pyodermas are secondary to an anatomical abnormality, the only curative procedure is to surgically ablate the folds along the lower jaw (see Chapter 10). Medical therapy (clipping, cleaning, and drying the area with a topical astringent, and topical or systemic corticosteroids) is often instituted before surgery to decrease the friability of the tissue and may be useful for longterm management in some animals. Once the infection is resolved, careful daily cleaning, especially after meals, may hold the condition in check without surgery, but relapses must be expected.

Congenital Ectodermal Defects

A variety of congenital ectodermal defects have been described in the dog and cat.[63] These animals are affected when young and present for either partial or near total hairlessness or baldness. Some of these animals also have abnormal dentition (Figs. 4–26 and 4–27). The combination of alopecia plus dental abnormalities in a young dog indicates a hereditary rather than an acquired alopecia. There is no treatment for the alopecia, and the animal should not be used for breeding.

Depigmentation Disorders

Depigmentation disorders, in which pigmentation is lost in apparently normal skin, are rare; they can be either focal or diffuse. Since inflammatory conditions such as discoid lupus erythematosus can cause hypopigmentation, it is important to recognize that idiopathic depigmentary processes do occur.

Spontaneous depigmentation (vitiligo) has been recognized in the dog, especially in the Belgian Tervuren and Rotweiler.[64] In these animals the site and extent of the depigmentation is variable. Usually the nose, lips, mouth, and eyelids are involved (Fig. 4–28), but the skin or toenails can also be affected. These animals are normal except for hypopigmentation. Diagnosis is confirmed by biopsy, which shows normal skin devoid of pigment or melanocytes. No therapy has proved effective. Apart from its cosmetic effect, vitiligo can predispose the dog to a second solar dermatitis, and intense solar exposure should be avoided.

The Vogt-Koyanagi-Harada syndrome is a condition of uncertain but probable autoimmune origin, tentatively recognized in the husky, Akita, and Samoyed.[65, 66] Afflicted animals have severe uveitis, and depigmentation of the skin, especially of the nose, lips, mouth, and eyelids. The condition appears to respond favorably to corticosteroids provided that the eyes have not been too severely damaged.

Cutaneous Lymphosarcoma

Cutaneous lymphosarcoma with or without systemic involvement occurs infrequently in the dog and rarely in the cat.[67] Cutaneous lymphomas can present as a nodular disease or as a bizarre dermatosis that mimics pemphigus, systemic lupus erythematosus, and a number of other disorders.[68] The most bizarre skin lesions tend to occur in a superficial epidermotrophic form called mycosis fungoides.

In the dog, mycosis fungoides usually presents as large, irregular areas of erythema, alopecia, and exfoliation combined with plaques of variable size, which may or may not be ulcerated.[69] Lesions can occur anyplace on the face and body. The lips and muzzle are usually depigmented and erythematous. Oral involvement is common (Fig. 4–29) and can take the form of discrete ulcers or a proliferative cheilitis and gingivitis, or both. Apart from the skin lesions, all other organ systems are usually normal except for a regional reactive lymphadenopathy. The animal is usually pruritic.

Diagnosis of a cutaneous neoplasm is difficult in the non-specific or early plaque stage. Skin biopsies are usually necessary to document the condition and differentiate it from inflammatory skin conditions.

Cutaneous lymphomas are not curable but may be controlled for a variable period of time with either systemic chemotherapy or topical nitrogen mustard application.[68, 69] Corticosteroids will usually not decrease the animal's pruritis unless they are combined with an appropriate chemotherapeutic regime. Because of the poor prognosis, many owners elect to euthanize the animal rather than treat it.

ANTIMICROBIAL THERAPY IN ORAL DISEASE

A variety of antimicrobial agents have proved useful in the symptomatic treatment of oral disease. It must be emphasized, however, that such therapy is usually adjunctive and there is little or no evidence for any primary oral bacterial infection in the dog and cat. The rationale behind most antimicrobial therapy is to depress oral flora that has overgrown as a result of a primary disease process. If possible, treatment should always be directed at correction or amelioration of the underlying disease. Indiscriminate use of antibiotics may predispose the animal to candidiasis. Antimicrobial agents, dosages, and indications are listed in Table 4–3.

Whether antibiotics are necessary at the time of periodontal examination or teeth cleaning has been the subject of much debate. There is ample evidence that invasion of the periodontal pocket with instruments causes a transient bacteremia,[70, 71] and that periodontal disease is common in dogs with clinically obvious bacterial endocarditis;[72] however, there is no direct evidence that treatment of dental disease in dogs causes endocarditis. Normal dogs clear oral bacteria from the blood within 20 minutes of onset of bacteremia.[73] When circumstances suggest that there is a greater than usual risk, such as an immunosuppressed animal or one with clinically evident chronic valvular disease and purulent debris in deep periodontal pockets, a single dose of a broad-spectrum bacteriocidal antibiotic given immediately before treatment seems prudent (ampicillin, 10 mg/kg intramuscularly is recommended). In general, the temptation to clean the teeth of an animal under anesthesia should be resisted if the major procedure performed creates deadspace in tissue planes in an otherwise clean wound. This is because the bacteremia associated with the teeth cleaning may seed infection in blood clots within the tissue spaces.[74]

SUPPORTIVE CARE OF THE PATIENT WITH ORAL DISEASE

Many oral diseases are extensive and painful, preclude grooming, and impair the appetite and the prehension or swallowing of

Table 4–3. Antimicrobials Used in the Treatment of Oral Disease

Compound	Indications	Dosage	Route
Lincocin	Ulcerative stomatitis	20 mg–45 mg/kg BID or TID	Oral, IM, IV
Cephalosporins Cephalexin	Ulcerative stomatitis	30 mg–40 mg/kg TID or QID	Oral, IM, IV, SC
Tetracycline	Ulcerative stomatitis Leptospirosis Maxillary or mandibular osteomyelitis	20 mg–60 mg/kg BID or TID	Oral, IM, IV
Procaine penicillin and	Leptospirosis	15,000–30,000 IU/kg BID	SC, IM
streptomycin	Leptospirosis	20 mg–40 mg/kg TID	SC, IM
Ampicillin	Supportive therapy in feline viral respiratory disease	20 mg–40 mg/kg TID	Oral, SC, IM, IV
Amoxicillin*	Supportive therapy in feline viral respiratory disease	20 mg–40 mg/kg TID	Oral, SC, IM, IV
Chloramphenicol	Supportive therapy in feline viral respiratory disease	60 mg–120 mg/kg TID	Oral, SC, IM, IV
Trimethoprim-sulfadiazine	Feline viral respiratory diseases gingivitis, ulcerative stomatitis	30 mg/kg TID	Oral
Metronidazole	Ulcerative stomatitis, gingivitis, periodontitis	50 mg/kg SID	Oral
Ketoconazole	Oral candidiasis, systemic fungal infections	10 mg/kg as single or divided dose	Oral
Chlorhexidine	Periodontal disease, oral cleansing	0.2% solution	As oral rinse or toothbrush solution

*As a single prophylactic IM injection before oral procedures, 10 mg/kg IM.
IM = intramuscularly; IV = intravenously; SC = subcutaneously.

food and water. Although treatment of the underlying lesion is most important, recovery is usually enhanced if it is accompanied by nursing and nutritional care. In some instances supportive care can be lifesaving.

Feeding

Provision of an adequate caloric intake is essential in patients that are unwilling or unable to eat. Injury and disease enhance

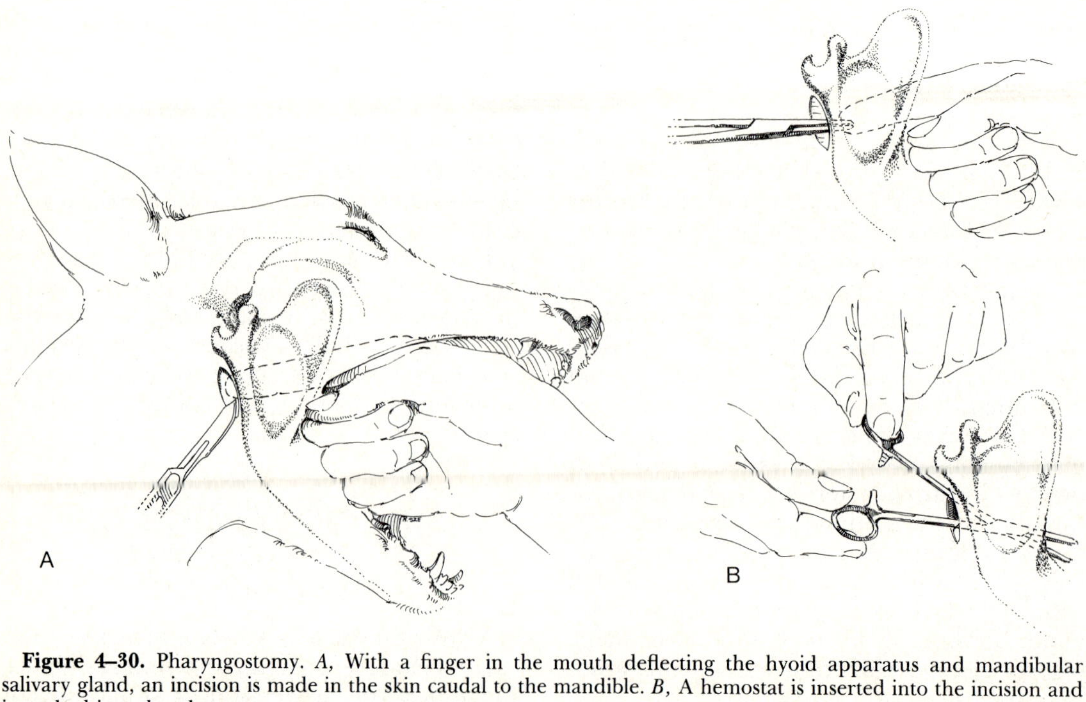

Figure 4–30. Pharyngostomy. *A,* With a finger in the mouth deflecting the hyoid apparatus and mandibular salivary gland, an incision is made in the skin caudal to the mandible. *B,* A hemostat is inserted into the incision and is pushed into the pharynx.

Illustration continued on opposite page

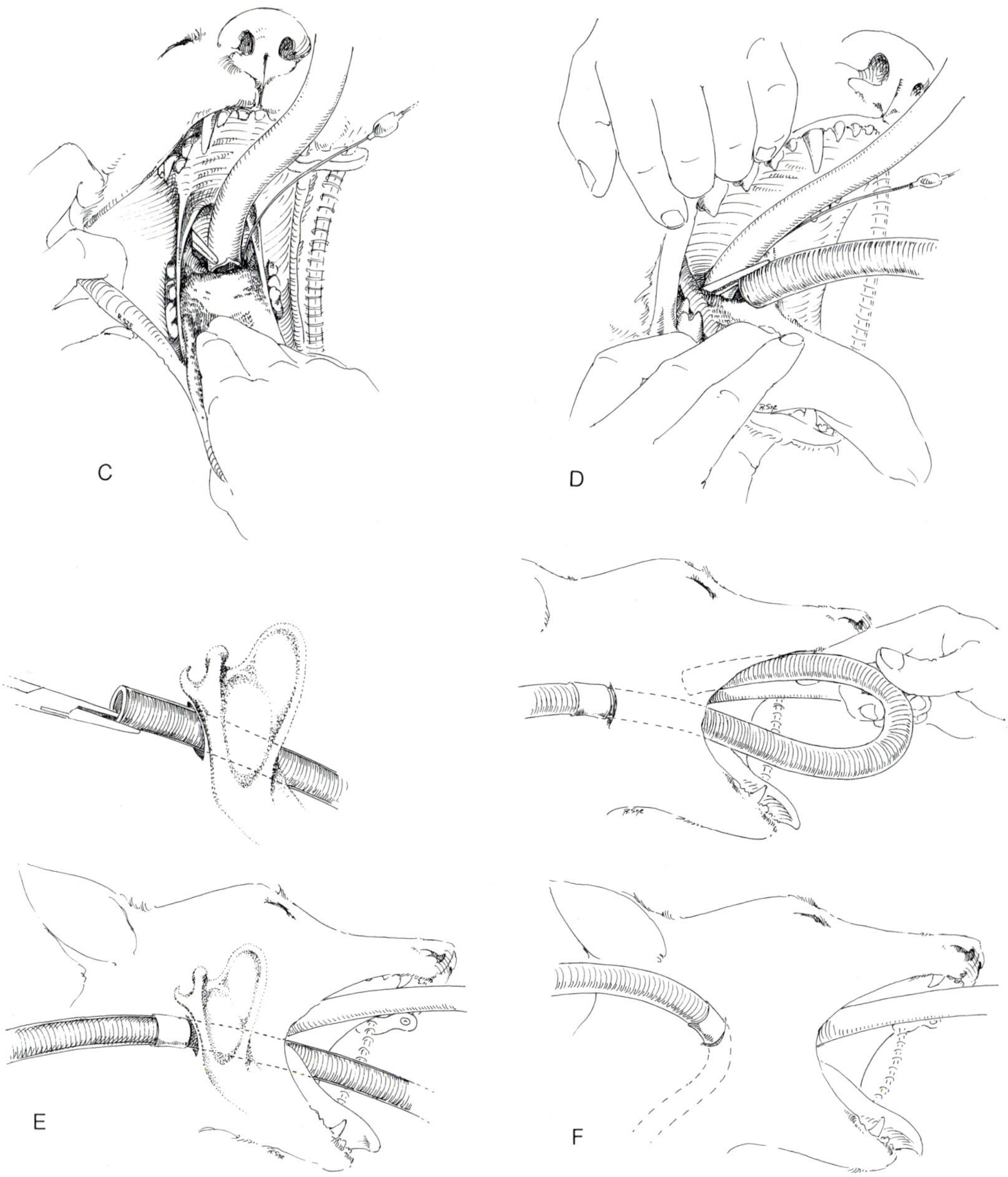

Figure 4–30. *Continued. C* and *D,* A feeding tube or endotracheal tube is placed between the jaws of the hemostat and is withdrawn through the incision. *E* and *F,* The tube is turned and inserted into the esophagus (as a feeding tube) or larynx (to bypass the oral cavity during oral or pharyngeal procedures). (From Slatter DH: Textbook of Small Animal Surgery. Philadelphia, W.B. Saunders Co., 1985.)

dietary protein requirements for tissue regeneration and repair, and immune function is depressed if food intake is decreased or protein loss is excessive.[54] Anorexic patients with mild oral disease frequently can be coaxed to eat if hand-fed one of the highly palatable canned meat-based foods. Dry cereal-based foods are best avoided in severe disease, since they are painful to chew and swallow and can prolong morbidity.[5] Dry food may be beneficial when oral lesions have healed, however, since it reduces the incidence and severity of gingivitis and related disorders.[46]

When oral lesions are severe or recovery is likely to be prolonged, feeding by a pharyngostomy tube is preferred. A pharyngostomy tube should always be used as an alternative to long-term force feeding in animals with painful oral lesions. Specific indications include mandibular and facial fractures, damage to the hyoid apparatus, diseases associated with severe stomatitis, glossitis, and gingivitis, and feline viral respiratory disease.

The only instruments required for the procedure are a mouth gag, a scalpel, a pair of curved hemostats, and appropriate tubing.[75] The tube may be made of rubber or polyethylene; soft rubber urinary catheters are ideal. The tube should not be so long that it passes through the caudal esophageal sphincter, since it predisposes to reflux esophagitis.[76] Tubes should always be removed as soon as practical, which means as soon as the animal begins to eat voluntarily. The presence of the tube does not impair the swallowing of solid food.

The lateral neck area on one side is clipped and prepared for surgery. Under general anesthesia, an index finger is inserted through the mouth into the pharynx and is then flexed to palpate and deflect the hyoid arch and mandibular salivary gland. The skin is incised directly over the finger tip (Fig. 4–30 *A*), and a large hemostat is pushed through the incision, intervening muscle, and mucosa, guided by the finger in the mouth (Fig. 4–30 *B*). A flexible feeding tube of suitable size is placed between the jaws of the hemostat and is pulled through the incision (Fig. 4–30 *C* and *D*). The tube is then turned in the mouth (Fig. 4–30 *E*) and inserted into the esophagus or trachea (Fig. 4–30 *F*).

Foods must be reduced to a liquid consistency before feeding. Canned food blended 1:1 with tap water, or prepared meat baby foods are good choices; supplemental vitamins may be added. The tube is also useful for administering liquid medication and to ensure adequate hydration. Feeding is best accomplished using a syringe and catheter adaptor, but the tube should be capped between feedings to preclude aerophagia. Food should be freshly prepared daily and fed frequently (at least four times daily). Clients can easily master the technique for continued tube feeding at home. The amount fed should approximate or preferably exceed normal daily caloric maintenance requirements.[77] The incision is allowed to granulate closed following removal of the tube.

Nursing

Nursing care is mainly common sense and involves ensuring the patients cleanliness, exercise, grooming, and comfort. Regular grooming is important, especially in cats.

Severe oral lesions may be cleaned with 0.2 percent chlorhexidine or dilute (1 to 3 percent) hydrogen peroxide solution. If carried out gently, animals readily accept this procedure, which facilitates the healing process. Accumulations of serum and necrotic tissue should be cleaned from the lips and commissures. Overvigorous cleaning is contraindicated if it leaves surfaces raw.

Competent and diligent nursing care by the veterinarian, staff, and client is an extremely important aspect of the treatment of oral lesions and must never be neglected.

References

1. Kaplan ML, Jeffcoat MJ: Acute necrotizing ulcerative gingivitis. *Canine Pract* 5:35–37, 1978.
2. Richardson RC, Jaeger LA, Wigle W: Treatment of systemic mycosis in dogs. *J Am Vet Med Assoc* 183:335–336, 1983.
3. Farrow BRH, Love DN: Bacterial, viral, and other infectious problems. *In* Ettinger SJ: Textbook of Veterinary Internal Medicine, 2nd ed., pp. 269–319. Philadelphia, WB Saunders Co., 1983.
4. Gaskell RM, Wardley RC: Feline viral respiratory disease: A review with particular reference to its epizootiology and control. *J Small Anim Pract* 18:1–16, 1978.
5. Johnson RP, Povey RC: Effect of diet on oral lesions of feline calicivirus infection. *Vet Rec* 110:106–107, 1982.
6. Gaskell RM, Povey RC: Experimental induction of feline viral rhinotracheitis virus: excretion in FVR-recovered cats. *Vet Rec* 100:128–133, 1977.
7. Barrett RE, Port JE, Schultz RD: Chronic relapsing stomatitis in a cat associated with feline leukemia virus infection. *Feline Pract* 5:34–38, 1975.
8. Cotter SM, Hardy WD, Essex M: Association of feline leukemia virus with lymphosarcoma and other disorders in the cat. *J Am Vet Med Assoc* 166:449–454, 1975.
9. Pyle RL, Dunbar M, Nelson PD, Hawkins JA, Turner LW: Canine blastomycosis. *Comp Cont Educ* 3:963–974, 1981.
10. Harvey CE, O'Brien JA: Nasal aspergillosis—penicillosis. *In* Kirk RW (ed): Current Veterinary Therapy 8, pp. 236–241. Philadelphia, WB Saunders Co., 1983.
11. Rosychuk, R.: Management of hypothyroidism. *In* Kirk RW (ed): Current Veterinary Therapy 8, pp. 869–876. Philadelphia, WB Saunders Co., 1983.
12. Connor S, Iranpoor B, Mills J: Alteration in parotid salivary flow in diabetes mellitus. *Oral Surg* 30:55–57, 1970.
13. Kornegay JN, Greene CN, Martin C, Gorgacz EJ, Melcon DK: Idiopathic hypocalcemia in four dogs. *J Am Anim Hosp Assoc* 16:723–734, 1980.
14. Hall DE: Blood coagulation and its disorders in the dog. Baltimore, Williams & Wilkins, 1972.
15. Osborne CA, Finco DR, Low, DG: Pathophysiology of renal disease, renal failure and uremia. *In* Ettinger SJ (ed): Textbook of Veterinary Internal Medicine, 2nd ed., pp. 1733–1792. Philadelphia, WB Saunders Co., 1983.
16. Oehme FW: Toxicological problems. *In* Ettinger SJ (ed): Textbook of Veterinary Internal Medicine, 2nd ed., pp. 173–207. Philadelphia, WB Saunders Co., 1983.

17. Cheville NF: The gray collie syndrome (cyclic neutropenia). *J Am Anim Hosp Assoc* 11:350–353, 1975.
18. Clark KA: Management of poisonous snakebites in dogs and cats. *Mod Vet Pract* 62:427–431, 1981.
19. Schaer M: A survey of Eastern Diamondback Rattlesnake envenomation in 20 dogs. Comp Cont Ed, in press.
20. Gaskell RM, Gruffydd-Jones TJ: Intractable feline stomatitis. *Vet Ann* 17:195–199, 1977.
21. Muller GH, Kirk RW: Small Animal Dermatology, 2nd ed. Philadelphia, WB Saunders Co., 1976.
22. Stannard AA, Gribble DH, Baker BB: A mucocutaneous disease in the dog resembling pemphigus vulgaris in man. *J Am Vet Med Assoc* 166:575–582, 1975.
23. Scott DW, Lewis RM: Pemphigus and pemphigoid in dog and man: comparative aspects. *J Am Acad Dermatol* 5:148–167, 1981.
24. Brown N, Hurvitz AI: A mucocutaneous disease in a cat resembling human pemphigus. *J Am Anim Hosp Assoc* 15:25–28, 1979.
25. Manning TO, Scott DW, Smith CA, Lewis RM: Pemphigus diseases in the feline: seven case reports and discussion. *J Am Anim Hosp Assoc* 18:433–443, 1982.
26. Halliwell REW: Skin diseases associated with autoimmunity. Part I. The bullous autoimmune skin diseases. *Comp Cont Ed* 2:911–918, 1980
27. Scott DW, Manning TO, Smith CA, Lewis RM: Pemphigus vulgaris without mucosal or mucocutaneous involvement in two dogs. *J Am Anim Hosp Assoc* 18:401–404, 1982.
28. Turnwald GH, Ochoa R, Barta O: Bullous pemphigoid refractory to recommended dosage of prednisolone in a dog. *J Am Vet Med Assoc* 179:587–591, 1981.
29. Griffin CE, MacDonald J: A case of bullous pemphigoid in a dog. *J Am Anim Hosp Assoc* 17:105–108, 1981.
30. Pederson NC: Immunosuppressive drugs and their role in the treatment of immunologic diseases of the dog. *Gaines Vet Symp* 28:13–20, 1978.
31. Manning TO, Scott DW, Kruth SA, Sozanski M, Lewis RM: Three cases of canine pemphigus foliaceous and observations on chrysotherapy. *J Am Anim Hosp Assoc* 16:189–202, 1980.
32. Fadok V: Thrombocytopenia and hemorrhage associated with gold salt therapy for bullous pemphigoid in a dog. *J Am Vet Med Assoc* 181:261–262, 1982.
33. Halliwell REW: Skin diseases associated with autoimmunity. Part II. The non-bullous autoimmune skin diseases. *Comp Con Ed* 3:156–162, 1981.
34. Matus RE, Scott RC, Saal S, Gordon BR, Hurvitz AI: Plasmaphoresis-immunoadsorption for treatment of systemic lupus erythematosus in a dog. *J Am Vet Med Assoc* 182:499–502, 1983.
35. Scott DW, Haupt KH, Knowlton BF, Lewis RM: A glucocorticoid-responsive dermatitis in cats resembling systemic lupus erythematosus in man. *J Am Anim Hosp Assoc* 15:157–171, 1979.
36. Scott DW: Immunologic skin disorders in the dog and cat. *Vet Clin North Am* 8:641–664, 1978.
37. Quimby FW, Smith CA, Brushwein M, Lewis RM: Efficacy of immunoserodiagnostic procedures in the recognition of canine immunologic diseases. *Am J Vet Res* 41:1662–1666, 1980.
38. Griffin GE, Stannard AA, Ihrke PJ, Ardans AA, Cello RM, Bjorling DR: Canine discoid lupus erythematosus. *Vet Immun Immunopathol* 1:79–87, 1979.
39. Walton DK, Scott DW, Smith CA, Lewis RM: Canine discoid lupus erythematosus. *J Am Anim Hosp Assoc* 17:851–858, 1981.
40. Miller WH Jr: Canine facial dermatoses. *Comp Cont Ed* 1:640–650, 1979.
41. Scott DW, Halliwell REW, Goldschmidt MH, DiBartola S: Toxic epidermal necrolysis in two dogs and a cat. *J Am Anim Hosp Assoc* 15:271–279, 1979.
42. Perryman LE: Mechanisms of immune deficiency diseases of animals. *J Am Vet Med Assoc* 181:1097–1101, 1982.
43. Hardy WD Jr: Feline leukemia virus non-neoplastic diseases. *J Am Anim Hosp Assoc* 17:941–949, 1981.
44. Theilen GH, Hills D: Comparative aspects of cancer immunotherapy: immunologic methods used for treatment of spontaneous cancer in animals. *J Am Vet Med Assoc* 181:1134–1141, 1982.
45. Johnessee JS, Hurvitz AI: Feline plasma cell gingivitis-pharyngitis. *J Am Anim Hosp Assoc* 19:179–181, 1983.
46. Egelberg J: Local effect of diet on plaque formation and development of gingivitis in dogs. 1. Effect of hard and soft diets. *Odont Rev* 16:31–41, 1965.
47. Hess PW, MacEwen EG: Feline eosinophilic granuloma. *In* Kirk RW: Current Veterinary Therapy 7, pp. 534–537. Philadelphia, WB Saunders Co., 1977.
48. Scott DW: Feline dermatology. Disorders of unknown or multiple origin. *J Am Anim Hosp Assoc* 16:406–416, 1980.
49. Chastain CB, Grahmann CL, Nichols CE: Adrenocortical suppression in cats given megestrol acetate. *Am J Vet Res* 42:2029–2035, 1981.
50. Willemese A, Lubberink AAME: Eosinophilic ulcers in cats. *Tijdschr Diergen* 103:1052–1056, 1978.
51. Madewell BR, Stannard AA, Pulley LT, Nelson VG: Oral eosinophilic granuloma in Siberian Husky dogs. *J Am Vet Med Assoc* 177:701–703, 1980.
52. Potter KA, Tucker RD, Carpenter JL: Oral eosinophilic granuloma of Siberian Huskies. *J Am Anim Hosp Assoc* 16:595–600, 1980.
53. Turnwald GH, Hoskins JD, Taylor HW: Cutaneous eosinophilic granuloma in a Labrador retriever. *J Am Vet Med Assoc* 179:799–802, 1981.
54. Sheffy BE, Williams AJ: Nutrition and the immune response. *J Am Vet Med Assoc* 180:1073–1076, 1982.
55. Jemmolt JB, Borysenko JZ, Borysenko M, McClelland C, et al: Academic stress, power motivation, and decrease in secretion rate of salivary secretory immunoglobulin A. *Lancet*: 1:1400–1402, 1983.
56. Borysenko M, Borysenko J: Stress, behavior and immunity: animal models and mediating mechanisms. *Gen Hosp Psychiatry* 4:59–67, 1982.
57. Lane JG: ENT and Oral Surgery in the Dog and Cat, p. 187. Bristol, England, Wright PSG, 1981.
58. Arnjberg J: Pasteurella multocida from canine and feline teeth, with a case report of *glossitis calcinosa* in a dog caused by *P. multocida*. *Nord Med Vet* 30:324–332, 1978.
59. Douglas SW, Kelly DF: Calcinosis circumscripta of the tongue. *J Small Anim Pract* 7:441–443, 1966.
60. Stedham MA, Jennings PB, Moe JB, Elwell PA, Perry LR, Montgomery CA: Glossitis of military working dogs in South Vietnam: history and clinical characteristics. *J Am Vet Med Assoc* 163:272–274, 1973.
61. Jennings PB, Lewis GE, Crumrine MH, Coppinger TS, Stedham MA: Glossitis of military working

dogs in Vietnam: experimental production of tongue lesions. *Am J Vet Res* 35:1795–1799, 1974.
62. Kunkle GA: Canine pyoderma. *Comp Cont Ed* 1:7–13, 1979.
63. O'Neill CS: Hereditary skin diseases in the dog and cat. *Comp Cont Ed* 3:791–798, 1981.
64. Mahaffey MB, Yarbrough KM, Munnell JF: Focal loss of pigment in the Belgian Tervuren dog. *J Am Vet Med Assoc* 173:390–396, 1978.
65. Bussanick MN, Rootman J, Dolman CL: Granulomatous panuveitis and dermal depigmentation in dogs. *J Am Anim Hosp Assoc* 18:131–138, 1982.
66. Halliwell REW: Autoimmune diseases in domestic animals. *J Am Vet Med Assoc* 181:1088–1096, 1982.
67. Goldschmidt MH: Skin tumors in the dog. Part III. Lymphohistiocytic and melanocytic tumors. *Comp Cont Ed* 2:588–594, 1981.
68. McKeever PJ, Grindem CB, Stevens JB, Osborne CA: Canine cutaneous lymphoma. *J Am Vet Med Assoc* 180:531–536, 1981.
69. Miller WH, Jr: Canine cutaneous lymphomas. *In* Kirk RW (ed): Current Veterinary Therapy 7. Philadelphia, WB Saunders Co., 1980.
70. Black AP, Crichlow AM, Saunders JR: Bacteremia during ultrasonic teeth cleaning and extraction in the dog. *J Am Anim Hosp Assoc* 16:611–616, 1980.
71. Jackson DA, Huse DC, Kissil MT: Bacteremia following ultrasonic scaling in the dog. Presentation at Ann Meet Am Coll Vet Surg 1981.
72. Calvert DA: Valvular bacterial endocarditis in the dog. *J Am Vet Med Assoc* 180:1080–1084, 1982.
73. Silver JG, Martin L, McBride BC: Recovery and clearance rates of oral microorganism following experimental bacteraemias in dogs. *Arch Oral Biol* 20:675–679, 1975.
74. Withrow SJ: Dental extraction as a probable cause of septicemia in a dog. *J Am Anim Hosp Assoc* 15:345–346, 1979.
75. Bohning RH, DeHoff WD, McElhinney A, Hofstra P: Pharyngostomy for maintenance of the anorexic animal. *J Am Vet Med Assoc* 156:611–615, 1970.
76. Lantz GC, Cantwell HD, Van Fleet JF, Blakemore JC, Newman S: Pharyngostomy tube induced esophagitis in the dog: an experimental study. *J Am Anim Hosp Assoc* 19:207–212, 1983.
77. Alpo Pet Center: Canine Nutrition and Feeding Management. Alpo Pet Foods, Allentown, Pennsylvania, 1984.
78. Riser WH, Parkes LJ, Shirer JF: Canine craniomandibular osteopathy. *J Am Rad Soc* 8:23–31, 1967.
79. Fox MW: Abnormalities of the canine skull. *Can J Comp Med Vet Sci* 9:219–222, 1963.
80. Fox MW: The otocephalic syndrome in the dog. *Cornell Vet* 54:250–259, 1964.
81. Gruneberg H, Lea AJ: An inherited jaw anomaly in long-haired Dachshunds. *J Genet* 30:285–296, 1940.
82. Ritter R: Konnen anomalien des begisses gezuchtet werden? *Dtsch Zahn Mund Kieferheik* 4:235–257, 1933.
83. Phillips, JM: "Pig jaw" in cocker spaniels. Retrognathia of the mandible in the cocker spaniel and its relationship to other deformities of the jaw. *J Hered* 36:177–181, 1945.
84. Stockard CR: The genetic and endocrinic basis for differences in form and behavior as elucidated by studies of contrasted pure-line dog breeds and hybrids. American Anatomical Memoirs. Philadelphia, Wistar Institute of Anatomy and Biology, 1941.
85. Cooper HK Jr, Mattern GW: Genetic studies of cleft lip and palate in dogs (a preliminary report). *Carnivore Genet Newsletter* 9:204–209, 1970.
86. Gardner JE Jr: Report of a survey on cleft palates in the English Bulldog. *Bulletin of the Bulldog Club of New Jersey*, September, 1954.
87. Horowitz SL, Chase HB: A microform of cleft palate in dogs. *J Dent Res* 49:892, 1970.
88. Jurkiewicz MJ: A genetic study of cleft lip and palate in dogs. *Surg Forum* 16:472–473, 1965.
89. Jurkiewicz MJ, Bryant DL: Cleft lip and palate in dogs: a progress report. *Cleft Palate J* 5:30–36, 1968.
90. Pearce RG: Anomalies of the English Bulldog. *Southwest Vet J* 22:218–220, 1969.
91. Aitchison J: Incisor dentition in short muzzled dogs. *Vet Rec* 76:165–169, 1964.
92. Golden AM, Stoller NH, Harvey CE: Survey of oral and dental disease in dogs anesthetized at a veterinary hospital. *J Am Anim Hosp Assoc* 18:891–899, 1982.
93. Arnall L: Some aspects of dental development in the dog. III Some common variations in their dentition. *J Small Anim Pract* 2:195–201.
94. Andrews AH: A case of partial anodontia in a dog. *Vet Rec* 90:144–145, 1972.
95. Bodingbauer J: Hochgradige zahnunterzahl (aplasie) beim hunde. *Wein Tierarzt Monaschr* 61:301–303, 1974.
96. Skrentary TT: Preliminary study of the inheritance of missing teeth in the dog. *Wein Tierarzt Monaschr* 51:231–245, 1964.
97. Burstone MS, Bond E, Litt R: Familial gingival hypertrophy in the dog (boxer breed). *Arch Pathol* 54:208–212, 1952.
98. Hutt FB, deLahunta A: A lethal glossopharyngeal defect in the dog. *J Hered* 62:291–293, 1971.
99. Ingham B: Aplasia of a ramus of the mandible in a cat. *Br Vet J* 126:iii–iv, 1970.
100. Elzay RP, Hughes RD: Anodontia in a cat. *J Am Vet Med Assoc* 154–667–670, 1969.
101. Kratochvil K: Oligodontia and pseudoligodontia in the domestic cat. *Acta Vet Brno* 44:291–296, 1975.
102. Loevy HT: Cytogenetic analysis of Siamese cats with cleft palate. *J Dent Res* 53:453–456, 1974.
103. Loevy H, Fenyes VL: Spontaneous cleft palate in a family of Siamese cats. *Cleft Palate J* 5:57–60, 1968.
104. Catcott EJ: Feline Medicine and Surgery. Wheaton, Illinois, American Veterinary Publications, 1964.
105. Robinson R: Genetics for Cat Breeders, p. 170. Oxford, Permagon Press, 1971.
106. Glenn BL: Feline porphyria. *Comp Pathol Bull* 2:2–3, 1970.
107. Glenn BL, Glenn HG, Omtvedt IT: Congenital porphyria in the domestic cat (Felis catus): preliminary investigation on inheritance pattern. *Am. J Vet Res* 29:1653–1657, 1958.
108. Tobias G: Congenital porphyria in a cat. *J Am Vet Med Assoc* 145:462, 463, 1964.
109. Patterson DF: Catalog of genetic disorders of the dog. *In* Kirk RW (ed): Current Veterinary Therapy 7, pp. 82–103. Philadelphia, WB Saunders Co., 1980.
110. Saperstein G, Harris S, Leipold HW: Congenital Defects in Domestic Cats. pp. 1–24. Ralston Purina Co., 1978.
111. Thompson RR, Wilcox GE, Clark WT, Jansen KL: Association of calicivirus infection with chronic gingivitis and pharyngitis in cats. *J Small Anim Pract* 25:207–210, 1984.

Chapter Five

Periodontal Disease

TK Grove

Periodontal disease is very common in dogs;[1] less is known of its incidence in cats. Almost all dogs more than 5 years of age have measurable gingival changes, whether the owner is aware of clinical signs of disease or not.[2]

STRUCTURE OF THE NORMAL PERIODONTIUM

The periodontal tissues surround and support the tooth in the mouth (Figs. 5–1 through 5–3). Clinically, the free gingival margin touches the tooth at the most coronal portion of the interface between tooth and periodontium. It should have a "knife edge" tip, be coral pink or physiologically pigmented, and tightly adapted to the tooth unless reflected away by an instrument. In the latter case, it should provide some resistance to displacement. The free gingival margin becomes part of the interdental papilla between the teeth. When adjacent teeth contact each other, there is a col, or slight depression, in the interdental papilla underneath the contact point between these teeth (e.g., between the lower fourth premolar and the first molar in dogs). When a physiological space exists between teeth, the free gingival margin encircles the tooth at approximately the same height circumferentially. A free gingival groove may or may not be present around normal teeth; in animals without previous periodontitis, this groove usually corresponds to the depth of the gingival sulcus. The attached gingivae are coral pink or physiologically pigmented, are tightly bound to periosteum, and are of variable width. The junction between the attached gingivae and alveolar mucosae is called the mucogingival junction. The alveolar mucosa is less firmly bound to the periosteum of the mandible and maxilla, contains muscle and elastic fibers, and is continuous with buccal and sublingual soft tissue.

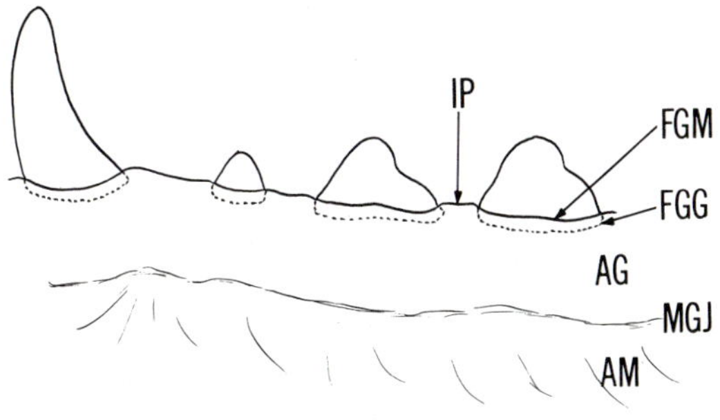

Figure 5–1. Gingival anatomical landmarks. FGM = free gingival margin; FGG = free gingival groove; AG = attached gingiva; MGJ = mucogingival junction; AM = alveolar (buccal or lingual) mucosa; IP = interdental papilla.

HISTOLOGICAL CHARACTERISTICS OF THE NORMAL PERIODONTIUM

The oral surface of the periodontium is covered by stratified squamous epithelium.

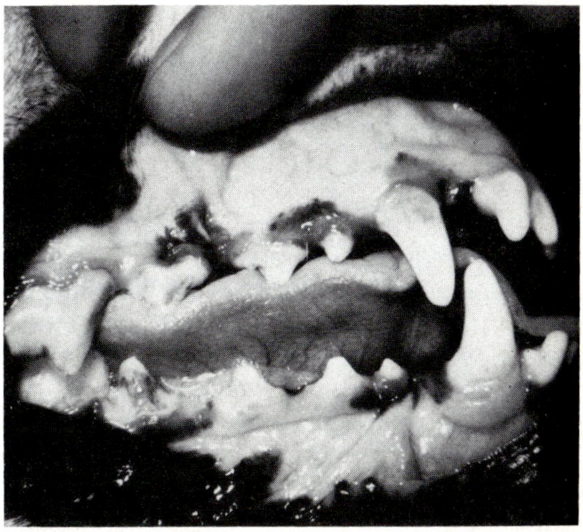

Figure 5–2. Mouth of a dog with gingivitis, plaque, and calculus deposition, showing gingivae surrounding the teeth.

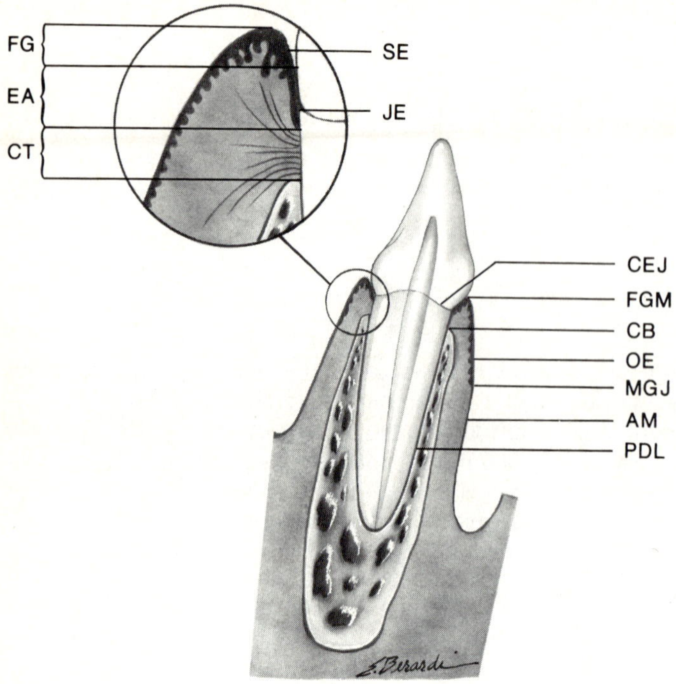

Figure 5–3. Diagrammatic cross section of a tooth in the mandible. AM = alveolar mucosa; CB = crestal bone; CEJ = cemento-enamel junction; CT = connective tissúe attachment; EA = epithelial attachment; FGM = free gingival margin; JE = junctional epithelium; MGJ = mucogingival junction; OE = oral epithelium; SE = sulcular epithelium; PDL = periodontal ligament.

This epithelium is made up of four layers: (1) basal, (2) spinous, (3) granular, and (4) cornified. The average renewal time of the gingival epithelium is about 10 days for monkeys[3] and may be similar for other animals.

The sulcular epithelium extends from the marginal gingivae to the epithelial attachment. It covers the subgingival soft tissues in a healthy animal. Epithelial projections and greater thickness distinguish this epithelium from that of the epithelial attachment (Fig. 5–4). The sulcular epithelium is two layers thick, consisting of a basal layer adjacent to connective tissue and a spinous layer adjacent to the tooth surface. Spinous epithelial cells are shed into the potential space between gingivae and teeth as the basal layer regenerates the sulcular epithelium. Leukocytes and gingival fluid migrate through this sulcular epithelium as a protective mechanism.[4]

The epithelial attachment is contiguous with the sulcular epithelium and the tooth. This epithelium, also termed the "junctional epithelium," is only a few cells thick and does not have projections into the gingival connective tissue. The epithelial attachment may end on enamel, dentin, or cementum, depending on the age of the animal and previous involvement with periodontal disease. In general, the epithelial attachment begins on enamel and, prior to maturity, migrates

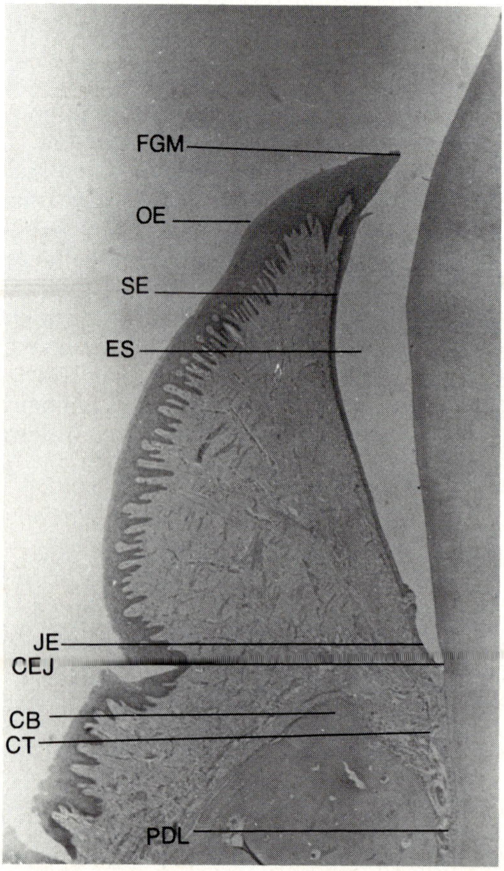

Figure 5–4. Histological section through the normal periodontium. ES = enamel space left after processing.

to the cemento-enamel junction, at which point it stays until trauma or disease moves it toward the end of the root (apex) of the tooth. This migration below the cemento-enamel junction signifies a pathological condition. Turnover time for the epithelial attachment is approximately 5 to 7 days.[5] Cuticle, fibrillar, or afibrillar cementum may be interposed between the epithelial attachment and the tooth.

Islands of epithelium associated with the periodontium are found in the periodontal membrane. Known as Malassez's epithelial rests, they are derived from remnants of Hertwig's epithelial root sheath during formation of the root of the tooth. They have no known function but may divide or become cystic on stimulation by inflammation.[6] Various cysts may originate from these rests. Without stimulation, these cells may persist as resting cells for the life of the individual with little or no mitosis.[7]

Underneath the periodontal epithelium there is connective tissue composed of bundles of collagen fibers that maintain the adaptation of the periodontal tissues of the teeth. These fiber bundles form along lines of stress, anchor the tooth to bone, adapt the gingivae to the teeth, and connect adjacent dental and periodontal structures.

The blood supply to the gingivae (connective tissue and epithelium combined) arises from the periosteum of the maxilla and mandible and also comes from the periodontal membrane space. The latter vessels are especially important in supplying the interdental and marginal gingivae.

The gingivae are innervated by the trigeminal nerve. Regional nerve blocks can be used to perform periodontal procedures[8] in very tractable animals; however, this method is usually impractical for all but the simplest procedures.

Space between the root of the tooth and the alveolar bone is filled by connective tissue bundles, which are termed the "periodontal membrane." These connective tissue bundles insert in the cementum on the root of the tooth and alveolar bone lining the alveolus, providing an organic union between tooth and bone. They also allow minor tooth movement when force is applied to teeth during external trauma or during normal mastication. The periodontal membrane is the chief determinant of proprioception during mandibular closing for prehension. The periodontal membrane contains nerve endings for pain perception.

The alveolar bone is a thin plate of cortical bone that lines the alveolus. It forms part of the alveolar process, which is that part of the mandible and maxilla containing the alveoli or sockets for the roots of the teeth. There is no definite boundary to the alveolar process in the normal animal; however, following tooth loss it resorbs.

EPIDEMIOLOGICAL FEATURES

Many breeds of dog develop periodontal disease naturally, some more severely than others.[1] In general, small dogs and dogs with abnormal occlusion (e.g., bulldogs with mandibular prognathism) have more severe problems than medium sized and larger dogs. Periodontal disease is an inflammatory condition of the tissues that surround and support the teeth. It is usually of bacterial origin. When there is only inflammation of the periodontium, the periodontal disease is called gingivitis. When there is inflammation plus detachment of the connective tissues from the root surfaces, the disease is called periodontitis. The disease begins as subclinical gingivitis, distinguished clinically primarily by an increase in the amount of fluid that exudes from the space between the gingivae and the teeth (the gingival crevice).[9] The disease progresses to gingivitis, which is clinically recognized by inflammation of the free gingival margin that, perhaps, extends to the attached gingivae as the disease becomes more longstanding. Later still, usually after years of inflammation (gingivitis), irreversible lesions occur, resulting in loss of the connection between periodontal tissues and the teeth (loss of attachment), and then the disease is called periodontitis. Without dental care, as dogs age they go through a sequence of the steps just described. Various indices are used to measure the severity of a given parameter for the measurement of periodontal problems and, when applied by an examiner, these indices result in scores. Higher values for these scores indicate more severe periodontal problems.

There is a tendency for subclinical and clinical gingivitis scores, plaque scores, and calculus scores to increase sharply between 1 and 3 years of age.[10] At 5 or 6 years of age, irreversible changes associated with periodontitis become evident. The severity of periodontal disease remains the same or increases thereafter; tooth loss, endodontic lesions, and periodontal abscesses occur in more severely affected animals. The disease does not regress or remit without treatment.

Dogs show clinical and histological signs of periodontal disease to a greater degree, and earlier, when maintained on a soft rather than a hard diet.[11, 12] A diet that is sticky, promoting accumulation of debris around the teeth, is more important in promoting periodontal disease than a nutritionally inadequate diet. If teeth are kept clean, periodontal disease will not develop even if the animal's diet is inadequate. Gingivitis is closely correlated with the development of bacterial plaque at the neck of the tooth. Periodontitis is closely correlated with longstanding gingivitis, plaque, and calculus. In both gingivitis and periodontitis measurements, upper teeth are slightly more severely affected than lower teeth.[10] Upper canine teeth are affected similarly to cheek teeth in disease severity. Lower canine teeth and incisors are usually less severely diseased than the rest of the mouth. Buccal surfaces are more severely affected by periodontitis than are lingual surfaces. Rostral and caudal surfaces of teeth are less diseased than are buccal surfaces but are more diseased than are lingual or palatal surfaces. The exception to this tendency occurs between the lower fourth and fifth cheek teeth. Disease in this location is often more severe than in other areas of the mouth, possibly because there is contact between these teeth.

ETIOLOGY AND PATHOGENESIS

Periodontal disease is caused by a change from a predominantly non-motile, gram-positive, aerobic, coccoid microbial flora on the neck of the tooth to a more motile gram-negative, rod-shaped, anaerobic flora. This change in bacterial composition can occur in 2 weeks when bacterial plaque is allowed to accumulate between teeth and gingivae. It appears that *Bacteroides asaccharolyticus* and *Fusobacterium nucleatum* may be especially important in the development of periodontal disease;[13, 14] however, many microbial forms are found around teeth in health and disease, making determination of the pathological role of each microbe difficult.

As plaque ages it calcifies, forming calculus. The surface of undisturbed calculus always is covered by plaque. Some investigators feel that without the mechanical effect of calculus, gingivitis would never progress to periodontitis. However, most feel that bacterial plaque is the primary and overwhelming reason for all forms of periodontal disease.[15–19] Calculus above the gingival margin is called supragingival calculus; calculus below the gingival margin is called subgingival calculus. There are differences in mineral content, thickness, density, and color between subgingival and supragingival calculus; however, the significance of these differences is unknown.

Other local factors, such as hair impaction and trauma from chewing foreign objects, probably play a role in the development of periodontal disease that is secondary to and dependent upon bacterial plaque for the initiation and progression of periodontal lesions. These cofactors have not been well investigated in veterinary dentistry.

Although neutrophils may participate in pathological processes that cause tissue destruction, it is likely that they are primarily protective of the host during the development of periodontal disease. Accordingly, diseases with neutrophil-compromising characteristics are often accompanied by more severe and aggressive periodontal lesions than those seen in other animals with similar local irritation around the teeth.[10] However, these compromised individuals are affected by periodontal disease only when bacterial plaque is present.

Periodontal disease is not inevitable as an animal ages. It is dependent on oral uncleanliness. Those animals who do not accumulate plaque or who have recurrent gingivitis treated will experience little or no periodontitis as they age.[20]

The accumulation of bacteria and their byproducts at the gingival margin causes an increase in the amount of fluid and leukocytes that normally exude from the gingival sulcus. This is called subclinical gingivitis and can be measured with filter paper strips placed in the gingival sulcus for a standardized period of time and stained with triketohydrindene hydrate (Ninhydrin). Gingivitis begins as a vasculitis of the marginal gingivae, and the intercellular spaces of the crevicular epithelium widen to allow enhanced emigration of polymorphonuclear neutrophils and gingival fluid into the sulcus. Later the acute inflammatory infiltrate is augmented by small and medium sized lymphocytes, macrophages, and plasma cells. More chronic gingivitis is characterized by predominantly plasma cells in the inflammatory infiltrate.

Calicivirus frequently can be isolated from cats with generalized gingivitis-stomatitis.[40] The significance of this observation in the etiology of periodontal disease in cats is unknown at present.

As already stated, periodontitis is the loss of attachment between periodontal tissue and the tooth, combined with inflammation of the periodontium. It is characterized by ulceration of the subgingival epithelium, loss of connective tissue attachment beneath the epithelial attachment, a decrease in the density and organization of collagen in the periodontal gingivae, and osteoclastic resorption of the marginal alveolar bone. Periodontitis that is not treated is usually progressive.[10, 21] In time, teeth become very mobile and are exfoliated. Frequently, there is abscessation of the periodontal or periapical tissues, an endodontic pathological condition of the pulp of the tooth, pain and difficulty masticating food, and occasionally severe bone resorption that will predispose the mandible to pathological fracture.

For additional reading on the etiology and pathogenesis of periodontal disease, see Grove TK, 1982.[22]

DIAGNOSIS

In practice, the diagnosis of periodontal disease is often suggested by the chief complaint or history that the client provides. Bad breath, yellow teeth, difficulty eating, loose teeth, and facial swellings are frequent problems related by the client that the veterinarian should regard as reasons for examining the mouth for a periodontal pathological condition. A cursory examination of the mouth during a visit for immunization or other routine veterinary service is always indicated. The presence of bad breath, inflammation of the gingivae, plaque, and calculus on the teeth (Fig. 5–5) warrants a more detailed examination. Dental cleaning (prophylaxis) is indicated once a year in many animals to treat recurrent gingivitis by removing plaque and calculus that would otherwise initiate the development of periodontitis. Extensive cleaning and detailed examination of the periodontium are probably best done concurrently at a single visit under general anesthesia.

Periodontal disease rarely requires emergency treatment. Initial therapy consisting of tooth cleaning will prevent further irreversible damage for several weeks if definitive treatment must be delayed.

Periodontal disease is basically inflammation caused by bacteria. Therefore, the cardinal signs of inflammation—heat, redness, swelling, pain, and loss of function—are a suggestion that the veterinarian may be dealing with periodontal disease. The presence of calculus and plaque on the teeth, migration of the attachment between tooth and periodontium toward the end of the root of the tooth, and exudate coming from beneath the gingival margin (Fig. 5–6) confirm the diagnosis in nearly all cases, especially when these findings are generalized rather than specifically localized to only one tooth or part of a tooth. Because periodontal disease is so common, it would be best to treat animals with these clinical findings as if they had periodontal disease, until proved otherwise

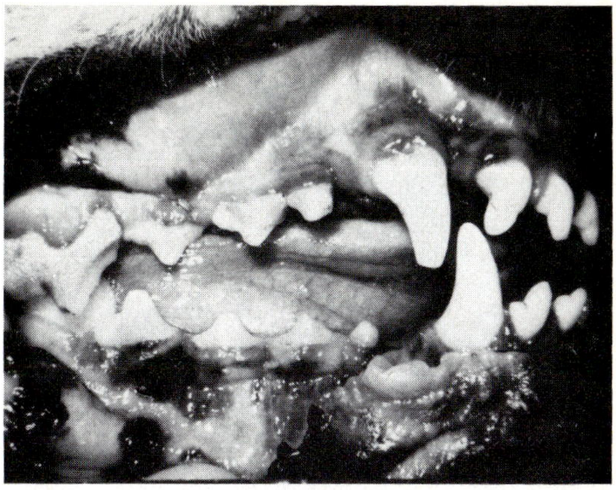

Figure 5–5. Inflammation and debris indicating the need for a comprehensive dental examination. This dog has gingivitis and periodontitis.

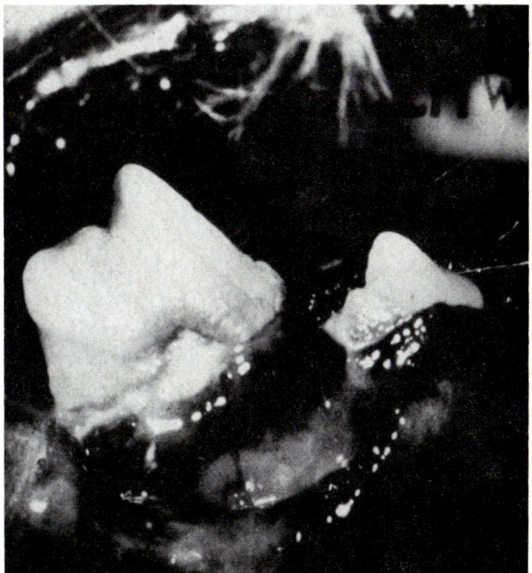

Figure 5–6. Purulent exudate coming from beneath the gingival margin.

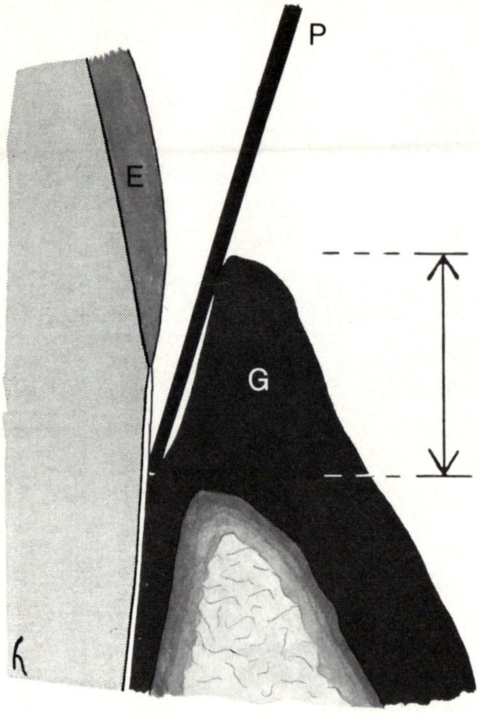

Figure 5–7. Probing the periodontal pocket. E = enamel; G = gingiva; P = probe.

by lack of response to meticulous tooth cleaning.

The primary objective in the diagnosis of periodontal disease is to distinguish between gingivitis and periodontitis. Animals with periodontitis may need surgery to optimize the life expectancy of the dentition. Gingivitis and periodontitis often look the same on unaided visual examination, especially when periodontitis is of the pocket-forming rather than the recessive variety. Radiographs and inspection of the gingival sulcus with a thin calibrated periodontal probe will readily distinguish between gingivitis and periodontitis.

The periodontal probe is held with the measuring tip parallel to the long axis of the tooth. The point of the probe is advanced gently below the gingival margin until soft tissue resistance is felt (Fig. 5–7). A notation is made of the depth of the pocket or sulcus at that point on the tooth. The presence of plaque, bleeding, and serous or purulent exudate and the presence and severity of inflammation in that location are also noted.[2] A chart for recording this information is shown in Figure 3–7. Color-coded periodontal probes graduated in millimeters facilitate speed and ease eye strain when the examination is made. Experienced examiners usually glide the probe along the tooth taking several measurements and recording the deepest areas on the rostral, buccal, caudal, and lingual surfaces when the recording is for clinical treatment planning. Research investigations usually require measurements to be made at predetermined points rather than at the location of the most severe lesion. The distance between the free gingival margin and the cemento-enamel junction is also recorded (Fig. 5–8). Using these two figures the attachment level can be calculated and recorded. This allows the examiner to determine which pockets represent loss of periodontal support ("true" pockets) and which pockets represent hyperplasia of the gingivae (pseudopockets). It tells the examiner when periodontal disease is present by demonstrating inflammation and loss of attachment despite the absence of periodontal pockets. Although this form of periodontal examination is quite tedious, it should be learned by the practitioner so that differentiation among pseudopockets, true pockets, and receding periodontal disease can quickly take place in everyday practice.

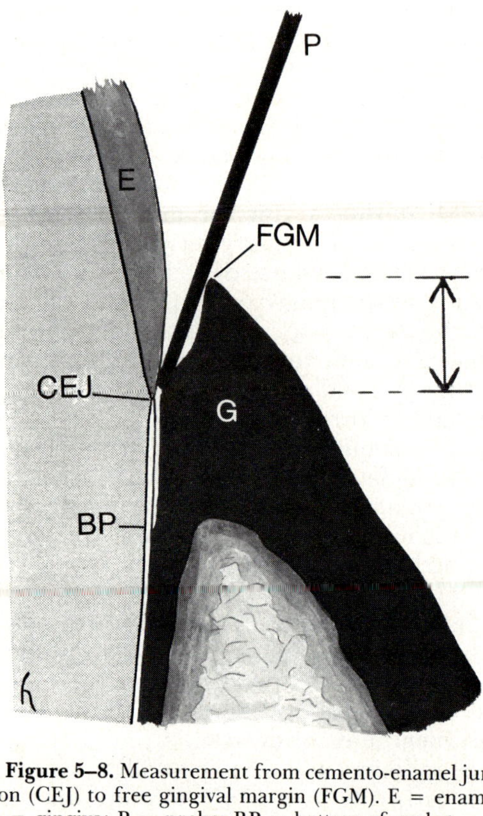

Figure 5–8. Measurement from cemento-enamel junction (CEJ) to free gingival margin (FGM). E = enamel; G = gingiva; P = probe; BP = bottom of pocket.

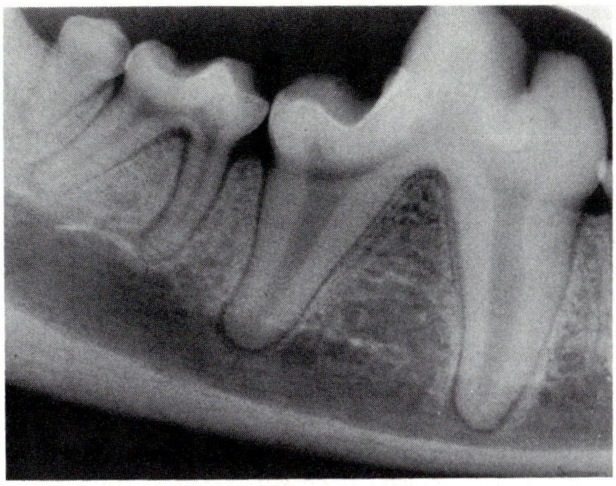

Figure 5–9. Radiograph showing normal relationship between tooth and alveolar bone.

Animals with pockets deeper than 3 mm, with concurrent attachment levels more than 2 mm below the cemento-enamel junction and inflammation, have periodontitis. Animals with attachment levels no greater than 2 mm below the cemento-enamel junction and inflammation have gingivitis no matter how deep the sulcus or pseudopockets. In both forms of periodontal disease, inflammation must be demonstrated to make the diagnosis, since postoperative periodontitis cases usually do not regain normal attachment levels.

Radiographs are useful in periodontal procedures[23, 24] (Fig. 5–9) primarily for assessing attachment levels on the rostral and caudal aspects of teeth; however, there may be connective tissue or epithelial attachment that does not show up on the radiograph. Normally, both pretreatment and posttreatment measurements show that these tissues each take up about 1 mm in an occlusal direction above the alveolar crest. Other diagnostic information gained from radiographs is almost entirely limited to hard tissues. Soft tissue inflammation, acute abscesses, and the presence or absence of active periodontal disease cannot be determined from radiographs. Use of parallel positioning technique is important to prevent loss of detail by foreshortening.

Radiolucency indicates bone loss or immature bone (Fig. 5–10). Early changes in the crest of the interdental septum in periodontitis cause radiolucency of the cortical plate on radiographs. Such changes are usually best seen on bite-wing radiographs, presumably because a more uniformly predictable parallel technique can be used.

The lamina dura represents a plate of bone lining the pocket through which x-rays must be absorbed in order to get a well-defined radiopaque line. In cases in which the root is curved, this structure will show up on the film only if sufficient bone is traversed in a straight line to create a radiopacity. Also, the degree of horizontal angulation of the x-ray beam may create an artifact, with the resulting appearance of a widened, narrowed, or lost periodontal ligament.

Cortical bone on the buccal and lingual surfaces of the teeth cannot be visualized well on radiographs. When resorption has occurred, the size of the rarefied area is usually underestimated, if seen at all, on radiographs. Generally, little information is gained regarding the configuration of bone on the buccal and lingual surfaces of teeth unless the pocket contains radiopaque material.

Bone defects can be detected on radiographs only if there is perforation or extensive destruction of cortical bone.[25] Loss of the trabecular pattern in radiolucent areas is primarily due to erosion at the junction of cancellous and cortical bone. Therefore, the radiographically visible area does not represent the lesion but only the extent of cortical erosion. Large defects in cancellous bone are often radiographically invisible.

The depth of intrabony pockets and interproximal craters, the degree of furcation (between the roots of a multirooted tooth) involvement (especially in occlusal projections), fenestration (a hole in the cortical plate of a jaw) and dehiscence (a cleft in the cortical plate of a jaw), and pocket shape can be recorded by clinical insertion of calibrated radiopaque points or contrast material. Large pieces of calculus can be seen when they are located on rostral or caudal surfaces on lat-

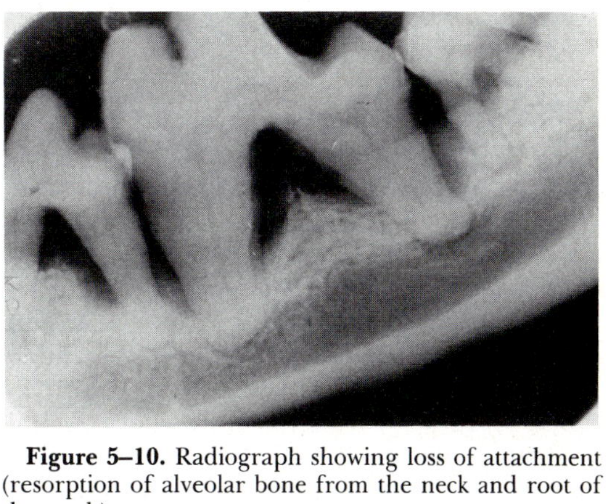

Figure 5–10. Radiograph showing loss of attachment (resorption of alveolar bone from the neck and root of the tooth).

eral projections, or occasionally on the buccal surface on occlusal projections; however, smaller and less mineralized calculus is often missed. Increased functional activity or disuse atrophy can be seen on radiographs as thickening of cortical bone or narrowing of periodontal ligament bone, respectively. The signs of trauma from occlusion (change in lamina dura or periodontal membrane space, root resorption, hypercementosis, osteosclerosis, pulp calcification, and root fracture) can be seen radiographically, but, as with other pathological conditions, they need to be correlated with clinical signs and history to make an adequate diagnosis.

SYSTEMIC PHASE OF PERIODONTAL THERAPY

Patients with systemic diseases, especially those that cause defects in neutrophil function, often show more severe signs of periodontal disease than a healthy patient would with the same amount of plaque and calculus.[10] This is also true of the severity of gingivitis in patients with vitamin deficiencies. The practitioner should remember that these conditions are aggravating, not causing, periodontal disease. Thus, controlling conditions such as diabetes will allow periodontal therapy to be more successful. In general, systemic disease states should be controlled as much as possible before periodontal therapy of an extensive nature is started.[20]

It is not usually necessary to premedicate patients with antibiotics when they are healthy and about to undergo periodontal surgery. However, patients with compromised systemic status (e.g., diabetes mellitus and valvular defects of the heart) should be premedicated with a broad-spectrum antibiotic so that a therapeutic blood level is present when surgery is in progress. This usually prevents infections caused by hematogenous seeding of oral flora. If surgery in addition to that performed in the mouth is to occur at the same appointment, it would be wise to premedicate these patients also because hematogenous seeding of oral flora can occur in these areas, which are relatively more avascular from surgery and are therefore more susceptible to infection. Ampicillin given as a single dose of 10 mg/kg intramuscularly 1 hour before surgery is effective. When surgery in addition to periodontal treatment has been provided on the same day, it may be wise to continue antibiotic therapy for 3 days from the time of surgery. Bacteremia associated with oral disease and treatment is discussed on page 53. All animals treated for periodontal problems benefit from a 2 week course of flushing the mouth daily for 1 minute with 0.2 percent chlorhexidine rinses to improve the results of periodontal therapy.

Animals with coagulation disorders should receive limited periodontal therapy of a conservative nature. Unless means to control bleeding, such as fresh whole blood, are available, surgery should not be performed. When teeth are periodontally involved and require surgical procedures to correct defects, it would be best to maintain them by scaling alone as long as possible. When they cannot be maintained any longer, creating an endodontic lesion by drilling into the pulp cavity will allow granulation tissue to encircle the root. The teeth will eventually become very mobile and will either come out themselves or can be extracted with light finger pressure. Little or no bleeding occurs using this technique and the teeth are not painful during the period after drilling into the pulp chamber.[26]

Although periodontal problems may seem worse during pregnancy, it is better to postpone periodontal treatment, other than scaling, until several months after delivery. Hormonal changes in pregnancy that make periodontal disease worse resolve after parturition, which may make treatment unnecessary. Risks to the fetus make it unwise to perform periodontal procedures other than simple scaling during pregnancy, especially considering that very little serious damage could be done to the dentition by periodontitis during the short gestation period of most domestic small animals.

TREATMENT OF PERIODONTAL DISEASE

A clean tooth will be surrounded by a healthy periodontium. All efforts in therapy are directed toward making the dentition biologically compatible with the surrounding soft and hard tissue.[20] Supplies and instruments used in periodontal treatment are shown in Figures 5–11 and 5–12 and are listed in Table 5–1.

Scaling and Root Planing

Either hand instruments or ultrasonic scalers plus hand instruments may be used for scaling and root planing. The procedure be-

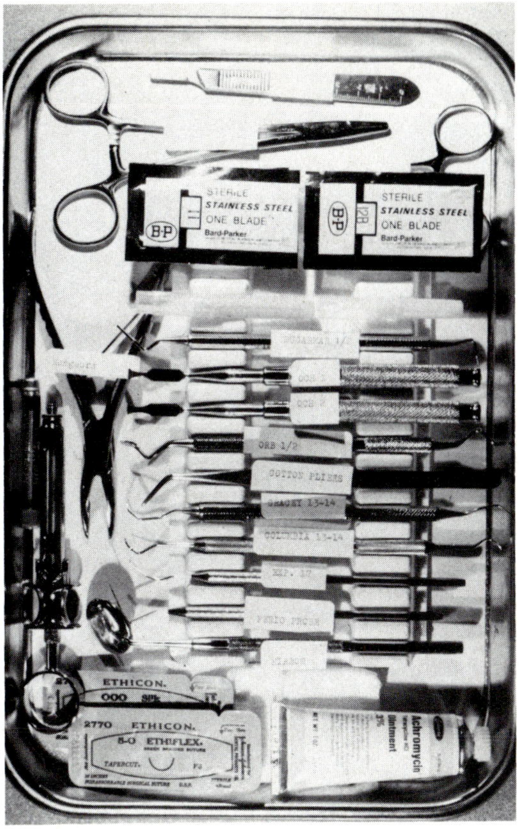

Figure 5–11. Instrument set for periodontal procedures (see also Table 5–1).

gins at the gingival margin using either a large scaler (e.g., Crane-Kaplan No. 6) (Fig. 5–13) or the side of a universal shape (e.g., Cavitron TFI-10 or PL) ultrasonic tip to dislodge supragingival calculus. If using hand instruments, a curette is then advanced below the gingival margin (see Fig. 5–14) to the bottom of the sulcus or pocket, the working edge is engaged (see Fig. 5–15), and the curette is drawn smoothly up the side of the tooth removing calculus as it advances. Several strikes may be necessary before all calculus is removed and the root feels smooth and hard.

If the operator is using an ultrasonic scaler, the same procedure is followed, but additional care must be exercised not to gouge the tooth. Because of the environmental contamination that results, a face mask should be worn during ultrasonic teeth cleaning. To avoid damage to the tooth, use only the side of the instrument, use copious water lavage during instrumentation, and use very little force when applying the instrument to the tooth. After using an ultrasonic instrument on the root surface, the surface should be smoothed with a hand curette (e.g., Columbia Nos. 13 and 14) and polished with prophylaxis paste (Fig. 5–16) containing fluoride to lessen dental hypersensitivity. Forced water or 0.2 percent chlorhexidine should be used to irrigate the gingival sulcus or pocket, and then the teeth should be dried with an air syringe or bulb to inspect for calculus. When dry, calculus will turn chalky white. Any deposits observed should be removed and the tooth repolished. A No. 17 explorer is used to probe below the gingival margin, inspecting the root surface all the way to the attachment apparatus. When roughness (indicating calculus or root resorption) is found, the area is curetted and polished again. Tooth cleaning, as already described, should be performed as soon as an accumulation of calculus is observed on the teeth. This usually occurs between 2 and 3 years of age. By

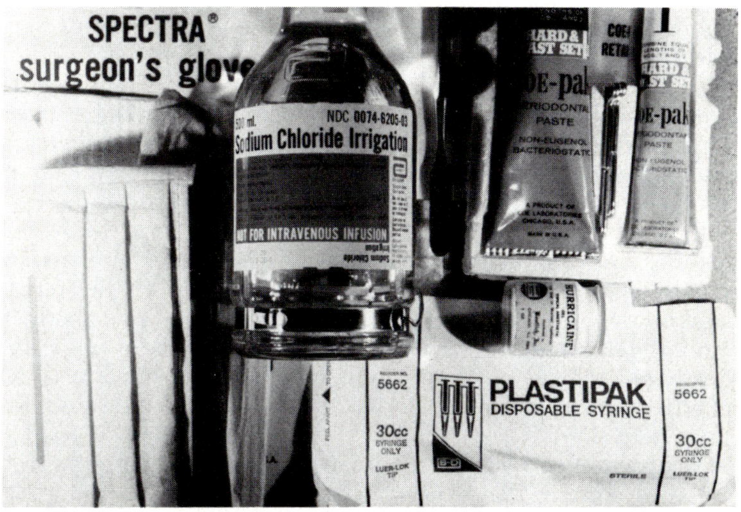

Figure 5–12. Supplies for periodontal procedures (see also Table 5–1).

Table 5–1. Instrument List for Periodontal Procedures

Hu-Friedy double-ended No. 3 explorer
Hu-Friedy single-ended No. 17 explorer
Hu-Friedy single-ended periodontal probe
Univ. of Mich. *color-coded*
Hu-Friedy Ochsenbein chisel No. 1
Hu-Friedy Ochsenbein chisel No. 2
Hu-Friedy Blumenthal rongeurs (standard)
Hu-Friedy double-ended periosteal elevator No. 9
Hu-Friedy double-ended Orban knife ½
Hu-Friedy Mayo-Hegar (Gardner 6) needle holder
Bard-Parker scalpel blades No. 11
Bard-Parker scalpel blades No. 12B
Box Ethicon sutures No. 2762 (5-0 Ethiflex)
Box Ethicon sutures No. 2770 (3-0 silk)
Kerr front-surface mirror and handle No. 5
Star double-ended MG Columbia curettes Nos. 13–14
Bunting files Nos. 14, 15, 16, 17, 18, and handles
Hu-Friedy double-ended Glickman scaler No. 3G/4G
Hu-Friedy double-ended Goldman-Fox scaler No. 4
Hu-Friedy double-ended Kramer scaler No. KRA2
Bard-Parker scalpel handle
Hu-Friedy surgical scissors S23
Cotton-tipped applicators
Slow-speed handpiece
Prophylaxis angle cups, coarse and fine polish
Saliva ejectors
Dental floss and tape
Col Pak—Hard and fast set, spatula, mixing pad
Dry foil
Achromycin 3 percent ointment
Iodine lotion and abscess syringe with curved cannula
Gauze sponges (sterile)
Cotton-tipped applicators
1:100,000 epinephrine 2 percent lidocaine local anesthetic
1:500,000 epinephrine 2 percent lidocaine local anesthetic
Dappen dishes
Headrest covers
Sharpening stones: mandryl mounted and needle sharpening stone (flat)
Tray covers
Paper cups and mouthwash
Soap
Towels
Handbrush
Electrosurgical instrument

removing this calculus and plaque, it is possible to slow or even halt the progress of periodontal disease. It would be wise to acclimate clients to the idea of periodic dental prophylaxis to prevent problems before they arise. Repeat visits for scaling and examination need to be tailored to the individual patient; most patients will benefit from one cleaning and examination each year. The frequency of repeated prophylaxis will depend on the owner's ability to clean the teeth regularly at home (see section on Preventive Measures); regular re-examination is recommended even if treatment under anesthesia is not necessary.

Cats present two difficulties during scaling and root planing that do not occur as frequently in dogs.[27] First, the teeth are much smaller, and the instruments available for cleaning teeth are not as concave on their working surfaces as they should be for extending below the gingival margin. The practitioner can compensate for this by using instruments that are thinner because they have been repeatedly sharpened. If these instruments are inserted below the gingivae with the edge kept parallel with the long axis of the tooth, the edge can be turned at a slight angle to engage and remove calculus when the attachment apparatus is reached. Whiteside No. 2, Younger No. 15, and Zerfing are scalers that work especially well for scaling the teeth of cats.

Second, root resorption appears to be more

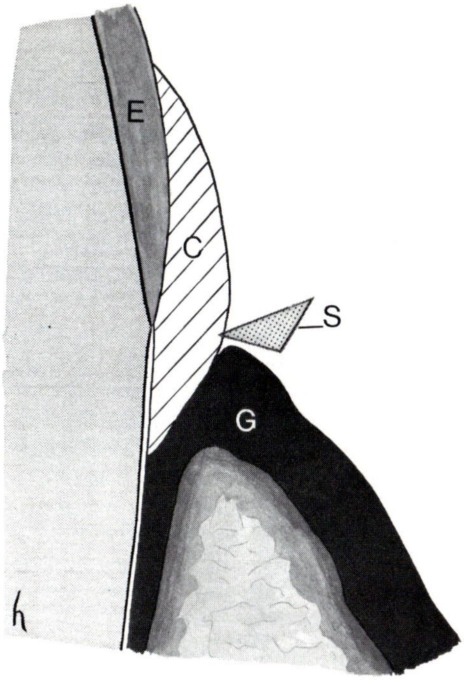

Figure 5–13. Removing large accumulations of supragingiva calculus with a scaler. C = calculus; S = scaler in cross section; E = enamel; G = gingiva.

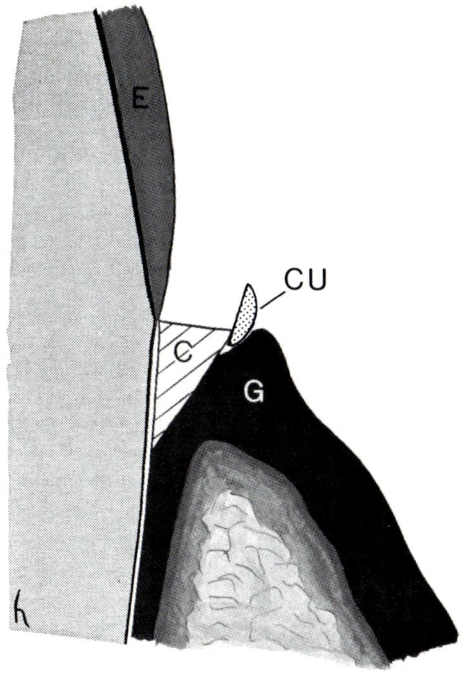

Figure 5–14. Inserting a periodontal curette below the gingival margin. CU = curette in cross section; E = enamel; C = calculus; G = gingiva.

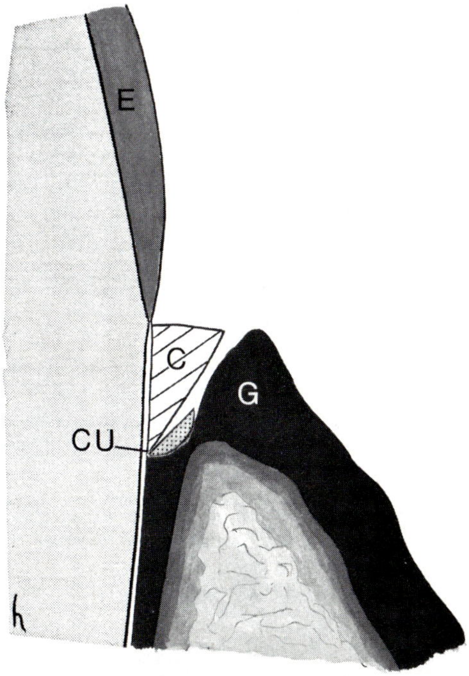

Figure 5–15. Engaging the root with the curette at the bottom of the pocket. E = enamel; C = calculus; G = gingiva; CU = curette.

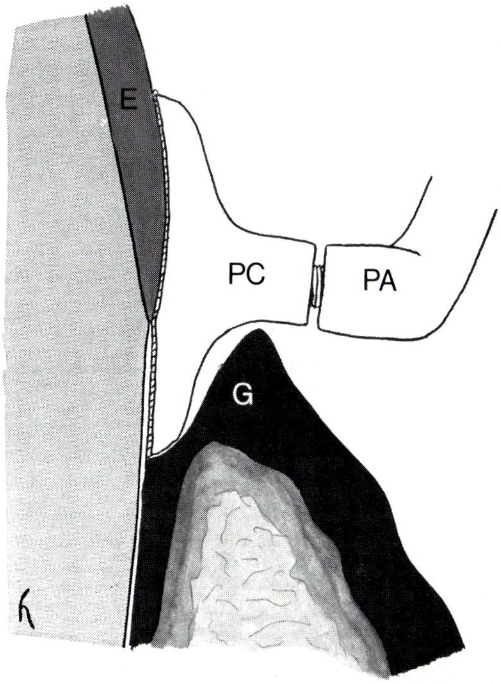

Figure 5–16. Polishing the root after cleaning with curettes and scalers. PA = prophylaxis angle; PC = polishing cup extending subgingivally; E = enamel; G = gingiva.

frequent in cats than in dogs.[28, 41] When the root feels abnormally rough or there are deficits in the structure of the root subgingivally, a radiograph should be taken of that tooth. The presence of extensive root resorption demonstrated on radiographs is an indication for extraction of the tooth. This phenomenon appears to be more frequent in cheek teeth in cats.

Preventive Methods

Periodontal disease is preventable. Numerous investigations have shown that chemoprophylaxis with chlorhexidine will prevent gingivitis and resolve simple gingivitis when deep pockets are not present.[29–34] Presumably, this is owing to the wide spectrum of antibacterial activity that chlorhexidine possesses; however, because the exact etiology of periodontal disease is unknown, the exact mechanism of action in the prevention and treatment of periodontal disease remains in question.

Postoperative use of chlorhexidine has been effective in preventing the re-establishment of gingivitis when no mechanical means of cleaning are used. It appears that 0.2 percent chlorhexidine flushed in a dog's mouth for 1 minute contact time daily is the easiest and most effective prophylactic measure. The effect of this prophylactic treatment is improved when all calculus and plaque are removed and pockets are made as shallow as possible before chlorhexidine rinses are instituted. Although chlorhexidine decreases the build-up of plaque and calculus, there will be a need for periodic mechanical prophylaxis by the veterinarian. This need is due to both staining by chlorhexidine and gradual development of small amounts of calculus even when rinsing is properly done.

A hard diet does not prevent the gradual accumulation of calculus over time but does seem to minimize plaque thickness and decrease the age of the plaque that is present by continually scraping it off. Although it is not of much benefit to humans because of the bell shape of their teeth, a hard diet does benefit dogs and cats because their teeth are more triangular.

Mechanically removing plaque daily with a toothbrush has been the most effective method of controlling dental disease in the human population, in which chemoprophylactic measures have not been approved by the Food and Drug Administration (FDA). The circular scrub method applied to the teeth with a soft, four-row, nylon brush once daily will remove supragingival plaque. This method of prophylaxis has not received much attention in veterinary medicine because few animals or owners are able to comply with such a rigid program. Some workers in the field of veterinary dentistry have found that using 0.2 percent chlorhexidine as a "medicine" on the toothbrush has a beneficial effect on client compliance with a tooth brushing program, and they report good cooperation from some owners.[35]

Preventive methods should be used before, during, and after periodontal treatment; combined with periodic scaling, they constitute the most effective conservative treatment of periodontal disease. Conservative treatment alone can produce very gratifying results when included in the preventive medicine package a practitioner presents to his clients. Surgery, when necessary, will work better if conservative therapy has been accomplished 1 month earlier.

Recognition of Surgical Cases

Animals with periodontal pockets no greater than 3 mm or 4 mm and with at least 2 mm attached gingivae on each surface of the tooth can usually be managed by regular scaling plus chemoprophylaxis or mechanical cleaning of the teeth at home. Patients with pockets greater than 4 mm 1 month after conservative therapy usually require surgery to gain access to subgingival calculus for thorough removal. When pockets are 5 mm or greater, scaling without surgical access to the root surface usually does not allow adequate calculus removal; this severely compromises attempts to control periodontitis.

Gingivectomy

In cases with pockets greater than 4 mm, *horizontal* (parallel to the cemento-enamel junction) bone loss, and adequate attached gingivae, the surgical procedure of choice[36] is gingivectomy (Fig. 5–17). When pockets end below the crest of adjacent bone (Fig. 5–20), bone loss is termed "*vertical.*"

Gingivectomy is performed under general anesthesia. Bleeding points corresponding to the level of attachment between periodontium and tooth are made in the gingivae with a periodontal probe (Fig. 5–18). The gingivae are cut off with cold steel or electroscalpel using a scalloped incision beginning below

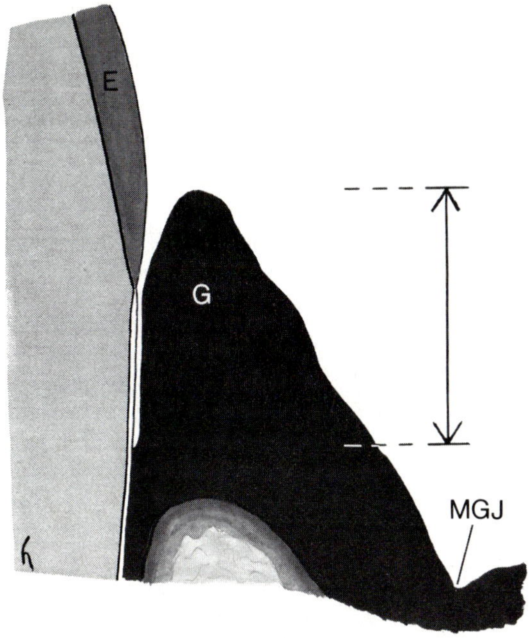

Figure 5–17. Horizontal bone loss with attached gingivae extending beyond the depth of the pocket; this patient is a gingivectomy candidate. MGJ = mucogingival junction; E = enamel; G = gingiva.

the bleeding point and aimed at the attachment. The cut is connected at the crestal bone between the teeth. When completed, the periphery of the incised area has a scal-

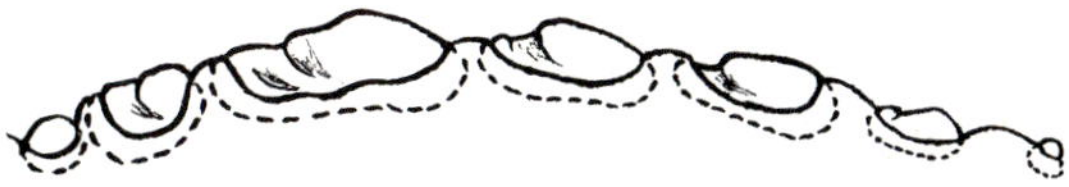

Figure 5–19. Outline of gingivectomy incision *(dotted line)* to remove gingivae covering crowns of mandibular teeth.

loped appearance (Fig. 5–19), and there is no pocket between the gingival margin and attachment. After the excised tissue is removed, the roots are planed smooth and free of calculus with curettes, as in the scaling procedure. Hemostasis is accomplished by pressure or commercial periodontal dressings, such as zinc oxide and eugenol or Col Pack, or both. Healing takes place by epithelial migration, mostly from the periphery of the incision. A guideline for estimating heaing time is one or two times (in days) the measured number of millimeters from the periphery of the incision to the attachement. During this time and for an additional week, the mouth should be irrigated for 1 minute daily with 0.2 percent chlorhexidine. Rubber ear syringes dispensed to the client make this chore easier and less traumatic.

Reverse Bevel Flap Surgery

When pockets are greater than 4 mm and bone loss is vertical (intrabony pockets) (Fig.

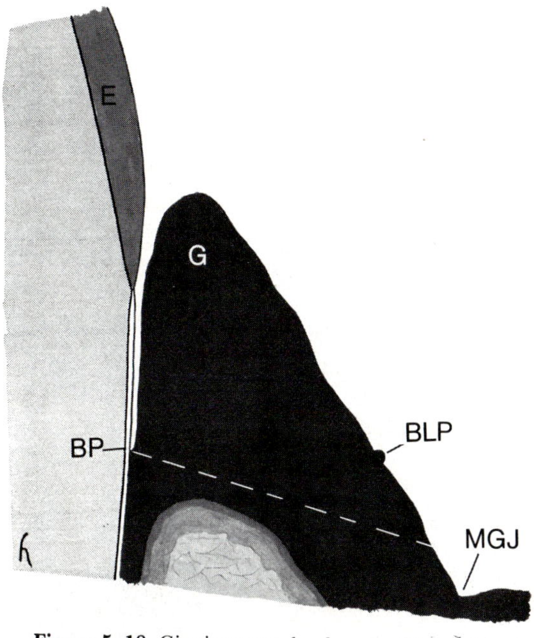

Figure 5–18. Gingivectomy landmarks. BLP = bleeding point; BP = bottom of pocket; E = enamel; G = gingiva; MGJ = mucogingival junction; dashed line = incision.

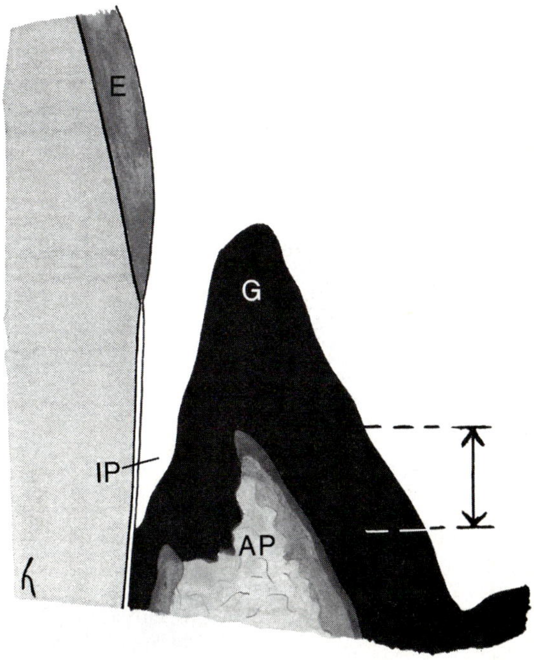

Figure 5–20. Intrabony pocket suitable for flap surgery. AP = alveolar process; IP = intrabony portion of pocket; E = enamel; G = gingiva.

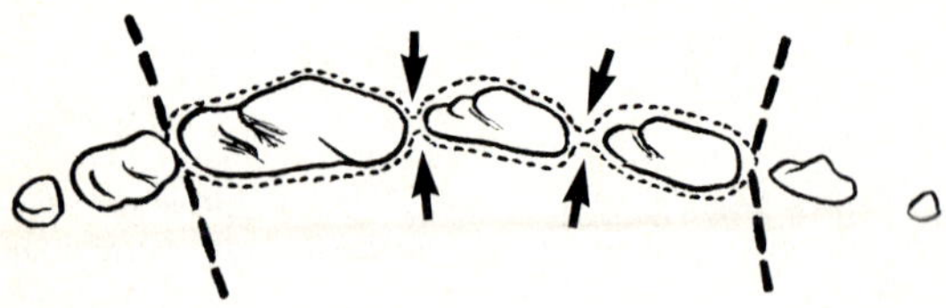

Figure 5–21. Preserving some interdental tissue *(arrows)* while making the incision *(dotted line)* for flap surgery. Releasing incisions *(dashed lines)* are seen at the ends of the flap section.

5–20), the procedure of choice is reverse bevel flap surgery.[20] Intrabony pockets can usually be appreciated easily on radiographs and by moving the periodontal probe away from the tooth in several directions to explore for a bony wall when checking pocket depth.

Flap surgery is performed under general anesthesia. An undermining incision is made in the attached gingivae through the periosteum of the alveolar process circumferentially around the tooth. The incision is designed so that most of the interdental tissue is preserved (Fig. 5–21). Next the flap is raised with a periosteal elevator, stopping short of the mucogingival junction. A second incision is then made, which severs the soft tissue attachment between tooth and gingivae (Fig. 5–22*A*). Using a curette or a rongeur, the soft tissue is removed between the tooth and flap margin (Fig. 5–22*B*). After removing this collar of soft tissue, the wound is irrigated with sterile normal saline, and the root is cleaned and smoothed with a curette. Meticulous cleaning and smoothing of the root is the most important step in the entire procedure. Some clinical judgment is required to decide whether to remove any of the alveolar process above the level of the pre-existing attachment apparatus (Figs. 5–23 and 5–24). Generally, alveolar process is removed when such removal will facilitate flap adaptation to the tooth. When the clinician believes that there will be unmanageable or progressive periodontal pockets postoperatively, some or all of the alveolar process above the attachment is removed. This can be done with rongeurs or bone chisels, avoiding the root. The tendency in periodontal surgery should be toward minimal bone removal.

The flaps are sutured between the teeth (Fig. 5–25) with interrupted sutures, attempting to get close adaptation between flap and tooth to promote first intention healing. Black silk suture, 3-0 or 4-0, is usually used if the animal is tractable and removal will be easy. Absorbable suture material is permissible but usually causes more irritation because it stays in the surgery site longer unless manually removed. The flap should not "climb" the tooth nor should it fall short of the tooth.

There is less problem with postoperative

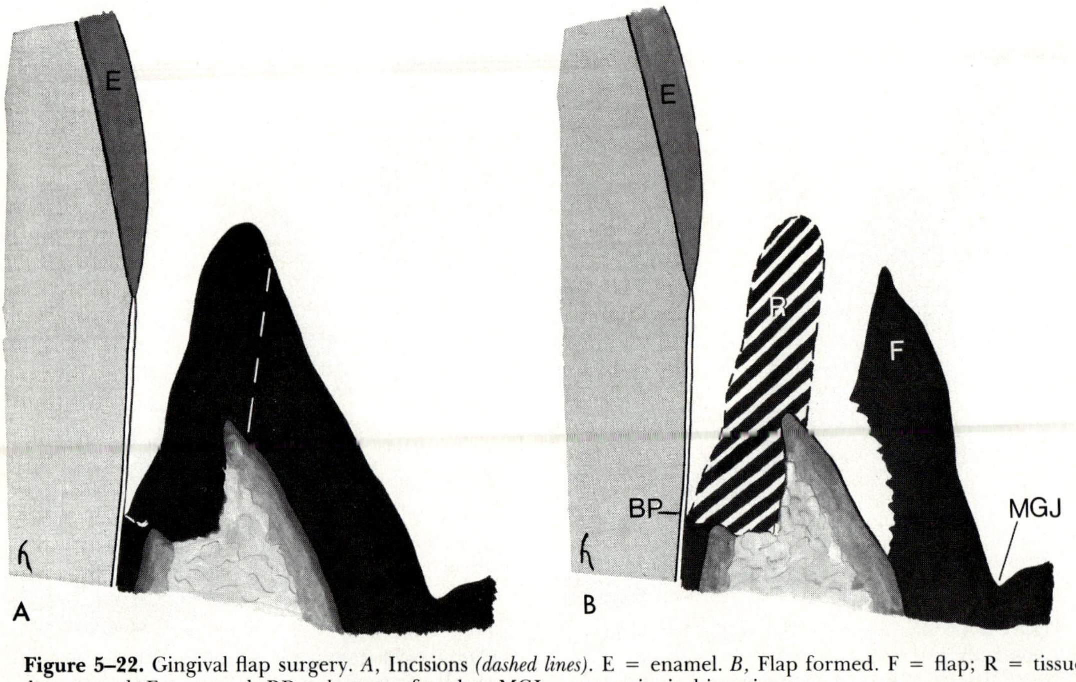

Figure 5–22. Gingival flap surgery. *A*, Incisions *(dashed lines)*. E = enamel. *B*, Flap formed. F = flap; R = tissue to be resected; E= enamel; BP = bottom of pocket; MGJ = mucogingival junction.

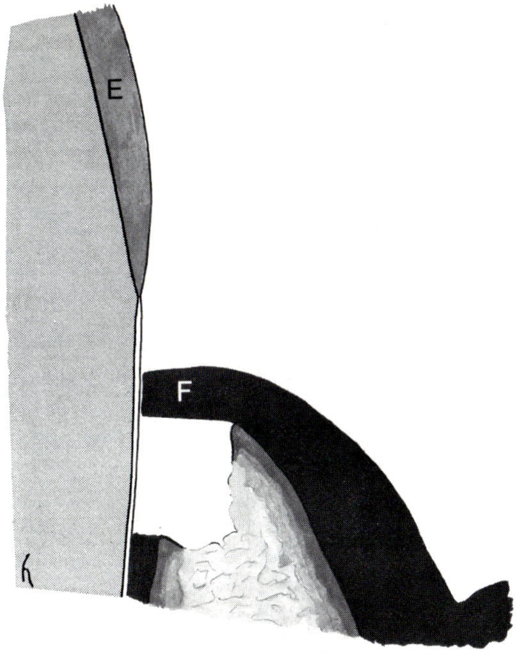

Figure 5–23. Proper flap adaptation to the tooth without alveolar process recontouring. E = enamel; F = flap.

hemorrhage with flap surgery than with gingivectomy; wet gauze compresses and periodontal dressings can be used to control the bleeding that does occur. The mouth should be irrigated daily with 0.2 percent chlorhexidine for at least 1 week. Sutures should be removed in 5 to 7 days to minimize irritation.

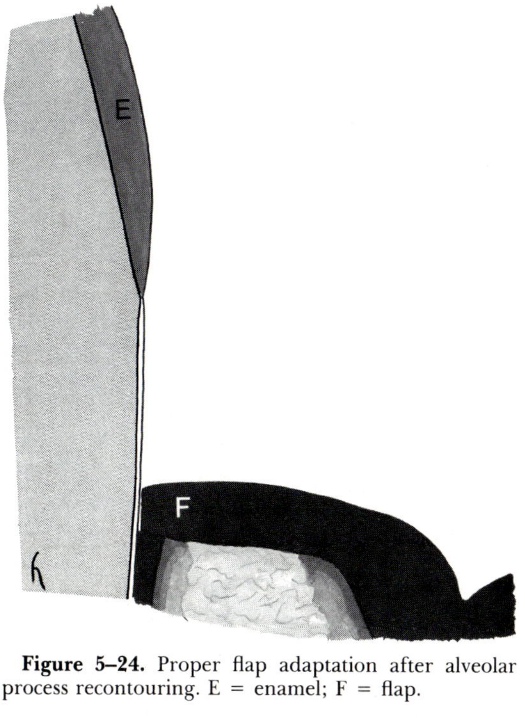

Figure 5–24. Proper flap adaptation after alveolar process recontouring. E = enamel; F = flap.

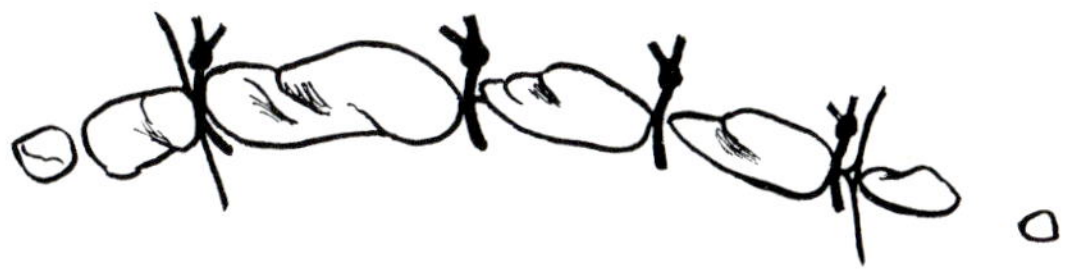

Figure 5–25. Interdental suturing to achieve close adaptation between gingival flaps and teeth.

Free Gingival Grafts

Free gingival grafts are used to increase the width of attached gingivae or to create a zone of attached gingivae when none exists.[37] They may also be used in the first part of a two-stage procedure to correct gingival defects when there are not enough attached gingivae to perform a pedicle graft.

One of the primary uses for free gingival grafts is when a cleft through the gingivae ends in alveolar mucosa (Fig. 5–26). A free gingival graft provides resistance to further extension of the cleft.

The procedure begins with careful scaling of the defect and the surroundng area of the involved tooth. Next a template of commercial "dry foil" or tinfoil is cut to the size of the proposed recipient site for the graft (Fig. 5–27). The clinician should try to place a graft that is approximately 20 percent larger than the healed site needs to be to accommodate shrinkage; the graft should blend smoothly with the surrounding gingivae.

The template is carried by cotton pliers to the proposed donor site and is allowed to adhere by the capillary action of saliva (Fig. 5–28). Donor sites should have thick (greater than 3 mm), wide bands of attached gingivae, should be free of rugae and pigmentation that is different from the recipient site if esthetics are important, and should not be

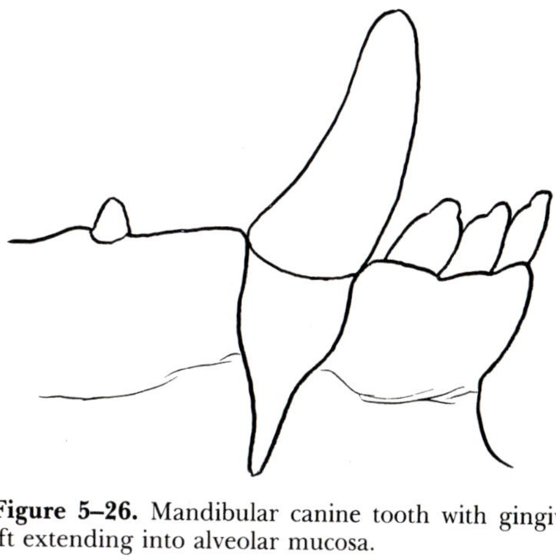

Figure 5–26. Mandibular canine tooth with gingival cleft extending into alveolar mucosa.

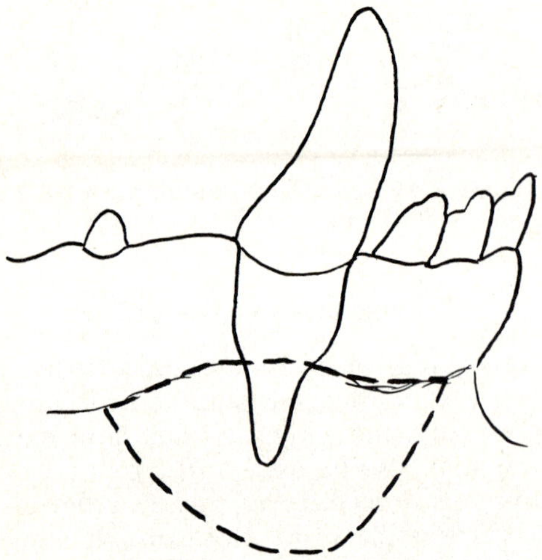

Figure 5–27. Tinfoil template *(dashed lines)* for proposed mucosal graft.

bony prominences if possible. A No. 12D or a No. 11 scalpel blade is convenient for tracing the template lightly on the attached gingivae; however, any thin, fine scalpel will do. The template is removed, and the surgeon deepens the incision to approximately 3 mm. The incision should be partial-thickness to protect the vascular supply of the donor site gingivae and avoid causing cortical bone resorption in that area. Usually there is a prominent edge on the proposed donor tissue someplace that can be slightly lifted by the scalpel blade while the surgeon begins to undermine the graft (Fig. 5–29). When this edge is lifted a sufficient distance for the needle to exit, a transfixing suture is placed using 5-0 Ethibond or other narrow-diameter suture and non-cutting needle. Absorbable suture is more irritating but can be used. Remember the direction of entry and exit that the needle made because once lifted, both sides of the graft look similar, and a graft placed with the epithelial surface to-

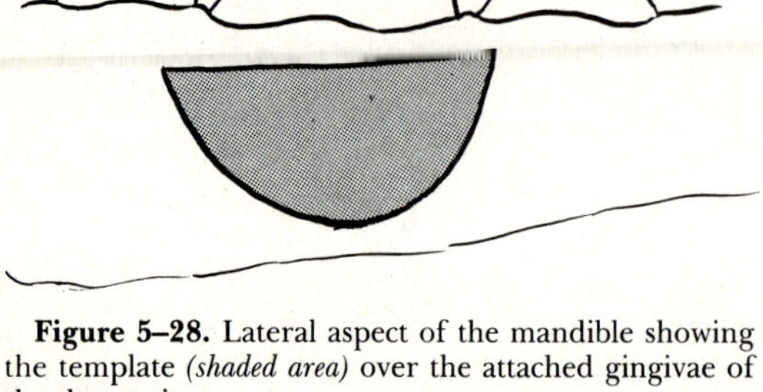

Figure 5–28. Lateral aspect of the mandible showing the template *(shaded area)* over the attached gingivae of the donor site.

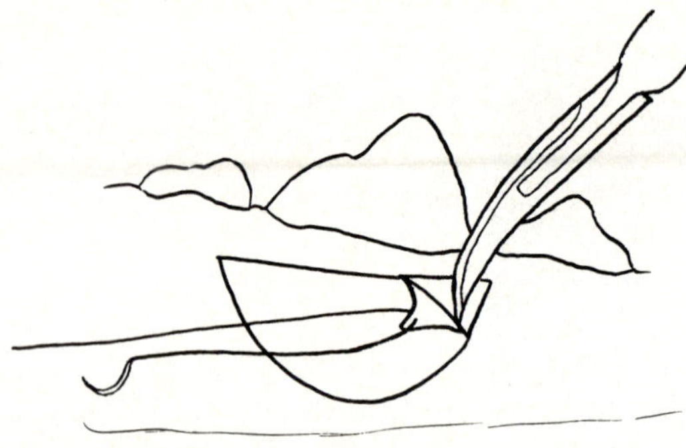

Figure 5–29. Split-thickness dissection of the graft.

ward the bed of the recipient site seldom survives. The transfixing suture can be used to manipulate the graft. While the recipient site is prepared, the free graft is placed in sterile normal saline or saline-soaked sponges.

The recipient site is prepared by placing the template used to harvest the donor tissue on the proposed graft site. The template is traced with a scalpel blade and then removed. The surgeon extends the incision to bone and removes the outlined alveolar mucosa overlying the graft site with a periosteal elevator or rongeurs (Fig. 5–30). The exposed tooth structure is planed smooth with curettes, and the graft (connective tissue side facing bone) is sutured in place (Fig. 5–31). Fine non-absorbable (e.g., 5-0 Ethiflex) suture attached around the periphery of the graft in an interrupted pattern is usually the most secure closure. A covering of commercial dry foil and periodontal dressing compressed against the graft for 1 minute encourages close adaptation between graft and

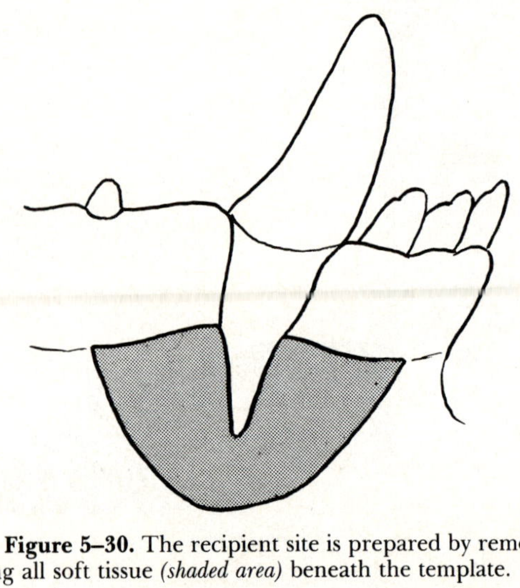

Figure 5–30. The recipient site is prepared by removing all soft tissue *(shaded area)* beneath the template.

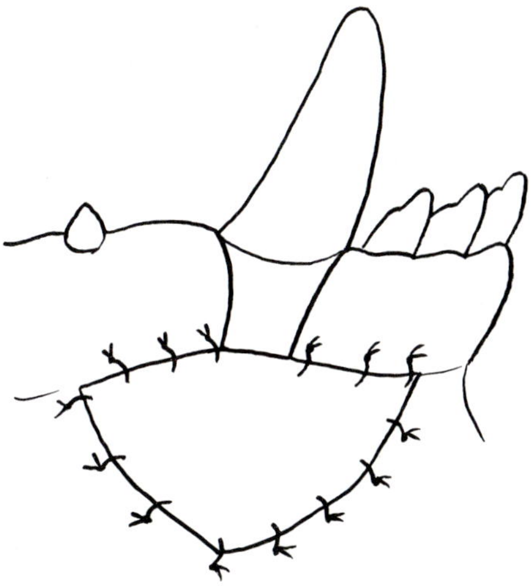

Figure 5–31. The graft is sutured in place.

bed, making proper healing more likely. The success rate of tissue transplants done in this fashion should be close to 100 percent. Additional protection might be gained by overlaying the dressing with an acrylic stent tied to the teeth when the surgeon anticipates trauma (such as stick biting) during the healing period.

Because grafts can easily be dislodged within the first week, it may be necessary to fit the patient with an Elizabethan collar, limit the diet to soft food, and prevent access to chew toys. The mouth should be rinsed once daily with 0.2 percent chlorhexidine and the sutures should be removed in 10 days. The graft will be solidly bound to the bed in 2 to 3 weeks in most cases. However, it would be wise to limit the chewing of hard food and objects for a month and continue rinsing with chlorhexidine during this period.

Pedicle Grafts

Pedicle grafts have an advantage over free gingival grafts because they take some of their blood supply with them when the tissue is transferred. This provides faster healing and a greater likelihood of the graft adhering to its new location. They cannot be used to transfer tissue between distant sites.

The procedure begins with the creation of a recipient bed of adequate size. Although split-thickness beds provide better vascular supply to the graft, they often allow motion in the graft, and motion sometimes allows further recession. Therefore, the bed is often created by removing periosteum and grafting to bone in the area of the tooth and to a split-thickness bed in the periphery (Fig. 5–32). The donor tissue is removed by split-thickness dissection in the area away from the recipient site and full-thickness dissection in the area adjacent to the graft site. The pedicle is rotated and sewn in position the same way a free gingival graft is secured (Fig. 5–33). The advantage of the split-thickness dissection is that the donor site is covered, preventing bone resorption. Healing and postoperative care for pedicle grafts is as for free gingival grafts.

Bone Grafts

When intrabony pockets exist that threaten to cause the loss of valued teeth, bone grafts have been used to stimulate osteogenesis and act as a scaffolding for the growth of new bone[38] designed to fill in such defects. These grafts are most successful when used in defects completely surrounded by bone ("three-walled defects") (Fig. 5–34), but may provide

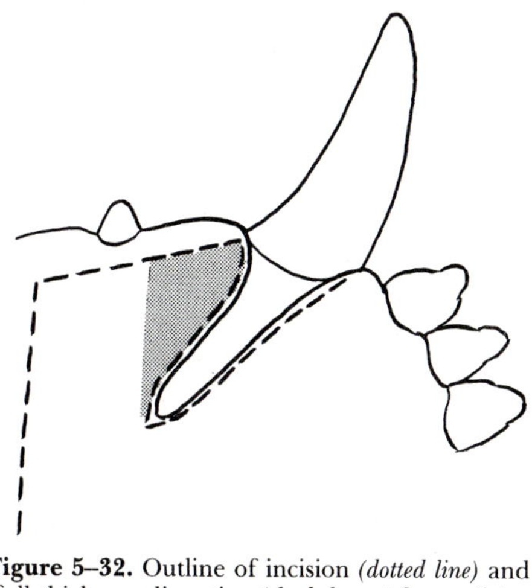

Figure 5–32. Outline of incision *(dotted line)* and area of full-thickness dissection *(shaded area)* for pedicle graft.

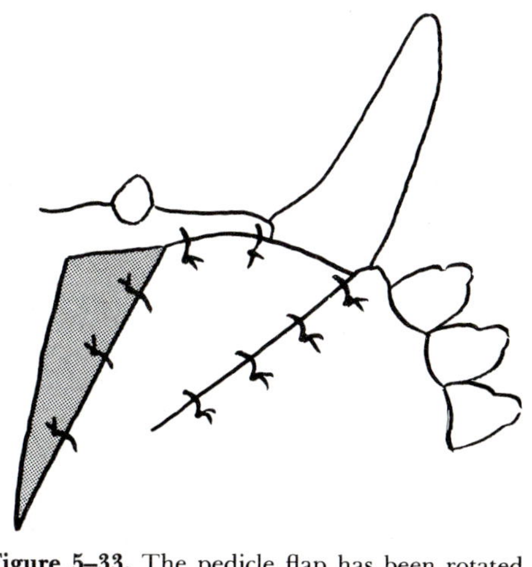

Figure 5–33. The pedicle flap has been rotated and sutured in place. The shaded area is left to granulate.

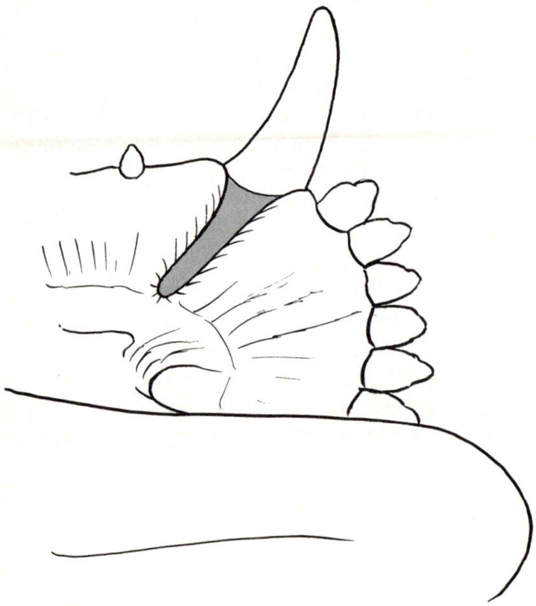

Figure 5–34. Mandibular canine tooth with a "three wall" defect *(shaded area)* on the medial surface. This area may be identifiable only on probing.

partial regeneration of bone in other intrabony pockets between teeth and defects in bone between roots of single teeth ("furcation defects"). Autogenous bone taken from intraoral sites provides the safest and best results; however, allografts and synthetic grafting material have been used with success.

Bone grafting procedures often are delayed for 1 month after thorough scaling and root planing. During this time it is advisable to maintain meticulous hygiene by chemoprophylaxis or mechanical cleaning, because bone grafted into inflamed and infected sites seldom gives the desired regenerative effect. Reverse bevel flap surgery is used to gain access to the surgical site. The defect is cleaned out, removing all soft tissue and planing the root smooth and clean. If the defect has been present for a long time, there may be cortical bone in the intrabony walls. This plate of bone is fenestrated with small, round burs to allow osteogenic elements to "bud" through from adjacent marrow into the defect. Bone is harvested from an intraoral site from which its removal will not jeopardize the level of attachment on other teeth. Edentulous spaces and healing extraction sites are often used to harvest bone; it may be taken with burs, trephines, or rongeurs. When bone is taken vertically from a hole (e.g., an extraction site or trephine hole), the donor site will regenerate with no permanent deformity. The bone removed is crushed with rongeurs into fine particles and is packed into the defect. The overlying tissue is closed, attempting to cover the defect tightly and eliminate communication between the oral cavity and the graft as much as possible. A free gingival graft may be placed over split-thickness reverse bevel flaps to provide close adaptation between soft tissue and tooth.[39] The free graft also retards epithelial migration into the defect when used in this manner. Healing is slow; there will not be much improvement within the first 6 months because all bone grafted must be removed before new bone can fill in the defect. The cleaner the mouth remains the more likely the bone graft will produce the desired regeneration of bone.

Combined Periodontic-Endodontic Procedures

When both periodontal and endodontic procedures are to be performed on the same tooth, it is usually best to complete the endodontic therapy first (page 88). Often with the resolution of the endodontic pathological condition, the periodontal tissues around an involved tooth show rapid and considerable improvement, and the prognosis for periodontal procedures done on that tooth is much better. This is especially true when there is communication between periodontal pockets and a periapical lesion. Intrabony defects that communicate with pathological periapical areas resulting from endodontic lesions show better bone regeneration following endodontic therapy and bone grafting than do intrabony defects that are strictly periodontal in origin.

Postoperative Complications

Bleeding and pain are managed as they would be in any other area of the body. When the periodontal dressing is dislodged, the flaps torn from their sutured position, and bone exposed around sutured sites, redressing the area and manipulating the flaps back to their former position is preferable to immediate surgery. Some healing by secondary intention usually does occur when the flaps are simply redressed in this manner, but the healing is usually adequate to avoid additional surgery. If additional surgery is required, it is best to wait until healing appears complete clinically; otherwise, the results of the second surgery are very unpredictable.

It is very unusual to have infection either in the soft or hard tissue following periodontal procedures. If infection does occur, it should be managed with antibiotics and the draining of abscess cavities.

Maintenance of Surgical Sites for Long-term Success

Treatment may cure periodontal disease in the patient; however, there remains a susceptibility to periodontal disease, and poor oral hygiene will cause gingivitis and periodontitis to return. Therefore, it is important to establish a regular recall program for periodontal prophylaxis and examination. People who have had periodontal disease and were treated are usually on a regular recall to the dental office every 3 months. The proper recall interval for veterinary patients has not been established; however, under optimum circumstances it is likely to be similar to that used for humans. When compromises must be made for financial reasons, lengthening the recall interval may be compensated for by changing to a hard diet, mechanical cleaning by the owner, or chemoprophylaxis. Clients need to be told that the success of periodontal treatment is directly related to continued cleanliness of the mouth.

The practitioner should not become discouraged by the presence of inflammation, plaque, and calculus on treated animals as they return for recall visits. This will frequently be the case either because of noncompliance by owners or because recall intervals have been lengthened for financial reasons. Practitioners should understand that treating recurrent gingivitis causes its resolution and prevents the irreversible lesions of periodontitis from occurring. Also, treated cases, despite the return of clinical signs of disease, have a better prognosis for long-term survival than do untreated cases.

References

1. Hamp SE, Viklands P, Farsomadsen K, Fornell J: Prevalence of periodontal disease in dogs. I. Clinical and roentgenographic observations. *IADR,* Abstract L 19, 1975.
2. Golden AM, Stoller N, Harvey CE: Survey of oral and dental diseases in dogs anesthetized at a veterinary hospital. *J Am Anim Hosp Assoc* 18:891, 1982.
3. Skougaard MR, Beagric GS: The renewal of gingival epithelium in marmosets (*Calithrix jacchus*) as determined through autoradiography with thymidine—H^3. *Acta Odont Scand* 20:467, 1962.
4. Egelberg J: Cellular elements in gingival pocket fluid. *Acta Odont Scand* 21:283, 1963.
5. Schroeder HE: Histopathology of the gingival sulcus. *In* Lehner T (ed): The Borderland Between Caries and Periodontal Disease. London, Academic Press, 1977.
6. Ramfjord SP, Engler WD, Hiniker JJ: A radioautographic study of healing following simple gingivectomy. II. The connective tissue. *J Periodont* 37:179, 1966.
7. Valderhaug JP, Nylen MU: Function of epithelial rests as suggested by their ultrastructure. *J Periodont Res* 1:69, 1966.
8. Monheim IM: Local Anesthesia and Pain Control in Dental Practice, 4th ed. St. Louis, The CV Mosby Co.,1969.
9. Loe H, Holm-Pederson P: Absence and presence of fluid from normal and inflamed gingivae. *Periodontics* 3:171, 1965.
10. Grove TK: The natural history of periodontal disease in beagle dogs—Gingival inflammation, debris, bifurcation involvement, and roentgenographic bone loss. Master's thesis, University of Michigan, 1975.
11. Burvasser P, Hill TJ: The effect of hard and soft diets on the gingival tissues of dogs. *J Dent Res* 18:389, 1939.
12. Egelberg J: Local effect of diet on early plaque formation and development of gingivitis in dogs. *Odont Rev* 16:31, 50, 1965.
13. Syed SA, Svanberg M, Svanberg G: The predominant cultivable dental plaque flora of beagle dogs with gingivitis. *J Periodont Res* 15:123, 1980.
14. Syed SA, Svanberg M, Svanberg G: The predominant cultivable dental plaque flora of beagle dogs with periodontitis. *J Clin Periodontol* 8:45, 1981.
15. Theilade E, Wright WH, Jensen SD, Loe H: Experimental gingivitis in man. *J Periodont Res* 1:13, 1966.
16. Loe H, Theilade E, Jensen SB: Experimental gingivitis in man. *J Periodont* 36:177, 1965.
17. Lindhe J, Hamp S, Loe H: Experimental periodontitis in the beagle dog. *J Periodont Res* 8:1–10, 1973.
18. Saxe SR, et al.: Oral debris, calculus, and periodontal disease in the beagle dog. *Periodontics* 5:217, 1967.
19. Lindhe J: Experimental periodontitis in the beagle dog. Lecture at University of Michigan, March 18, 1974.
20. Ramfjord SP, Ash MM: Periodontology and Periodontics. Philadelphia, WB Saunders Co., 1980.
21. Sorensen WP, Loe H, Ramfjord SP: Periodontal disease in the beagle dog—a cross sectional clinical study. *J Periodont Res* 15:380, 1980.
22. Grove TK: Periodontal disease. *Comp Cont Ed Pract Vet* 4(7):564, 1982.
23. Kelly GP: Relationship of radiographic bone height, pocket depth, and attachment level in a longitudinal study of periodontal disease. University of Michigan Thesis No. 759, 1973. School of Dentistry.
24. Cain RJ: Radiographic determination of bone height in a longitudinal study of periodontal therapy. University of Michigan Thesis No. 662, 1971. School of Dentistry.
25. Pauls V, Trott JR: A radiological study of experimentally produced lesions in bone. *Dent Practit* 16:254, 1966.
26. Kerr DA: Personal communication. University of Michigan School of Dentistry, 1974.
27. Durr UM, Reichart P: Gingivitis der Katze—mediakamentose und chirurgishe Therapie. *Kleinter Prax* 23:231, 1978.

28. Schneck G, Osborn JW: Neck lesions in the teeth of cats. *Vet Rec* 99:100, 1976.
29. Lindhe J, Hamp SE, Loe H, Schiott CR: Influence of topical appication of chlorhexidine on chronic gingivitis and gingival wound healing in the dog. *Scand J Dent Res* 78:471, 1970.
30. Hamp S, Lindhe J, Loe H: Long term effect of chlorhexidine on developing gingivitis in the beagle dog. *J Periodont Res* 8:63, 1973.
31. Foulkes D: Some toxicological observations on chlorhexidine. *J Periodont Res* 12(Suppl 8):55, 1973.
32. Davies RM, Jensen SB, Schiott CR, Loe H: The effect of mouth rinses and topical application of chlorhexidine on the bacterial colonization of the teeth and gingiva. *J Periodont Res* 5:96, 1970.
33. Schiott CR, Loe H, Jensen SB, Kilian M, Davies RM, Glavind K: The effect of chlorhexidine mouth rinses on human oral flora. *J Periodont Res* 5:84, 1970.
34. Listgarten MA, Ellegaard B: Electronmicroscopic evidence of a cellular attachment between junctional epithelium and dental calculus. *J Periodont Res* 8:143, 1973.
35. Harvey CE: Personal communication, 1983.
36. Loe H, Wright W II: Gingivectomy. *Odont Tidskr* 73:501, 1965.
37. Sullivan HC, Atkins JH: The role of free gingival grafts in periodontal therapy. *Dent Clin North Am* 13:133, 1969.
38. Patterson RL, Collings CK, Zimmerman ER: Autogenous grafts in the alveolar process of the dog with induced periodontitis. *Periodontics* 19, 1967.
39. Ellegaard B, Karring T, Loe H: New periodontal attachment procedure based on retardation of epithelial migration. *J Clin Periodont* 1:75, 1974.
40. Thompson RR, Wilcox GE, Clark WT, Jansen KL: Association of calicivirus infection with chronic gingivitis and pharyngitis in cats. *J Small Anim Pract* 25:207, 1984.
41. Reichart PA, Durr UM, Triadan H, Vickendey G: Periodontal disease in the domestic cat. A histopathologic study. *J Periodont Res* 19:67, 1984.

Chapter Six

Disorders of Teeth

LE Rossman, DA Garber, and CE Harvey

CONGENITAL ANOMALIES

Dental anomalies, either inherited or resulting from external interference with fetal or neonatal development, are common, but are rarely of clinical importance in dogs and cats.

Anodontia

Anodontia is the absence of one or more teeth; it can be either total (no teeth present) or partial. This condition is common in dogs and cats.[1–7] Congenital absence of teeth is more common in the permanent dentition than in the deciduous dentition; if deciduous teeth are missing, the permanent teeth in that location usually will be missing also.

Supernumerary Teeth

More than the number normally found is common in the dog, 10 percent of dogs having one or more extra teeth. There is considerable variation in the incidence among various breeds of dogs, from 2 percent in huskies to 19 percent in spaniels in one study.[8] There is some evidence that this condition is inherited in some dogs.[5]

The supernumerary teeth may crowd other teeth, causing malposition, malocclusion, or incomplete eruption of adjacent teeth and periodontal disease. The teeth causing crowding should be removed. The permanent tooth may erupt to one side of the deciduous tooth at that location, thus preventing the eruption pressure that normally causes exfoliation of deciduous teeth, and causing permanent retention of the deciduous tooth as a supernumerary tooth.

Retained Deciduous Teeth

The deciduous teeth are an interim dentition that is in place during the growth of the jaws. If a deciduous tooth is retained when the permanent tooth in that location has erupted, there is inevitably a change in the direction of eruption, and crowding or malocclusion may result.[9] Retained deciduous teeth are particularly common in toy dogs[10] and have been observed in the cat.[11] The incisor and canine teeth are affected most commonly (Fig. 6–1). Early recognition and strategic extraction (see Fig. 6–34) may allow the development of a normal permanent occlusion. Extraction of deciduous teeth is usually simple but is not always successful because the slender root may fragment. The root fragments may cause subgingival inflammation affecting the developing permanent tooth. The technique in which the crown is snapped off with forceps close to the gingivae is more likely to cause this complication, though it has been used successfully for many years.[12] Retention of deciduous teeth may follow distemper infection in dogs.[13]

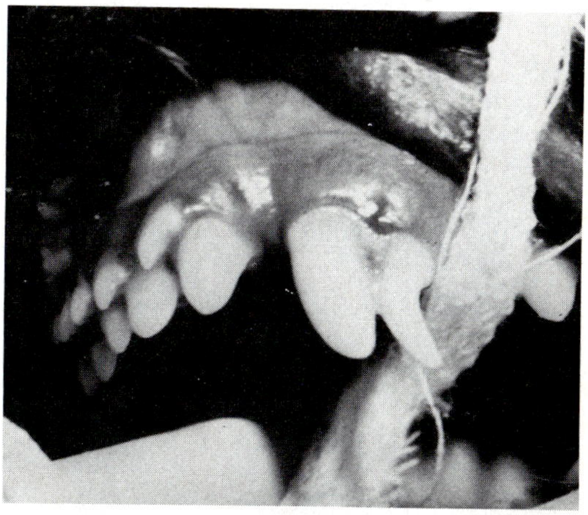

Figure 6–1. Retained deciduous canine and incisor teeth in a 10 month old dog. (From Harvey CE, O'Brien JA, Rossman LE, Stoller NH. *In* Ettinger SJ (ed): Textbook of Veterinary Internal Medicine, 2nd ed, Ch. 55. Philadelphia, WB Saunders Co., 1983.)

Rotation and Crowding of Teeth

Rotation (twisting of a tooth of normal shape away from its normal alignment with the jaw) is very common in dogs,[1,8] particularly in brachycephalic breeds (Fig. 6–2). Crowding of several teeth in the same area of the jaw is less common but more severe (Fig. 6–3), since periodontal disease is likely to develop at the distorted gingival margin. Treatment is not usually necessary; however, judicious extraction to reduce crowding, or orthodontic movement of affected teeth, is indicated if the owner wishes to ensure lifelong retention of the teeth.

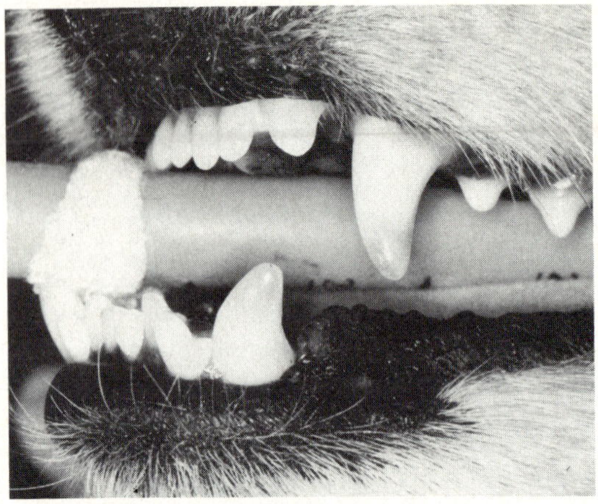

Figure 6–3. Crowded incisor teeth in the mandible of a dog, predisposing to periodontal disease. The dog is also prognathic.

Impacted Teeth

Impacted teeth fail to erupt because of a barrier in the normal eruption path. This condition is rarely recognized in dogs and cats. The cause is either lack of space or misalignment of the tooth bud, resulting in an eruptive path that is blocked by adjacent teeth. A completely impacted tooth is recognized by its absence in the dental arcade but its presence radiographically; such teeth rarely cause signs of disease unless they are in the maxilla and interfere with nasal function, in which case nasal discharge can result.[14] Partial eruption can lead to abscessation or cyst formation;[15] partially erupted teeth can also cause nasal discharge (Fig. 6–4). The treatment for impacted teeth is extraction if the impaction is affecting the position of or causing resorption of the roots of the peranent teeth adjacent to it, or if they are causing abscessation. Surgical removal of bone and soft tissue overlying an impacted vital tooth may allow it to erupt.

Abnormalities in the Shape of Teeth

Developmental anomalies in the shape of the teeth are rare and are of little clinical relevance. Extraction is indicated for esthetic reasons or if gingival disease results. Abnor-

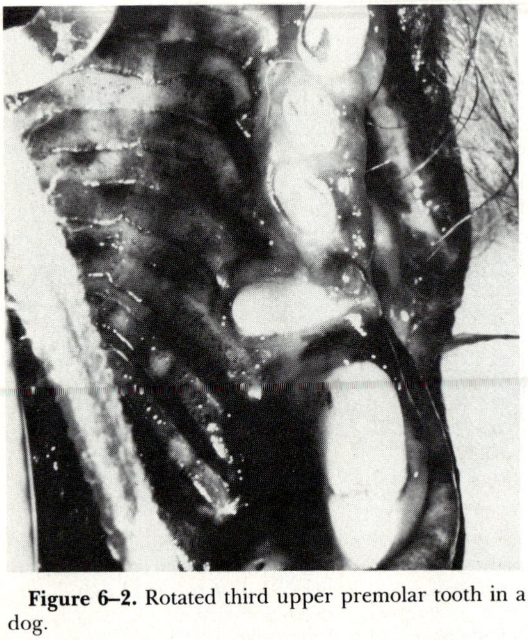

Figure 6–2. Rotated third upper premolar tooth in a dog.

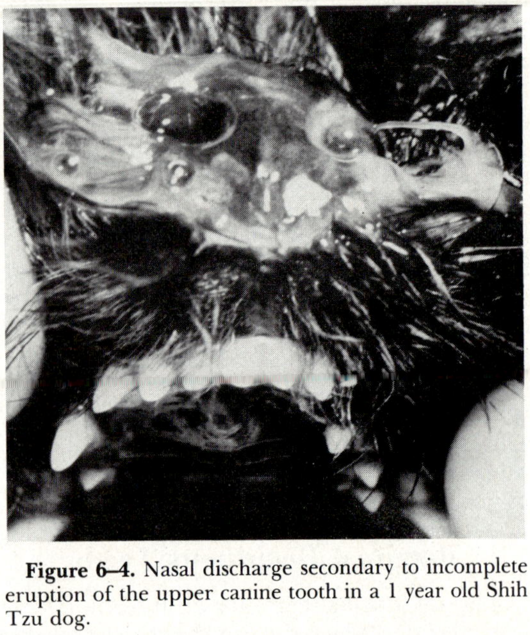

Figure 6–4. Nasal discharge secondary to incomplete eruption of the upper canine tooth in a 1 year old Shih Tzu dog.

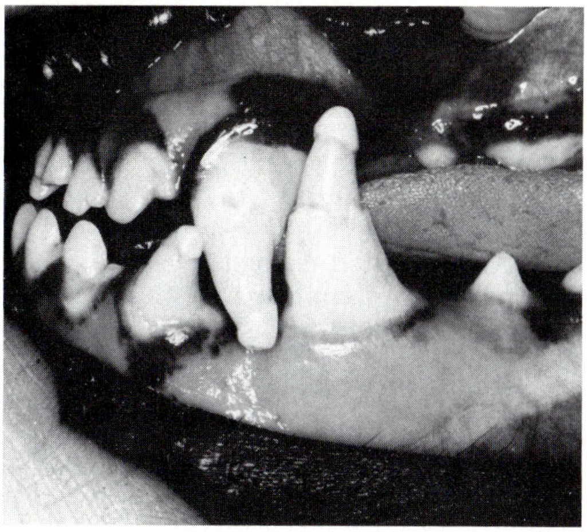

Figure 6–5. Enamel hypoplasia on the canine and incisor teeth of a dog.

malities that may be seen include dens in dente (an area of enamel within the dentin, which may expose the pulp cavity to bacterial contamination);[16] gemination (division of a single tooth bud, resulting in a single root with two crowns); tooth fusion (the joining of two normally separate tooth buds); dilaceration (an abnormally sharp curvature of a root); supernumerary roots; and enamel pearls (areas of enamel formed on a root that prevent normal periodontal attachment).[17]

Enamel Formation Abnormalities

Defects in the enamel, known as enamel hypoplasia, can occur during tooth development or as a result of exposure of the formed enamel surface to a corrosive irritant. The usual cause is distemper infection early in life,[18] which disrupts the enamel-forming ameloblasts. As a result of the efficiency of present-day vaccines, this lesion is now rare. The lesions appear as opaque or brown-stained irregularities in the enamel surface (Fig. 6–5). The defects rarely put the tooth at risk of caries or pulpal infection. A normal appearance can be restored by an acid-etched bonding of composite resin material (see Fig. 6–25).[19, 20] Other possible causes of enamel hypoplasia are periapical inflammation or trauma affecting the permanent tooth bud, nutritional deficiencies, and generalized systemic infections or endocrine dysfunctions early in life. Hypocalcification of the enamel can occur if there is excessive fluoride intake during tooth development.

Tetracycline Staining

Tetracycline bonds with any tissue undergoing calcification, including enamel and dentin, creating a permanent discoloration that appears brown, yellow-orange, or gray.[21] External bleaching techniques using heated hydrogen peroxide are not effective in correcting the staining. Resin bonding (page 94) over affected enamel can restore a normal appearance.

TRAUMA TO TEETH

Attrition

The crowns of the permanent teeth should not lose appreciable health over the life of a dog or cat on a "normal" diet. Slight wear is considered normal; however, attrition (in which the rate of crown height loss is rapid) is abnormal but common in dogs;[1] it is rare in cats. Diet and chewing habits account for most instances of severe attrition (Fig. 6–6). Attrition may occur because one tooth wears abnormally against another in a dog with malocclusion (Fig. 6–7).

Grooming is a major function of the incisor teeth; pathological grooming (as a result of flea bite dermatitis, for example) may wear the teeth completely down to the gingivae (Fig. 6–8).

The dental pulp responds to rapid wear by laying down reparative dentin, which is

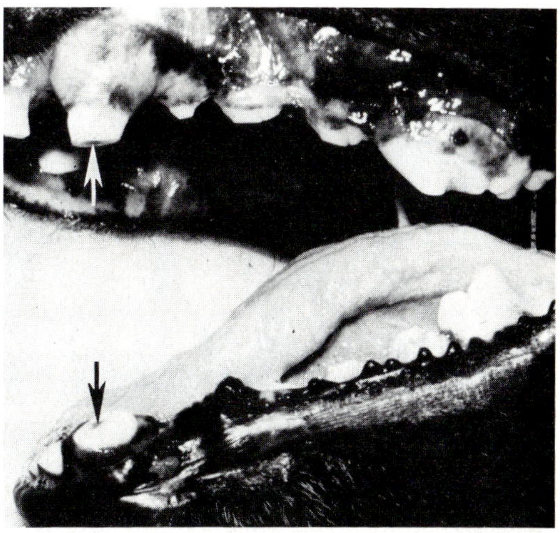

Figure 6–6. Severe generalized attrition of teeth in the mouth of a dog. Secondary dentin is visible as a dark mark *(arrows)* on the canine teeth. (From Harvey CE, O'Brien JA, Rossman LE, Stoller NH. *In* Ettinger SJ (ed): Textbook of Veterinary Internal Medicine, 2nd ed, Ch. 55. Philadelphia, WB Saunders Co., 1983.)

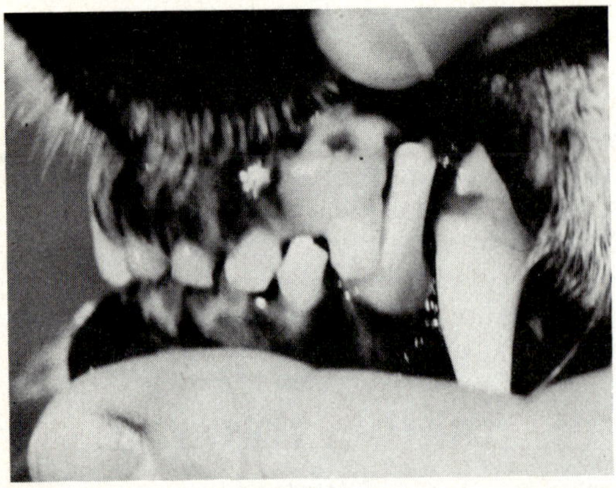

Figure 6–7. Attrition of a canine tooth caused by the canine tooth in the lower jaw wearing against the upper canine tooth. (From Harvey CE, O'Brien JA, Rossman LE, Stoller NH. *In* Ettinger SJ (ed): Textbook of Veterinary Internal Medicine, 2nd ed., Ch. 55. Philadelphia, WB Saunders Co., 1983.)

visible as a dark brown mark on affected teeth (see Fig. 6–6). Occasionally, the rate of wear may be too rapid for the reparative process to keep pace with, and pulp exposure occurs.

Treatment of teeth with worn crowns is usually not necessary unless pulp exposure has occurred (page 86). The permanent teeth of the dog and cat do not erupt continuously, so the crown will not grow back into occlusion once the cause of the abnormal wear is eliminated. If appearance is important, crown height can be restored (page 92).

Fracture

Fractured teeth are common in the dog and cat; the fracture is often noted as an incidental finding. Causes are external and occlusal trauma. The teeth most frequently noted to be fractured are the canine and upper carnassial teeth.[22]

Cleavage of the enamel surface without exposure of the pulp cavity (as happens frequently with upper carnassial teeth (Fig. 6–9) does not require treatment unless there are rough edges that could lacerate the cheek; these edges are smoothed off as necessary (see Fig. 6–23). The extremely hard enamel protects the dentin from occlusive force; once enamel is removed, the odontoblastic processes in the dentin are stimulated and cause the pulp adjacent to the fracture site to form reparative dentin over the next several weeks.[23] If odontoblastic processes in the exposed dentinal tubules are stimulated by heat, cold, or pressure, the animal may cry or howl in pain.

If the fracture exposes the pulp cavity (Fig. 6–10), endodontic therapy is necessary to prevent the possibility of eventual tooth loss. Pulpotomy is an alternative if the tooth is available for treatment within several hours of fracture. These procedures are described further on.

A fractured tooth does not require restoration of full crown height for useful function and acceptable appearance. Endodontic treatment and sealing the access cavity will leave sufficient height in many cases. There

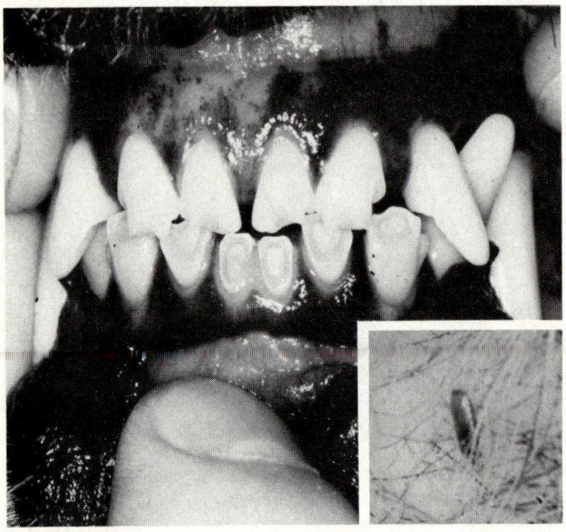

Figure 6–8. Severe attrition of the lower incisor teeth of a dog caused by gnawing. *Inset,* Flea causing the dermatitis in this dog.

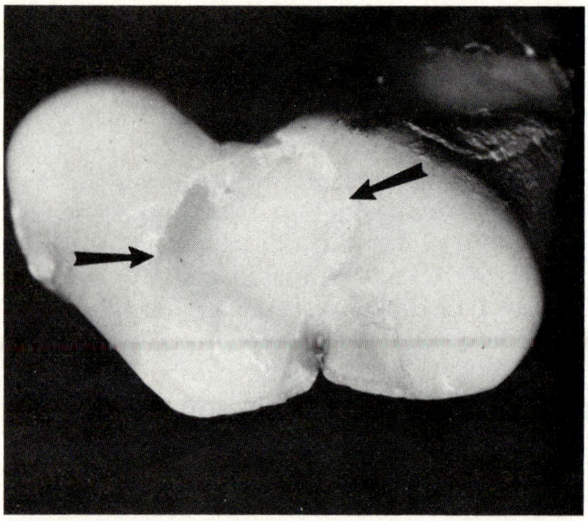

Figure 6–9. Fracture of the crown *(arrows)* of an upper carnassial tooth of a dog without penetration into the pulp cavity.

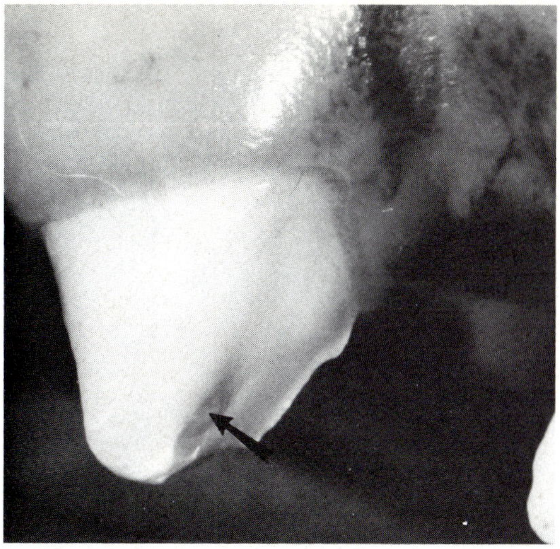

Figure 6–10. Fracture of an upper canine tooth of a dog with exposure of the pulp *(arrow)*.

is no appreciable shifting of other teeth in the mouth of the dog or cat following loss of crown height or loss of a whole tooth.

A horizontal fracture at the alveolar bone crest or root requires extraction. The animal favors the other side of the mouth when chewing or biting, and there is marked mobility of the crown. The pain in this case emanates from the surrounding gingival tissue. If the root is intact, the tooth can be salvaged by removing the crown and resecting gingiva and bone to expose enough of the root for endodontic treatment and placement of a post, core, and crown restoration.

Horizontal fractures below the alveolar crest may not be recognized or may not require treatment, since the surrounding bone may stabilize the fragments.[24] Pulp vitality may be maintained, and eventually a cementoid material is deposited that unites both fragments, especially with more apical fractures. There is no sign of this type of injury unless the dental pulp dies, in which case the crown takes on a dark gray or brown color. If the crown is discolored, indicating pulp death, the options are to extract the tooth including the apical segment, to perform root canal therapy, or to leave the tooth alone. Once periodontal communication is established, the tooth is doomed to eventual loss, so the prognosis in this situation depends on the position of the fracture.

Sometimes trauma does not cause a fracture but is severe enough to distort the pulpal blood supply, causing hemorrhage into the dentinal tubules or pulpal necrosis. The result is discoloration of the crown from white to gray or brown (Fig. 6–11); extraction or root canal therapy is indicated to eliminate the pathological tissue in the pulp cavity and prevent a periapical abscess. Normal tooth coloration rarely is restored as a result of endodontic treatment; composite resin bonded to the enamel (page 94) can be used to return the tooth to normal appearance.

If a fracture occurs through the long axis of a tooth, restoration is rarely possible, because occlusal forces are likely to cause separation of the fragments. Treatment by small pin restoration has been used successfully in occasional cases.[25]

Avulsion

Avulsion of a tooth from its socket may be partial or total (Fig. 6–12). Treatment is to reposition the tooth as quickly as possible if the owner wishes to retain a normal appearance. Ideally, the owner should put the tooth back into the socket immediately if the animal is cooperative. If this is not possible, the tooth is placed in a container of milk and is brought to the hospital with the animal; milk retards bacterial growth and keeps the periodontal ligament tissue nourished. The tooth should be repositioned within 1 hour for the best chance of maintaining vitality of the peri-

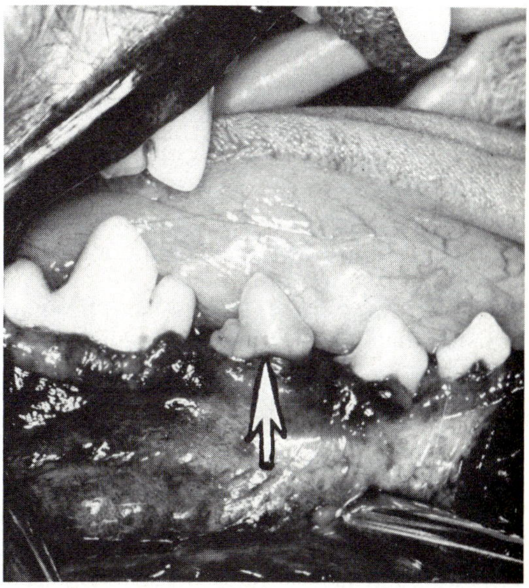

Figure 6–11. Discoloration of a lower fourth premolar tooth *(arrow)* caused by trauma, resulting in the death of the pulpal tissues.

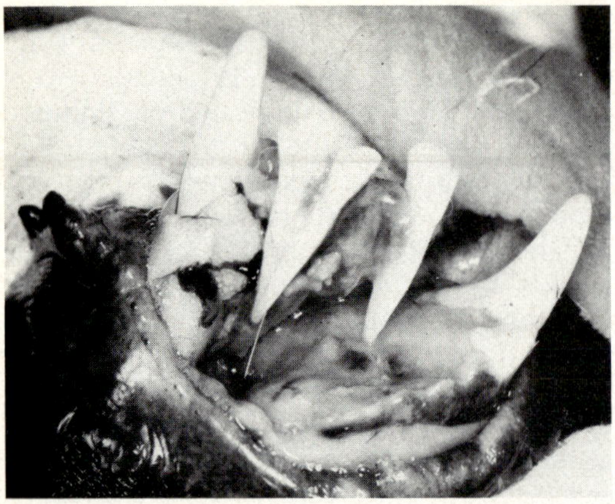

Figure 6–12. Avulsion of incisor teeth in a dog. Some are completely and some are incompletely avulsed.

odontal ligament; this usually precludes performing root canal therapy at that time. The tooth is repositioned (without cleaning off any attached soft tissue),[26] and is held in place with orthodontic brackets. About a week later, root canal therapy is performed and the brackets are removed; leaving the brackets in place longer may induce ankylosis and eventual resorption.[27] Resorption also occurs if there has been any destruction of the periodontal ligament,[27] which can occur at such a rapid rate that the tooth is lost within a year. The periodontal ligament acts as a double periosteum; once it is removed or becomes necrotic, the bone recognizes the tooth as a foreign body, and osteoclastic resorption commences.

Resorption of Teeth

Resorption is either internal or external. Internal resorption occurs when the dental pulp has become pathological and is eating away tooth substance from within. External resorption occurs as a result of odontoclastic activity of the periosteum of the alveolar bone. The usual cause is trauma. The diagnosis is made by clinical and radiographic examination.

Internal resorption may be recognized by the red coloration it gives to the crown (Fig. 6–13). To retain the tooth, internal resorption must be treated as soon as it is recognized. Excellent results can be expected if root canal therapy is performed before the resorption process erodes through the root or crown and communicates with the external environment.

Several categories of external root resorption are recognized in human dentistry following replacement of avulsed teeth or other severe trauma to the periodontal ligament. Most of these conditions have not been recognized in veterinary patients. Resorption of the entire root, similar to inflammatory resorption of human teeth, is seen occasionally

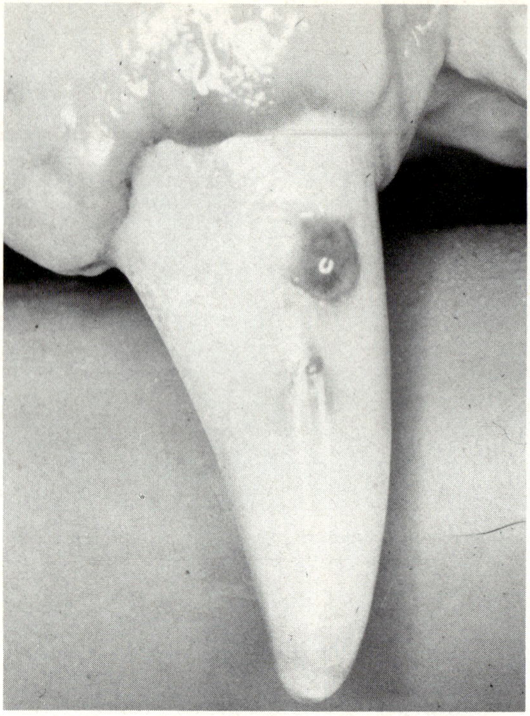

Figure 6–13. Internal resorption of tooth substance causing discoloration and penetration of the enamel of the canine tooth of a dog.

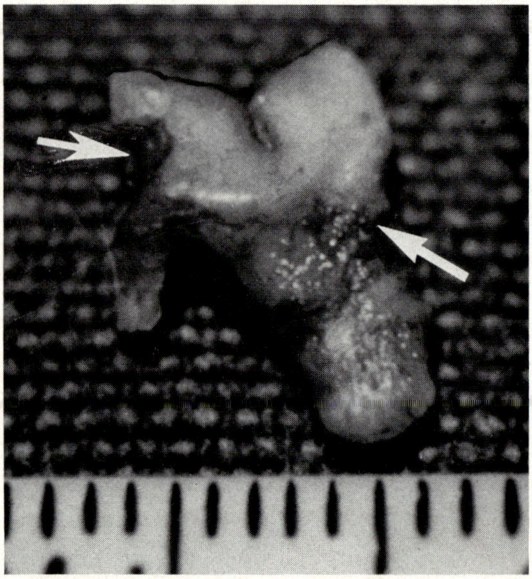

Figure 6–14. Osteoclastic resorption *(arrows)* of the cemento-enamel junction area of a premolar tooth of a cat with periodontal disease.

in dogs,[28] as is localized root resorption.[78] Localized root resorption is seen more commonly in cats;[29, 79] the lesions occur in cats with periodontal disease, and they grossly resemble caries (Fig. 6–14). Since several teeth often are involved, treatment is usually extraction.

Caries

Caries is demineralization of tooth enamel by toxins produced by carbohydrate-fermenting bacteria. If allowed to continue, the decay can reach the pulp cavity and cause endodontic disease. Caries is uncommon in both dogs and cats for several reasons.[8, 30, 31] A coarse diet helps to clean the teeth. A diet low in fermentable carbohydrate does not promote development of cariogenic flora. The shape of the teeth and the large interdental spaces do not promote clinging of food material (the exception is the plateaued, crushing crown of the first upper molar tooth, which is the tooth most often affected by caries in the dog). The alkaline saliva of carnivores also inhibits cariogenesis. It is difficult to cause caries in the dog even when a cariogenic diet is fed for long periods to dogs inoculated with a cariogenic flora.[32]

Presenting signs include reluctance to eat and jaw chattering. Diagnosis is by inspection (Fig. 6–15*A*) and requires sedation or anesthesia because of the discomfort that the procedure may cause even in a cooperative dog. The lesion is scratched with a sharp dental explorer (Fig. 6–15*B*); caries lesions are soft and sticky compared with most other lesions of the enamel, such as enamel hypoplasia.

Treatment is either extraction of the affected tooth (esthetically important teeth are rarely affected) or resection of the lesion. The diseased tissue and a thin layer of normal dentin is removed with a carbide bur in a dental handpiece, and the tooth is restored with amalgam if an occluding surface is involved (see Fig. 6–24). If the depth of removal is close to the pulp cavity, a sedative dressing such as zinc oxide and eugenol is applied prior to restoration of the enamel. Endodontic treatment must be performed if the lesion has eroded into the pulp cavity or if the pulp cavity is penetrated during treatment.

Carnassial Abscess

Carnassial abscess (facial sinus, malar abscess) is the most common form of chronic osteomyelitis of the maxilla. This condition is an infection or fistula arising from the

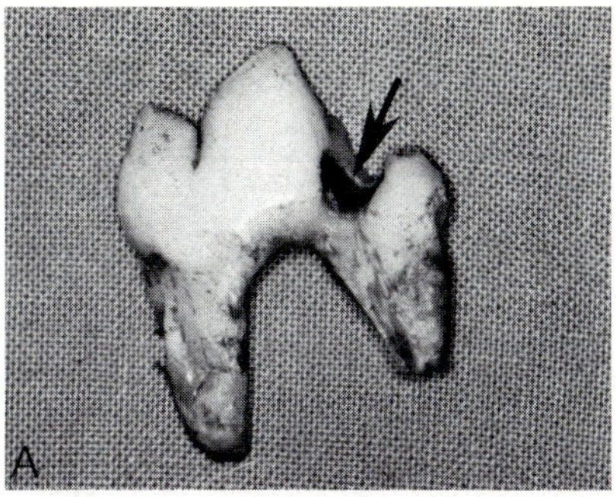

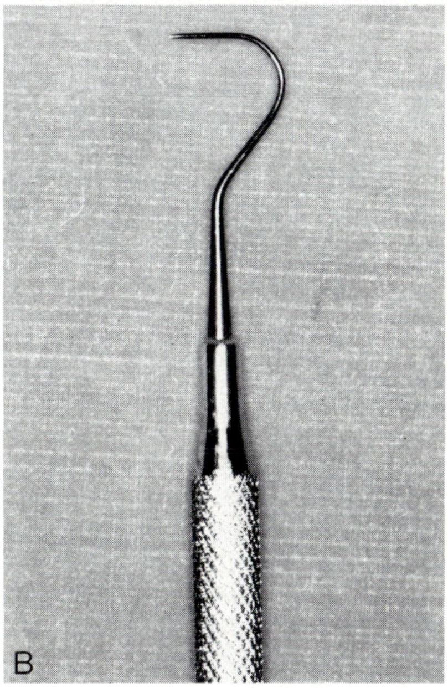

Figure 6–15. *A*, Caries cavity in the lower first molar tooth of a dog *(arrow)*. *B*, Pointed dental explorer used to diagnose caries.

upper carnassial (fourth premolar) tooth and less often from the upper first molar tooth. It is seen in dogs of any breed, but most often in middle aged or older animals. It is rare in cats.[33] A similar syndrome occurs less often around the first molar tooth in the mandible.[34]

The maxillary bone is eroded over the root of the tooth, and a swelling, which often goes on to rupture (Fig. 6–16), results on the side of the face. Typically, the swelling is ventral and slightly rostral to or level with the medial canthus of the eye. Occasionally the fistula may open into the conjunctival sac.[33, 35] The discharge produced is rarely grossly purulent; more often it is serosanguineous. Crown fracture, root abscess, or periodontal disease are obvious on some but not all affected teeth.[36] It has not yet been established with certainty whether the condition results from periodontal disease or endodontic disease, or both; pressure necrosis from occlusive

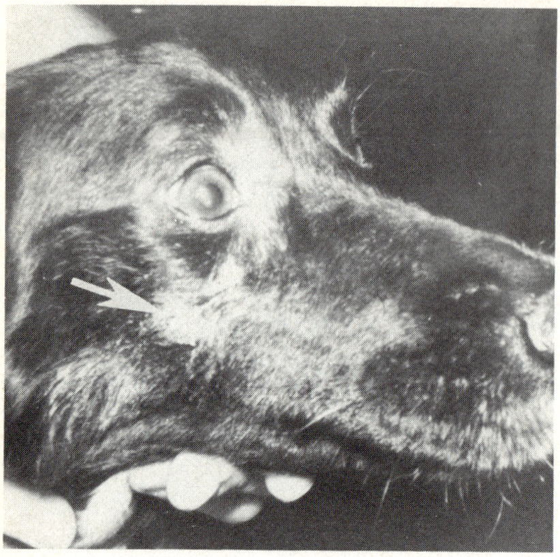

Figure 6–16. Carnassial abscess *(arrow)* on the side of the face of a dog.

trauma has been suggested as a cause.[37] When a mandibular tooth is affected, the fistula opens either into the buccal fold or onto the skin surface (Fig. 6–17).

Treatment of carnassial abscess consists of extraction of the tooth immediately beneath the lesion. Endodontic treatment also has been used successfully,[38] though the root structure of the upper carnassial tooth makes this a rather demanding procedure (page 91). Carnassial abscess is a localized condition that can be treated successfully in almost all affected animals.

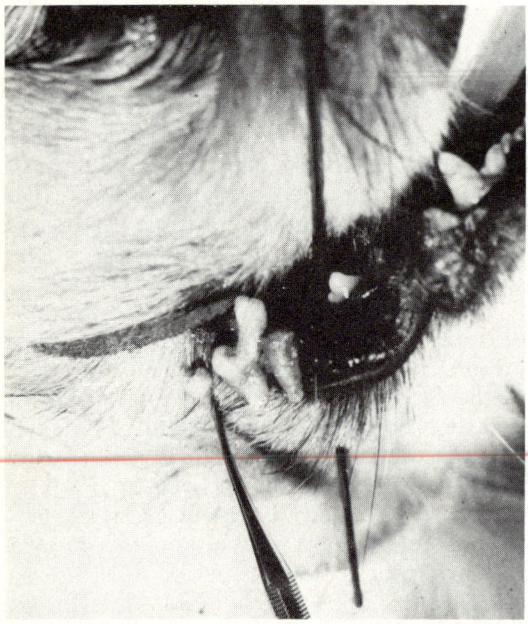

Figure 6–17. Dental fistula arising from a lower carnassial tooth of a dog. A probe has been passed from the alveolus to the fistula. The extracted tooth is lying on the lower lip.

PULPAL (ENDODONTIC) AND PERIAPICAL DISEASE

The dental pulp is the embryological organ for tooth development. Once the tooth has formed, the pulp becomes a physiological organ encased in hard tooth structure. Because of the presence of the dentinal tubules, the pulp responds to dentinal irritation. Caries, if detected early and removed, will cause reversible inflammation in the pulp; however caries deep in the dentin that has exposed the pulp will infect it beyond recovery. A tooth fracture that is severe enough to expose the pulp also creates an irreversible clinical problem, since it leaves the pulp with no potential for healing. If a restoration is placed over an exposed pulp, degeneration of the blood supply and subsequent autolysis of the tissue will occur.

The root canal is essentially a blind sac that communicates directly with the supporting alveolar bone at the root apex. Once the pulp tissue degenerates, it fuels an apical inflammatory response. Unless the source is removed either by extraction or endodontic treatment, the cells in the bone and apical periodontal ligament erect a barricade against the insult; the result is apical periodontitis. This will persist until the abnormal environment is corrected. Endodontic treatment should be performed before apical periodontitis has had time to develop.

The periapical response proceeds in one of three directions:

1. *Abscess formation,* which is usually rapid, creates pain and swelling. The presenting signs are lethargy, favoring one side during eating, or loss of appetite. The tooth is painful if touched, though this often is not observed in the dog and cat. If the abscess is allowed to develop, bone erosion may continue until a fistula is formed, relieving the pressure.[39] A radiograph taken with a probe inserted into the fistula reveals its source (Fig. 6–18), which is not always the tooth directly above the fistula.[40] Tooth extraction or endodontic treatment avoids the needs for surgical exploration and curettage, drains, and antibiotic administration.

The acute abscess also may become chronic, with the establishment of a connective tissue wall. Factors that may be important in determining whether an abscess becomes acute or chronic include resistance of the

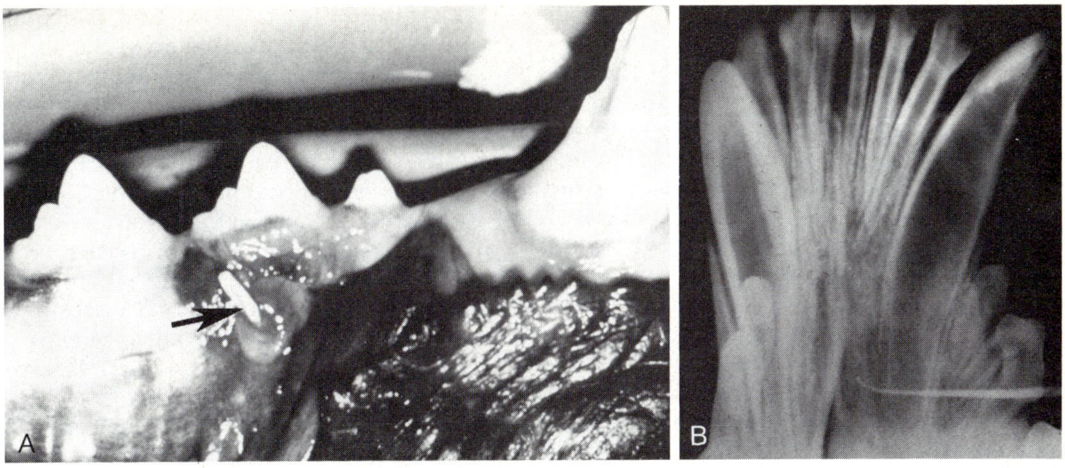

Figure 6–18. *A*, A radiodense gutta percha point has been inserted into a dental fistula to identify the source of the fistula *(arrow)*. *B*, Radiograph showing the probe leading to a radiolucent area adjacent to the open apex of the canine tooth in this young dog.

host, the bacterial organisms present, and the cause of the original insult.[41] The acute abscess is composed of infiltrating inflammatory cells; a chronic abscess resembles the lesion of periodontal disease, an inflammatory infiltrate surrounded by a cell-rich zone of fibroblasts and collagen.[42] Chronic abscess is more easily seen radiographically because enough calcium has been removed to expose a radiolucent periapical area (Fig. 6–19).[43]

2. *Cyst formation* appears as a radiolucent lesion surrounded by a well-differentiated cortical plate of bone (Fig. 6–20). Diagnosis can be confirmed only by histological examination. Treatment is extraction, conservative

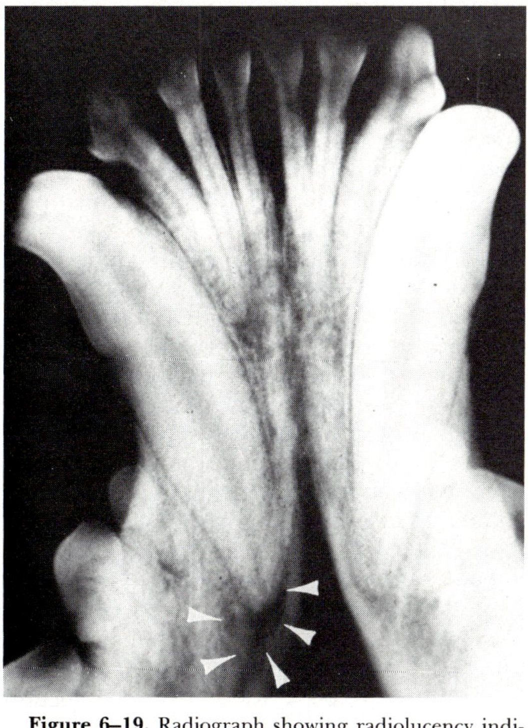

Figure 6–19. Radiograph showing radiolucency indicating a periapical abscess *(arrows)*.

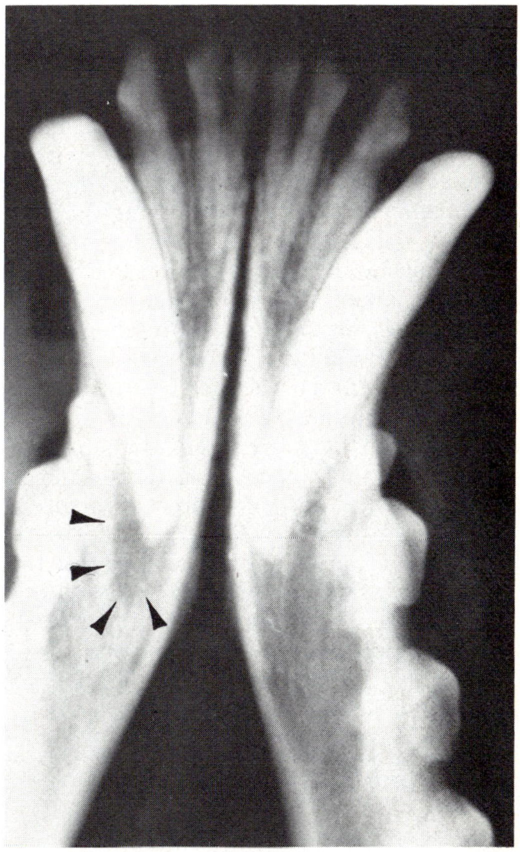

Figure 6–20. Radiograph showing a possible periapical cyst at the root apex of a lower canine tooth; a radiolucent center is surrounded by a sclerotic margin *(arrows)*.

endodontic treatment, or endodontic treatment and apicoectomy. Cyst formation occurs as a result of the activation of the epithelial cell rests in the periodontal ligament that remain after root formation; initiating factors have not been identified. Like chronic abscess, cyst formation can be viewed as the body's attempt to externalize a periapical irritation. The cells on the healthy side of the lining are normal.

3. *Cellulitis.* Infection can spread beyond the primary contamination site in some cases to infect adjacent tissues. Spread of infection is regulated by the pathogenicity of the organism. Release of streptokinase or lysozymal enzymes from degranulating polymorphonuclear leukocytes may aid the spread of infection. The limiting factor appears to be the relation of muscle insertions with respect to the root apex, causing most infections taking the path of least resistance to create a swelling or fistula within the confines of the oral cavity rather than to spread to other fascial planes of the head or neck.

Diagnosis of Endodontic Disease

The diagnosis of diseases in tooth structure in dogs is sometimes very simple by observing pulp exposure in a fractured tooth, but in other cases it may be difficult. The veterinary patient's response to heat, cold, and electrical stimulation of the teeth or gingivae is of dubious value. Observation is often the only tool available, though palpation and percussion are sometimes useful. Signs such as favoring one side of the mouth when eating, rubbing the mouth with the paws, lethargy, and fever indicate the need to inspect the animal's dentition, searching for signs of trauma such as a fractured tooth or tooth discoloration or abscess or fistula around the teeth. Radiographs may show a fracture or periapical bone loss (see Fig. 6–20).

A radiograph made while a radiopaque probe is present in a fistula usually will indicate whether the origin of the tract is endodontic, since fistulae of endodontic origin almost invariably develop from the root apex (see Fig. 6–18*B*).

Endodontic (Root Canal) Treatment

The purpose of endodontic treatment is to remove the infected pulp cavity contents and seal off a sterile and dead, but functional, tooth that will last the lifetime of the animal.

Proper endodontic treatment requires some specialized equipment and instruments. An x-ray machine is mandatory; radiographic technique is described in Chapter 3, page 30. The approximate length of the root of the tooth can be obtained from measuring the radiographic image. For access to the pulp cavity, the ideal handpiece is a cool running dental unit that directs a water spray toward the tooth. The bench engine or Dremmel motor tools often used to power handpieces in veterinary dental practice are less desirable because they become hot, are more difficult to control, revolve with such high torque that the standard dental carbide burs lose their cutting efficiency very quickly, and may not be able to accept the contra-angle handpiece necessary for some endodontic access preparations. They are useful as an initial low-cost instrument and for teeth polishing following scaling.

General anesthesia is essential; a deep surgical plane is required during removal of vital pulp tissue. The endotracheal tube can be placed through the mouth unless the tube interferes with access for the bite impressions that are necessary for crown restoration or with occlusion assessment and adjustment; tube placement through a pharyngotomy or tracheotomy incision is used in these latter situations.

Pulpotomy

If the animal is available for treatment immediately following traumatic exposure of the pulp, pulpotomy can be considered. The dental pulp is removed from the crown portion of the tooth, and calcium hydroxide paste is placed over the remaining pulp tissue and is covered by a zinc oxide and eugenol dental cement. A filling of dental amalgam is formed in the crown defect, and the crown is smoothed off with a dental bur.

A longterm failure rate of 20 percent has been reported when using this technique in dogs.[44] Full endodontic treatment can be completed in one procedure, takes little longer than pulpotomy, and is less likely to fail. Pulpotomy is therefore not recommended for use in mature dogs. The advantage of pulpotomy is its potential use in immature animals, because it may permit continued tooth development. The high pH within the pulp cavity caused by calcium hydroxide will inhibit osteoclastic activity and tend to induce odontoblastic activity.[45, 46] Full endodontic treatment usually is necessary to ensure retention of the tooth once tooth development has ceased; this is assessed from periodic radiographic examination.

Full Endodontic Treatment

All endodontic treatment procedures require proper access to the tooth, mechanical instrumentation and control of bacteria within the canal, and careful three-dimensional obturation of the canal.

Access must be obtained in a dry aseptic field. The surface of the tooth is bathed with an antiseptic and isolated from surrounding structures prior to making the access hole. Knowledge of root anatomy is essential in order to obtain direct access into the cavity; an opening must be made that avoids any overhang that would prevent the root canal instruments from gaining access to the entire wall of the canal.

Canine teeth are treated most commonly. The incisal edge usually is fractured, and the tooth is therefore shorter than the opposite canine. A large, round bur mounted in a dental handpiece is used to obtain access (Fig. 6–21*A*). Since these teeth have long, curved roots, instrumentation of the canal can be difficult. An additional opening madethrough the buccal or rostral wall of the tooth just above the gingivae provides more direct access (Fig. 6–21*B*). When planning this passage, the tooth should be considered in three dimensions to prevent creation of an unwanted opening or perforation through the side of the tooth; radiographs made from two different views permit accurate orientation.

After gaining access, an instrument is passed through the length of the canal until it meets the resistance of the apical delta (Fig. 6–21*C*), and a radiograph is made to determine the length of the canal. Root canal instruments include files and reamers, which are arranged in widths that increase in 0.01-mm increments. Since canine teeth in the dog are longer than the standard 25-mm human endodontic files, 55-mm (H. Schein Co., Fig. 6–21*D*) or 40-mm (Syntex Dental Corp.) files are used. If greater length is necessary (such as for the canine teeth of large exotic cats; see Chapter 20), the blades of the shorter instruments are soldered to orthodontic wire.

The endodontic file is worked and twisted along the canal wall to debrde adherent soft tissue (Fig. 6–21*E*). Some organic dentin is removed so as to reduce the amount of organic substrate subsequently available for bacterial growth. Proceeding to a wider instrument, more surface area is reamed, ensuring that the critical concentration of contaminants is removed. Barbed broaches are introduced intermittently to remove accumulating tissue fragments.

The pulp in the canine tooth of a dog is large, particularly in immature animals (Fig. 6–21*F*); tissue that is not removed may be packed into the apical portion of the canal, leading to a failure requiring subsequent extraction or periapical surgery.

Sodium hypochlorite diluted to 2.5 percent, and 3 percent hydrogen peroxide solutions are used in addition to instrumentation (Fig. 6–21*G*). Sodium hypochlorite dissolves organic tissue and is used as a final rinse to neutralize the peroxide and prevent oxygen liberation in the periapical tissue, resulting in emphysema. Excess solution is removed through a narrow metal suction tip attached to a surgical aspirator.

After thorough instrumentation of the canal, and multiple irrigations, a clean root canal is indicated by delivering white dentinal shavings on the file (Fig. 6–21*H*). After drying with sterilized paper points (Fig. 6–21*I*), the canal is ready for closure and sealing.

There are two main methods in use for filling and sealing a root canal. Our preference is to insert a core of gutta percha (Fig. 6–21*J*), which is compressed into place with a root canal spreader (Fig. 6–21*K*), and is followed by the insertion and compression of additional cones. The cones are dipped in root canal sealer or cement (Fig. 6–21*L*) to fill any spaces betwen the gutta percha cones and the root canal walls. We prefer to use gutta percha for obturation because it can be condensed three-dimensionally and can be removed easily if any corrections or retreatments are required. It also has the advantages of not dissolving in oral fluids and being well tolerated by adjacent tissues. The gutta percha is covered by a layer of dental cement, and the crown is restored (page 92).

The alternative obturation technique uses root canal cement only, which is injected through a syringe and long needle directly into the clean and dry root canal as the needle is slowly withdrawn.[47, 48] The filling material is gently tamped down and allowed to set for a few minutes; then the access opening is

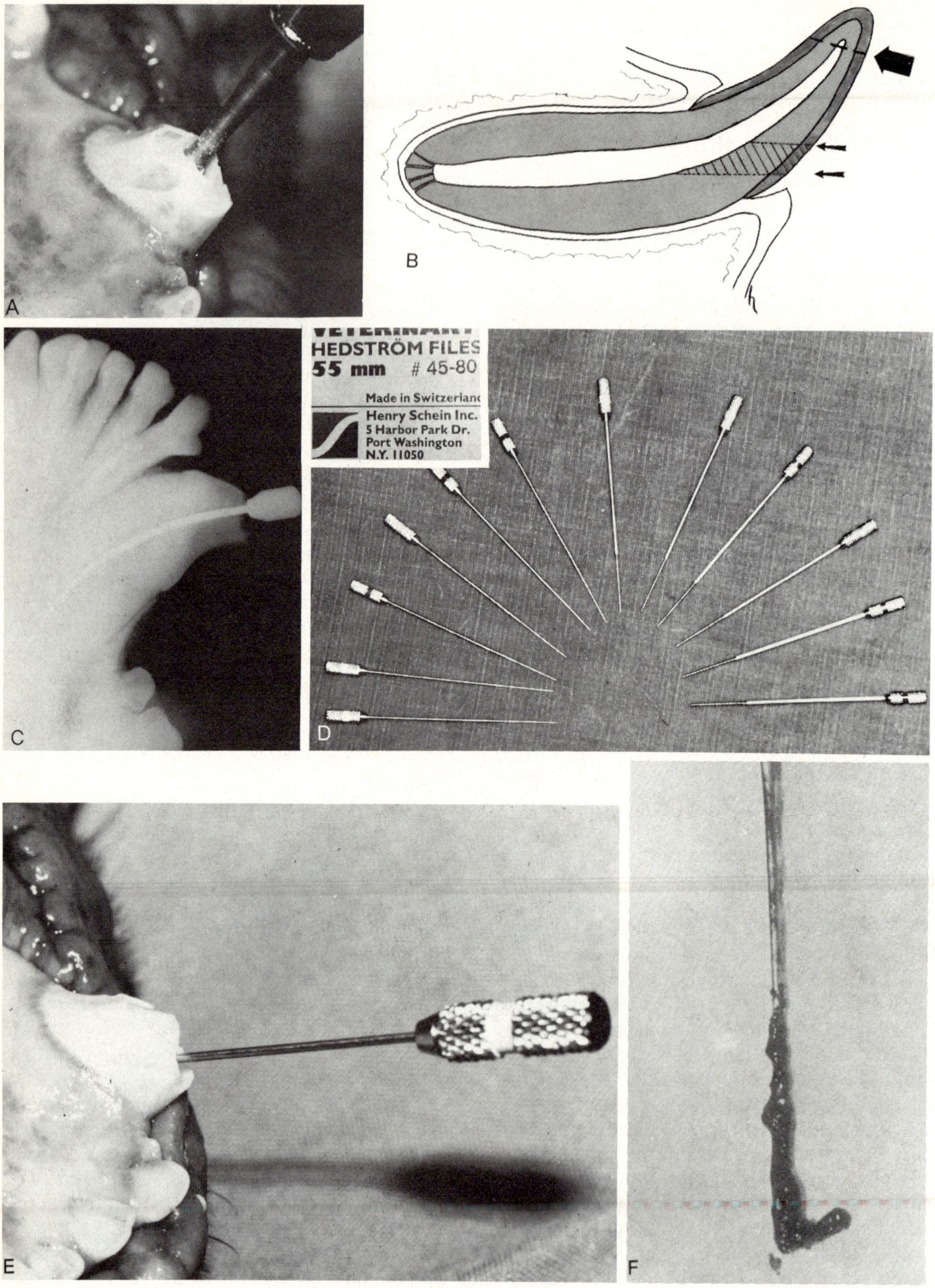

Figure 6–21. Endodontic treatment of the canine tooth of a dog. *A*, The pulp exposure at the fracture site is enlarged with a dental bur. *B*, A second access site is made with the bur above the gingivae *(small arrows)* if the fracture is at the tip of the crown *(large arrow)*. *C*, Radiograph showing a small-diameter endodontic file fully inserted to measure the depth of the canal. *D*, Endodontic files (55 mm). *Inset*, Photograph of endodontic file package. *E*, The endodontic file is used to enlarge and clean the side of the canal. *F*, Pulpal tissue extracted by the file or broach.

Illustration continued on opposite page

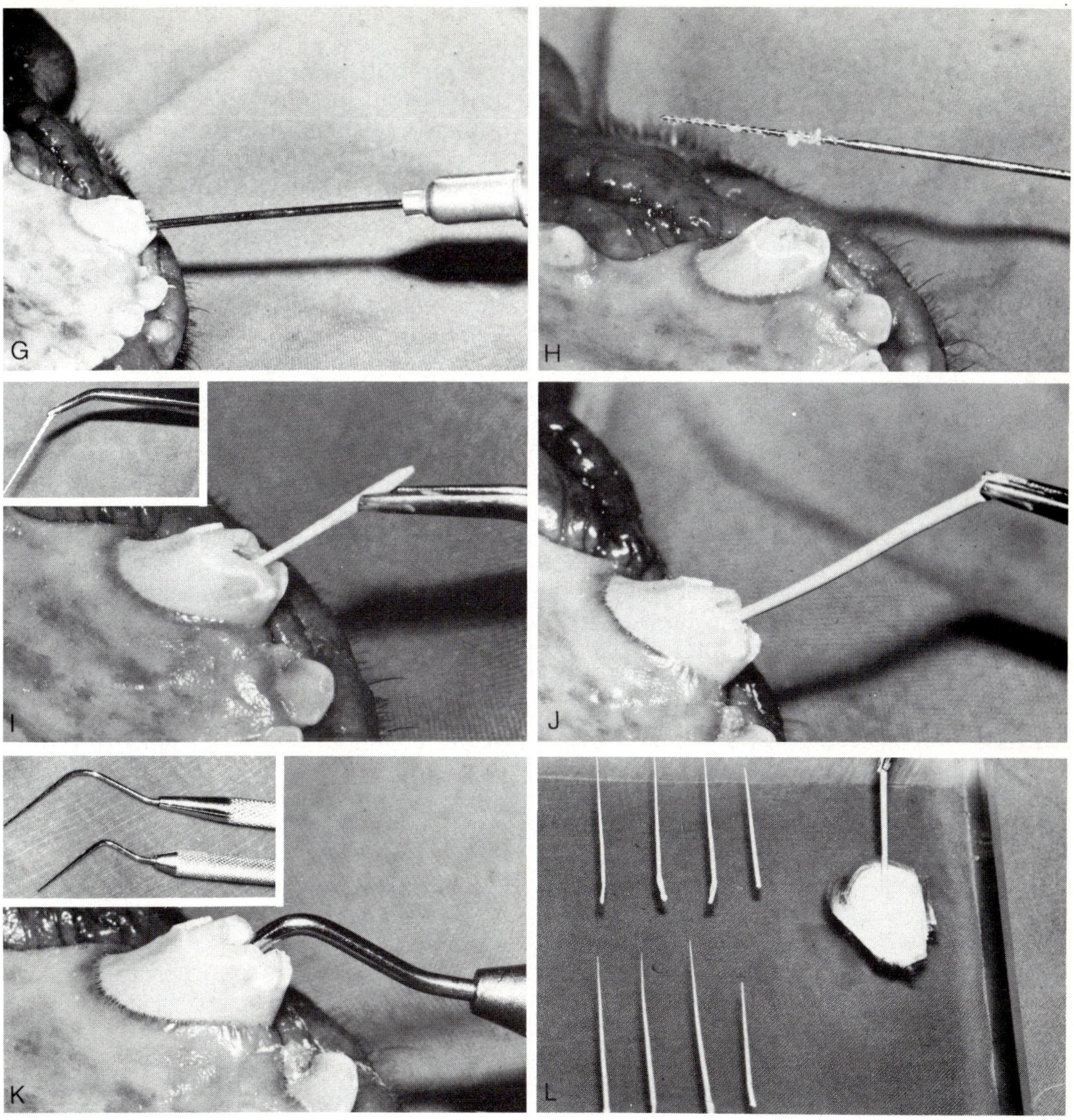

Figure 6–21 *Continued. G,* Irrigation of the canal with hydrogen peroxide or sodium hypochlorite. *H,* Dentin shavings on a file indicating that all soft tissue has been removed. *I,* Sterile paper points used to dry the canal. *J,* Gutta percha core inserted into the canal. *K,* The gutta percha core is condensed with a root canal spreader *(inset). L,* Additional gutta percha points are covered with root canal cement before insertion. (Restoration of crown shown in Figs. 6–24, 6–25, and 6–27).

restored. This technique requires fewer instruments and supplies. There are no long-term follow-up studies on teeth of dogs comparing the two techniques; both have been used for several years with success.

It should not be necessary to perform any other procedure as long as the source of the infection has been removed thoroughly. Biological repair occurs at the apex of the tooth even if an apical delta exists.[49, 50] Healing will occur even if a stump of pulp tissue is left. If fistulation occurs, surgical apicoectomy can be performed subsequently.

Treatment of Multirooted Teeth

The single-rooted canine tooth is the tooth most often treated; however, the same technique can be used on other teeth. Access to the roots of multirooted teeth in dogs may require removal of a large part of the crown.[38] Endodontic treatment of the upper carnassial tooth in a dog is much easier if the small rostromedial root is transected with a bur or diamond wheel and removed.[48] Instrumentation of the two large roots is performed as described previously, and the hemisection defect is sealed with an amalgam restoration prior to filling and sealing the canals.

Apicoectomy

It has been suggested that satisfactory endodontic treatment of canine teeth in dogs requires apicoectomy (surgical access to the apex of the root)[51] combined with an approach to the canal through the crown. In our experience, apicoectomy is necessary only if an approach through the crown fails to permit removal of all pulpal tissue or if a necrotic root is visible on a radiograph.

To perform an apicoectomy, a gingival flap overlying the root apex (which usually is easily palpable) is formed and reflected (Fig. 6–22*A*,*B*). The bone over the root, and the apex of the root, are removed carefully, using a high-speed handpiece and carbide bur (Fig. 6–22*C*). The success of this procedure depends on leaving some bone intact between the gingival margin and the apicoectomy site to seal off the periapical region during healing. Abnormal periapical tissue is curetted, and the pulp cavity is cleaned with files inserted from the crown access site. The canal is then filled and sealed as for a standard endodontic procedure. An amalgam filling is placed to seal the root apex (Fig. 6–22*D*). The mucosal incision is closed with absorbable sutures (Fig. 6–22*E*).

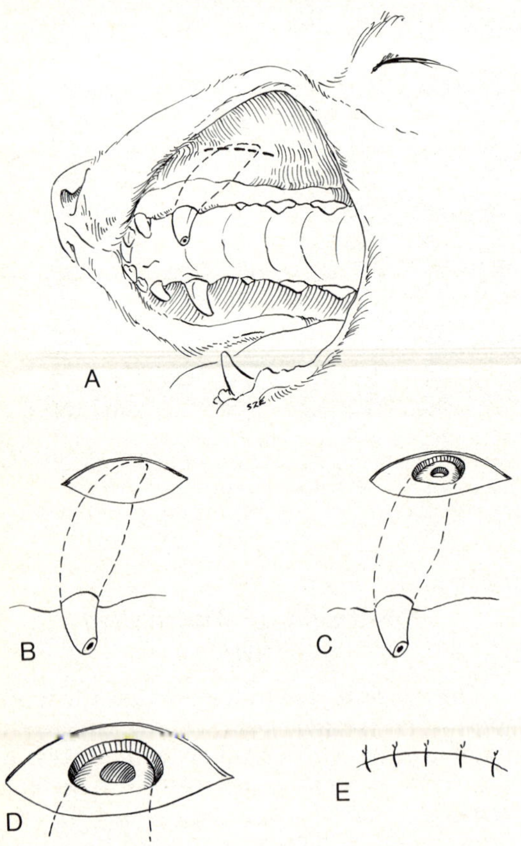

Figure 6–22. Apicoectomy of an upper canine tooth. *A* and *B*, Gingival flap created over root apex. *C*, The bone overlying the root and the apex of the root have been removed with a dental bur. *D*, Amalgam restoration of the apicoectomy. *E*, The gingival mucosa is sutured.

Endodontic treatment performed through an apicoectomy without a crown access site will result in eventual loss of the tooth because an apical plug cannot adequately seal off the noxious contents of the root canal.

Whether apicoectomy is necessary during root canal therapy in canine teeth of dogs remains controversial.[51–55] Thorough reaming of the root canal to the apex of the tooth and coronal sealing are the most critical factors preventing reinfection.[49, 50] There are few documented longterm follow-up reports of results in clinical patients. A success rate of 95 percent at a mean period of 2½ years was found in one study of 92 teeth in 75 dogs treated by filling the canal with zinc oxide, eugenol, and formaldehyde without apicoectomy.[56] An undocumented failure rate of 30 percent following conventional nonapicoectomy endodontic treatment has been mentioned.[57] In studies in which apicoectomy was performed, a failure rate of 20 to 25 percent at 18 to 24 months in an unstated number of dogs was reported; however, this report also stated that no failures occurred in 20 dogs treated by apicoectomy, retrograde amalgam filling, zinc oxide and eugenol filling of the root canal, and amalgam crown restoration.[51]

RESTORATIVE DENTISTRY

Restorative techniques can be used to reform the surface of a tooth, or to replace sections of crown that have been lost. Simple defects not affecting the pulp cavity can be smoothed and rounded off with a dental bur (Fig. 6–23*A*,*B*). More sophisticated restoration usually is not required unless the tooth is functionally important, as in guard or attack dogs, or esthetically important to the owner.

Restorative Materials and Techniques[58–62]

Selection of the appropriate restorative dental material depends on several factors,

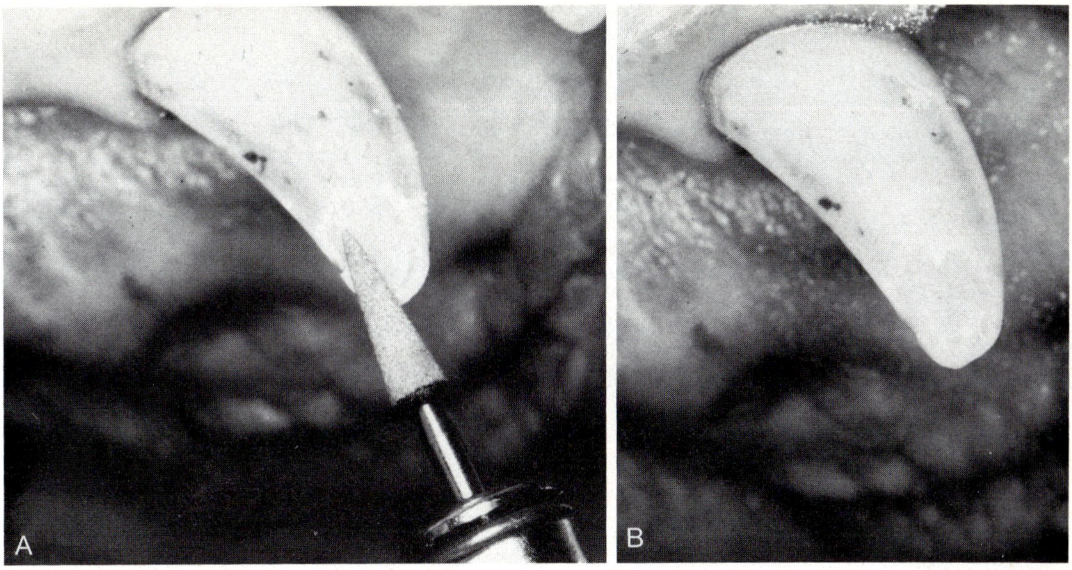

Figure 6–23. Smoothing down the jagged edges of enamel of a fractured tooth in which the fracture did not extend into the pulp cavity.

including consideration of the forces to which the teeth are subjected. The pH of oral fluids fluctuates constantly with the ingestion of food. The temperature range in a meal may vary, and constant exposure to the wet oral cavity with its associated enzymes and microbial plaque additionally complicates the requirements of a permanent restoration.

The dental materials generally used are amalgam, composite resin systems, cast metals, and cements and bases.

Amalgam

Amalgam is an alloy of silver and mercury with other metals added in small amounts to control its functional properties. The finished restoration has a dark metallic coloration. It is useful for sealing apicoectomy openings and for restoring caries cavity preparations in caudal teeth. Amalgam alloys come preproportioned in capsules that require mechanical trituration with a rapid oscillatory motion to mix the alloy (Fig. 6–24*A*). The length of trituration time depends on the type of material and is specified by the manufacturer. The material is removed from the capsule after trituration and is placed and condensed in the prepared cavity (Fig. 6–24*B* and *C*) by hand or by a mechanical condenser (Fig. 6–24*D*). While still in the plastic state, it is carved and fashioned into a facsimile of the original tooth form (Fig. 6–24*E*).

Because of the lack of adhesiveness of amalgam, cavity preparation for an amalgam restoration must be undercut to retain the filling (see Fig. 6–24*C*). If the carious lesion extends toward the pulp, a pulp sedative material such as zinc oxide and eugenol is placed between the amalgam and the underlying freshly cut dentin. Moisture contamination should be avoided until the amalgam has set, since zinc in the alloy reacts with water, producing a marked expansion of the material. For that reason, alloys that do not contain zinc are preferred.

Resin Materials[58, 59, 62]

Several plastic resin materials have been developed as dental restoratives. Methylmethacrylate, the original material, produces considerable heat and expands during polymerization.

A more recent material is a monomer based on the BIS-GMA molecule. This formulation has become the most widely used dental composite resin material. To the resin various types of fillers are added, such as glass beads, quartz, and silica, resulting in a material with lower polymerization shrinkage, less volatility, and a less traumatic effect on the pulp, since it produces less heat during polymerization. Its lower coefficient of thermal expansion results in less volumetric changes in the mouth and less microleakage.

A second breakthrough was the development of the acid etch technique, in which orthophosphoric acid changes the enamel surface configuration to promote adhesion

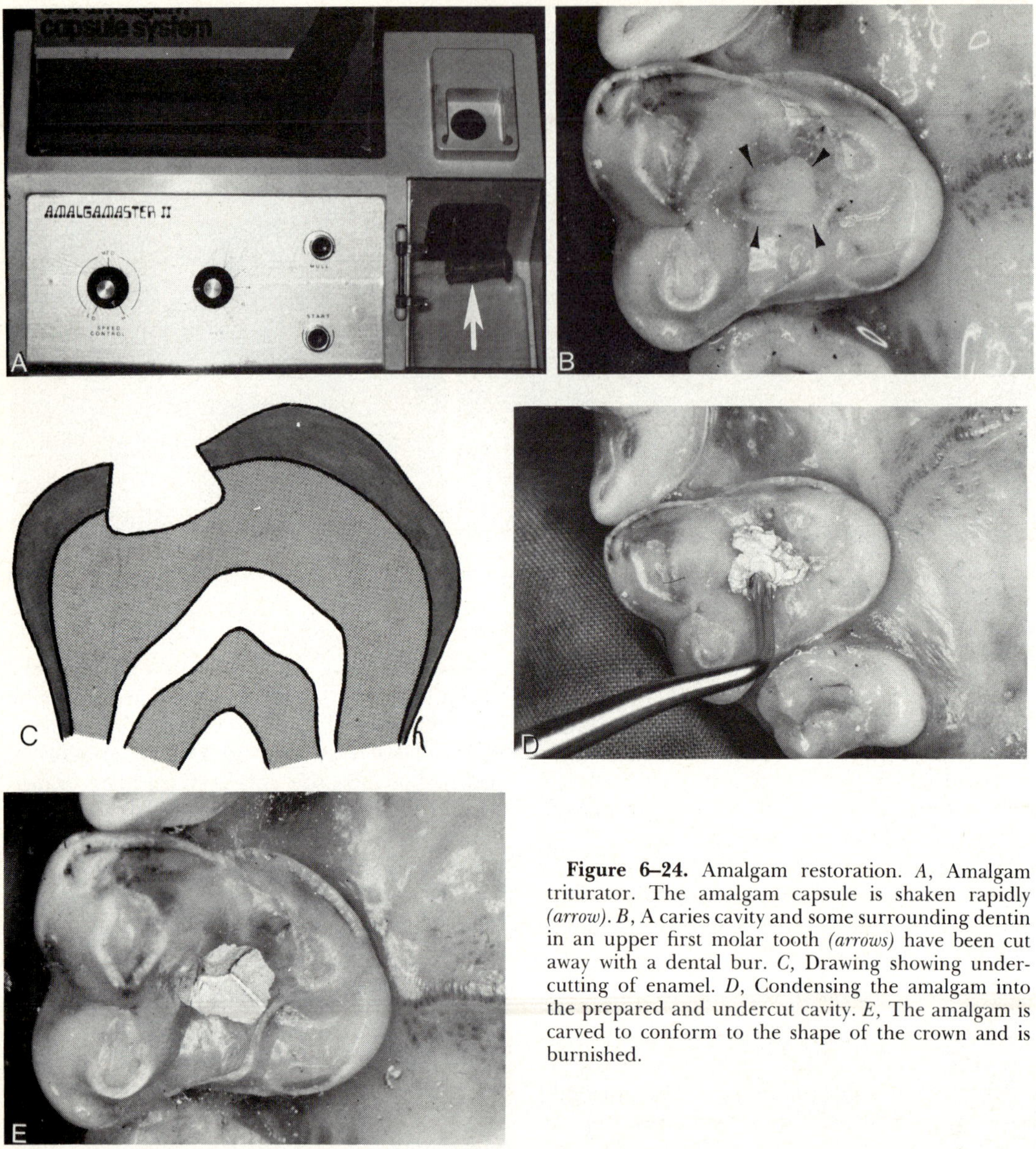

Figure 6–24. Amalgam restoration. *A*, Amalgam triturator. The amalgam capsule is shaken rapidly *(arrow)*. *B*, A caries cavity and some surrounding dentin in an upper first molar tooth *(arrows)* have been cut away with a dental bur. *C*, Drawing showing undercutting of enamel. *D*, Condensing the amalgam into the prepared and undercut cavity. *E*, The amalgam is carved to conform to the shape of the crown and is burnished.

of the restorative material to the underlying tooth structure. The acid selectively erodes part of the enamel surface in a series of three distinct patterns, creating micropores into which the resin flows, hardens, and interlocks.

After application of the acid, the enamel appears chalky white. The basic BIS-GMA resin is very viscous and will not flow into the micropores of the etched enamel. All kits of the material now come in two parts, the filled BIS-GMA resin and an unfilled bonding material that is made less viscous by the addition of various thinning agents.

A further development leading to widespread use of the resin system was light activation of the polymerization process, providing unlimited time for placing and shaping the material into the desired form. The lights used for this process are expensive, however. It may be more practical to use the time-limited mixed-resin polymerization materials in veterinary patients.

Resin Bonding—Clinical Technique

Mechanical cleaning of the enamel is the first step in the bonding procedure. Calculus and plaque are removed, and the enamel is prepared with a non-fluoridated pumice in a polishing cup to remove all enamel contaminants (Fig. 6–25*A*,*B*). The tooth is dried with

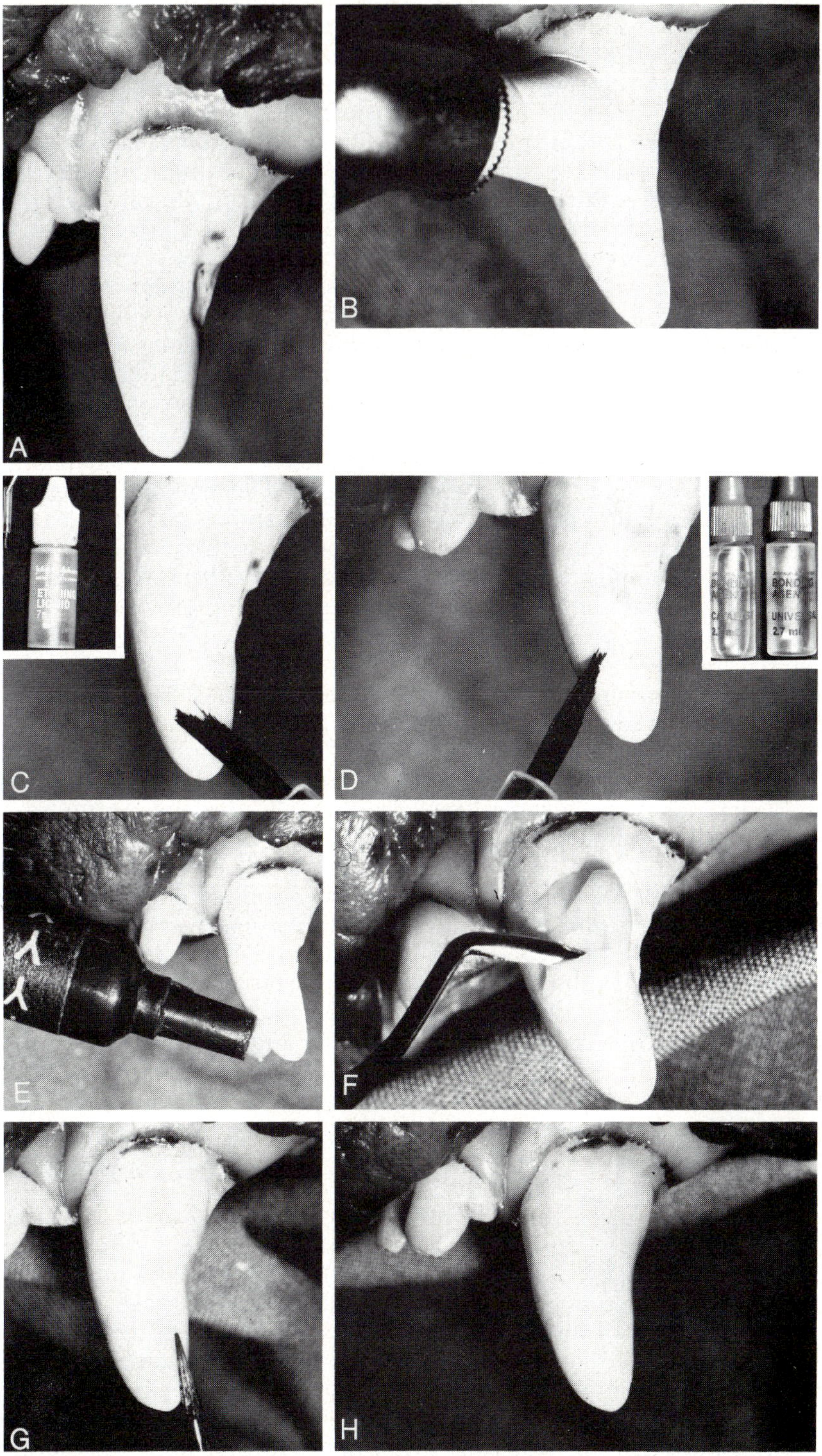

Figure 6–25. Bonded resin restoration. *A,* Enamel irregularity on a canine tooth. *B,* The surface of the tooth is cleaned thoroughly with a mild abrasive pumice and prophylaxis cup. *C,* Orthophosphoric acid is painted onto the enamel. *D,* Unfilled resin is applied to the site. *E,* Filled resin is layered on top of the unfilled resin. *F,* The resin is shaped with a spatula. *G,* Excess material is removed with a dental bur. *H,* The finished, polished tooth.

a warm stream of air and is isolated from the rest of the mouth. The 30 percent orthophosphoric acid is applied with a small, soft brush gently swabbed over the area for 1 to 2 minutes (Fig. 6–25*C*). Hard pressure or the use of cotton should be avoided, since this may fracture the friable etched enamel rods and destroy bonding capability.

The enamel is washed free of the acid with water for about 20 seconds. It is critical to remove the acid and reactive products so that the dried micropores are available for bonding. After washing, it is also critical to keep the prepared tooth free of saliva to prevent contamination by salivary mucoproteins. The washed enamel is dried with a stream of warm air.

The filled resins are available in two forms. The light-cured material consists of a single paste, whereas the chemically catalyzed material consists of two pastes, one containing the resin and one containing the catalyst. Both systems require that the less-viscous unfilled resin be painted on the etched tooth first; this material spreads across the surface, entering the enlarged enamel micropores (Fig. 6–25*D*). The filled resin is placed (Fig. 6–25*E*) and is shaped with a spatula (Fig. 6–25*F*). The light-cured material should be added in small increments to allow the light to penetrate the full depth of the added material.

Oxygen interferes with the free radical polymerization of the resins; thus, there usually is a surface layer of resin that is not completely polymerized. This should not be removed because the subsequent application of the filled resin makes this combination a chemical bond.

The restoration can be shaped with diamond burs in varying grades, or with 12-fluted carbide burs (Fig. 6–25*G*). The finishing is done with impregnated polishing discs operating at low speed, and progressing from a coarse to a medium and ultimately to a superfine grit (Fig. 6–25*H*).

A new series of restorative resin composites based upon particularly small filler particles has been available for only a short time. The advantage of these microfill or microfine resins (particle size approximately 0.04 μ) is that they can be polished to a very smooth surface. One of the problems with the traditional composites is the inability to polish them adequately. The smaller particle size in the microfill resin systems results in an increase in the resin content, and the final composite is somewhat weaker than the conventional composites. The decision as to which resin to use depends on the occlusal stress that the restoration will be subjected to.

Composite resins are particularly useful in restoring appearance and function to fractured teeth. They are also useful for masking esthetic deformities, such as enamel hypoplasia and dental abrasions (see Fig. 6–25),[19, 20, 60] as well as for altering deformed teeth or teeth with color abberations.

When a tooth is fractured to the extent that dentin is exposed, a new material (Scotch Bond, 3M Co.) that bonds directly to dentin can be used; etching with acid, which could compromise the underlying pulp, is not necessary. The surrounding enamel margin should be etched, since this increases the bond strength on the enamel and seals the margin. The bonding agents are mixed in equal quantities and are painted onto the prepared tooth structure. They are then air dried, and other layers are painted on as necessary. One of the BIS-GMA composites is then applied in the usual manner. Quite large fractures can be repaired with this system, which has eliminated the need to fabricate a cast metal cap[64, 65] in most instances.

With the resin systems now available, there is little need to place smooth or threaded pins[24, 66–68] into the dentin to increase the likelihood of retention (Fig. 6–26). In situations in which only part of the crown is missing and endodontic treatment has been done, a stainless steel post can be placed in the canal (Fig. 6–26*A* and *B*), then composite resin material acid-etched into the surrounding enamel is built up around the post to restore the normal tooth form (Fig. 6–26*C* and *D*). Fractures of teeth subjected to great occlusal stress should be restored with a full post, core, and crown system.

Cast Crown Restoration

In a fractured tooth in which most of the crown has broken off and the pulp is exposed, it is necessary to first perform endodontic treatment (page 88). Once the root is sealed, a cast metal restoration is placed to protect the remaining tooth structure and restore function. Given the occlusive force that large working dogs can generate on their canine teeth, these restorations must be meticulously prepared. Access to a well-equipped dental laboratory is essential. These techniques are successful (see Fig. 6–27),[65, 67] but probably are best left to personnel experienced in restorative dentistry.

After obturation of the root canal and

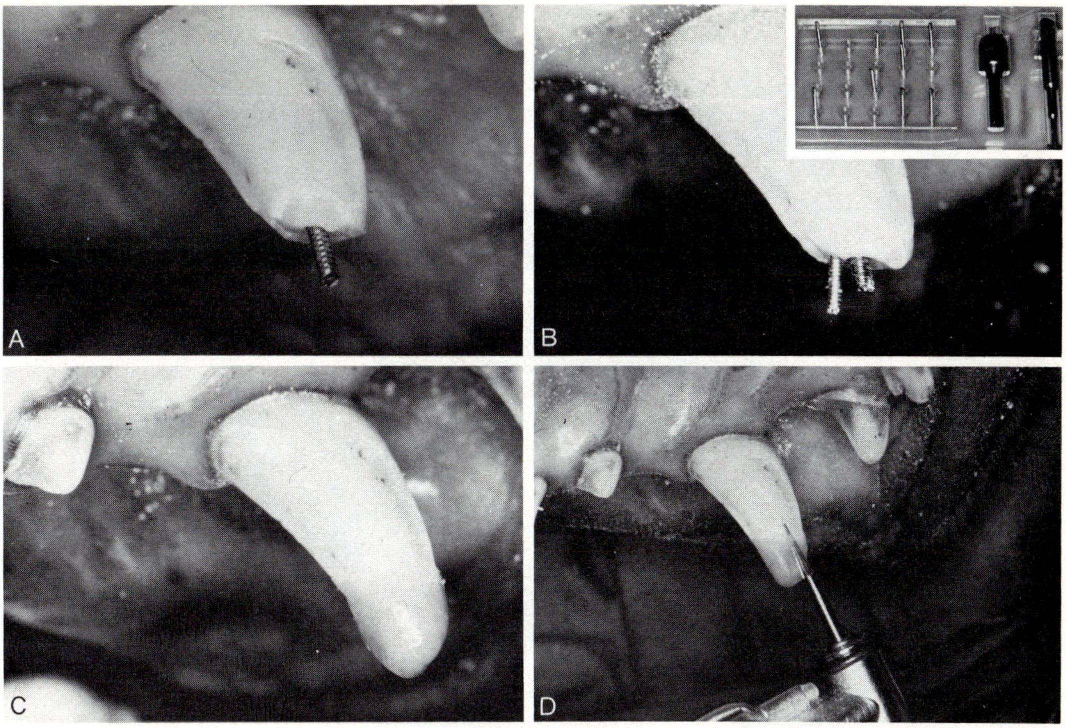

Figure 6–26. *A,* Threaded steel post inserted into a predrilled hole in a fractured crown of a canine tooth. *B,* A smaller, threaded pin is inserted to prevent rotation of the restoration. *Inset,* The Thread Mate system. Threaded pins, drill, and pin driver. *C,* Composite resin material has been layered over the pins. *D,* A dental bur is used to remove excess resin material.

setting of the root canal filler, about two thirds of the filling is removed. The canal is shaped with a dental bur to a smooth, parallel-sided or slightly tapered form to receive a post and core. This is necessary because there is often insufficient supragingival tooth structure remaining to retain a cast restoration. It also adds strength to the compromised tooth. Retention for the restoration is obtained from this post system to which a cast core is attached.

This type of restoration is somewhat difficult to implement in a dog because the root curves away from the crown; in humans, the post, core, and crown are for the most part in the same plane. In the dog, the cast metal post is placed into the root canal along its long axis, and the core is attached to the post at an angle of 100°. The system must be designed so that a crown placed over the core will prevent the displacement of the post and core from within the body of the root.

The internal surface of the root is smoothed into the desired shape, compromising the remaining dentin as little as possible. The prepared root canal must have no undercuts. The root face itself is prepared with a 2-mm × 3-mm antirotation notch in the dentin. The core will jut up at an angle of 100° to the post, and the crown will be cemented over the core and the remaining prepared root structure in such a way as to prevent displacement of the post and core horizontally.Two vertical grooves are placed in the buccal and lingual aspects of the remaining root structure so that the crown slides over the core and into the grooves. In a dog's incisor tooth, the root canal and crown lie essentially in the same plane and do not require these antidisplacement grooves.

A crown is cast in a dental laboratory from a model of the tooth. It is necesary to have an accurate impression of the tooth structure remaining in the mouth. There are many materials that can be used for the impression. We prefer one of the rubber base or polyether (polysulfide) materials. An impression tray is made by taking an alginate impression of the jaw and fabricating a model in stone. The acrylic tray for the impression material is then made on this model.

To make the impression, the two components of the material are mixed in equal

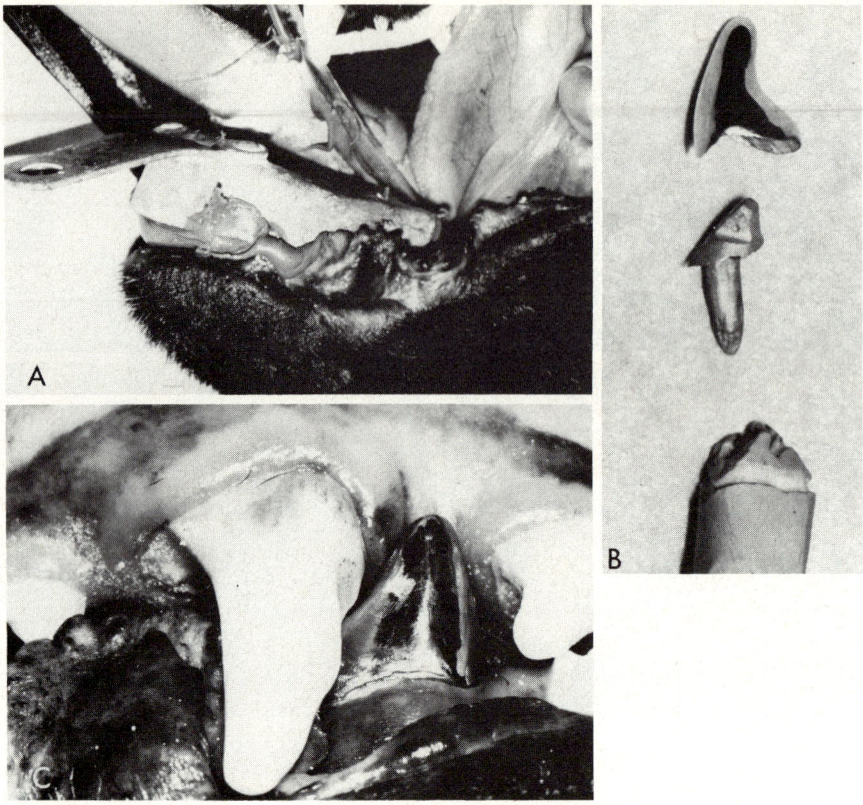

Figure 6–27. Cast crown restoration. *A*, Rubber-base impression material is used to form an impression of the tooth preparation. *B*, A metal post, core, and crown are fabricated from models trial-fitted onto a stone model. *C*, The post, core, and crown are cemented in place after a trial fitting in the mouth.

quantities and are introduced into the prepared root canal by means of a syringe. It is necessary to support the material within the canal with some form of metal or plastic bar that is notched, coated with adhesive, and placed into the canal following injection of the impression material. The rest of the impression material is placed in the tray, which is itself placed over the root stump and adjacent teeth (Fig. 6–27*A*).

After the material has set and the complete impression is removed from the mouth, it is checked for accuracy and the presence of the crown margin. This impression is poured into a die stone, and a wax pattern is developed and cast in metal. Many metals can be used; the strongest and least expensive is a nickel chromium alloy (Fig. 6–27*B*). The cast post and core is tried on the die, and a crown replicating the original is made to fit over the core. The length of the crown should be somewhat shorter than that of the original crown.

To obtain a normal occlusal relationship, it is necessary for the laboratory to closely duplicate the relative positions of the teeth in both jaws. It is difficult to take an occlusal registration of a dog and place it on an articulator as is done for humans. Instead, a self-curing acrylic is placed on the lateral aspects of the teeth, with the jaws in normal full occlusion. The result is sufficiently accurate as a duplication of the occlusion, and can be made for both sides to obtain a model of normal tooth height on the opposite, unfractured side. In order to observe occlusion, it may be necessary to remove the endotracheal tube for a short period or to intubate the animal via a pharyngostomy or tracheotomy incision, since with oral intubation it is impossible to completely shut the jaws.

The crown is cast in the steel alloy (Fig. 6–27*B*). The ceramometal can be coated with porcelain to duplicate the color of the animal's natural tooth; however this is not recommended for working dogs, since the shearing strength of porcelain is relatively low, and the potential for fracture following unsupervised occlusal trauma is high.

After the crown is fabricated, the animal is

reanesthetized, and the post and core are tried in the canal for size and fit, followed, in turn, by the crown. If everything fits, the occlusion is checked, and any interfering contacts are smoothed off.

The restoration is then cemented to the tooth to retain the restoration in place and prevent ingress of bacteria. The most commonly used cement for this purpose is zinc oxyphosphate, which is available as a powder and liquid that are mixed together. Recently a glass ionomer cement was developed that bonds to dentin and the oxidized surface of the cast metal restoration; it is an equally strong cementing medium with the added advantage that it constantly leeches out fluoride ions, preventing decay at the restorative interface.

It is essential that the cement be placed both in the canal and on the post and core. Cement placed only on the post results in loss of cementing medium as the post scrapes against the side of the canal during placement. There should also be a venting mechanism to provide for release of the cement and pressure caused by the plunger effect of the post; a groove is made that runs along the length of the post.

Once the post and core are in position and are locked by the antirotation wedge, the crown is cemented, is slipped over the core into the locks in the remaining root structure, and is held in place for 5 minutes. Excess cement is removed with a scaler or curette (Fig. 6–27*C*). Dry food and chewing on hard surfaces should be avoided if possible for 48 hours.

Cements and Bases

A cement base is designed to induce changes in the underlying pulpal tissue and minimize inflammatory activity in a vital tooth. It is also useful as an effective thermal insulating medium. The strength of the base must be sufficient to withstand the placement of the overlying composite or amalgam. With amalgam, in particular, the condensing activity may fracture the base; it is useful to have a zinc oxide–eugenol base material when using amalgam, since the eugenol also acts as a sedative to the pulp.

In composite systems, eugenol retards the setting process and is therefore contraindicated. In such cases, a base of calcium hydroxide is placed beneath the resin material. This also serves to isolate the dentin from the acid during the etching process.

The most commonly used dental cements are zinc oxyphosphate, glass ionomer, and Resis systems. Zinc oxyphosphate is useful if there is sufficient dentin between the cementing medium and the underlying pulp. It also works well when endodontic therapy has been performed, because there is no risk of developing pulpal inflammation associated with the acidic activity of the cement.

The newer cements, which are aluminum silicate polyacrylic materials, are of value in that they appear to bond to tooth structure by physico-chemical and ionic activity.

TEETH EXTRACTION

Teeth require extraction for many reasons; however, the technique used is generally the same. The tooth is loosened with a root elevator before extraction forceps are placed or wedge leverage is applied. Particularly in small dogs, or in cats, in whom the jaw can be fractured by excessive use of force, the fingers and the palm of the hand are used to provide as much support to the jaw as possible in order to limit the force applied to any one point on the jaw (Fig. 6–28). Teeth with a considerable amount of root exposure will often still be firmly adherent to the jaw; this is particulary true of canine and carnassial teeth. The narrow teeth of cats are prone to fracture during extraction; the use of a

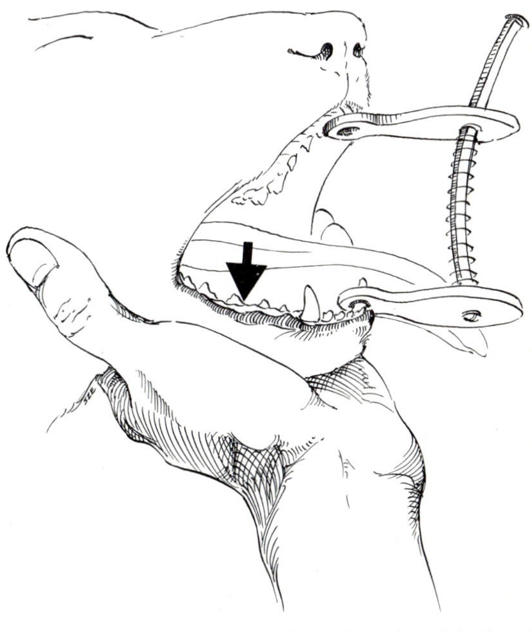

Figure 6–28. Tooth extraction. The palm of the hand is used to distribute the pressure created by the root elevator *(arrow)* to reduce the risk of jaw fracture.

narrow-pointed scalpel blade to sever the periodontal fibers has been suggested.[37]

Single-root teeth (in the dog, the incisors, the canines, the first premolars in both jaws, and the second and third lower molar teeth; in the cat, the canines, and the upper first premolar and molar teeth) are removed by inserting the root elevator between the gingival margin and the crown or exposed root. Pressure is applied while rotating the elevator through a small arc (Fig. 6–29*A*, and *B*). The instrument should be kept at a 30° to 45° angle to the long axis of the root to avoid allowing it to slip off and injure the gingiva. A finger is kept extended along the blade of the elevator to act as a stop if the instrument slips. Considerable force is necessary to break down the periodontal ligament. The root elevator is used against all available surfaces of the root until it begins to loosen. At that point, the tooth is grasped with an extraction forceps (Fig. 6–29*C*) and is removed by rotating the forceps while pulling. If the tooth resists pulling, it can be further loosened by rapidly pushing it into and pulling it out of the socket while twisting.

The canine teeth have massive roots (see Fig. 2–4, page 15). In large dogs, it is often quicker and less traumatic to incise and reflect the gingiva on the lateral surface of the tooth (Fig. 6–30*A* and *B*), then resect the alveolar bone overlying the root with a bone chisel or orthopedic or dental bur (Fig. 6–30*C*). The root is loosened with a root elevator (Fig. 6–30*D*), allowing the tooth to be pulled with an extraction forceps (Fig. 6–30*E*). The gingival flaps are sutured with simple interrupted absorbable sutures (Fig. 6–30*F*). An alternative technique is to incise the gingiva away from the bone to be removed when creating the mucoperiosteal flap, so that following extraction the suture line is not located over the space left by the resected bone.[69, 70] In narrow-nosed dogs with extensive periodontal disease, in whom the risk of creating an oronasal fistula following

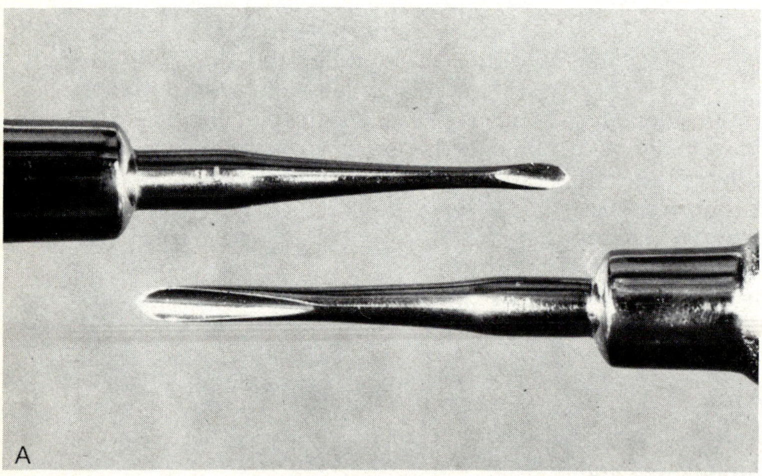

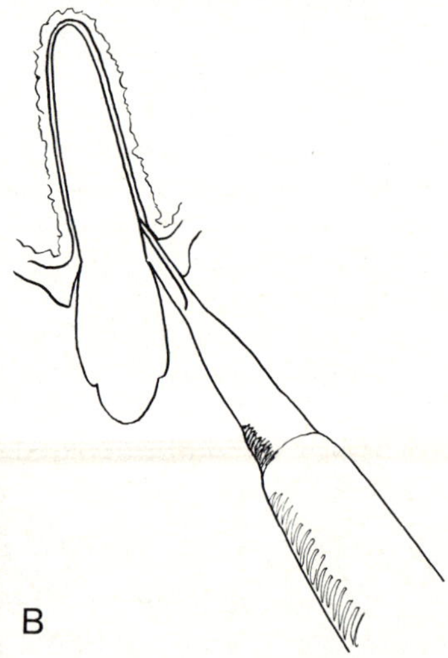

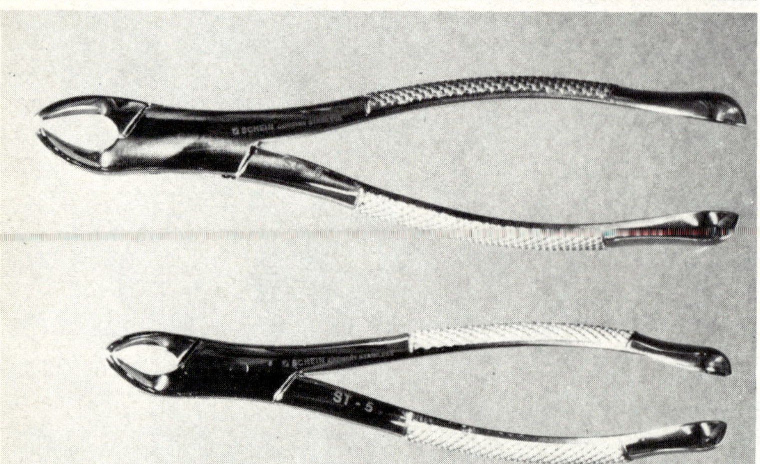

Figure 6–29. Extraction of an incisor tooth. *A*, Root elevators. *B*, The root elevator is rotated over a small arc while being pushed firmly against the tooth-bone junction. *C*, Extraction forceps.

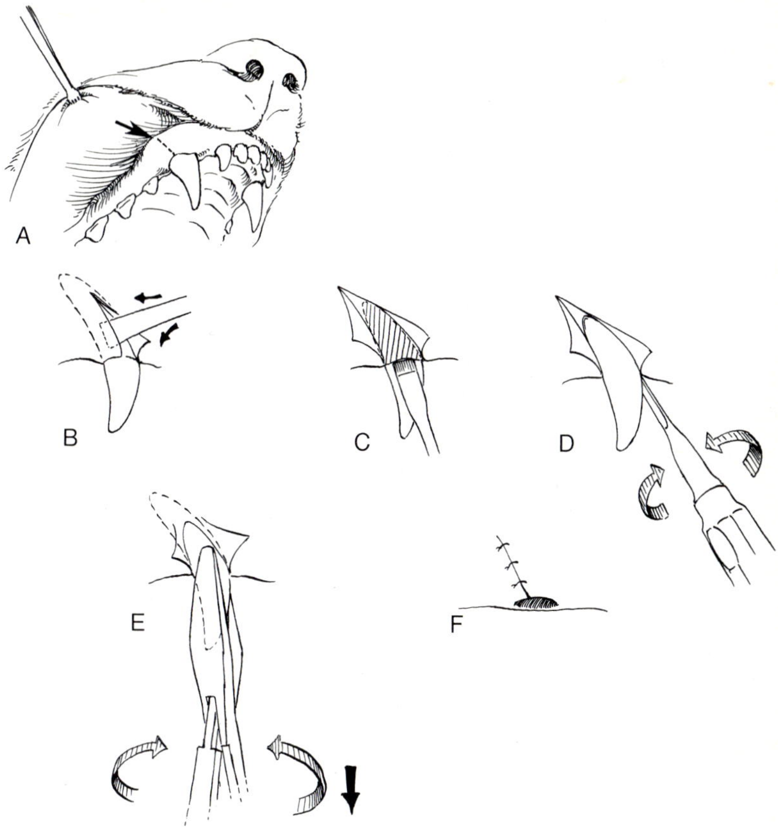

Figure 6–30. Extraction of a canine tooth. *A*, Gingival incision over the root *(arrow)*. *B*, The gingival tissue is reflected. *C*, The lateral alveolar bone is removed. *D*, The tooth is loosened with the root elevator. *E*, Extraction forceps deliver the tooth. *F*, The gingival incision is closed.

canine tooth extraction is greatest, particular care is taken to avoid damaging the bone medial to the root. When using forceps, the crown should not be levered laterally, since this pushes the root medially into the nasal cavity.

Two-root teeth (in the dog, the second and third upper premolar, the second, third, and fourth lower premolars, and the first and second lower molars; in the cat, the second and third upper premolars, the first and second lower premolars, and the first lower molar) can be removed in similar fashion, or the tooth can be separated into single-root sections by sawing or fracturing the crown into two pieces. Each piece is then taken out as a separate one-root tooth.

The three-root tooth that is most frequently extracted is the upper fourth premolar (carnassial) tooth. This tooth has roots second only to the canine tooth in size (see Fig. 2–4, page 15). It can be removed intact by using the root elevator to free as much of the periodontal attachment as can be reached, including making a passage through the furcation between the roots. The root elevator is then passed through the channel between the roots and is rotated, forcing the angled handle of the instrument into the furcation as a wedge, thus forcing the intact tooth from its sockets (Fig. 6–31).[71] An alternative method is to saw or fracture the tooth into two or three sections, using a tooth cutter, hack saw, wire saw, or dental cutting disc (Figure 6–32*A* and *B*),[72, 73] and to remove each root separately (Figure 6–32 *C* and *D*). This technique works most conveniently if the entire crown is removed, because each root is then exposed, allowing accurate placement of the root elevator. When working on the upper carnassial and first molar teeth, the elevator should be kept under firm control to prevent the instrument from dislodging and slipping into the facial tissues or the orbit.

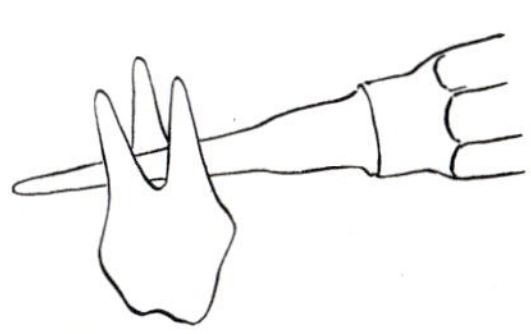

Figure 6–31. Tooth extraction. Using the neck of the root elevator as a wedge between the roots (furcation area) of a multirooted tooth.

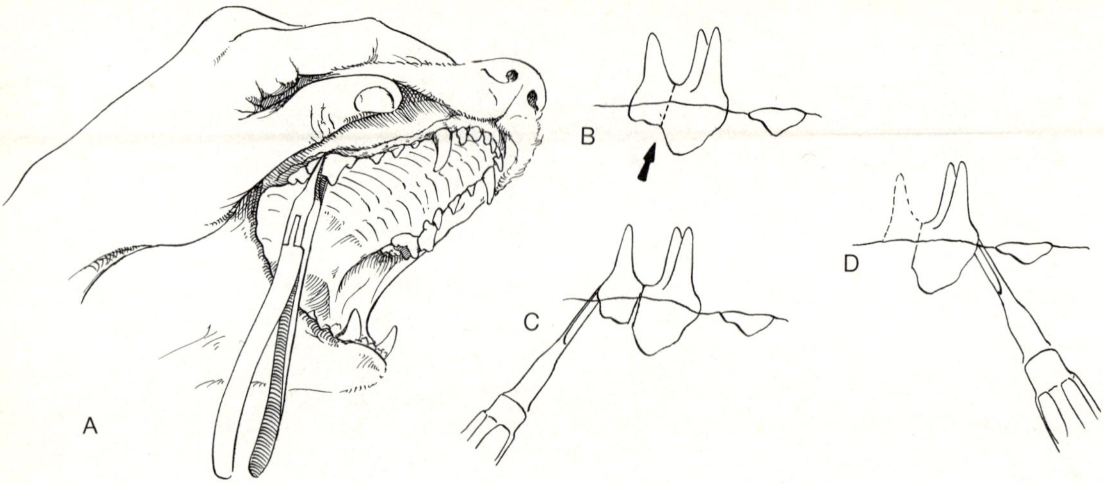

Figure 6–32. Carnassial tooth extraction. *A* and *B*, The tooth is cut or sawn into one- and two-root sections. *C* and *D*, The separated sections are removed in turn. (Figure 6–31 shows an alternative technique.)

With any tooth, an effort should be made to search for fractured root fragments if the roots do not come out intact; these fragments can be loosened with a root tip pick (Fig. 6–33).

Following extraction, the alveolus is left empty. If hemorrhage does not stop within a minute of completing removal of the tooth, a piece of gauze sponge can be inserted into the alveolus; the sponge will fall out 1 or 2 days later.

Extraction of deciduous teeth is usually easy, since the roots are shorter and narrower than those of the equivalent permanent teeth (Fig. 6–34). Care is taken so that the root elevator does not penetrate into the area of the erupting permanent teeth, since this may disturb their normal development. Removal of the entire tooth is not necessary; the crown can be snapped off with an extraction forceps,[12] avoiding the need for anesthesia in some dogs.

A gas-driven oscillating forceps can be used to remove teeth in dogs, requiring less time and causing less alveolar bone trauma than standard techniques.[74]

Most dogs and cats tolerate extraction of teeth very well: sedation may be necessary during the recovery stage from anesthesia, but most animals start eating without pain the next day. New bone fills the empty socket in 21 to 28 days in dogs; packing the socket with gauze delays healing considerably.[75]

Complications of tooth extraction include the following;

1. *Hemorrhage,* which could be severe in animals with chronic kidney disease or with undetected clotting abnormalities. Some bleeding often continues for 1 or 2 days following extraction; the owner should be warned to expect some blood mixed with water in the animal's water bowl.

2. *Fracture of the mandible,* particularly in old, small-breed dogs. This condition should be prevented by careful extraction technique,

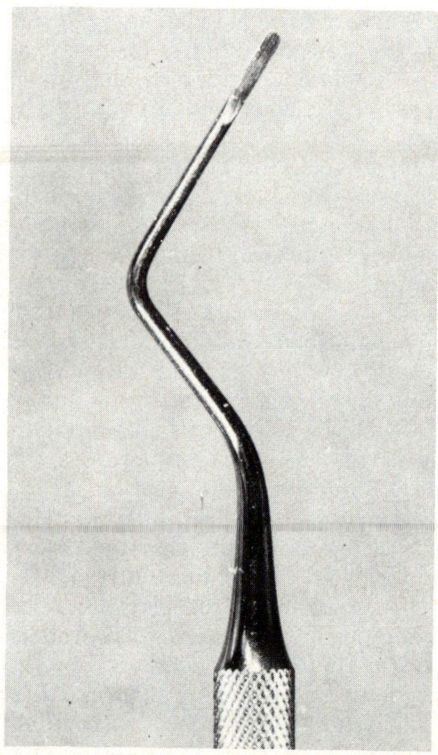

Figure 6–33. Root tip pick for freeing root fragments.

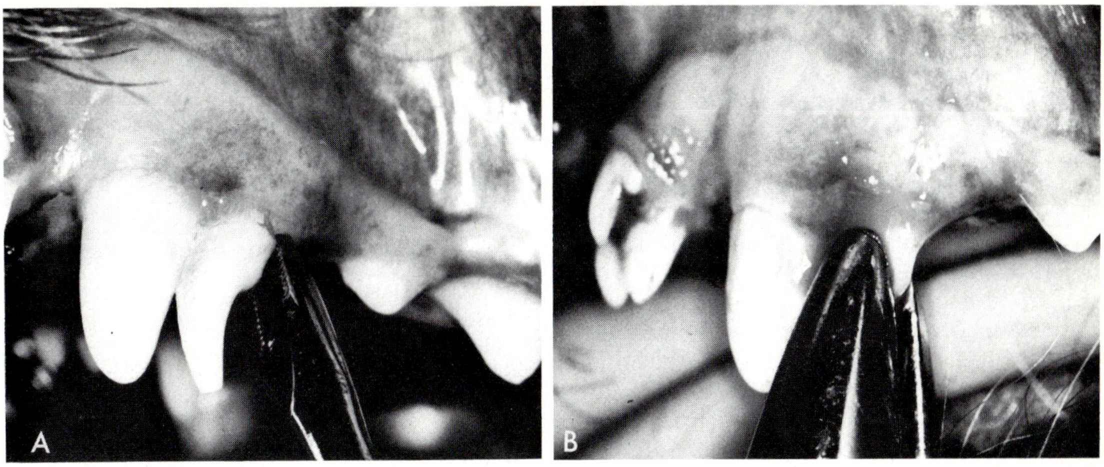

Figure 6–34. Extraction of retained deciduous canine tooth. *A*, The tooth is loosened with a root elevator. *B*, The tooth is removed with an extraction forceps.

because dogs with the highest risk of fracture of the jaw during tooth extraction are also those with the least desirable features for fracture healing. Repair of mandibular fractures is described in Chapter 9, page 142.

3. *Retention of part of a root that was fractured during extraction.* This may cause no obvious abnormality, or it may lead to a root abscess with subsequent fistula formation (Fig. 6–35*A*). Treatment of a diseased retained root is by radiographic location of the root and extraction (Figure 6–35*B–D*), which may

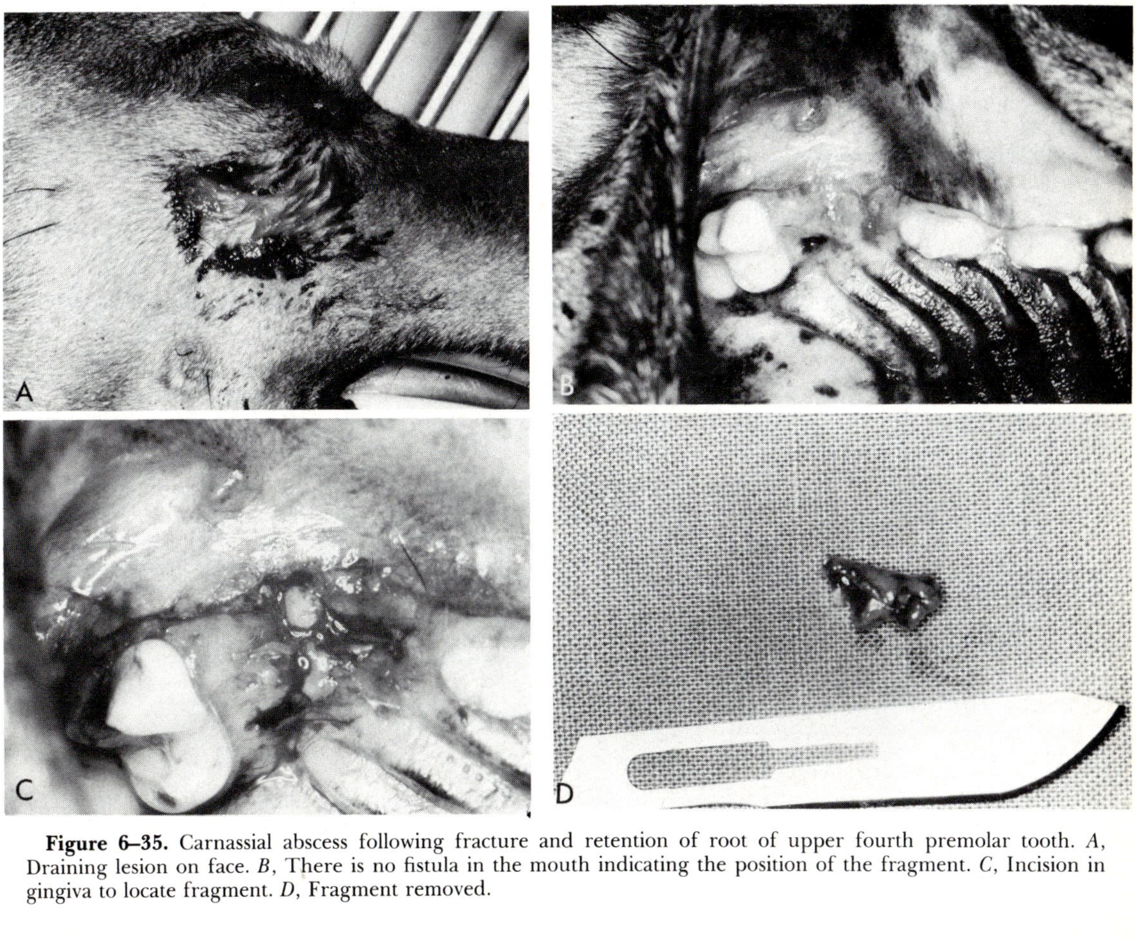

Figure 6–35. Carnassial abscess following fracture and retention of root of upper fourth premolar tooth. *A*, Draining lesion on face. *B*, There is no fistula in the mouth indicating the position of the fragment. *C*, Incision in gingiva to locate fragment. *D*, Fragment removed.

require surgical removal of overlying bone.[76] Isolated normal vital roots that are below the level of surrounding bone will be covered by bone and gingiva following healing.[77]

4. *Necrosis of bone* around the extraction site occurs occasionally (see Fig. 10–25, page 171). The socket does not heal, fills with food, and becomes an area of potent bacterial activity. Osteomyelitis may spread from the original site, though this is rare. Conservative treatment is unlikely to be effective. Surgical treatment consists of removal of the affected bone with a rongeur until healthy bleeding bone is reached (see Fig. 10–25*B*). The surgical site is left uncovered. With well-established osteomyelitis, oral tetracycline therapy (20 mg/kg TID for a minimum of 4 weeks) is recommended.

5. *Oronasal fistula.* Extraction of the upper canine teeth, and occasionally of other upper jaw teeth, can result in loss of alveolar bone. The nasal and oral epithelia heal together to form a permanent fistula. This is particularly common in narrow-nosed, small dogs with extensive periodontal disease. Treatment consists of closure of the fistula by creating a flap of buccal epithelium. The buccal flap can be created and sutured in place at the time of extraction if the opening into the nasal cavity is large, or the tissues can be allowed to heal, and any remaining fistulous opening is repaired 2 weeks or more later. Buccal flap surgery for closure of an oronasal fistula is described in Chapter 10, page 167.

6. *Functional abnormalities* following extraction of teeth are rare, even if all the teeth are removed. Both dogs and cats adapt well and learn to prehend food of varying consistency with the tongue. The owner should provide several types of food to see which the animal can manage best. If both mandibular canine teeth are removed, the tongue may hang out of the mouth on one side when relaxed.

References

1. Golden AM, Stoller NH, Harvey CE: Survey of oral and dental disease in dogs anesthetized at a veterinary hospital. *J Am Anim Hosp Assoc* 18:801–800, 1982.
2. Arnall L: Some aspects of dental development in the dog. III Some common variations in their dentition. *J Small Animal Pract* 2:195–201, 1961.
3. Andrews AH: A case of partial anodontia in a dog. *Vet Rec* 90:144–145, 1972.
4. Bodingbauer J: Hochgradige zahnunterzahl (aplasie) beim hunde. *Wein Tierarzt Monaschr* 61:301–303, 1974.
5. Skrentary TT: Preliminary study of the inheritance of missing teeth in thė dog. *Wien Tierarzt Monaschr* 51:231–245, 1964.
6. Elzay RP, Hughes RD: Anodontia in a cat. *J Am Vet Med Assoc* 154:667–670, 1969.
7. Kratochvil Z: Oligodontia and pseudoligodontia in the domestic cat. *Acta Vet Brno* 44:291–296, 1975.
8. Colyer F: Variations and Diseases of the Teeth in Animals. London, John Bale, 1936.
9. Bodingbauer J: Milchzahnpersistenz beim hund. *Kleinter Prax* 23:339–334, 1978.
10. Bell AF: Dental disease in the dog. *J Small Anim Pract* 6:421–428, 1965.
11. Wisdorf H, Hermanns W: Persistierende milchhakenzahne im oberkiefer einer hauskatze. *Kleinter Prax* 19:14–16, 1974.
12. Whitney GD: Removal of retained deciduous teeth in dogs. *Mod Vet Pract* 54:46, 1973.
13. Bodingbauer J: Retention of teeth in dogs as a sequel to distemper infection. *Vet Rec* 72:636–638, 1960.
14. Christensen HC, Morgan SD: What is your diagnosis? *J Am Vet Med Assoc* 176:649–650, 1980.
15. Field EA, Speechley JA, Jones DE: The removal of an impacted maxillary canine and associated dentigerous cyst in a Chow. *J Small Anim Pract* 23:159–163, 1982.
16. Ross DL: Veterinary dentistry. *In* Ettinger SJ: Textbook of Veterinary Internal Medicine, 2nd ed. WB Saunders Co., 1983.
17. Schneck GW: A case of enamel pearls in a dog. *Vet Rec* 92:115–117, 1973.
18. Dubielzig RR: The effect of canine distemper virus on the ameloblastic layer of the developing tooth. *Vet Pathol* 16:268–270, 1979.
19. Bedford PGC, Heaton MG: A repair technique for dental abrasion in the dog. *Vet Rec* 101:327, 1977.
20. Marvich JM: Repair of enamel hypoplasia in the dog. *Vet Med Small Anim Clin* 70:697–699, 1975.
21. Bennett IC, Law DB: Incorporation of tetracycline into developing dog enamel and dentin. *J Dent Res* 44:780–793, 1965.
22. Eisenmenger E: Konservierende behandlung von zahnfrakturen des hundes. *Wien Tierarzt Monaschr* 58:30–40, 1970.
23. Sveen OB, Hawes RR: Differentiation of new odontoblasts and dentin bridge formation in rat molar teeth after tooth grinding. *Arch Oral Biol* 13:1399–1412, 1968.
24. Bender IB, Freedland JB: Clinical considerations in the diagnosis and treatment of intra-alveolar root fractures. *J Am Dent Assoc* 107:595–600, 1983.
25. Klein H: Schienung einer caninus langsfraktur beimn hund. *Kleinter Prax* 24:144, 1979.
26. Sherman P: Intentional replantation of teeth in dogs and monkeys. *J Dent Res* 47:1066–1071, 1968.
27. Andreason JO: Relationship between surface and inflammatory resorption and changes in the pulp after replantation of permanent incisors in monkeys. *J Endodont* 7:294–301, 1981.
28. Kaplan B: Root resorption of the permanent teeth of a dog. *J Am Vet Med Assoc* 151:708—709, 1967.
29. Schneck G, Osborn JW: Neck lesions in the teeth of cats. *Vet Rec* 99:100, 1976.
30. Gardner AF, Darke BH, Keary GT: Dental caries in domesticated dogs. *J Am Vet Med Assoc* 140:433–436, 1962.
31. Schneck GW: Caries in the dog. *J Am Vet Med Assoc* 150:1142–1143, 1969.
32. Lewis TM: Resistance of dogs to dental caries; a two year study. *J Dent Res* 44:1254–1257, 1965.

33. Teague HD, Toombs JP: Infraocular fistula secondary to an upper canine tooth abscess. *Feline Pract* 9:32–33, 1979.
34. Holmberg DL: Abscessation of the mandibular carnassial tooth in the dog. *J Am Anim Hosp Assoc* 15:347–350, 1979.
35. Neuman NB: Chronic ocular discharge associated with a carnassial tooth abscess. *Can Vet J* 15:128, 1974.
36. Wright JG: Some observations on dental disease in the dog. *Vet Rec* 51:409–422, 1939.
37. Lane JG: Small animal dentistry. *In Pract* 3:23–30, 1981.
38. Franceschini G: Traitement des fistulaires dentaires chez le chien par obturation des canaux. *Rec Med Vet* 150:675–685, 1974.
39. Bender IB, Seltzer S: Roentgenographic and direct observation of experimental lesions in bone, Parts I and II. *J Am Dent Assoc* 62:152–160, 708–716, 1961.
40. Rossman LE, Rossman SR, Garber DA: The endodontic periodontic fistula. *Oral Surg Oral Med Oral Pathol* 53:78–81, 1982.
41. Sundquist G: Bacteriological studies of necrotic dental pulps. Odontol Diss 7, Univ Umea, Sweden 1976.
42. Bergenholtz G, Lekholm U, Liljenberg B, Lindhe J: Morphometric analysis of chronic inflammatory periapical lesions in root filled teeth. *Oral Surg* 55:295–301, 1983.
43. Seltzer S, Bender IB: The Dental Pulp. Philadelphia, J. B. Lippincott Co., 1975, pp. 162–178.
44. Kostlin R, Schebitz H: Zur endodontischen behandlung der zahnfraktur beim hund. *Kleinter Prax* 25:187–196, 1980.
45. Cvek M: Clinical procedures promoting apical closure and arrest of external root resorption in nonvital permanent incisors. Fifth International Conference on Endodontics. Philadelphia, University of Pennsylvania, 1973, pp. 30–41.
46. Tronstad L, Anreasen J, Hasselgren G, Kristerson L, Piis I: pH changes in dental tissues after root canal filling with calcium hydroxide. *J Endodont* 7:17–21, 1981.
47. Tholen MA: Concepts of Veterinary Dentistry. Edwardsville, Kansas, Veterinary Medicine Pub. Co., 1983.
48. Colmery B: Presentation at Eastern States Veterinarian Association Meeting, 1984.
49. Davis MS, Joseph SU, Bucher JF: Periapical and intracanal healing following incomplete root canal fillings in dogs. *Oral Surg* 31:667–675, 1971.
50. Bhaskar SN, Rappaport HM: Histologic evaluation of endodontic procedures in dogs. *Oral Surg* 31:526–535, 1971.
51. Ross DL, Myers JW: Endodontic therapy for canine teeth in the dog. *J Am Vet Met Assoc* 157:1713–1718, 1970.
52. Bellizzi R: Veterinary endodontics. *J Am Vet Med Assoc* 180:6, 1981.
53. Bellizi R, Worsing J, Woody RD, Keller DL, Drobotij E: Nonsurgical endodontic therapy, utilizing lingual coronal access on the mandibular canine tooth of dogs. *J Am Vet Med Assoc* 179:370–374, 1981.
54. Ross DL: Canine endodontic therapy. *J Am Vet Med Assoc* 180:356–357, 1981.
55. Tholen M: Veterinary endodontics. *J Am Vet Med Assoc* 180:4–6, 1981.
56. Bigler B: Experimentelle und klinische untersuchung zur frage der endodontischen therapie des hundegebisses. *Zbl Vet Med* 25:794–813, 1978.
57. Lawer DR: Root canal with retrograde amalgam filling. *Calif Vet* 33:11–15, 1979.
58. Goldstein RE: Esthetics in Dentistry. Philadelphia, JB Lippincott Co., 1976.
59. Phillips RW: Dental materials. *Dent Clin North Am* 27:643–830, 1983.
60. Moffa JP: Physical and mechanical properties of gold and cast metal alloys; alternatives to gold in dentistry. *Dept Health Educ Welfare Pub.* NIH 77–1227, 1977.
61. McLean JW: The Science and Art of Dental Ceramics, Vol 1. Nature of dental ceramics and their clinical use. Chicago, Quintessence Pub. Co., 1979.
62. Winkler S: Resins in dentistry. *Dent Clin North Am* 19:211–427, 1975.
63. Ashton AP, Howard D: Repair technique for dental abrasion in the dog. *Vet Rec* 101:372, 1977.
64. Jirava E, Krepleka V, Fagos Z: Uber die behandlung von frakturierten zahnen bei hunden. *Berl Munch Tierartz Woch* 12:235–237, 1966.
65. Scheffler VKH: Restitution des dens caninus beim diensthund. *Much Vet Med* 34:504–507, 1979.
66. Dorn AS: Crown restoration of canine teeth with composite bonding. Annual Meeting of American College Veterinary Surgeons, 1983.
67. Klein H: Vergleich verschiedener uber kronungstechniken am kunstlich frakturierten caninus des hundes. Diss Tierartz Hochscule Hannover 1–88, 1979.
68. Zetner K: Die prosthetische versorgung von zahnfrankturen mit adhesivkunstoffen. *Kleinter Prax* 21:271–277, 1976.
69. Boulton J: Dental flap operation for tooth extraction. *Can Vet J* 1:167–169, 1960.
70. Richman S, Schunick W: Flap operation for removal of the canine tooth. *In* La Croix JV, Hoskins HP (eds.): Canine Surgery. Evanston, North Am Vet, pp. 46–48, 1939.
71. Peddie JF: Extraction of a dog's carnassial tooth. *Mod Vet Pract* 62:129–131, 1981.
72. Currey JR: Canine exodontia. Proc Ann Meet Am Vet Med Assoc, pp. 178–180, 1963.
73. Jones RS, Thordal-Christensen A: Extraction of the upper carnassial tooth in the dog. *Mod Vet Pract* 43:68, 1962.
74. Mumaw ED, Miller AS: The application of a frequency oscillation method for tooth extraction in dogs. *Lab Anim Sci* 25:228–231, 1975.
75. Huebsch RF, Hansen LS: A histopathologic study of extraction wounds in dogs. *Oral Surg Oral Med Oral Pathol* 28:187–196, 1969.
76. Blogg R: Exodontia in the dog. *Aust Vet J* 39:57–61, 1963.
77. Plata RL, Kelln EE: Intentional retention of vital submerged roots in dogs. *Oral Surg Oral Med Oral Pathol* 42:100–108, 1976.
78. Hamp SE, Olsson SE, Farso-Madsen K, Viklands P, Fornell J: A macroscopic and radiologic investigation of dental diseases in the dog. *Vet Radiol* 25:86–92, 1984.
79. Reichart PA, Durr UM, Triadan H, Vickendey G: Periodontal disease in the domestic cat. *J Periodont Res* 19:67–75, 1984.

Chapter Seven

Diseases of the Jaws and Abnormal Occlusion

JP Weigel and AS Dorn

OCCLUSIVE PATTERNS

Normal occlusive patterns are described in Chapter Two. Most abnormal occlusal patterns can be classified in two general categories. The first category consists of the condition in which there is a long mandible and a short maxilla, which is referred to as prognathism or "undershot jaw" (Fig. 7–1). The brachycephalic breeds, such as the Boston terrier, English bulldog, and pug, show this pattern as a "normal" anatomical feature. As a result of this abnormality, these breeds develop overcrowding of teeth and early periodontal disease.

The second category of abnormal occlusion is characterized by a short mandible and a long maxilla and is referred to as brachygnathia or "overshot jaw" (Fig. 7–2). This anomalous occlusion is not "normal" in any breed, but it has been seen in a variety of dogs. It has been reported as having an autosomal recessive mode of inheritance in long-haired dachshunds.[1] In this condition growth of the rostral portion of the mandible is retarded. The resultant "overshot" pattern accentuates the occlusive problem by allowing the length of the maxilla to grow unrestricted. Other recognized occlusive patterns include anterior crossbite, wry jaw, level bite, lingually displaced canine teeth, and retained deciduous teeth.

Prognathism

The determination of prognathism is derived from the position of the lower canine and premolar teeth. In the prognathic pat-

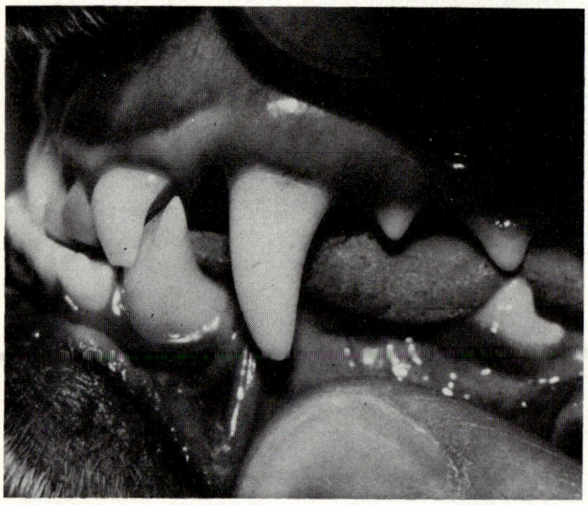

Figure 7–1. Prognathic occlusion. The lower canine tooth is wearing against the upper lateral incisor tooth. The lower incisor teeth are rostral to the upper incisor teeth.

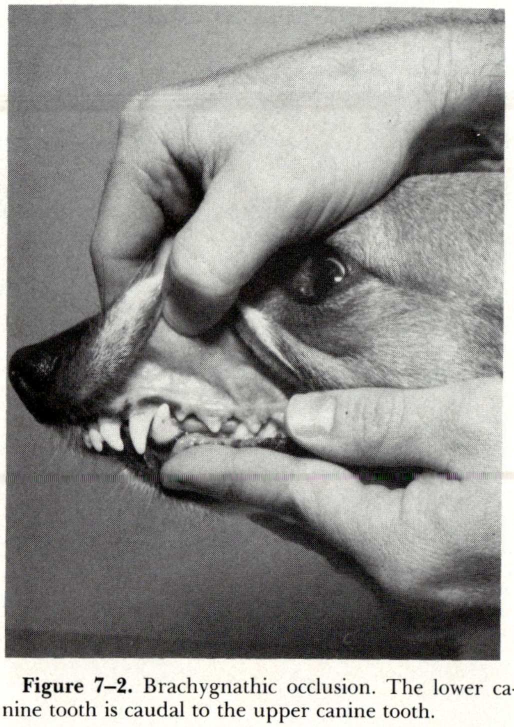

Figure 7–2. Brachygnathic occlusion. The lower canine tooth is caudal to the upper canine tooth.

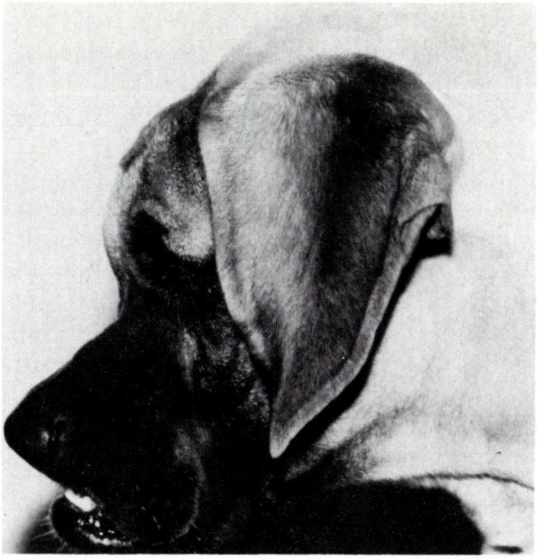

Figure 7–3. This adult Great Dane suffered severe bite injuries to the maxillary and nasal region, resulting in severe retardation of maxillary growth and prognathic occlusion.

tern, these teeth are rostral to their normal position in relation to the maxillary dentition. This condition is often very obvious, with gross disparity of jaw length.

The causes of prognathism are not clearly understood. Hereditary factors are important in many cases, but the modes of inheritance are unknown. The development of proper occlusion is complex, and it is dependent on multiple factors. In the brachycephalic breeds, the prognathic deformity results from an inherited defect in development of the bones in the base of the skull. The length of the mandible is determined by a set of genetic factors that are different from those affecting skull development.[2] Tooth position and the resulting dental interlock also affect occlusive patterns. Some of these factors are not inherited defects, but are caused by trauma[3] (Fig. 7–3). All genetic and environmental factors interplay to produce the phenotype.

Dental interlock is important in guiding the longitudinal growth of the maxilla and mandible, particularly when animals are 3 to 9 months of age. The most significant teeth involved are the canines and incisors. Because of the conical shape of the teeth, slight alterations in tooth position can quickly affect how the mandibular and maxillary dentitions interlock. The loss of dental interlock, or the presence of abnormal interlock, results in a worsening of tooth position, which affects the development of the rest of the arcade. Poor tooth position and an abnormal interlock result in a loss of the forces required to maintain correct jaw length. Developmental defects or trauma can cause slight tooth malposition, initiating a cascade of events that result in malocclusion.[4]

Two types of prognathism are seen. The first type occurs early in life and is evident before the permanent dentition appears. The second type of prognathism occurs in immature dogs after the permanent teeth have erupted. It has been suggested that extracting the lower deciduous canine and incisor teeth at a very young age will correct the early onset of prognathism, the theory being that the caudal position of these teeth in relation to the position of the corresponding upper teeth blocks the normal rostral growth of the mandible. Extraction should be performed by the time the animal is 6 to 8 weeks of age. If a puppy's occlusion corrects itself after extraction of the deciduous teeth, one can be reasonably assured that the defect was not inherited. However, if no improvement occurs, breeding of the affected animal should be discouraged.[5]

Extracting deciduous teeth can be difficult because the roots of these teeth are thin and very long. The roots should be removed intact when possible; however, if breakage occurs, it is not advisable to explore for the root remnants. Exploration of the deciduous alveolar pocket risks damaging the developing permanent tooth bud. Extraction techniques are described in Chapter Six.

Dental interlock is not a causal factor in the second type of prognathism, since it appears after the eruption of the permanent teeth. Once the malocclusion is present, the interlock is lost, and the prognathism is worsened because of the altered occlusal forces.[4] This type of prognathism appears when the animal is around 8 to 10 months of age, and there is no known breed susceptibility for this rare anomaly (Fig. 7–4). It has been stated that this form of prognathism is genetic.[3]

Other Forms of Prognathism

Displaced Canine Teeth. The diagnosis of prognathism is based on the canine and premolar occlusion. One form of prognathism with a normal incisal relationship is characterized by a slightly longer mandible. In this condition the lower canine comes in contact with the upper lateral incisor. In addition, the lower fourth premolar crown tip comes in contact with the upper third premolar. Level bite is a more severe expression of this

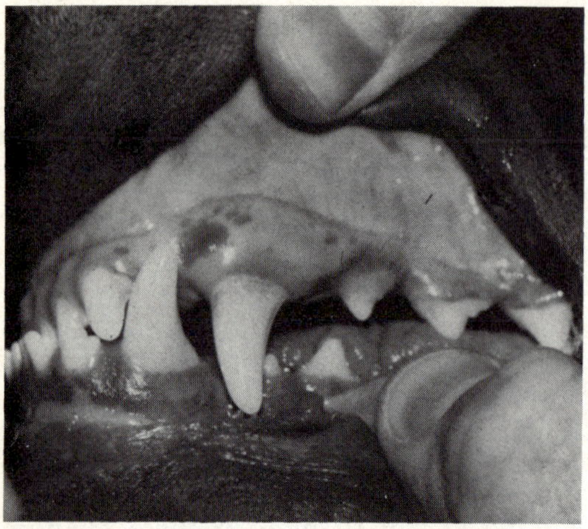

Figure 7–4. Prognathic occlusion that developed in a Weimaraner after eruption of permanent teeth.

form of malocclusion, in that the crown tips of the lower incisors are in direct contact with the tips of the upper incisors. Another subtle form of prognathism is that in which the crown tips of the upper and lower premolar teeth do not intersect in the same horizontal plane. The slightly long mandible bows ventrally, thus allowing proper canine occlusion[3] (Fig. 7–5).

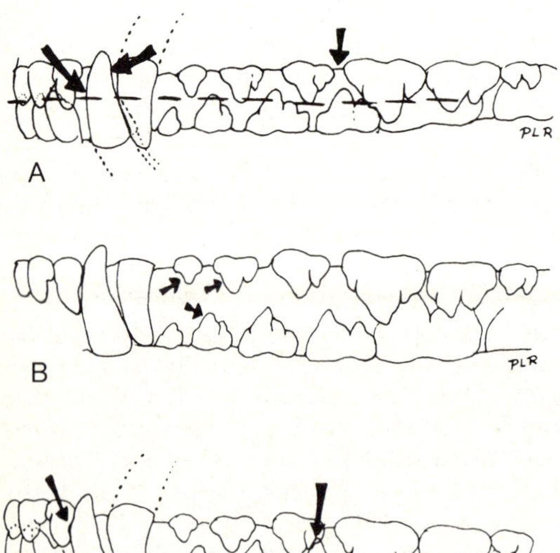

Figure 7–5. *A*, Normal occlusion in the dog. Note the relationships of the lower canine and the fourth premolar with the upper arch and the occlusal plane formed by the cusp tips (*arrows*). *B*, Prognathism evidenced by a ventral deviation of the mandible, creating space between the premolar cusp tips *(arrows)*. *C*, A slight degree of prognathism, with the lower canine resting on the distal surface of the upper lateral incisor and the face along with a shift of the lower fourth premolar *(arrows)*. Incisal relationships are unreliable guides for evaluation of jaw structure. (From Ross DL: Occlusion in the Dog. *Southwestern Vet* 28:249, 1975.)

Wry Mouth

An abnormal occlusal pattern in which one side of the mandible is longer than the other is called wry mouth. This condition is considered to be an inherited defect. When the primary defect is in the maxilla, the mandible is secondarily involved because of the influence of dental interlock, in which case the occlusion of the rostral teeth is normal. When the primary defect is in the mandible there is malocclusion of the rostral teeth.[3]

Anterior Crossbite

When there is a rostral displacement of the lower incisors the condition is called anterior crossbite. The rest of the dentition is normal. This is not considered to be a true prognathism and is not usually thought to be genetic. The condition is apparent in 4 to 7 month old puppies. Orthodontic manipulation, as discussed later in this chapter, has been reasonably successful in the management of this problem.

CORRECTION OF OCCLUSIVE ABNORMALITIES

Treatment of malocclusion in the dog and cat is neither sophisticated nor common in veterinary dentistry. No inherited defect should be corrected in dogs shown for conformation or in dogs used for breeding. However, when malocclusion is severe, treatment would be helpful in preventing or helping secondary problems, such as heavy dental calculus accumulation, early periodontal disease and subsequent loss of teeth, abnormal wear, and severe halitosis.

Orthodontic techniques are discussed further on. Corrective osteotomies and major facial reconstruction in the dog are mostly experimental at this time, though they can be used with success to correct malocclusion.[6] Experimental osteotomies on the mandible and maxilla in the dog show that both can be lengthened by up to 1 cm (Fig. 7–6).[6–8] The mandibular alveolar nerve can be stretched to accommodate this increased length without loss of function; it also can be accommodated within a surgically shortened mandible.[9] It is helpful in these lengthening

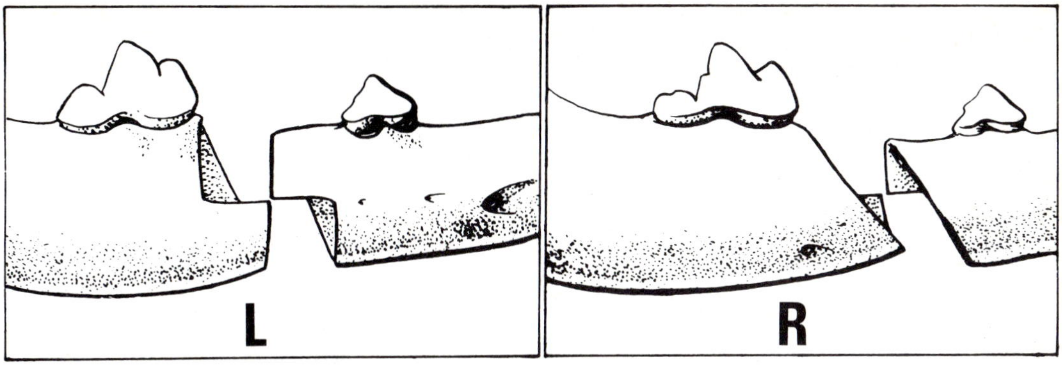

Figure 7–6. Dry specimen showing the combined cortical sections of a mandibular ramus with a step buccally (L) and an oblique cut lingually (R). (From Michieli S, et al: Surgical Lengthening of the Mandible: A Laboratory Model. *Oral Surg* 50:208, 1980.)

procedures to use an autogenous cancellous bone graft and a stablizing implant such as a Dacron-urethane basket or similar biocompatible material to hold the graft[7] (Fig. 7–7).

At present, the discussion of occlusive defects in dogs and cats is based on clinical impression, anecdotal information, and extrapolation from human dentistry. Scientific study of these problems, including extensive cephalometric analysis of the developing canine and feline skulls, is needed before definitive statements can be made about pathogenesis and treatment in these animals.

OTHER JAW ABNORMALITIES

The management of jaw injuries is described in Chapter Nine. Periodontal disease (Chapter Five), and, occasionally, defects in teeth (Chapter Six), can cause disease in the deeper bone tissue of the jaws. Tumors affecting the jaws are described in Chapter Eight.

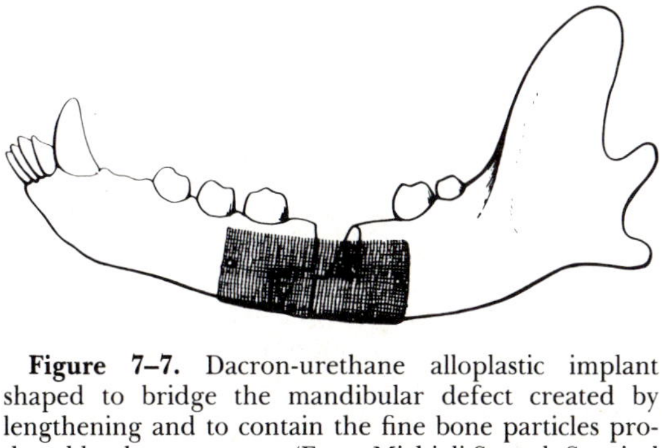

Figure 7–7. Dacron-urethane alloplastic implant shaped to bridge the mandibular defect created by lengthening and to contain the fine bone particles produced by the osteotomy. (From Michieli S, et al: Surgical Lengthening of the Mandible: A Laboratory Model. *Oral Surg* 50:209, 1980.)

Cartilaginous Mandibular Symphysis

Cartilaginous mandibular symphysis, in which the rostral angle of the mandible does not ossify, occurs in newborn dogs. It is an inherited condition. The teeth do not have strong support and will loosen with occlusive trauma. The breakdown of tooth attachment results in periodontal disease and premature loss of affected teeth. There is no known primary treatment for this rare condition.[4] Treatment of the secondary periodontal disease is indicated (Chapter 5).

Craniomandibular Osteopathy

Craniomandibular osteopathy is an uncommon disease that affects a variety of breeds, including the Scottish, Cairn, Boston, and West Highland white terriers; Labrador retrievers; Great Danes; and Doberman pinschers.[10–12] This disease is considered to be a non-neoplastic developmental condition that is characterized by protuberant exostosis of the caudal mandible and tympanic bullae. Usually, these dogs are presented with fever, depression, pain, and reduced range of motion of the temporomandibular joint. The bony exostosis may be palpable. Diagnosis of craniomandibular osteopathy is made from clinical signs and radiographic examination. It has been reported that treatment with prednisone is helpful in relieving clinical signs but not in curing the disease.[12] Surgical removal of the exostosis temporarily relieves the osseous restriction of the temporomandibular joint; however, the lesions grow back. Genetic factors are suspected because the disease occurs more commonly in closely related terrier breeds. The presence of inflammatory cells suggests a reactive cause;[10] however, the etiology is unknown. The prognosis is guarded at best, since severe exostosis prevents the dog from eating. The extensive bone growth ceases spontaneously when the dog reaches skeletal maturity at 11 to 13 months of age.[12]

Infections of the Mandible

Infections of the mandible are more common than is generally believed and usually arise from extension of periodontal disease. Extensive resorption of bone can occur from chronic infection of the periodontal pocket. Periapical abscesses seen in severe periodontal disease can lead to resorption of the mandibular cortex. In some affected animals, the infection of the mandible may be so severe that it drains through an opening in the skin.

Primary infection of the mandible can also occur. Recent reports have indicated the relatively common frequency of anaerobic infections (particularly *Bacteroides* spp.) in small animals and, in particular, their role in chronic osteomyelitis.[13, 14] In the mandible, severe progressive osteomyelitis, with destruction of bone and adjacent soft tissue, can be seen (Fig. 7–8). A putrid odor accompanies these infections. Diagnosis is confirmed by aerobic and anaerobic cultures of the lesions. Treatment includes thorough debridement of all visible necrotic tissue, lavage, drainage, and antibiotic therapy. Most anaerobic bacteria are suspectible to beta-lactam antibiotics, such as penicillin and the cephalosporins. However, some species of anaerobes, such as *Bacteroides,* produce beta-lactamases. Also, some anaerobic infections occur in concert with aerobic bacteria, such as *Staphylococcus aureus,* and some of these bacteria produce beta-lactamases. Sensitivity analysis should be included with the cultures. In the case of beta-lactamase–producing infections, a bactericidal antimetabolite, such as metronidazole, or chloramphenicol and clindamycin can be used (see Table 4–2).[13] It may be necessary to continue antibiotic therapy for several months. Some anaerobic infections tend to recur after cessation of antibiotic therapy.

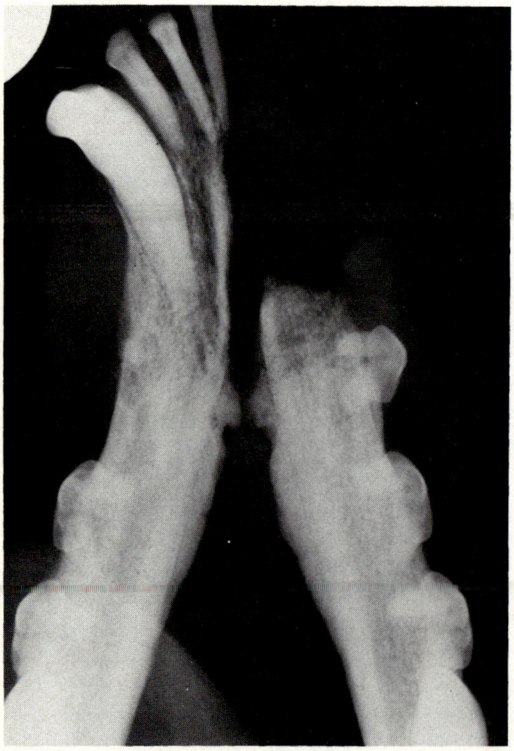

Figure 7–8. Severe destruction of mandibular bone seen radiographically. Mixed cultures of aerobic and anaerobic bacteria were obtained from this dog. There was no histological evidence of tumor.

Systemic Metabolic Disease Affecting the Mandible

Nutritional secondary hyperparathyroidism, also known as "rubber jaw," can lead to a softening of the mandibular bone. Nutritional hyperparathyroidism is usually associated with low levels of calcium or excessive levels of phosphorus in the diet; however, with the advent of well-balanced commercial animal foods, this disease is seen infrequently. The maladjusted diets lead to a calcium-phosphorus imbalance or to an absolute or relative hypocalcemia that triggers the release of parathyroid hormone. This causes an increase in osteoclastic resorption of bone and a raised serum calcium concentration. The resorption of bone leads to a softening of the mandible and, thus, to the name "rubber jaw." The classic radiographic sign of hyperparathyroidism is resorption of the lamina dura surrounding the teeth in the mandible. The disease is corrected by dietary adjustment and supplementation with calcium.[15]

Renal secondary hyperparathyroidism can cause a similar lesion. However, in this case the primary diseased organ is the kidney, which fails to eliminate phosphate because of a reduced glomerular filtration rate and impaired renal tubular function. The serum phosphorus level increases and exceeds the serum calcium level. The resulting calcium-phosphorus imbalance stimulates parathyroid hormone release to counter the hypocalcemia.[16] In addition, the kidney's production of the active vitamin D compound hydroxycholecalciferol is reduced, resulting in a lowered intestinal absorption of calcium. Vitamin D is important in the production of a carrier protein that facilitates the transport of calcium across the mucosal barrier of the intestine. Serum calcium levels drop, increasing the need for parathyroid hormone. The resulting increased level of parathyroid hormone causes osteoclastic bone resorption, which is seen throughout the skeleton and can be advanced in the mandible.

THE TEMPOROMANDIBULAR JOINT

Temporomandibular Joint Dysplasia

Temporomandibular joint dysplasia, also known as "open-mouth jaw-locking," has been documented in a variety of breeds, including the Irish setter,[17,18] the bassett hound,[19,20] the Saint Bernard,[21] and the American cocker spaniel.[22] The etiology of the condition is unknown, but it is thought to originate from a combination of factors, including increased mobility of the mandibular symphysis[19] and dysplasia of the glenoid cavity and condyloid process, causing laxity of the joint.[17]

This disease appears during early adulthood. Locking of the mandible in an open position, usually after the animal has yawned, is the major clinical sign. The jaw-locking occurs because the coronoid process slips laterad to the zygomatic arch. Generally, these dogs do not exhibit pain or arthralgia.

Several osseous abnormalities may be present, causing the joint laxity. A shallow glenoid fossa, with an abnormally positioned retroglenoid process, and an abnormally shaped condyloid process may lead to increased mobility within the temporomandibular joint (Fig. 7–9). This increased laxity allows the coronoid process of the mandible to move laterally. There has to be increased mobility of the mandibular symphysis to allow rotation and independent movement by one hemimandible. Laxity of the collateral ligaments

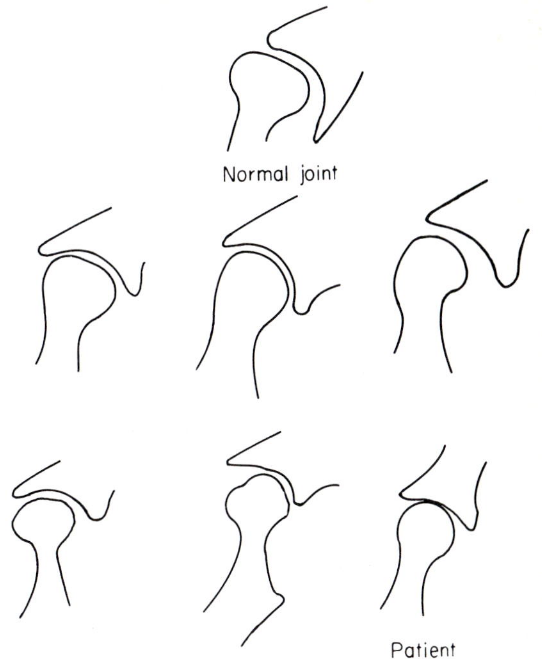

Figure 7–9. The temporomandibular joints of six dogs with temporomandibular dysplasia and of one dog with a normal joint. (From Hoppe E, Svalastoga E: Temporomandibular dysplasia in American cocker spaniels. *J Small Anim Pract* 21:67, 1980.)

is also found, which allows increased rotation and lateral movement of the ramus of the mandible. When the mandible is opened to an extreme position, the coronoid process displaces laterally, engages the ventral border of the zygomatic arch, and slips laterad to the arch, preventing closure of the mouth (Fig. 7–10). The side of the mouth that locks

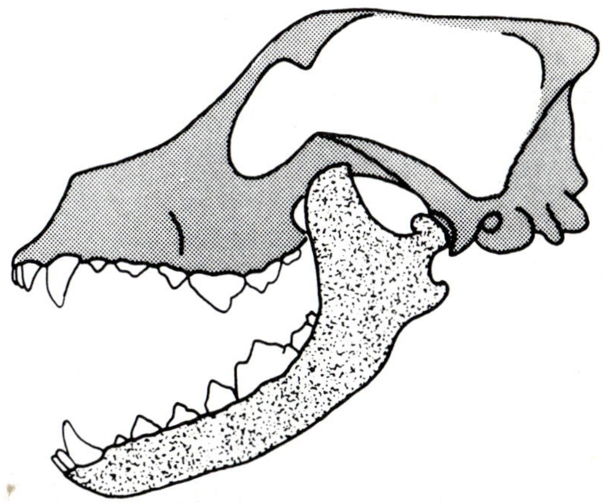

Figure 7–10. The coronoid process is displaced laterad to the rostral part of the zygomatic arch, preventing closure of the mouth. (From Robbins G, Grandage J: Temporomandibular joint dysplasia and open-mouth jaw-locking in the dog. *J Am Vet Med Assoc* 171:1073, 1977.)

open is opposite the most dysplastic temporomandibular joint.

Treatment consists of surgically removing a portion of the ventral border of the zygomatic arch. The incision is made through the skin of the cheek. The periosteum of the zygoma is incised and reflected, and the bone is removed with a rongeur. The mandible is manipulated to ensure that sufficient bone has been removed. The periosteum and the aponeurosis of the masseter muscle are sutured. It may be necessary to remove the full thickness of the zygoma, which does not result in any orbital defect.[23]

Arthritis of the Temporomandibular Joint

Degenerative arthrosis of the temporomandibular joint can occur in the dog; however, it is not common. Most cases of degenerative arthrosis are the result of trauma. The cat also can be affected with severe degenerative arthrosis of the temporomandibular joint. Primary inflammatory or immunological arthritis of the temporomandibular joint has been suspected in the dog. Temporomandibular arthralgia occurs in dogs with multiple polyarthritides. However, a specific diagnosis of rheumatoid arthritis or systemic lupus erythematosus has not been made. Samples of synovial fluid from other joints have confirmed the presence of a primary inflammatory arthritis, but synovial fluid samples were not taken from the temporomandibular joint. Treatment consists of anti-inflammatory or analgesic medications, or condylectomy if necessary (see further on).

Traumatic Conditions of the Temporomandibular Joint

Fractures and dislocations are the most common traumatic conditions seen in the dog and cat. Temporomandibular dislocation is usually unilateral and occurs in a rostrodorsal direction, but occasionally it can be bilateral. The retroglenoid process must be fractured for the mandibular condyloid process to dislocate in a caudal direction. Most dislocations are caused by blunt trauma from the lateral aspect, forcing the mandibular condyloid process on that side to become displaced rostrally. The contralateral condyloid process is pushed caudally against the retroglenoid process. When the condyloid process is displaced cranially from the site of the trauma, the temporal and masseter muscles pull the condyle dorsally against the zygomatic arch. On clinical presentation, the mandible is offset to the side opposite the dislocated joint.

Reduction is accomplished by forcing the condyle ventrally. The tension of the muscles and the surrounding tissues will then pull the condyle back into place. The downward movement of the condyle can be accomplished by inserting a fulcrum, such as a tubular structure (plastic pen or wood dowel), into the caudal recess of the oral cavity and gently forcing the mouth closed (Fig. 7–11). Although this method is very satisfactory in cats, traction may be necessary as an initial maneuver in large dogs. In most cases open reduction is unnecessary and should be avoided to prevent fibrous ankylosis of the temporomandibular joint.

Occasionally, reduction is incomplete, and

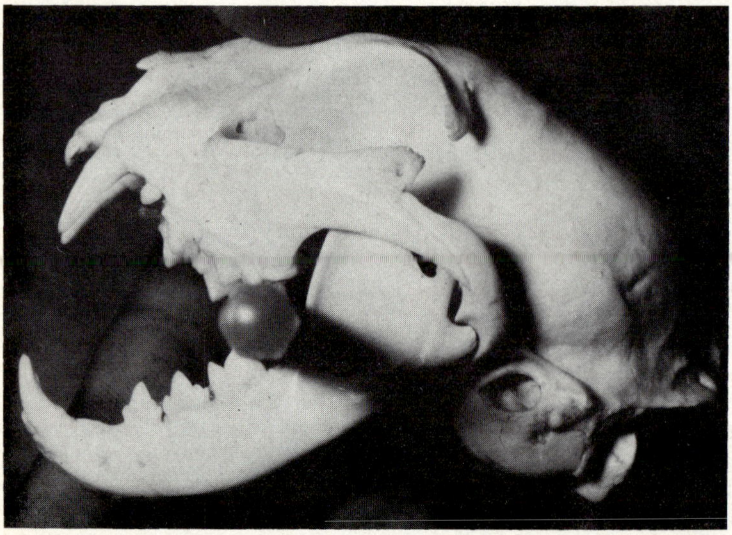

Figure 7–11. Correct positioning of a fulcrum (an ink pen) in the caudal recess of the mouth to assist in the reduction of a temporomandibular dislocation.

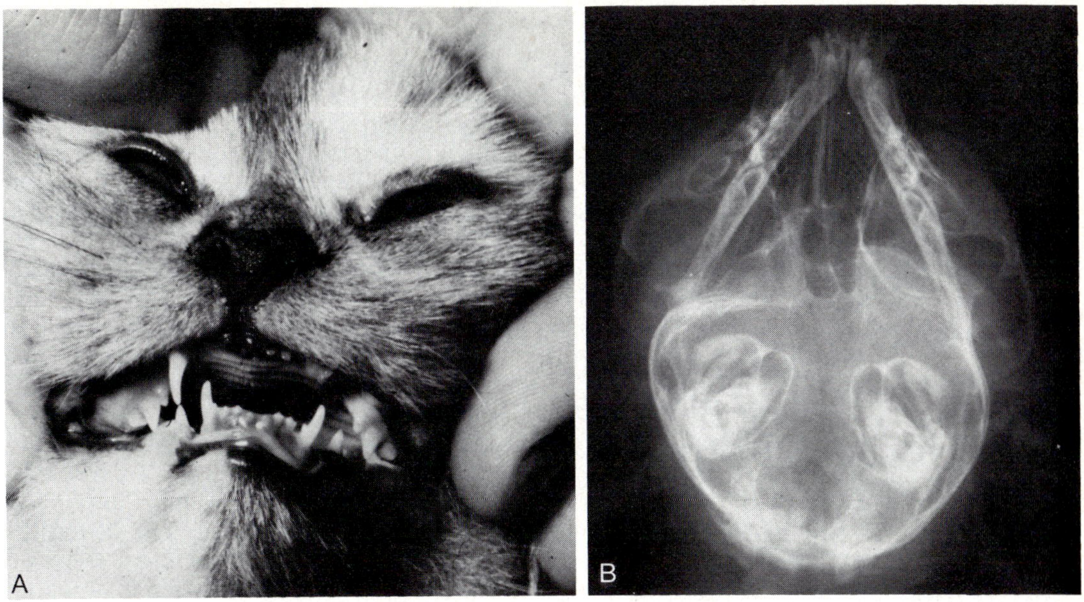

Figure 7–12. *A*, Persian cat with a suspected temporomandibular dislocation. *B*, Radiographs of the skull and mandible show no dislocation, but there is asymmetry of the skull.

subluxation remains because of a folded articular disc. Surgery may be indicated to repair or remove the disc, which allows reduction of the mandible to a normal position. When the mandible is reduced, it is unnecessary to immobilize the joint. Rest and a liquid diet, to prevent additional trauma, are helpful. In animals with severe instability or bilateral dislocations, muzzling with tape to limit movement may be necessary for 2 to 3 weeks.

Caudal dislocations are more common in young puppies and require particular attention. Unrecognized fractures of the retroglenoid process and subsequent mandibular displacement can result in arthritis and ankylosis. Unrestricted function in normal occlusion must be maintained whenever possible in these patients.

In cases of temporomandibular dislocation, radiographs must be taken to confirm the diagnosis. In some cases, the clinical appearance may be misleading. Radiographs will eliminate other causes for mandibular displacement, such as fractures or congenital deformities of the maxilla or other bones of the skull[24] (Fig. 7–12).

Fractures of the temporomandibular joint most frequently involve the medial portion of the condyloid process of the mandible. Occasionally, these fractures occur bilaterally and are associated with other fractures of the mandible. Temporomandibular joint fractures require little treatment. Surgical invasion of the joint, even to remove small articular fragments, should be avoided, since this would increase the chance of ankylosis.

Temporomandibular Joint Condylectomy

Bony ankylosis of the temporomandibular joint can occur as a posttraumatic complication. The treatment for ankylosis and an inhibited range of motion of the temporomandibular joint consists of condylectomy, with subsequent development of a fibrous pseudarthrosis. Condylectomy is performed through an incision that parallels the ventral border of the zygomatic arch. The caudal origin of the masseter muscle is lifted subperiosteally, exposing the joint capsule. The joint capsule is incised both cranially and laterally, and the lateral one half of the condyle is removed with a rongeur. The articular disc is incised with a scalpel, and the medial portion of the condyloid process is removed by means of a wire saw. Good results have been reported following unilateral condylectomy, whereas temporary, mild malocclusion has been noted following bilateral condylectomy.[25]

The initial clinical results of condylectomy for ankylosis and temporomandibular joint inhibited range of motion have been encouraging. Chronic cases with exuberant fibrous ankylosis do not respond as favorably. At this time, it would be advisable to suggest condylectomy early in the course of irreversible and progressive degenerative arthrosis of the temporomandibular joint.[26]

Osteoarthritis of the temporomandibular joint can be secondary to severe osteitis of the temporal bone in the tympanic bullae and external acoustic meatus. This osteitis is caused by chronic otitis externa.[27] The function of the temporomandibular joint can be compromised, and in such cases condylectomy is the only treatment that is likely to benefit the animal.

MISCELLANEOUS CONDITIONS OF THE MASTICATORY APPARATUS

Eosinophilic Myositis. This occurs most frequently in the German shepherd and in similar large breed dogs. The affected dogs are usually young. Swelling is a clinical sign, along with pain in the temporal pterygoid and masseter muscles. Severe swelling will result in exophthalmus and secondary corneal irritation. The condition has an acute onset, and there may be a peripheral eosinophilia. The condition is confirmed if histopathological examination demonstrates cellular infiltration of the muscle by eosinophils and mononuclear cells and necrosis of muscles; however, clinical signs are confined to the muscles of mastication. The condition has a tendency to relapse, and the more it recurs the more likely it is that trismus will occur.[28] Treatment is palliative and consists of reducing the inflammation with corticosteroids such as prednisolone, starting at 2 mg to 4 mg/kg BID, and decreasing the dose steadily over 4 weeks. The prognosis is not uniformly grave, but it is generally guarded. Not all affected dogs will lose complete function of the temporomandibular joint.

Atrophic Myositis. Atrophic myositis may be a sequela of eosinophilic myositis, but it occurs in different breeds and at different ages. It may occur unilaterally or bilaterally and is characterized by the inability to open the jaws normally. Atrophy of the temporal and masseter muscles is obvious on physical examination. There is usually little or no pain, no swelling, and an insidious onset. Diagnosis is confirmed when the histopathological examination demonstrates muscle atrophy and lymphocytic infiltration. This disease does not necessarily result in complete trismus, but it will in progressive cases.

Idiopathic Trigeminal Neurapraxia or Neuropathy. This has been described in the dog. The major clinical sign is failure to close the mouth. The mandible is very lax, and the muscles of mastication are paralyzed. This condition does not directly affect the temporomandibular joint and is idiopathic and generally self-limiting. There is no known treatment except loosely muzzling the mouth to prevent drying of the oral mucosa. Spontaneous recovery takes approximately 2 to 3 weeks.[29]

Tetanus and Retrobulbar Abscess. These are other conditions that can affect the function of the temporomandibular joint. Tetanus typically affects the muscles of mastication, as well as other skeletal muscles. Normal function of the temporomandibular joint is inhibited. This disease is not common, but it does occur in both the dog and the cat. A retrobulbar abscess does not directly affect the temporomandibular joint; however, because there is swelling and inflammation, joint motion causes severe pain. Once the abscess is drained and the infection is treated with antibiotics, pain-free motion of the joint returns.

ORTHODONTICS

Types of Tooth Movement

Orthodontics is that branch of dentistry that is concerned with studying the growth of the craniofacial complex, the development of occlusion, and the treatment of dentofacial abnormalities. The most popular method of correcting dentofacial and occlusal abnormalities in veterinary medicine is to move teeth, using a variety of techniques.[30–32]

Methods of Movement

Intrusion. This method consists of moving the tooth directly into the alveolus surrounding the tooth. It is the most difficult movement to accomplish because one tries to move the tooth in the same direction that it is stressed when in occlusion. The supporting structure of the tooth is geared to resist this type of force in the form of the direction of the periodontal fibers and the hydraulic action of the root and socket. Very light force is used, and when done properly little relapse is seen. If excessive force is used to accomplish intrusion, absorption of the apex of the root may result. Intrusion is a relative movement in relation to surrounding teeth and is rarely used in veterinary orthodontics.

Extrusion. This method consists of moving the tooth in the direction that an erupting tooth normally follows. This is one of the easiest types of movement to accomplish provided that there is no occlusal interference. Extrusion is best carried out with light, continuous force during rapid periods of alveolar growth. Excessive force may result in the loss of the tooth or in damage to the alveolus, with subsequent loosening of the tooth.

Tipping. When a force is applied to a tooth at a single point on the crown, a tipping movement will occur. As this type of force is applied, the tooth pivots against the alveolar crest, and the apex moves in the opposite direction. This creates a center of rotation, or fulcrum, at approximately the junction of the middle and the apical thirds of the root. The lighter the force that is applied to the crown, the further the fulcrum moves toward the apex. Areas of compression and tension are created on opposite sides of the periodontal ligament, reducing the undesirable reverse movement of the apex of the tooth. Tipping is best accomplished with a light, continuous force. Usually the crown moves more than the root.

Translation. When a fixed attachment is placed on the crown of a tooth, and leverage principles are applied to move the tooth so that the crown and root move in the same direction without a change in axial inclination, bodily movement, or translation, is achieved. There is a great deal of resistance to this type of movement from the periodontium. Accordingly, bodily movement of a tooth is considerably more difficult to achieve than are simple tipping movements. Initially, light force is preferred; however, greater force may be necessary later.

Root Movement. In this situation, the root moves, with no appreciable movement of the crown. Examples of this principle are seen in the uprighting of the tipped tooth when the crown is held stationary and in torquing procedures in which the root is moved in a labiolingual direction. This type of movement has limited application in veterinary orthodontics.

Rotation. This movement consists of pivoting a tooth around a long axis of the root. The periodontal fibers, which attach the tooth to the alveolus, are stretched in one direction. This is a complicated tooth movement that is difficult to effect and difficult to retain. Upon releasing the force on the tooth, the fibers have a tendency to recoil, causing the tooth to revert to its original position, especially if the rotation is rapid with strong, continuous force. For this reason, it is wise to retain the corrected position of the rotated tooth for a time sufficient to allow the fibers to accommodate to the new position. Rotation is best effected by alternating periods of stabilization and movement.

Anchorage in Tooth Movement

Anchorage is an important concept in orthodontic practice.[30] Since teeth are moved by applying a direct force to the tooth, there must be an anchor or a point of resistance from which this force originates. Normally, other teeth are used as anchor units. Since there is as much force exerted against the anchor unit as against the tooth to be moved, the anchor tooth may move more than the target tooth if the procedure is not planned correctly.

In veterinary orthodontics, intraoral anchorage is usually applied and may be categorized as simple, stationary, or reciprocal. Simple anchorage means that the anchor teeth will be tipped during movement. This technique is the most widely practiced in veterinary orthodontics. Stationary anchorage refers to resistance of body movement; in this case, anchor teeth would have to move entirely or translate if there is any movement. The term "stationary anchorage" is considered to be orthodontic jargon. Reciprocal anchorage is the ideal tooth moving situation; one tooth is moved against another to allow both of them to move more or less equally.

There may not be enough anchor units within the mouth to provide the desired resistance. In this case, it may be necessary to reinforce the anchorage provided by the teeth, using devices such as lingual arches and hollow appliances that use the palate and mandible for additional support. In humans, it is possible to supplement anchorage with a cranial extraoral appliance, but this is not a practical technique in veterinary orthodontics.

Tissue Damage Associated with Orthodontic Tooth Movement

The three major adverse effects of orthodontic tooth movement are root resorption, crystal bone loss, and pulpal damage.[32, 33]

In root resorption, damage to the cementum and the dentin occurs. Trauma to root structures results in the laying down of secondary dentin and additional cementum. Prolonged tipping of teeth may cause root resorption. The magnitude of force exerted on the tooth may be an important causative factor in this problem. One hypothesis is that fluid transfer is blocked as a result of the build-up of pressure against the tooth. The disruptive process occurs along the alveolar wall on the contralateral aspect of the alveolus. If root resorption is not accompanied by adequate position response, crystal bone may also be lost. A second hypothesis suggests that forces that occlude vessels lead to ligament destruction and resorption of part of the crystal bone.

Pulpal damage occurs rarely. The usual cause is extreme force applied over a short period of time. The pathological response of the pulpal tissue is described in Chapter Six.

Materials and Techniques in Orthodontics

The two major types of orthodontic technique are removable (Hawley) appliances and fixed appliances. Both techniques provide the practitioner with various options and possibilities.[31]

Removable Appliances

Removable appliances consist of three parts—the active force, the baseplate, and the retentive device.[34]

The active force is usually obtained with springs, elastic bands, or jackscrews. These materials provide light, continuous force, whch is most desirable in the adult patient. Springs allow the appliance to be seated in the mouth. They require meticulous preparation, since the spring must come in contact with the tooth at a specific location, and the direction of tooth movement is determined by the contact point of the spring. Elastic bands offer continuous reciprocal force. Because they lose elasticity with use, replacement at regular intervals is necessary. Jackscrews are available in a variety of types. They are embedded into the baseplate to provide either local or generalized force for use on single or multiple teeth.

The main function of the baseplate is to hold the active forces and retaining devices together. It is usually constructed of acrylic resin and is custom-made for each patient. The baseplate anchors the appliance by coming into close contact with surrounding teeth. Sufficient thickness must be allowed to provide strength to the baseplate.

The retentive device is the part of the appliance that provides attachment and stability to intraoral structures. The usual retentive devices are clasps and labial arch wires, which may be built into the buccal and labial sides of the baseplate. The retentive devices are anchored to the teeth to force specific movement or to secure the baseplate in the oral cavity. Additional retention may be obtained by contouring the baseplate around the teeth to resist dislodging forces.

Fixed Appliances

The fixed appliance is the other major type of orthodontic technique in common use. The basis of fixed techniques is the dental bracket, which is bonded directly to affected or surrounding teeth.

Brackets are available in both metal and plastic.[35] For very small dogs and cats, plastic brackets may be used. They are slightly softer and will flex and bend slightly. Because of this feature, they are less effective than metal brackets. This is probably a positive feature when considering orthodontic treatment for very small animals, since major tooth movements may result in root and alveolar resorption, with eventual tooth loss. A metal bracket is more desirable if extensive orthodontic treatment requiring considerable movement or rotation of teeth is anticipated.

Some brackets have solid, perforated bases. The bonding adhesive is squeezed through the perforations and provides a mechanical bond between the bracket and the resin. If this type of bracket base is used, excessive adhesive should not be allowed to accumulate under the wings of the bracket. Brackets with a wire mesh base appear to attach better to canine or feline teeth. As with the perforated base, there is the danger of excessive adhesive spoiling the bracket if adhesive is allowed to accumulate under the bracket wings during bonding. Once a bracket is fastened directly to the teeth, it can be used to hold an elastic band or wire retainer, it can serve as an anchorage point for movement of another tooth, or it can hold a removable appliance in place.

Construction of a Removable Appliance

When constructing a removable appliance, an alginate* impression is made of the mouth[5, 36] (Fig. 7–13). The alginate is mixed in a rubber bowl and is placed in an impression tray before being inserted in the mouth. An impression tray may be custom-built with boxing wax, but a plastic drug bottle that is cut to accommodate the dental arcade works very well (Fig. 7–14). The alginate impression requires about 1 minute to make; general anesthesia usually is necessary to keep the patient absolutely still (Fig. 7–15). A stone model is made from dental casting stone† that is liquified and poured into the alginate mold (Fig. 7–16). Bubbles and air spaces will develop in deep impressions unless each area is carefully filled or unless a vibrator is used to release trapped air (Fig. 7–17). The cast stone is allowed to dry and the alginate is removed. The resultant casting should be a perfect impression of the upper or lower dental arcade, or of both (Fig. 7–18). The removable appliance baseplate is made from this impression using self-curing orthodontic acrylic resin* (Fig. 7–19).

*Jeltrate, LD Caulk Co., Milford, Delaware.
†Castone, Ranson and Randolph Co., Toledo, Ohio.

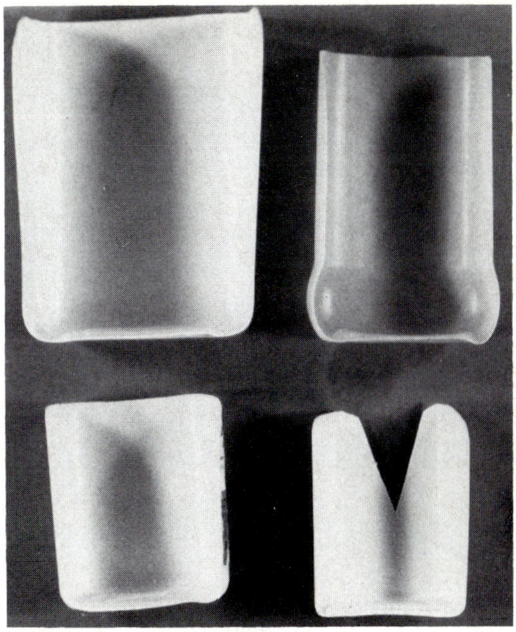

Figure 7–14. Impression trays cut from plastic containers.

The cast stone impression is placed on a flat surface and a separating medium (Modern Foil)† is painted over the surface (Fig. 7–20) to prevent the acrylic from adhering to the stone. The liquid and powder compo- .

*Orthodontic Resin, LD Caulk Co., Milford, Delaware.
†Modern Foil, Modern Materials Manufacturing Co., St. Louis, Missouri.

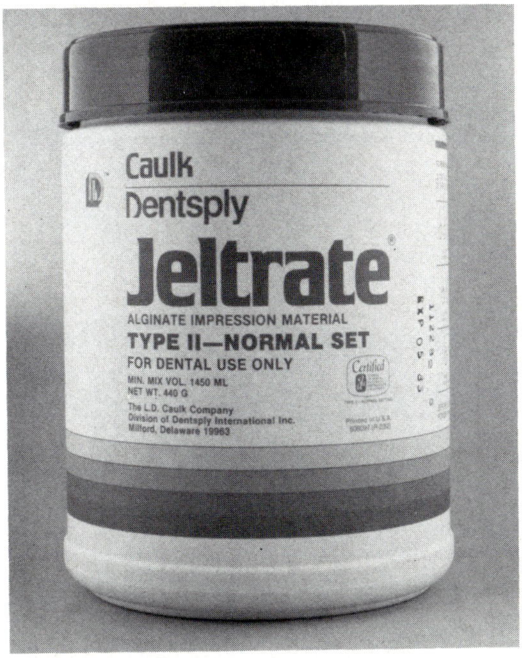

Figure 7–13. Alginate impression material.

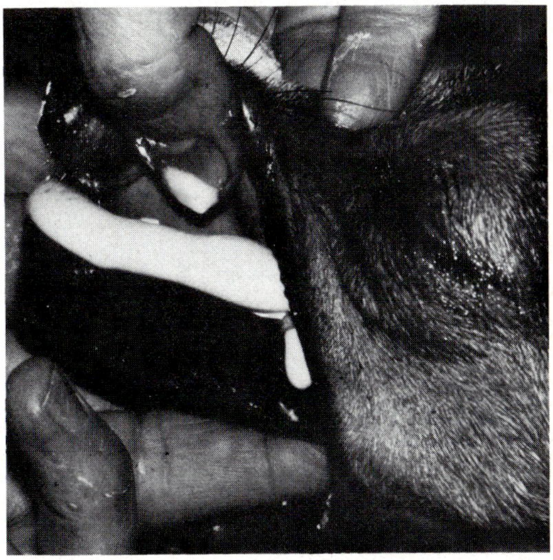

Figure 7–15. Alginate impression being taken.

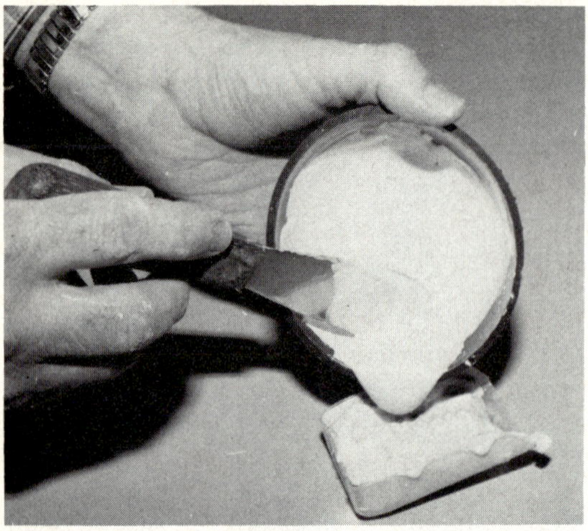

Figure 7–16. Cast stone is mixed with water to the desired consistency and is then poured into the alginate impression.

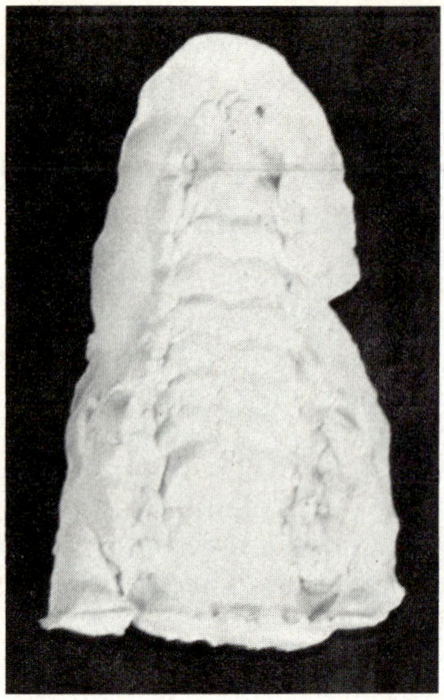

Figure 7–18. A cast stone reproduction of the upper dental arcade of a dog.

nents of the self-curing acrylic are applied slowly in small amounts to reduce the porosity of the completed appliance (Fig. 7–21). During the application of the acrylic, wires and jackscrews may be incorporated to provide active forces for displacement and retention in the oral cavity. The edges should reach the teeth rather than the gingival margins to avoid food impaction and irritation of soft tissues. After sufficient acrylic has been applied, the appliance is dried and cured in hot water for about 30 minutes. It is then polished and fitted to the patient. Minor adjustments in the shape of the appliance may be made with a dental handpiece and finishing stones.

The cast stone impression should be kept on file until the orthodontic manipulations are completed. It may be appropriate to cast another impression after the orthodontic treatment is completed in order to assess the progress of treatment.

Techniques for Bonding Brackets

Prior to bonding any brackets, the teeth should be thoroughly cleaned and pol-

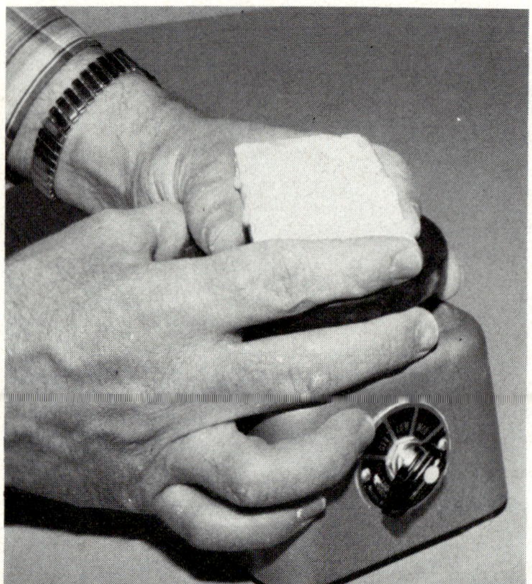

Figure 7–17. Immediately after pouring the cast stone mix into the impression, it is set on a vibrator for 1 minute in order to remove trapped air.

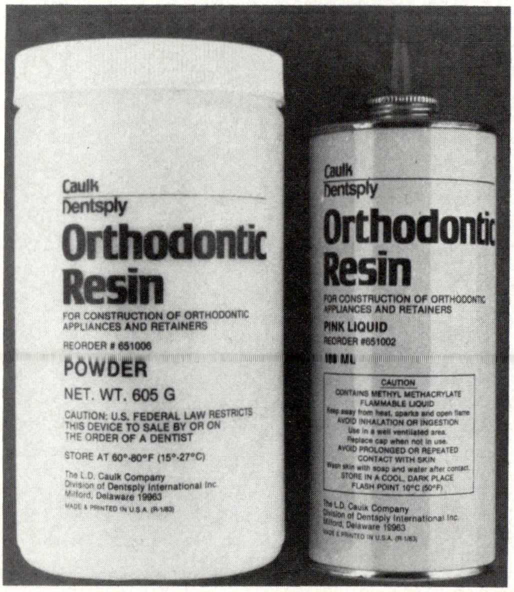

Figure 7–19. Common orthodontic resins.

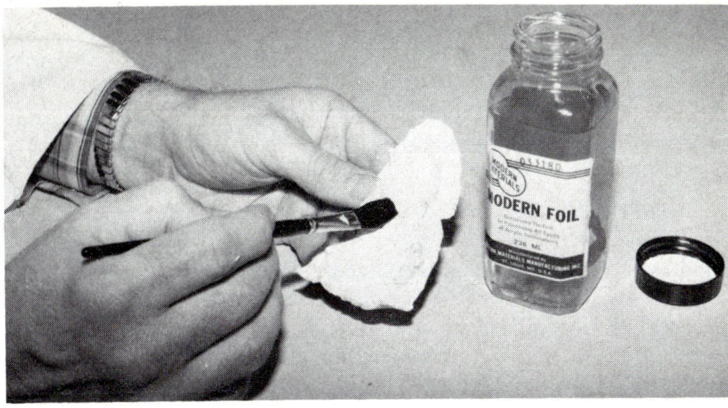

Figure 7–20. Modern Foil is brushed onto the dry cast.

ished.[5, 35] It may be necessary to remove calculus deposits by hand scaling or ultrasonic scaling. The teeth to be bracketed are polished with a plain dental polish or pumice. It is important that this paste be free of any oil or chemicals that might interfere with adhesion of the bonding paste.

The newly polished teeth are rinsed with water and are isolated, thoroughly dried, and etched with phosphoric acid. Although most manufacturers recommend etching for 1 minute, 2 or 3 minutes are more satisfactory in the dog and cat. The teeth are thoroughly rinsed and dried. The bonding cement is carefully applied to the teeth as well as to the bracket base, and the bracket is held in position on the tooth for at least 1 to 1½ minutes to ensure an adequate bond. Orthodontic pliers can be used to hold the two elements together. Excess bonding paste is removed from around the bracket to permit attachment of wires or elastic bands. Available bonding systems are described in Chapter Six.

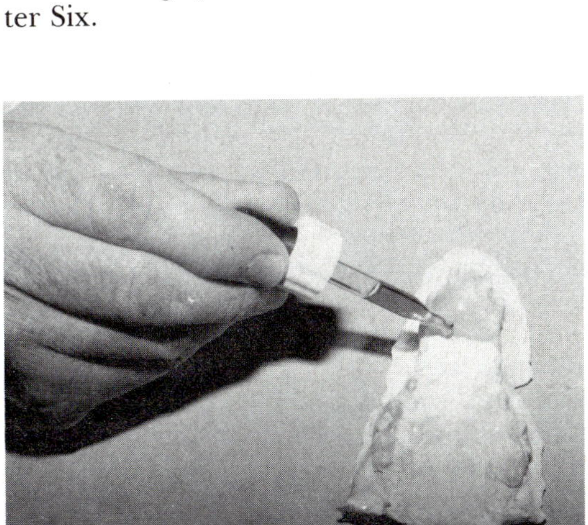

Figure 7–21. The intraoral acrylic appliance is constructed gradually by the intermittent application of powder and fluid resins.

The evidence to date suggests that etching enamel is not a harmful procedure.[35] Although it is believed that 10 μ of enamel thickness are lost each time a tooth is etched, this is not significant given that the total enamel thickness is 1500 μ to 2000 μ. If the etched area is left untouched *in vivo,* remineralization takes place very rapidly. It has been suggested that etched enamel wears more rapidly than does normal enamel, particularly in the first 28 days following an acid etching procedure. An average of 55.6 μ of enamel loss was noted following bracket removal, after which the enamel was smoothed and then polished. The remaining tooth surface appeared clinically and microscopically similar to unetched enamel. It remains to be established whether this new surface is more prone to caries formation and abrasion.

Extensive use of acid etching in restorative dentistry has convinced most practitioners that a strong bond between tooth and resin can be achieved, and that this bond is similar to that obtained by the banding of teeth.

Most orthodontic manipulations in veterinary medicine require 6 to 10 weeks to complete.[5] When satisfactory tooth movement has been obtained, the brackets are removed, the excess cement is scraped off, and the enamel surface of the tooth is polished. Removal of the resin that remains on the surface of the tooth may be a tedious and time-consuming task. The use of special pliers that have a chisel-like beak may be helpful, and a finishing tool on a straight handpiece may help remove excess resin before the teeth are polished.

Because of the availability of brackets that can be bonded directly to teeth, the use of orthodontic bands fixed around teeth is no longer necessary. The advent of direct-bonding orthodontic brackets has revolutionized orthodontic practice and has permitted the practical development of veterinary orthodontics.

Corrective Orthodontics for Specific Conditions

As stated previously, anterior crossbite is an abnormal occlusal relationship in which the lower incisors are located rostral to the upper central incisors.[3, 30] The anterior crossbite usually is caused by an abnormal axial inclination of one or more upper incisors, which can result from any of the following: trauma to the primary dentition, a retained pulpaceous deciduous tooth root, an abnormally situated supernumerary tooth, a bony or fibrous tissue barrier resulting from a deciduous tooth that has been permanently lost, inadequate arch length, biting habits, or cleft lip.

In humans, untreated anterior crossbite of dental origin results in the following unfavorable sequelae: (1) loss of arch length owing to adjacent teeth drifting into the space; (2) abnormal wear of the teeth; (3) traumatic occlusion of end locked incisors, leading to apical migration; (4) development of malocclusion, leading to adverse mandibular and maxillary growth; (5) excessive tension on the temporomandibular joint; and (6) interference with normal muscular function and mastication.

Specific long-term sequelae to anterior crossbite in veterinary patients have not been described, but some of the sequelae that occur in humans also occur in dogs and cats, including abnormal tooth wear and the development of malocclusion. Patients with anterior crossbite may have excessive calculus deposition on their teeth, leading to periodontal disease later in life. Malocclusion that leads to adverse mandibular and maxillary growth is a problem when anterior crossbite occurs in deciduous teeth because abnormally positioned deciduous teeth often result in abnormally positioned permanent teeth. Adverse mandibular and maxillary growth may be avoided by extraction of the deciduous teeth when the animal is 6 to 8 weeks of age.

Two methods of treatment for anterior crossbite are used in veterinary orthodontics.[5] In the first method, the upper incisors are forced in a rostral direction with a removable intraoral appliance. The second, more common method is to force the lower incisors in a caudal direction. In this technique, brackets are cemented on the lateral lower incisors.

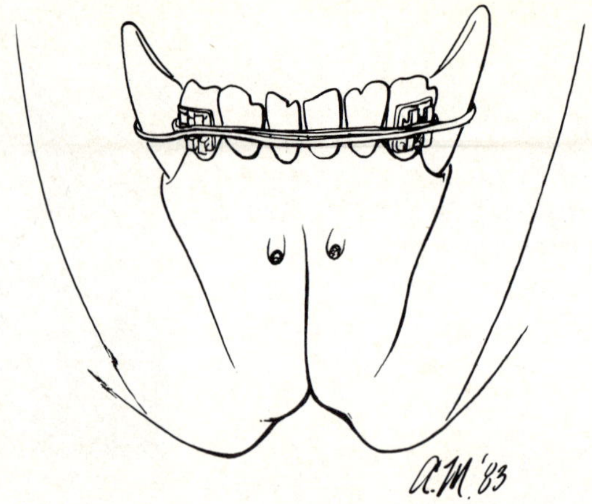

Figure 7–22. Incisors of the lower arcade are moved caudally with an elastic around the canine teeth and in front of the incisors. The elastic is held in place by brackets on the lateral incisors.

An orthodontic elastic band is placed in a figure-eight pattern around the lower canine teeth and through the brackets on the lateral incisors, providing a small amount of force that tips the lower incisors caudally so that they occlude behind the upper incisors (Fig. 7–22).

A removable intraoral appliance is useful for moving individual upper incisors.[34] Appropriate active forces may be exerted with screws or springs. The intraoral appliance is held in the mouth with elastic bands and brackets cemented on the upper canine and lateral incisor teeth. The appliance usually extends caudad to the upper canine teeth. Major expansion of a maxillary appliance may be achieved by using a jackscrew or expansion devices to move all of the incisors of the maxillary arcade (Fig. 7–23). The use of microscrews* or conventional springs may cause specific incisor teeth to move in a rostral direction (Fig. 7–24). Mandibular wedge osteotomy can be used for moving multiple lower incisor teeth.[37]

Another common type of orthodontic abnormality is rostral deviation of upper or lower canine teeth. This condition may be unilateral or bilateral and may occur in association with wry mouth. If correction of wry mouth is not possible, orthodontic manipulation of the affected canine teeth is an acceptable alternative.

*Erel Microscrews, Rocky Mountain Orthodontics, Denver, Colorado.

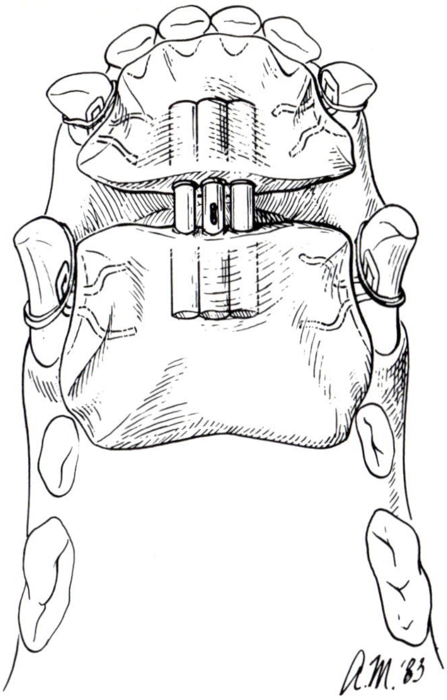

Figure 7–23. The incisors of the upper arcade are forced rostrally with a removable intraoral appliance and expansion screw. The spring-loaded expansion device is adjusted regularly to separate the two parts of the appliance. The appliance is held in the mouth with brackets on the upper canine teeth and lateral incisors and small elastics fastened to retention hooks in the appliance.

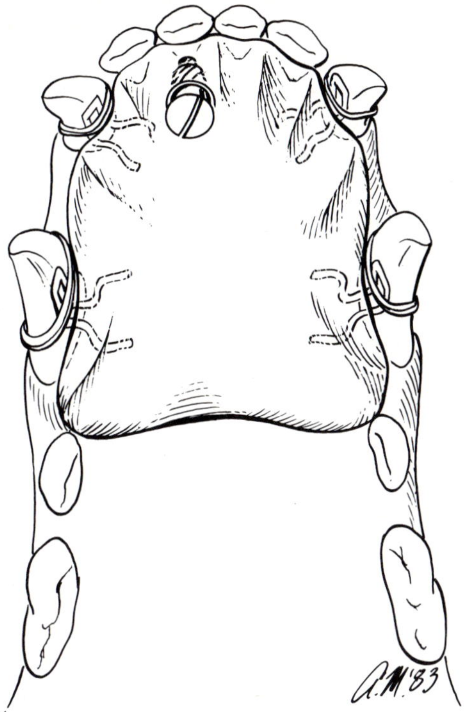

Figure 7–24. Upper incisors may be moved by building a single screw or wire into the removable appliance. An Erel microscrew is placed in the appliance and is adjusted regularly. The intraoral appliance is held in the mouth with elastics fastened to brackets on the upper canine teeth and lateral incisors.

Movement of a single canine tooth is fairly simple. A bracket is bonded to the tooth on the rostral or lateral side, depending on the desired direction of movement. An anchor consisting of another bracket or wire is attached to the cheek teeth in the same arcade on the same side. Usually, carnassial and molar teeth are used because of their size and multiple roots. An elastic band is used to pull the canine tooth toward the anchor (Fig. 7–25). Rostral movement of a single canine tooth can be achieved by application of the inclined plane principle; a plastic wedge is fitted to the opposite jaw to force the tooth forward each time the mouth is closed.[38]

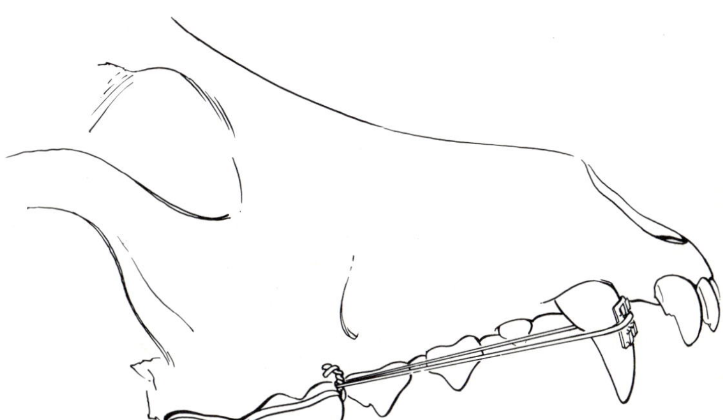

Figure 7–25. An upper or lower canine tooth may be moved caudally by pulling the tooth toward an anchorage of wire on the premolar and molar teeth. A hook is made from the wire and an elastic band may be secured around the hook. A bracket placed on the canine tooth will prevent slippage of the elastic.

Equipment

A variety of manufacturing companies and dental suppliers sell orthodontic equipment. Collaboration with local orthodontists is useful in building appliances and attaching brackets and elastics to teeth. Local dental laboratories may be helpful in building appliances and obtaining expansion devices. The veterinarian starting orthodontic practice must be willing to work with a variety of individuals and obtain information from a variety of sources to ensure success in the developing discipline of veterinary orthodontics.

References

1. Gruneberg H, Lea AJ: An inherited jaw anomaly in long-haired dachshunds. *J Genet* 39:285–297, 1940.
2. Evans HE, Christensen GC: Miller's Anatomy of the Dog, 2nd ed. Philadelphia, WB Saunders Co., 1979, p. 129.
3. Ross DL: Occlusion in the dog. *Southwest Vet* 28:247–250, 1975.
4. Ross DL: Veterinary dentistry. *In* Ettinger SJ (ed): Textbook of Veterinary Internal Medicine, Philadelphia, WB Saunders Co., 1975, pp. 1053–1054.
5. Ross DL: Veterinary orthodontics. Personal communication, 1983.
6. Brass W: Zur Korrektur von Zahnstellungs und Kieferanomalien des Hundes mit Dehnungsplatten und durch kieferchirurgische Masnahmen. *Kleinter Prax* 21:79–82, 1976.
7. Michieli S, Pizzoferrato A, Freeman S, Leake D: Surgical lengthening of the mandible: A laboratory model. *Oral Surg* 50:207–213, 1980.
8. Calabrese CT, Winslow RB, Lathan RA: Altering the dimensions of the canine face by the induction of new bone formation. *Plast Reconstr Surg* 54:467–470, 1974.
9. Leighton RL: Surgical correction of prognathous inferior in a dog. *Vet Med Small Anim Clin* 72:401–405, 1977.
10. Brinker WO, Piermattei DL, Flo GL: Handbook of Small Animal Orthopedics and Fracture Treatment. Philadelphia, WB Saunders Co., 1983, pp. 415–417.
11. Pool RR, Leighton RL: Craniomandibular osteopathy in a dog. *J Am Vet Med Assoc* 154:657–660, 1969.
12. Watson ADJ, Huxtable CRR, Farrow BRH: Craniomandibular osteopathy in Doberman pinschers. *J Small Anim Pract* 16:11–19, 1975.
13. Walker RD, Richardson DC, Bryant MJ, Draper CS: Anaerobic bacteria associated with osteomyelitis in domestic animals. *J Am Vet Med Assoc* 182:814–816, 1983.
14. Walker RD, Richardson DC. Anaerobic bacterial infections. *Mod Vet Pract* 62:289–292.
15. Rowland GN, Fetter AW: Nutritional secondary hyperparathyroidism. *In* Bojrab MJ (ed): Pathophysiology in Small Animal Surgery. Philadelphia, Lea & Febiger, 1981, pp. 677–680.
16. Cavanagh PG: Secondary renal hyperparathyroidism. *In* Bojrab MJ (ed): Pathophysiology in Small Animal Surgery. Philadelphia, Lea & Febiger, 1981, pp. 681–684.
17. Johnson KA: Temporomandibular joint dysplasia in an Irish setter. *J Small Anim Pract* 20:209–218, 1979.
18. Stewart WC, Baker GJ, Lee R: Temporomandibular subluxation in the dog. A case report. *J Small Anim Pract* 16:345–349, 1975.
19. Robins G, Grandage J: Temporomandibular joint dysplasia and open-mouth jaw locking in the dog. *J Am Vet Med Assoc* 171:1072–1076, 1977.
20. Thomas RE: Temporo-mandibular joint dysplasia and open-mouth jaw locking in a basset hound: A case report. *J Small Anim Pract* 20:697–701, 1979.
21. Culvenor JA: What is your diagnosis? *J Am Vet Med Assoc* 172:719–720, 1978.
22. Hoppe F, Svalastoga E: Temporomandibular dysplasia in American cocker spaniels. *J Small Anim Pract* 21:675–678, 1980.
23. Harvey CE: Presentation at Annual Meeting, Am Coll Vet Surg 1977.
24. Ticer JW, Spencer CP: Injury of the feline temporomandibular joint: Radiographic signs. *Vet Radiol* 19:146–156, 1978.
25. Tomlinson J, Presnell KR: Mandibular condylectomy: Effects in normal dogs. *Vet Surg* 12:148–154, 1983.
26. Lantz GC, Cantwell HD, Van Vleet JF, Cechner PE: Unilateral mandibular condylectomy: Experimental and clinical results. *J Am Anim Hosp Assoc* 18:883–890, 1982.
27. Lane JG: Disorders of the canine temporomandibular joint. *Vet Ann* 22:175–187, 1982.
28. Chrisman CL, Averill DR: Focal myositis of head musculature. *In* Ettinger SS (ed): Textbook of Veterinary Internal Medicine, 2nd ed. Philadelphia, WB Saunders Co., 1983.
29. Robins GM: Dropped jaw—mandibular neurapraxia in the dog. *J Small Anim Pract* 17:753–758, 1976.
30. Moyers RE: Biomechanics of Tooth Movements. *In* Moyers RE (ed): Handbook of Orthodontics, 3rd ed. Chicago, Yearbook Medical Publishers, 1973, pp. 430–444.
31. Seiders GW: Orthodontic principles. *Dent Clin North Am* 16:459–466, 1972.
32. Selhorst F: Orthodontische Behandlungen an Hunden. *Tierartz Umschau* 20:166–176, 1965.
33. Goldman HM, Gianelly AA: Histology of tooth movement. *Dent Clin North Am* 16:439–448, 1972.
34. Schlossberg A: The removable orthodontic appliance. *Dent Clin North Am* 16:487–495, 1972.
35. Way DC: Direct bonding and its application to minor tooth movement. *Dent Clin North Am* 22:757–770, 1978.
36. Tholen MA: Concepts in Veterinary Dentistry. Edwardsville, Kansas, Veterinary Medicine Publishing Co., 1983, pp. 44–46; pp. 148–154.
37. Yamagata J: Dental malocclusion and odontorthosis in dogs. *J Jap Vet Med Assoc* 32:194–199, 1979.
38. Kind RE, Mays RA: Use of an inclined plane for correction of ectopic mandibular canine tooth in a dog. *Vet Med Small Anim Pract* 71:52–55, 1976.

Chapter Eight

Oropharyngeal Neoplasms

AM Norris, SJ Withrow, and RR Dubielzig

TYPES OF NEOPLASMS OCCURRING IN THE DOG AND CAT

Oropharyngeal neoplasms occur frequently in the dog and cat, the oropharynx being the fourth most common site of malignant neoplasia in these species.[1–4] Both benign and malignant tumors are encountered, with the latter type predominating.[4,5] Malignant melanoma, squamous cell carcinoma, and fibrosarcoma are the most common malignant tumors of the canine oral cavity.[4–11] Squamous cell carcinoma occurs with regularity in the mouth of the cat, whereas malignant melanoma and fibrosarcoma are rare.[4,12]

Benign tumors in dogs are common, with the tumors of periodontal origin predominating.[13] A standard nomenclature for the canine epulides has been suggested, and three types are recognized. They are fibromatous epulis, ossifying epulis, and the locally aggressive acanthomatous epulis.[14,15] Canine oral papillomatosis is a viral disease of young dogs that is seen occasionally.[11] Benign oropharyngeal tumors are rare in cats, though fibroma and papilloma have been noted.[4,5] Transmissible venereal tumors occasionally occur in the canine oropharynx and are transplanted there by licking.

Tumors of the dental laminar epithelium are rare in both dogs and cats. Ameloblastoma is the most frequently diagnosed tumor of this sort;[14,15] ameloblastic fibro-odontoma and complex and compound odontoma are very rare.[15,16] Dental tumors described in the cat include inductive fibroameloblastoma[15,17] and ameloblastoma.[12]

Myoblastoma and hemangioma occur very occasionally in or on the tongue of the dog.

HISTORY AND CLINICAL SIGNS

Animals with oropharyngeal neoplasms are presented to veterinarians because of excessive salivation, bleeding from the mouth, difficulty in mastication, dysphagia, halitosis, or an obvious oral mass (Fig. 8–1). Often the oral mass is quite small, whereas metastases from the primary tumor may result in cervical lymph node enlargement, a cough re-

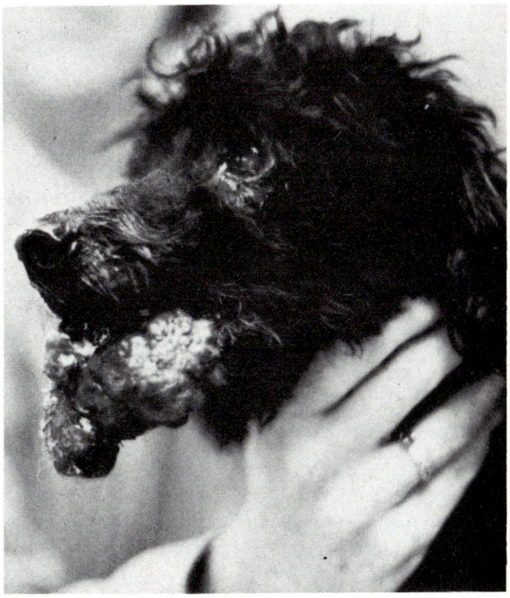

Figure 8–1. An advanced gingival melanoma of the rostral mandible in a 14 year old black poodle.

Table 8–1. Comparison of the Common Oral Tumors[3, 5, 8, 10]

	Malignant Melanoma	Squamous Cell Carcinoma (SCC)	Fibrosarcoma	Epulis
Dogs	30%–40%	20%–40%	10%–20%	60% of benign tumors
Cats	Rare	65%	20%	Rare
Average age (yr)	11	9	8	8
Male:female ratio	4:1	1:1	2:1	1:1
Common location of lesion	Gingivae, labial mucosae, buccal mucosae, palate	Gingivae or tonsils	Gingivae	Gingivae
Radiographic evidence of pulmonary metastases at autopsy	14%	8% of tonsillar SCC 3% of non-tonsillar SCC	10%	—
Animals with metastases at necropsy	81%	77% of tonsillar SCC	35%	—

sulting from pulmonary metastases, anorexia because of mechanical interference with mastication, or systemic tumor cachexia.

Oral tumors are most prevalent in older dogs. Exceptions include oral papillomatosis in young dogs (mean age of 1 year) and inductive fibroameloblastoma in young cats (less than 18 months of age).[11, 17]

Male dogs are at an increased risk for developing malignant oral tumors when compared with females.[2–4, 9] This sex distribution is most pronounced with malignant melanoma, which, according to one study, occurs four times as frequently in males as in females. Fibrosarcoma occurs twice as commonly in males.[10] A sex predilection seems to exist for squamous cell carcinoma if one examines the site of origin of the tumor, with tonsillar squamous cell carcinoma occurring most frequently in males and non-tonsillar squamous cell carcinoma occurring with equal frequency in both sexes.[10]

Breeds that are at a significantly higher risk of developing oropharyngeal cancer include the golden retriever, German shorthaired pointer, weimaraner, Saint Bernard, and cocker spaniel.[3, 4, 6, 10] It is generally believed that breeds with heavily pigmented oral mucosae develop melanomata more frequently.[5, 7, 9]

The specific site of involvement depends, in part, on the tumor type (Table 8–1). The gingivae are the most frequent sites of involvement for fibrosarcoma (87 percent), non-tonsillar squamous cell carcinoma (81 percent), and malignant melanoma (55 percent). The majority of tumors (76 percent) of buccal or labial mucosa are melanomata, whereas 66 percent of hard palate tumors are melanomata.[10] Tumors of tonsillar origin are most likely to be squamous cell carcinoma or lymphosarcoma.

INCIDENCE AND CLINICAL DESCRIPTION

Malignant Melanoma

Malignant melanoma is a common oropharyngeal neoplasm and is regarded by some authors as the most common type.[3–5] Melanomata are rare in cats.[4] Although a clinical correlation has been made between the amount of oral and skin pigmentation and the risk of developing melanoma, this hypothesis has yet to be proved. The cocker spaniel is at an increased risk for developing malignant melanoma,[5, 6, 9] with some authors

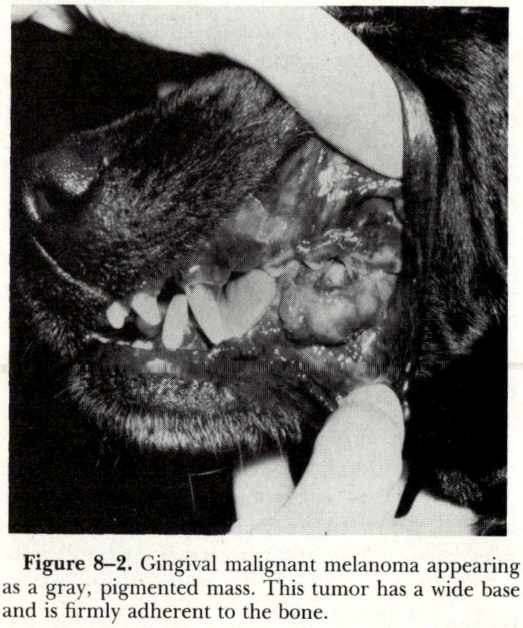

Figure 8–2. Gingival malignant melanoma appearing as a gray, pigmented mass. This tumor has a wide base and is firmly adherent to the bone.

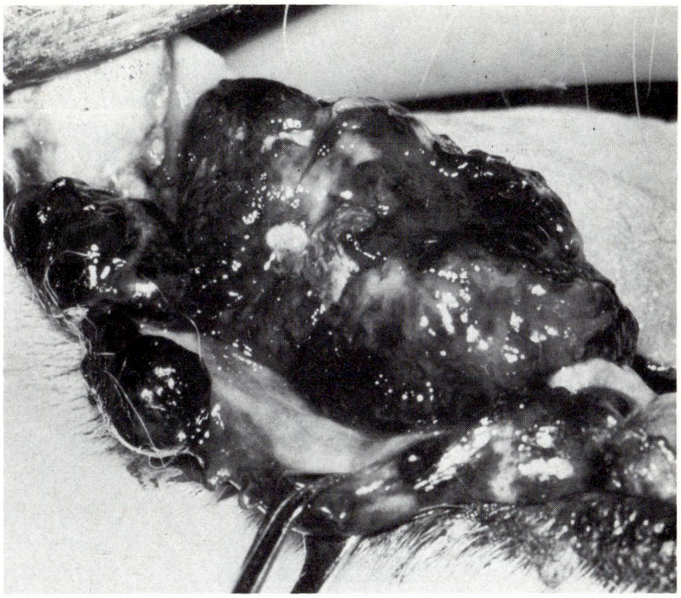

Figure 8–3. Malignant melanomata often undergo necrosis, ulceration, and hemorrhage as shown in this middle aged dog.

stating that the black cocker spaniel is at a still higher risk.[5] Malignant melanomata occur two to four times as frequently in males as in females.[4–7, 10] Melanomata occur most frequently on the gingivae (55 percent), labial mucosae (20 percent), hard palate (10 percent), and buccal mucosae (10 percent).[6, 10]

On visual examination, melanomata may be intensely pigmented or non-pigmented, with a variety of intermediate forms existing (Fig. 8–2). The result is that many tumors have a gray or mottled appearance. Ulceration and hemorrhage commonly are seen (Fig. 8–3). Melanomata often undergo very rapid growth. Thorough palpation of the regional lymph node is essential, since 60 percent of necropsied dogs had involvement of the regional lymph node.[10]

The histological classification of melanomata in dogs is an enigma to pathologists. The biological behavior of melanomata in these animals seems to depend more on the site of the primary lesion than on the histological appearance of the primary tumor.[18] This observation, considered with the fact that melanomata of the oral cavity most frequently are malignant, leads pathologists to believe that melanocytic neoplasms of the oral cavity have poor prognoses regardless of the histological types. The only morphological criterion that is useful in evaluating the expected behavior of oral melanomata is the mitotic index. Tumors with a mitotic index greater than 3 are significantly more likely to cause the death of the animal than are tumors with a mitotic index of less than 2.[19]

Squamous Cell Carcinoma

Squamous cell carcinoma is common in the dog and is by far the most prevalent oral tumor in the cat.[3–5] The tumor should be classified anatomically as tonsillar or non-tonsillar because of the differing biological behavior of the two types. In the dog, tonsillar and non-tonsillar squamous cell carcinomata occur with approximately equal fre-

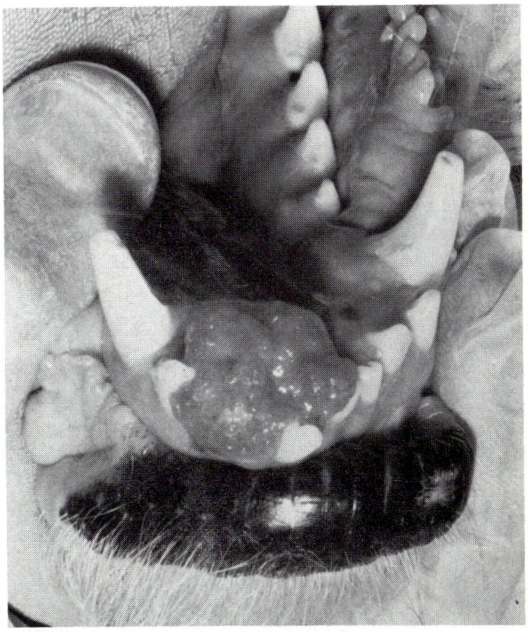

Figure 8–4. Lower jaw of a dog with a squamous cell carcinoma. The gingivae are the most common sites of non-tonsillar squamous cell carcinoma.

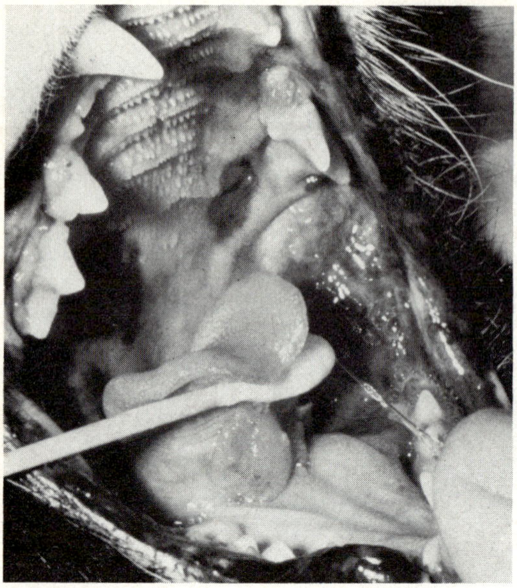

Figure 8–5. Sublingual squamous cell carcinoma in a cat. This type of neoplasm often invades the musculature of the tongue.

quency. Eighty-one percent of non-tonsillar squamous cell carcinomata arise from the gingivae, with the lips and tongue being the next most common site of involvement (Fig. 8–4).[10] Non-tonsillar squamous cell carcinoma in dogs occurs with equal frequency in males and females, whereas tonsillar squamous cell carcinoma occurs more frequently in males.[6, 9] It has been suggested that tonsillar carcinomata occur with a high frequency in industrialized metropolitan areas, such as London and Philadelphia, where carcinogens are at a greater concentration.[7, 9] Studies comparing the rural *versus* urban frequency of tonsillar carcinoma are not available.

In the cat, squamous cell carcinoma occurs most commonly along the ventrolateral aspect of the tongue or in the tonsil (Fig. 8–5), with gingival tumors being less frequent.[4, 5, 12, 15, 20] The gross appearance of oral squamous cell carcinoma in cats is similar to its appearance in dogs. Ulceration and secondary infection are common. The tumor tends to deeply invade the musculature of the tongue, with metastasis to the regional lymph nodes occurring late in the disease.[20] Although histological grading has been used for feline squamous cell carcinoma, it does not appear to be of prognostic value.[20]

Gingival Squamous Cell Carcinoma

Gingival squamous cell carcinoma originates from the gingivae adjacent to the teeth. These tumors are usually proliferative and are almost always ulcerative in the dog, resulting in excessive salivation and halitosis. They are usually red and quite friable.[7] The neoplasms are locally invasive, resulting in lysis of bone and loosening of the teeth (Fig. 8–6). Gingival squamous cell carcinoma in cats may not be ulcerative or proliferative, but it can cause lysis of bone and may mimic a primary bone tumor or chronic osteomyelitis. Dogs are often initially treated for dental disease by tooth extraction, with the subsequent appearance of an oral mass.[7] Gingival squamous cell carcinoma bears a better prognosis than does tonsillar squamous cell carcinoma because of a lower rate of metastasis (see section on Prognosis).

Histologically, gingival squamous cell carcinomata in both dogs and cats have a variable appearance, depending upon the degree

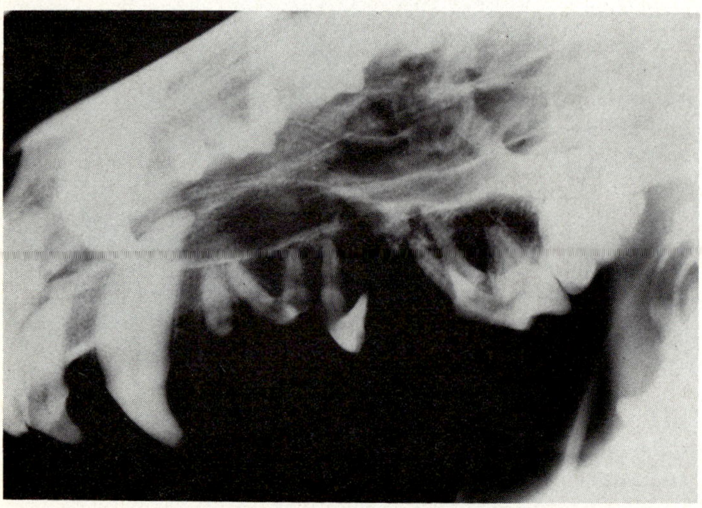

Figure 8–6. Radiograph of maxillary squamous cell carcinoma demonstrating extensive bone loss.

of tumor differentiation. Well-differentiated tumors have a more clearly defined basement membrane, and there is evidence of stratification and differentiation in the proliferative downgrowths. Nevertheless, even well-differentiated tumors have a tendency to locally invade soft tissue and bone. The histomorphological characteristics of squamous cell carcinomata and their relationship to the expected biological behavior and response to therapy need to be studied in a large number of cases in which both the histological criteria and the treatment modalities are carefully controlled.

Tonsillar Squamous Cell Carcinoma

Tonsillar carcinoma is a highly aggressive tumor that carries a very poor prognosis for the patient. The clinical signs reflect oropharyngeal obstruction and include dysphagia, cervical enlargement, dyspnea, anorexia, cough, and drooling.[7, 10] The tonsils may be small, and on initial inspection they may appear normal, whereas the regional lymph nodes (usually mandibular) are often dramatically enlarged. Thus, clinicians may incorrectly diagnose the cervical mass as a primary thyroid carcinoma or a lymphosarcoma and fail to appreciate the primary tumor. Careful inspection and biopsy of the tonsils under anesthesia are often required to ensure a correct diagnosis. If a fine-needle aspirate of the mandibular lymph nodes yields a diagnosis of carcinoma, a diagnostic tonsillectomy should be performed, regardless of the gross appearance of the tonsils.

Squamous cell carcinoma of the tonsil may appear as a large, proliferative or ulcerative tumor that results in oropharyngeal obstruction (Fig. 8–7), or the tonsil may be only minimally enlarged, firm, and slightly nodular in appearance. Occasionally, the tonsil may be destroyed and replaced with a red or gray, granular plaque that has invaded the surrounding tissue.[7] About 10 percent of tonsillar squamous cell carcinomata are bilateral.[10] The mandibular lymph nodes are usually enlarged, reflecting the high incidence of metastatic disease.[7, 10] The ipsilateral lymph node is usually affected, though the contralateral node may also have metastases. Spread to retropharyngeal lymph nodes is frequent.[7] In one study, 96 percent of dogs with tonsillar squamous cell carcinoma had metastases to regional lymph nodes.[7]

Histologically, squamous cell carcinoma of the tonsil in dogs is usually a poorly differentiated and locally invasive neoplasm. In cases of chronic inflammatory disease of the tonsil, the epithelium will sometimes show a proliferative change that has to be differentiated from tonsillar carcinoma. The tonsillar epithelium basement membrane may appear to be disrupted in inflammatory disease. Little is known about the prognostic significance of the histological appearance of tonsillar squamous cell carcinoma in dogs.

Fibrosarcoma

Fibrosarcoma is the third most common malignant neoplasm of the oral cavity in the

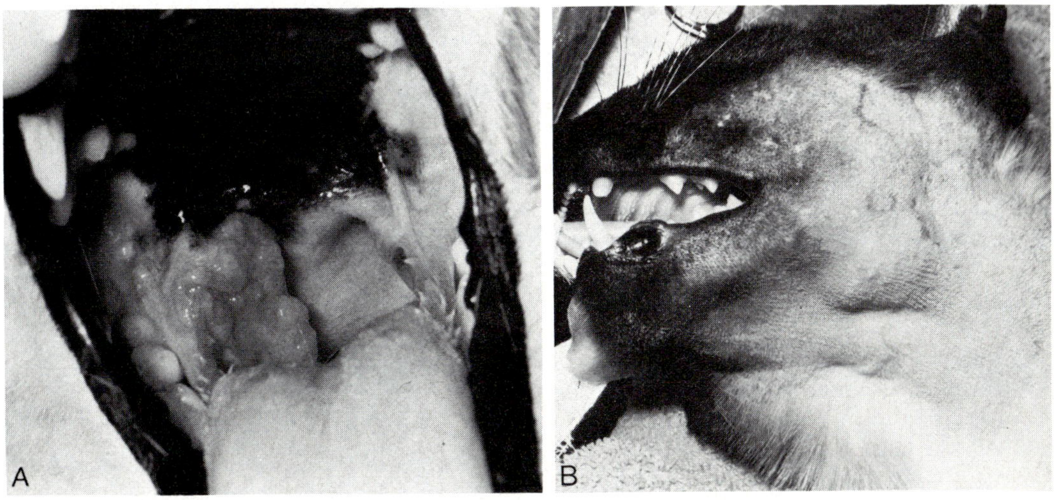

Figure 8–7. *A*, A proliferative tonsillar squamous cell carcinoma of the right tonsil in a cat. These tumors have a very high incidence of metastasis. *B*, The tumor has metastasized to the mandibular lymph nodes.

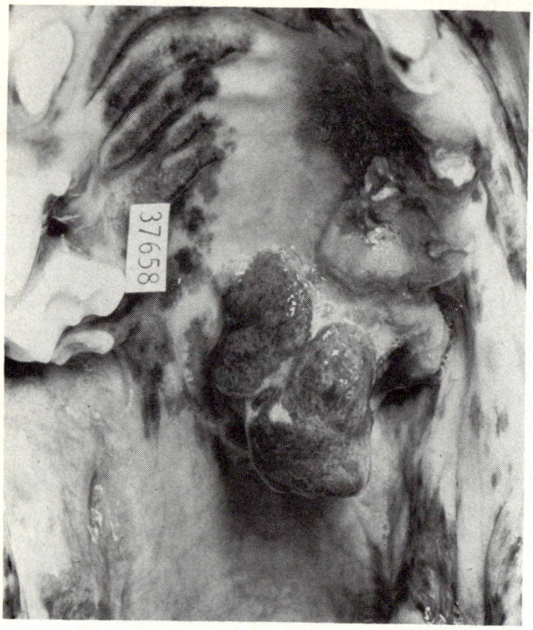

Figure 8–8. Fibrosarcoma of the hard palate is demonstrated in this photograph, though a gingival location is more common.

dog.[3,4,9,10] Although it is the second most frequently diagnosed oral neoplasm in cats, it remains uncommon.[3,4,6,8] This tumor occurs in slightly younger dogs (average age of 8 years) than melanoma (11 years) or carcinoma (9 years).[10] Fibrosarcoma is twice as common in males as in females.[4,10] Larger breeds of dogs tend to develop fibrosarcoma more frequently than do small breeds.[10] The gingivae are the most common sites for fibrosarcoma formation (87 percent), though fibrosarcoma of the hard palate is also seen (Fig. 8–8).[10]

The tumors are firm and are often deeply attached to the underlying tissue. They are usually smooth and multilobulated, with ulceration being more uncommon than with other malignancies. Regional lymph nodes are rarely enlarged, reflecting the low tendency for metastases. Fibrosarcoma is locally invasive, resulting in early bone destruction.[5,7–10]

As with other malignant oral neoplasms, fibrosarcomata vary in their histomorphological characteristics. The degree of differentiation or anaplasia does not correlate well with the expected biological behavior and the response to therapy. The establishment of a histological diagnosis of oral fibrosarcoma can be difficult if the biopsy is poorly taken; the most common mistake is to remove an inadequate sample. The morphological features of the superficial portions of the soft tissue tumor are often complicated and changed by a superficial inflammatory reaction. Edema and neovascularization disrupt the characteristic pattern of connective tissue growth that is diagnostic of fibrosarcoma. Sometimes oral fibrosarcomata appear to be extremely edematous throughout the tumor. Some oral fibrosarcomata are extremely well-differentiated, tempting the pathologist to diagnose fibroma. In these instances, it is useful to refer to the clinical aspects of the case, which will usually suggest a malignant rather than a benign disease.

Lymphosarcoma

On gross examination, lymphosarcoma of the tonsils may be confused with squamous cell carcinoma (Fig. 8–9). In lymphosarcoma, the tonsils are bilaterally involved and are quite large and pink. The appearance of the tonsil is smooth and uniform. There is usually generalized lymphadenopathy, though isolated tonsillar enlargement is occasionally encountered. Histologically, lymphosarcoma of the tonsils resembles lymphosarcoma of other lymphoid organs. The normal architecture of the tonsil is replaced by a homogenous sheet of neoplastic lymphocytes.

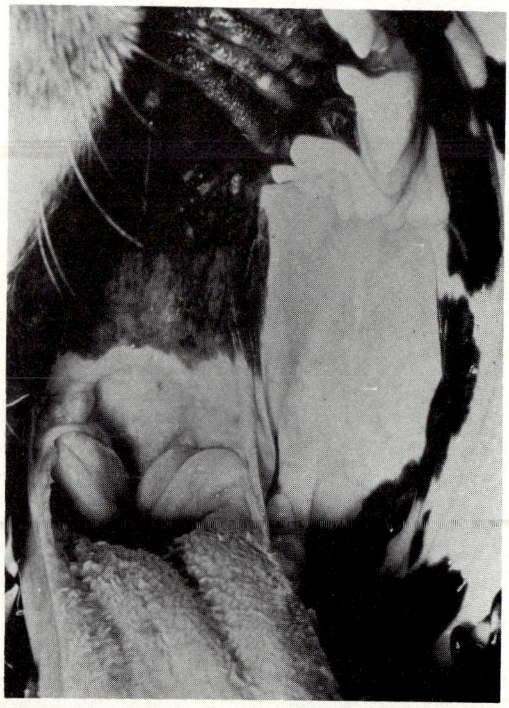

Figure 8–9. Tonsillar lymphosarcoma appears as a bilateral enlargement of the tonsils, being firm and pink in color.

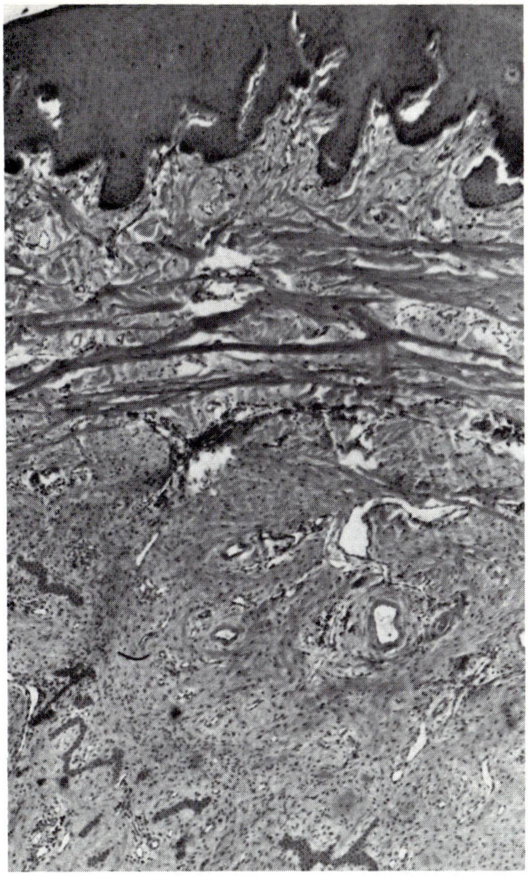

Figure 8–10. Photomicrograph of gingivae, showing gingival epithelium with normal subgingival stroma invaded by a fibromatous epulis. Notice the qualitative difference in the stroma of the epulis compared with the normal gingival stroma. Strands of epithelial cells are seen in the fibromatous epulis stroma.

Epulis

As already stated, tumors of the periodontal ligament (epulides) are the most common benign oral tumors in dogs.[5, 14, 21] One author reports that 25 percent of all canine oral neoplasms are of periodontal origin.[5] The three types of recognized epulides include fibromatous epulis, ossifying epulis, and acanthomatous epulis.[14] The average age of dogs with epulides is about 8 years, though these tumors may be seen in young dogs. The incidence among males and females is equal.[14] A familial predisposition has been reported in boxer dogs.[21]

The morphological hallmark of the epulides is the presence of periodontal ligament–type stroma (Fig. 8–10). Other features that may or may not be present in all types of epulides are long strands of interconnecting epithelium reminiscent of dental laminar epithelium and collagenous hard matrix substance. The collagenous matrix can be of three types: osseous, dentinous, or cementoid. They are difficult for the morphologist to differentiate (Fig. 8–11). If a major portion of the tumor is made up of collagenous hard matrix, particularly if it is osteoid, the tumor should be classified as ossifying epulis of periodontal origin. The hallmark of acanthomatous epulis is interbranching sheets of epithelial cells (Fig. 8–12). These cells are large and polyhedral in the central portions of the sheets and usually display prominent intracellular bridges. They have the morphological characteristics of acanthocytes, hence, the name acanthomatous epulis. Peripherally, the epithelial cells tend to palisade in a manner reminiscent of ameloblasts. The epithelial portion of acanthomatous epulis has the potential for local invasion in a manner very similar to that of squamous cell

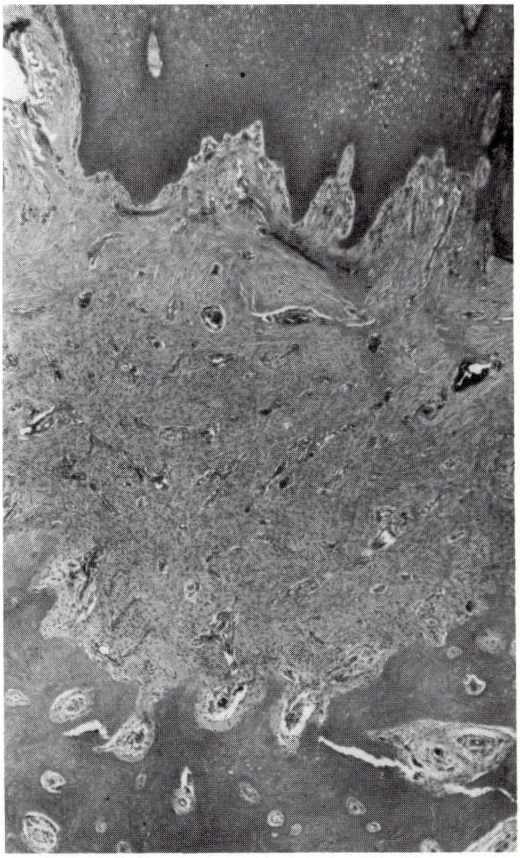

Figure 8–11. Photomicrograph of ossifying epulis of periodontal origin. Periodontal ligament–type stroma is seen abutting against the gingival epithelium. Collagenous hard matrix reminiscent of osteoid is seen deep in the epulis.

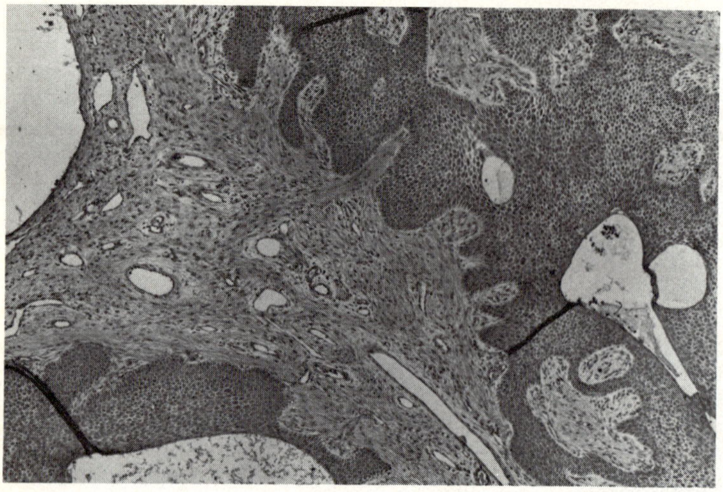

Figure 8–12. Photomicrograph of an acanthomatous epulis, showing interbranching sheets of epithelial cells with smooth basement membranes and intercellular separation within the sheets. The stroma has the characteristics of periodontal ligament–type stroma.

carcinoma. Keratinization is never seen with acanthomatous epulis, and the basement membrane surfaces tend to be smooth and intact. These features, plus the presence of periodontal ligament–type stroma, are important in differentiating squamous cell carcinoma from acanthomatous epulis.

Fibromatous epulis is a firm, smooth-surfaced, pedunculated or sessile mass at the gingival recess (Fig. 8–13). The tumor may be single, but multiple tumors are more usual. Although they are benign and noninvasive growths, they can become rather extensive and envelop the teeth. This tumor has been called by a variety of names, including epulis, fibromatous epulis of periodontal origin, and gingival hypertrophy or hyperplasia. The dense cellular stroma and collagen resemble the periodontal membrane, but remnants of dental laminar epithelium and small amounts of osteoid, dentin, or cementum are also present.[14, 15] Therapy is not necessary unless the tumor interferes with mastication, in which case surgery is curative if the site of origin is resected. Recurrence is common following superficial resection.

If the epulis has a prominent osteoid component, the tumor is classified as an ossifying epulis. The biological behavior of this tumor is identical to that of the fibromatous epulis.[14, 15]

Acanthomatous epulis is also of perio-

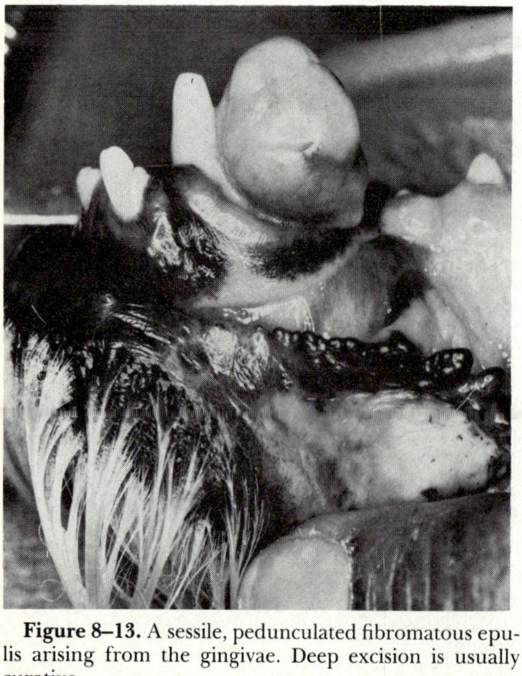

Figure 8–13. A sessile, pedunculated fibromatous epulis arising from the gingivae. Deep excision is usually curative.

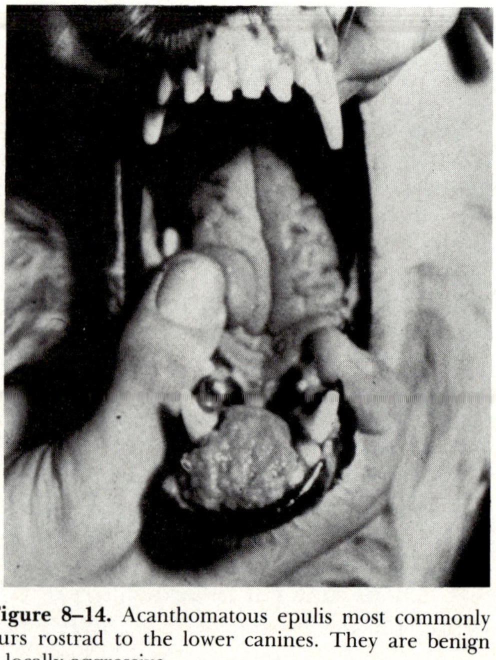

Figure 8–14. Acanthomatous epulis most commonly occurs rostrad to the lower canines. They are benign but locally aggressive.

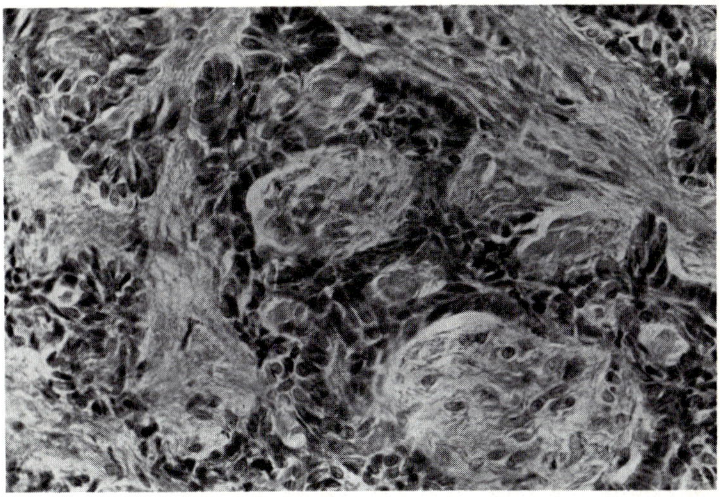

Figure 8–15. Photomicrograph of an ameloblastoma, showing interbranching strands of epithelial cells.

dontal origin, but it is characterized by large amounts of acanthomatous epithelium in cords or solid sheets with prominent intracellular bridges.[14, 15] Earlier reports classified this tumor as an adamantinoma,[22] though this term should be abandoned and the tumor referred to as an acanthomatous epulis.[14] These tumors occur most frequently on the mandible, rostral to the incisors (Fig. 8–14), but they can occur anyplace in the dental arcade. The behavior of acanthomatous epulis is that of a locally aggressive tumor with resulting bone lysis.[13, 14, 22]

Tumors of Dental Epithelial Origin

Ameloblastoma (keratinizing ameloblastoma) is the most frequent of the rather rare tumors of dental laminar epithelium.[14, 15, 23] There is no association among sex, breed, and anatomical site for these tumors.[23] They are soft, fleshy tumors that are visible on the gingivae, but they originate from the deeper dental epithelium.[23, 24] Ameloblastoma can be quite cystic or solid and can often result in osteolysis and production of new bone. Teeth become loose and if not extracted will fall out. The histological finding of enamel inclusions is highly suggestive of an ameloblastic tumor.

Several histological features are important in diagnosing ameloblastoma. Epithelial cells exist in either long strands or broad sheets. Palisading is common at the periphery, and separation with prominent intracellular bridges occurs centrally in the sheets of epithelial cells (Fig. 8–15). There may be collagenous matrix reminiscent of osteoid, cementum, or dentin. Often, there is an intimate association of the epithelial cells and the collagenous matrix, suggesting an inductive effect. Keratinization frequently occurs in the epithelial cells, and is seen as the formation

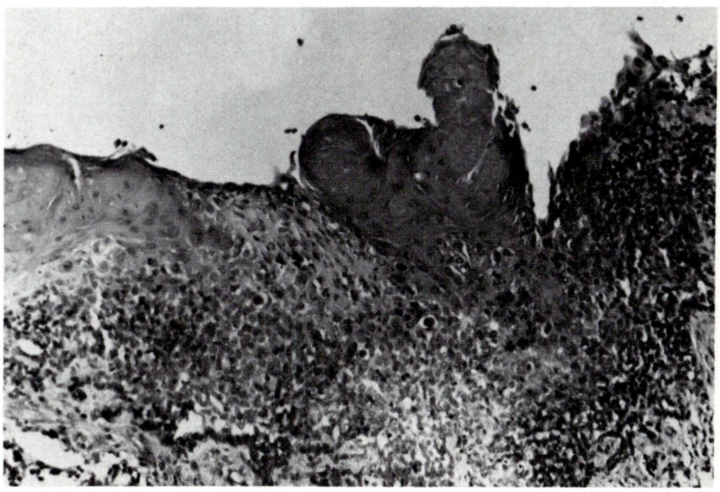

Figure 8–16. Photomicrograph of a keratinizing ameloblastoma. The large, ballooning keratinocytes are characteristic.

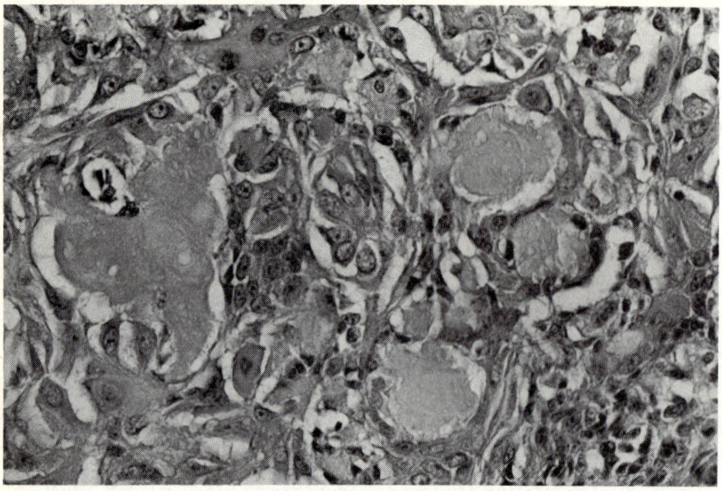

Figure 8–17. Photomicrograph of an ameloblastoma showing intercellular hyaline inclusions.

of large ballooning keratocytes (Fig. 8–16). The stroma does not have the characteristics of periodontal ligament–type stroma. Another common feature of ameloblastoma is the presence of intracellular hyaline inclusions (Fig. 8–17). Recently, it has been shown in some cases that these inclusions have characteristics of amyloid. Ameloblastoma is differentiated from acanthomatous epulis by the presence and nature of the keratinization, the lack of periodontal ligament–type stroma, and the presence of intracellular hyaline deposits. Ameloblastoma is differentiated from squamous cell carcinoma by the nature of the keratinization; the presence of induced collagenous matrices, such as osteoid, dentin or cementum; and the presence of intracellular hyaline inclusions.

Odontomata (complex and compound) are very rare in dogs.[6, 13] The cells of these tumors are capable of making all the dental tissues, including enamel, cementum, dentin, and pulp. There must be epithelium reminiscent of ameloblastic epithelium and a matrix reminiscent of dentin, with an intimate approximation of the two tissues that can be called inductive (Fig. 8–18). The adjectives, complex or compound, are applied based on whether the tumor is poorly differentiated or well differentiated.[11, 15, 16] The compound odontoma may have a number of tooth-like structures reflecting its high degree of differentiation (Fig. 8–19).[16]

Ameloblastic odontomata have features of both ameloblastomata and odontomata. These tumors have ameloblastic cells that are typical of ameloblastoma, but they also have an enamel matrix and dentin.[11, 15, 16]

Oral Papilloma

Oral papillomatosis in dogs is caused by infection with a papovavirus. The tumor affects young animals of any breed and either

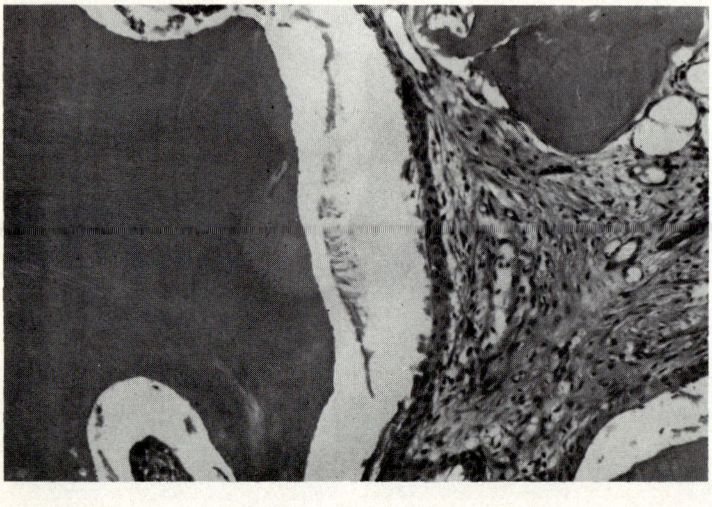

Figure 8–18. Photomicrograph of a complex odontoma, showing well-formed dentin, ameloblastic-like epithelium, and partially decalcified enamel matrix. Although all the elements of normal odontogenesis are present, they are not organized into tooth-like structures as would be seen in a compound odontoma.

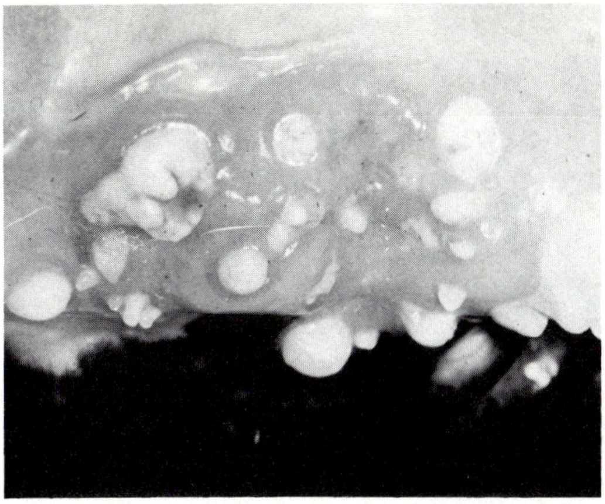

Figure 8–19. Compound odontoma in the maxilla of a dog producing many tooth-like structures.

sex.[6] Initially, papillomata are smooth, white, and slightly elevated, and occur around the lips or tongue. They then become more cauliflower-like, and fine villous projections are noted on the surface of the tumors (Figs. 8–20 and 8–21). The warts may be single or multiple and can extend to the palate, buccal cavity, or oropharynx. The incubation period is 5 weeks.[25] Lesions persist for 4 to 8 weeks, with spontaneous regression commonly occurring.[25] Histologically, oral papillomata are characterized by a verrucous proliferation of both epithelium and stroma. The basement membrane of the epithelial component is

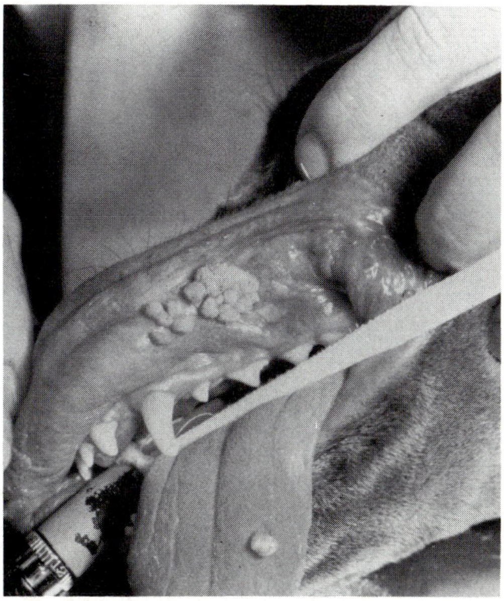

Figure 8–20. Papillomatosis appearing as a small cauliflower-like growth on the tongue and gingiva.

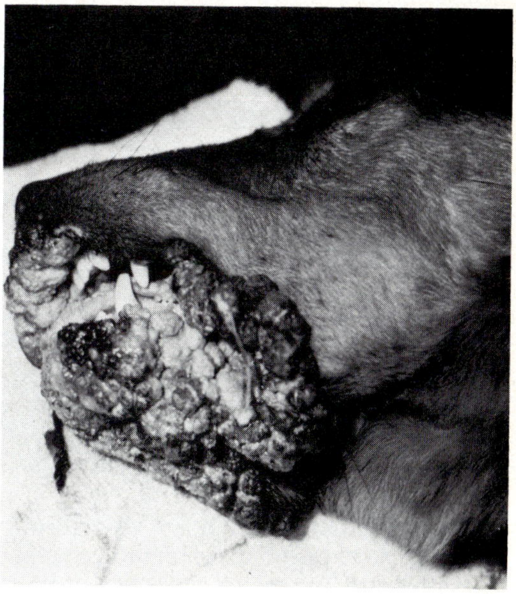

Figure 8–21. An advanced case of papillomatosis invading the lower and upper jaw. The papillomata have coalesced into one mass.

smooth and intact, and there is little or no tendency for this component to infiltrate.

Benign Oral Tumors in Cats

Benign oral tumors are rare in the cat, and though retrospective studies note the occurrence of fibromata, ameloblastomata, and odontomata, there are few detailed reports on the epidemiology of benign feline oral tumors.[3–6, 8, 26] Six cats with inductive fibroameloblastoma were reported recently. All of the cats were young, and the tumor affected the rostral maxilla.[15, 17]

Inductive fibroameloblastomata contain ameloblastic epithelium and dental pulp–like stroma. The ameloblastic epithelium exists in cup-like structures containing dental pulp–like differentiation of the stroma in their center (Fig. 8–22). This arrangement suggests an inductive relationship between the ameloblastic cells and the stroma, hence, the term "inductive fibroameloblastoma." Metastatic disease has not been recorded. Ameloblastomata also occur in cats, and their behavior is similar to the disease described in dogs.[2, 12, 26]

DIAGNOSTIC TECHNIQUES

Considering the advanced age of most animals having oropharyngeal neoplasms, a

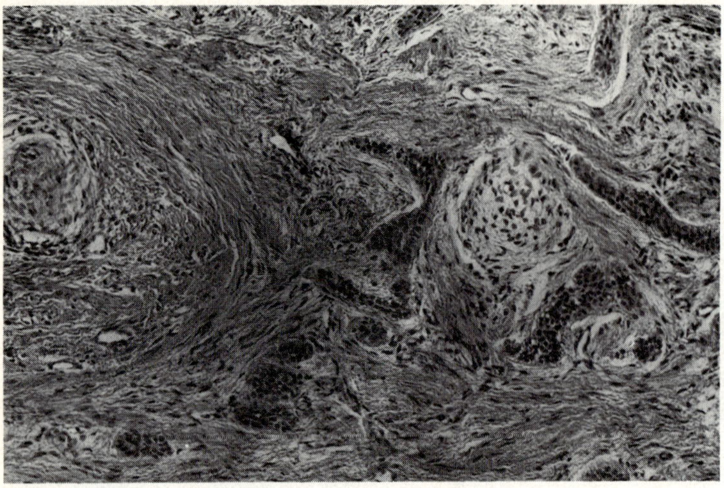

Figure 8–22. Photomicrograph of an inductive fibroameloblastoma from a young cat. Strands of epithelial cells are seen surrounding nests of stromal tissue that have the appearance of dental pulp–like stroma.

thorough geriatric evaluation to determine the medical status of the patient is essential. In addition to a thorough history and physical examination, a minimum data base is required, and consists of the following: a complete blood count (CBC), a urinalysis, liver and kidney function tests (serum glutamic pyruvic transaminase [SGPT], serum alkaline phosphatase, blood urea nitrogen [BUN], and creatinine determinations), a blood glucose determination, and a total serum protein (albumin:globulin ratio) determination (Table 8–2). This data may reveal impending organ failure and will allow the clinician to select the most appropriate therapy. Radiotherapy requiring numerous anesthetic episodes may not be advisable if significant kidney or liver dysfunction is evident. When planning chemotherapy, drugs that are activated by the liver, such as cyclophosphamide, should be avoided if hepatic disease is present.

Skull radiographs should be taken in all animals with gingival or palatine tumors or when any tumor is fixed to bone, in order to determine the presence and extent of bone invasion. Lateral, oblique, and intraoral projections may be needed to demonstrate bone invasion. Radiographic evidence of an osteolytic or osteoblastic reaction was present in 77 percent of dogs with squamous cell carcinoma, 68 percent of dogs with fibrosarcoma, and 57 percent of dogs with malignant melanoma.[10] The actual incidence of bone invasion is probably higher than reported, since 40 percent of existing bone must be destroyed before lesions are seen radiographically.

Table 8–2. Minimum Data Base in the Evaluation of Patients with Oropharyngeal Neoplasms

Complete blood count (CBC)
Liver function tests (SGPT, serum alkaline phosphatase)
Renal function tests (BUN, creatinine determinations)
Blood glucose determination
Total serum protein (A:G ratio)
Urinalysis
Skull radiographs
Thoracic radiographs
Biopsy and histopathological evaluation of the lesion
Lymph node aspirate or biopsy

Thoracic radiographs are essential for all animals with oropharyngeal tumors. Based on the interpretation of chest radiographs, 14 percent of dogs with malignant melanoma, 10 percent of dogs with fibrosarcoma, 8 percent of dogs with tonsillar squamous cell carcinoma, and 3 percent of dogs with non-tonsillar carcinoma had lung metastases.[10] The incidence of false-negative thoracic radiographs is high; at least 13 percent of dogs with malignant melanoma have lung metastases at autopsy, despite negative chest radiographs.[10]

The most critical procedure in the evaluation of a patient with oropharyngeal neoplasia is a biopsy. It allows the clinician to establish the diagnosis, formulate a treatment regime, and give the owner an accurate prognosis. Tissue may be procured through an excisional biopsy, a wedge biopsy, or a needle punch. The only guideline is that the biopsy must avoid areas of superficial necrosis and must sample the deeper, viable tissue. Electrocautery should not be used on small samples because the entire biopsy will be coagulated. If the results of the biopsy do not correlate with the gross appearance of the oral mass, it is advisable to obtain a second biopsy.

Based on necropsy findings from 139 dogs with oropharyngeal neoplasms, it seems reasonable to recommend surgical removal or biopsy of regional lymph nodes for purposes of staging the disease.[10] Although necropsy results may represent a biased sample because they reflect animals with advanced disease or recurrence of disease, 73 percent of dogs with tonsillar squamous cell carcinoma, 60 percent of dogs with melanoma, and 19 percent of dogs with fibrosarcoma had metastases to regional lymph nodes at autopsy.[10] Cytological examination of lymph node aspirates may be adequate for diagnosing metastatic melanomata and tonsillar squamous cell carcinomata. Nodes that test positive for tumor can be treated with radiotherapy or radiotherapy and adjuvant chemotherapy.

STAGING

The World Health Organization has formulated the TNM (tumor-node-metastases) classification for canine and feline tumors of the lips, oral cavity, and oropharynx. Stage

Table 8–3. WHO Staging System for Tumors of the Oral Cavity

Feline or Canine Tumors of the Oral Cavity (Buccal Cavity) Clinical Stages T N M

Date__________ Dog/Cat__________

Case Number__________

Name of Owner__________

Age _____ Sex_____ Breed__________

Body Weight__________ lbs__________ kgs
(1 kg = 2.2 lbs)

The following classification applies to the rostral two thirds of the tongue, the floor of the mouth, the buccal mucosa, the alveolus, and the hard palate.

Circle appropriate classification for each category:

T-Primary Tumor

- Tis Preinvasive carcinoma (carcinoma *in situ*)
- T0
- T1 Tumor 2 cm or less maximum diameter
  (a) without bone involvement (b) with bone involvement
- T2 Tumor 2–4 cm maximum diameter
  (a) without bone involvement (b) with bone involvement
- T3 Tumor more than 4 cm maximum diameter
  (a) without bone involvement (b) with bone involvement

N-Regional Lymph Nodes

- N0 Regional lymph nodes not palpable
- N1 Movable ipsilateral nodes
  - $N1_a$ Nodes not considered to contain growth*
  - $N1_b$ Nodes considered to contain growth*†
- N2 Movable contralateral or bilateral nodes
  - $N2_a$ Nodes not considered to contain growth*
  - $N2_b$ Nodes not considered to contain growth*†
- N3 Fixed nodes

M-Distant Metastasis

- M0 No evidence of distant metastases
- M1† Distant metastases present—specify sites:

Stage Grouping

Stage	T	N	M
I	T1	N0, $N1_a$, or $N2_a$	M0
II	T2	N0, $N1_a$, or $N2_a$	M0
III*	T3	N0, $N1_a$, or $N2_a$	
IV	Any T	$N1_b$	M0
	Any T	Any $N2_b$ or N3	M0
	Any T	Any N	M1

*Histologically negative, †histologically positive.
†Distant nodes to be included.

grouping has been suggested for oral cavity tumors and will allow large cooperative prospective studies to be performed (Table 8–3)[27] and should provide prognostic information as well as accurate comparison of treatment results among different investigators.

TREATMENT PRINCIPLES

The management of oropharyngeal neoplasms is dependent upon accurately diagnosing and staging the disease. This information, in conjunction with the known biological behavior of individual tumors, allows one to plan therapy rationally. There is no protocol available that is adequate for all tumors, and therapy should be individualized. The following list outlines the treatment principles for oropharyngeal tumors.

1. The first surgical procedure offers the best chance for cure.
2. Wide local excision should include 1 cm of healthy tissue.
3. Aggressive surgical techniques may improve survival times, especially in epulides and dental tumors.
4. Squamous cell carcinomata appear to be radiosensitive, whereas fibrosarcomata and melanomata respond poorly.
5. Radiation of acanthomatous epulides and ameloblastomata has resulted in prolonged survival times.
6. Malignant melanomata and tonsillar squamous cell carcinomata have a guarded prognosis. Adjuvant therapy may be helpful, but see No. 7.
7. No recommendation can be made regarding the use of chemotherapy or immunotherapy because available data is insufficient at present.

Surgery

Surgery has been and remains the most important modality for treating oropharyngeal neoplasms. Unfortunately, conservative scalpel incision often fails to control local disease, either because of inadequate soft tissue removal or because of unknown bone invasion. The anatomical site of the tumor (e.g., the hard palate) often precludes complete surgical extirpation using conservative techniques. In some cases, local control can be achieved, but the presence of metastatic disease results in treatment failure.

The first operation provides the best opportunity to cure a malignant tumor, therefore casual removal of an oral mass or a quick biopsy is contraindicated. The biopsy procedure and tumor removal may be combined for small lesions, whereas larger lesions needing extensive surgery may require separate surgical procedures. The tumor should be widely excised, including at least 1 cm of surrounding healthy tissue.[28, 29] This rule is often difficult to adhere to with oropharyngeal neoplasms and is a major cause of treatment failure.[10, 20] With the advent of more aggressive surgical techniques, including hemimandibulectomy and partial maxillectomy, the potential for long-term control and cure by surgical means has increased.[30, 31] These techniques are described in Chapter 10. Multimodality therapy for the management of oropharyngeal neoplasms may be preferable to simple surgical excision. In the case of gingival squamous cell carcinoma, surgical resection of most of the mass, combined with radiation, can be effective.

Cryosurgery

Cryosurgery for oropharyngeal neoplasms has been used as a primary treatment modality or as an adjunct to scalpel excision. Advantages of cryosurgery in the treatment of oral neoplasms include (1) ease of application, (2) shortened surgical time, (3) low postoperative morbidity in high-risk patients, (4) good hemostasis, (5) rapid relief of discomfort and odor, (6) destruction of tumor cells in the bone that are inaccessible to scalpel excision, and (7) normal anatomy and function are preserved because dead bone behaves as an allograft and becomes revascularized.[32, 33]

The best use of cryosurgery is when minimal bone invasion is present, on small oral masses, or for freezing the bony tumor bed after the bulk of the neoplasm has been removed by electrosurgery. Cryosurgery is often misused in advanced cases of oral neoplasia, in which freezing causes further weakening of the bone, and pathological fractures may result. It also precludes histological examination of the margins. A study of 149 dogs with oral cancers treated by cryosurgery alone yielded mean survival times of 147 days for melanoma, 154 days for fibrosarcoma, and 240 days for squamous cell carcinoma.[33] Complications resulting from cryosurgery include severe hemorrhage (though this is rare), edema of the oral cavity, air embolism resulting in death, mandibular fracture, and oronasal fistula.[32] Although cryosurgery probably has a role in the management of oropharyngeal neoplasms, controlled studies comparing the results with other treatment methods are needed before specific recommendations for its use can be made.

Hyperthermia

Hyperthermia is an investigational treatment modality in managing human and animal cancer patients that has applicability in oropharyngeal tumors.[34–37] Temperatures greater than 45 degrees C cause protein denaturaton of both normal and neoplastic cells, and host damage ensues at this temperature.[35] Temperatures between 41 degrees C and 45 degrees C have a tumoricidal effect, but the mechanism of action is poorly understood.[38, 39] Cellular hypoxia and acidosis are felt to be important factors that result in cellular damage.[38] Methods of achieving hyperthermia include radiofrequency current or ultrasound.[35] Hyperthermia is probably of most value in combination with radiation therapy.[34, 35, 37] A mean survival time of 13 months was reported in 10 dogs with oral fibrosarcoma managed by radiotherapy and hyperthermia,[37] which is better than radiation alone.[40, 41]

Electrosurgery

Electrosurgery is used primarily for debulking large tumors prior to cryosurgery or radiotherapy. It is also useful for highly vascular tumors in which the coagulating effects of electrical current are needed.

Radiotherapy

Radiotherapy is playing an increasingly important role in the management of oropharyngeal neoplasms. It may be used as the sole form of therapy or in an adjuvant role following incomplete surgical resection. Therapeutic x-ray machines (orthovoltage or megavoltage) or radioactive compounds ^{60}Co and ^{137}Cs are suitable sources of radiation. Diagnostic machines should never be used. Orthovoltage x-rays are most effective for treating superficial tumors with little bone involvement. Bone absorbs more radiation at its surface than does soft tissue, resulting in a reduced dose of radiation beneath the bone surface. As a result, oropharyngeal tumors with extensive bone involvement may be resistant to low-energy x-rays.

A total radiation dose of 4000 rad to 4500 rad (40 Gy to 45 Gy) is recommended, and should be given in ten fractions on a Monday, Wednesday, and Friday schedule.[42–44] Tumor response is dependent on vascularity and oxygenation, size, and histological type. Two studies have determined that the response of oral fibrosarcomata to radiation is poor, with fewer than 10 percent of irradiated animals being free of signs of tumor at 18 months.[40, 41] Severe side effects, consisting of osteonecrosis, were observed in 2 of 13 dogs irradiated;[41] both studies used orthovoltage x-rays. The use of ^{60}Co gamma radiation may improve survival times. Misonidazole (a radiosensitizer of hypoxic cells) has been used in conjunction with orthovoltage radiotherapy for the treatment of oral fibrosarcoma in dogs. There was no significant improvement in results when compared with radiation alone.[45] The use of radioprotectors,[46, 47] radiosensitizers,[45, 47] and hyperthermia[34, 37] may improve the effectiveness of radiotherapy in the future. Radiotherapy can also be used for therapeutic or prophylactic treatment of regional lymph nodes in tonsillar squamous cell carcinoma and tonsillar melanoma, and it is probably more effective than lymphadenectomy in preventing tumor spread.

Treatment Modalities for Specific Tumors

Carcinomata appear to be more radiosensitive than do mesenchymal tumors.[44, 48] Radiation (3750 rad) provided tumor control for 12 months in 50 percent of dogs with gingival squamous cell carcinoma, with increased control at higher doses.[49] Recent clinical experience with the treatment of both gingival and tonsillar squamous cell carcinomata suggests that results are not as good as would be expected from *in vitro* tumor response curves.[50] Tonsillectomy followed by ^{60}Co gamma-radiation resulted in a mean survival time of 150 days in eight dogs treated.[51]

Acanthomatous epulis at the rostral mandible is best treated by surgical excision. If located elsewhere in the mouth, surgical resection may not be practical, and irradiation is the preferred treatment. It is not necessary to surgically reduce the size of the tumor before irradiating.[52] The response of acanthomatous epulis to radiation therapy is very good, with a mean survival time of 21 to 24 months.[52, 53] Malignant tumor formation at the site of previously irradiated acanthomatous epulis has been noted.[52]

The preferred method of treatment for

ameloblastoma is radical resection of bone (i.e., mandibulectomy or subtotal maxillectomy), which can result in cure. Less radical surgery, such as curettage, will afford prolonged remission (greater than 1 year), but recurrence is the rule.[23] In a small number of cases, radiotherapy has resulted in the prolonged remission of ameloblastoma.[23, 53]

There are no controlled clinical trials evaluating the efficacy of chemotherapy in the treatment of oropharyngeal neoplasms in animals. Anecdotal reports concerning the use of chemotherapy are encountered in the literature, but no recommendations can be made at this time. A preliminary evaluation of bleomycin in feline and canine squamous cell carcinomata showed that this antibiotic may cause temporary remissions in dermal tumors of low-grade malignancy, but that it was of limited value in highly invasive tumors.[54]

Published data from controlled trials on the role of immunotherapy in treating oral cancer are not available. A number of studies are being performed at veterinary institutions, and results should be available in the near future. Autogenous vaccines have been used in the treatment of canine oral papillomatosis with excellent results. This form of therapy is rarely needed, because spontaneous remission is the rule, with scalpel excision, cryosurgery, or electrocautery being used on refractory cases.

PROGNOSIS

The prognosis for any malignant tumor of the oropharynx is poor. Non-tonsillar squamous cell carcinomata have the best prognosis because they remain localized, with metastases developing late in the course of the disease. They are amenable to both surgery and radiation. Fibrosarcoma, though a localized disease, has a poorer prognosis. This reflects the local aggressiveness, radioresistance, and palatine location typical of this tumor, making surgical resection difficult. Melanomata have the poorest prognosis, with only 20 percent of patients surviving 1 year following surgical resection.[55] Metastases from the primary tumor site and local recurrence are responsible for treatment failures.

More aggressive surgical procedures, in conjunction with radiotherapy, should allow better prognosis for animals with non-tonsillar squamous cell carcinoma and fibrosarcoma. Chemotherapy, immunotherapy, and hyperthermia are areas that should be investigated through prospective studies for the treatment of melanoma and tonsillar squamous cell carcinoma.

Benign oropharyngeal tumors have a good prognosis. The prognosis for papillomatosis is excellent, as this tumor undergoes spontaneous remission or responds to simple surgical excision or cryosurgery. Epulides are often surgically curable, except for acanthomatous epulis, which may require radiotherapy. Dental tumors have a very good prognosis when aggressive surgery or irradiation, or both of these modalities, are used. Failures result because of inadequate surgical resection.

References

1. Dorn CR, Taylor DON, Frye FL, Hibbard HH: Survey of animal neoplasms in Alameda and Contra Costa Counties, California. I. Methodology and description of cases. *J Natl Cancer Inst* 40:295–305, 1968.
2. Dorn CR, Taylor DON, Schneider R, Hibbard HH, Klauber MR: Survey of animal neoplasms in Alameda and Contra Costa Counties, California. II. Cancer morbidity in dogs and cats from Alameda County. *J Natl Cancer Inst* 40:307–318, 1968.
3. Dorn CR, Priester WA: Epidemiologic analysis of oral and pharyngeal cancer in dogs, cats, horses and cattle. *J Am Vet Med Assoc* 169:802–806, 1976.
4. Priester WA, McKay FW: The occurrence of tumors in domestic animals. *Natl Cancer Inst Monographs,* NIH Publication No. 80–2046, Bethesda, Maryland.
5. Gorlin RJ, Barron C, Chaulhry AP, Clark AJ: The oral and pharyngeal pathology of domestic animals. A study of 487 cases. *Am J Vet Res* 20:1032–1061, 1959.
6. Gorlin RJ, Peterson WC: Oral disease in man and animals. *Arch Dermatol* 96:390–403, 1967.
7. Brodey RS: A clinical and pathologic study of 130 neoplasms of the mouth and pharynx in the dog. *Am J Vet Res* 21:787–788, 1960.
8. Brodey RS: A clinico-pathological study of 200 cases of oral and pharyngeal cancer in the dog. *In* New Knowledge about Dogs. New York, Gaines Dog Research Center, 1961, pp. 5–11.
9. Cohen D, Brodey RS, Chen MS: Epidemiology aspects of oral and pharyngeal neoplasms of the dog. *Am J Vet Res* 25:1776–1779, 1964.
10. Todoroff RJ, Brodey RS: Oral and pharyngeal neoplasia in the dog: A retrospective survey of 361 cases. *J Am Vet Med Assoc* 175:567–571, 1979.
11. Moulton JE: Tumors in domestic animals. Berkeley, University of California Press, 1978, pp. 240–250.
12. Cotter SM: Oral pharyngeal neoplasms in the cat. *J Am Anim Hosp Assoc* 17:917–920, 1981.
13. Gorlin RJ, Meskin LH, Brodey R: Odontogenic tumors in man and animals: Pathological classification and clinical behaviour. *NY Acad Sci* 108: 722–771, 1963.
14. Dubielzig RR, Goldschmidt MH, Brodey RS: The nomenclature of periodontal epulides in dogs. *Vet Pathol* 16:209–214, 1979.
15. Dubielzig RR: Proliferative dental and gingival disease of dogs and cats. *J Am Anim Hosp Assoc* 18:577–584, 1982.

16. Figueiredo C, Barros HM, Alvaros LE, Damanto JH: Composed complex odontoma in a dog. *Vet Med/Small Anim Clin* 69:268–270, 1974.
17. Dubielzig RR, Adams WM, Brodey RS: Inductive fibroameloblastoma, an unusual dental tumor of young cats. *J Am Vet Med Assoc* 174:220–222, 1975.
18. Weiss E, Frese K: Histological classification and nomenclature of tumors of the skin. Bull WHO 50:79–100, 1974.
19. Bostock DE: Prognosis after surgical excision of canine melanomas. *Vet Pathol* 16:32–40, 1979.
20. Bostock DE: The prognosis in cats bearing squamous cell carcinoma. *J Small Anim Pract* 13:111–125, 1972.
21. Burstone MS, Bond E, Lih R: Familial gingival hypertrophy in the dog (Boxer breed). *Arch Pathol* 54:208–212, 1952.
22. Langham RF, Keahey KK, Mostosky UV, Schirmer RG: Oral adamantinoma in the dog. *J Am Vet Med Assoc* 146:475–480, 1965.
23. Dubielzig RR, Thrall DE: Ameloblastoma and keratinizing ameloblastoma in dogs. *Vet Pathol* 19:596–607, 1982.
24. Langham RF, Mostosky UV, Schirmer RG: Ameloblastic odontoma in the dog. *Am J Vet Res* 30:1873–1876, 1969.
25. Konishi S, Tokita H: Studies of canine oral papillomatosis. I. Transmission and characterization of the virus. *Jap J Vet Sci* 34:263–268, 1974.
26. Brodey RS: Alimentary tract neoplasms in the cat. A clinicopathological survey of 46 cats. *Am J Vet Res* 27:74–80, 1966.
27. Owen LN (ed): TNM Classification of Tumors in Domestic Animals. Bulletin of the World Health Organization, 1st ed., 1980, pp. 21–25.
28. Withrow SJ: Surgical management of cancer. *In* MacEwen EG (ed): Vet Clin North Am: Small Animal Practice, Veterinary Clinical Oncology. Philadelphia: W. B. Saunders 1977; 7:13–20.
29. Brodey RS: Surgery. *In* Theilen GH, Madewell BR (eds): Veterinary Cancer Medicine. Philadelphia, Lea & Febiger, 1979.
30. Withrow SJ, Holmberg DL: Mandibulectomy in the treatment of oral cancer. *J Am Anim Hosp Assoc* 19:273–286, 1983.
31. Withrow SJ: Partial maxillectomy in the treatment of oral cancer. *J Am Anim Hosp Assoc.* In press.
32. Withrow SJ, Griener TP, Liska W: Cryosurgery: Veterinary considerations. *J Am Anim Hosp Assoc* 11:271–282, 1975.
33. Harvey HJ: Cryosurgery of oral tumors in dogs and cats. *In* Withrow SJ (ed): *Vet Clin North Am:* Cryosurgery, 1980; 10:821–830.
34. Lord PF, Kapp DS: Hyperthermia and radiation therapy in cancer treatment. *Vet Radiol* 23:203–210, 1982.
35. Core DN: Hyperthermia and cancer. *Comp Cont Ed Small Anim* 4:719–725, 1982.
36. Grier RL, Brewer WG, Theilen AH: Hyperthermic treatment of superficial tumors in cats and dogs. *J Am Vet Med Assoc* 177:227–233, 1980.
37. Brewer JG, Turrell JM: Radiotherapy in the treatment of fibrosarcomas in the dog. *J Am Vet Med Assoc* 1881:146–150, 1982.
38. Overgaard J, Bichol P: The influence of hypoxia and acidity on the hyperthermic response of malignant cells in vitro. *Radiology* 123:511–514, 1977.
39. Overgaard J: Effect of hyperthermia on malignant cells in vitro: A review and a hypothesis. *Cancer* 39:2637–2646, 1977.
40. Hilmas DE, Gillette EL: Radiotherapy of spontaneous fibrous connective tissue sarcomas in animals. *J Natl Cancer Inst* 56:365–368, 1976.
41. Thrall DE: Orthovoltage radiotherapy of oral fibrosarcomas in dogs. *J Am Vet Med Assoc* 179:159–162, 1981.
42. Silver IA: Use of radiotherapy for the treatment of malignant neoplasms. *J Small Anim Pract* 13:351–358, 1972.
43. Gillette EL: Radiation therapy of canine and feline tumors. *J Am Anim Hosp Assoc* 8:359–362, 1976.
44. Gillette EL: Radiotherapy. *In* Theilen GH, Madewell BR: Veterinary Cancer Medicine. Philadelphia, Lea & Febiger, 1979, pp. 85–94.
45. Creasey WA, Phil D, Thrall DE: Pharmacokinetic and antitumor studies with the radiosensitizer misonidazole in dogs with spontaneous fibrosarcomas. *Am J Vet Res* 43:1015–1018, 1982.
46. Walker MA: A review of drugs that may be used in conjunction with radiotherapy. *Vet Radiol* 23: 220–222, 1982.
47. Thrall DE, Beiry DN, Girardi AJ: Evaluation of radiation and WR-2721 in dogs with spontaneous tumors. *In* Brady L (ed): Radiation Sensitizers: Their Use in the Clinical Management of Cancer. New York, Masson Publishing, USA Inc., 1980, pp. 343–347.
48. Banks WC, Morris CE: Results of radiation treatment of naturally occurring animal tumors. *J Am Vet Med Assoc* 166:1063–1065, 1975.
49. Gillette EL: Large animal studies of hyperthermia and irradiation. *Cancer Res* 37:2242–2244, 1971.
50. Thrall DE, Jeglum A: Personal communication, 1983.
51. MacMillan R, Withrow SJ, Gillette EL: Surgery and regional radiation for tonsillar squamous cell carcinoma: retrospective review of eight cases. *J Am Anim Hosp Assoc* 18:311–314, 1982.
52. Thrall DE, Goldschmidt MH, Biery DN: Malignant tumor formation at the site of previously irradiated acanthomatous epulides in four dogs. *J Am Vet Med Assoc* 178:127–132, 1981.
53. Langham RF, Mostosky UV, Schirmer RC: X-ray therapy of selected odontogenic neoplasms in the dog. *J Am Vet Med Assoc* 170:320–322, 1977.
54. Buhles WC, Theilen JH: Preliminary evaluation of bleomycin in feline and canine squamous cell carcinoma. *Am J Vet Res* 34:289–291, 1973.
55. Harvey HJ, MacEwen EB, Brown D, Paitnaik AK, Withrow SJ, Jongeward S: Prognostic criteria for dogs with oral melanoma. *J Am Vet Med Assoc* 178:580–582, 1980.

Chapter Nine

Trauma to Oral Structures

JP Weigel

INTRODUCTION

Healing of oral wounds is similar to wound healing elsewhere in the body. However, there are modifying factors within the oral cavity that affect healing. The following factors all play a role in the healing process: the unique biomechanical and anatomical function of the bones of the face and jaw; the protruding teeth; specialized tissue such as the gingivae; the constant exposure to contamination; and the specialized medium of saliva, food, and foreign material. Although these factors might retard healing in other areas of the body, healing in the oral cavity usually progresses rapidly, the major reason being the abundant vascular supply.

Oral wounds are frequently contaminated, but if the immune system is normal the resident organisms do not affect the oral cavity. The persistent presence of organisms results in a low-grade, chronic inflammatory response of the gingivae, which may, in fact, stimulate healing.[1] However, if a drug or an abnormal condition reduces body defenses, or if a wound is necrotic, infection can be established.

Moisture will affect the condition of the oral mucosa. An exposed and traumatized oral mucosa becomes dehydrated rapidly and is easily invaded by organisms.

Injury to oral structures is often associated with other bodily injury. Head trauma is evidenced by central neural deficits, palpable fractures, and subcutaneous emphysema from fractured nasal or frontal bones. The neurological status of such patients should be evaluated and monitored. An important consideration for the emergency clinician is a patent airway. The oral cavity ends at the pharynx, which can be compromised by hemorrhage, bone fragments, and edema. In treating and examining such individuals, the emergency clinician must be ready to place an endotracheal tube or to perform a tracheostomy quickly if upper respiratory obstruction occurs.

Suture selection is important in oral surgery. Sutures without stiff, irritating ends are preferable. Surgical gut loses strength quickly and cannot withstand the trauma and moist environment of the oral cavity. In general, braided sutures are preferred for intraoral surgery because they are well tolerated by the patient and do not untie during wound healing (see also page 156).

Suturing of oral wounds may be unnecessary because they granulate well. If the wound has exposed bone or a fistula communicating with the nasal cavity, second intention healing may be prolonged or inhibited, resulting in a sequestrum or fistula. In general, the principles of open, contaminated wound treatment apply to oral structures.

MAXILLARY FRACTURES

Fractures of the facial bones, the hard palate, and the upper arcade of dentition do not require surgical treatment. Most fractures of these bones do not cause severe displacement and will heal quickly with conservative measures. Exceptions include malocclusion, large areas of oronasal communication, malalignment with facial deformity, and obstruction to airflow through the nasal cavity.

Simple maxillary fractures are easy to realign soon after injury, but realignment is difficult if they are multiple or comminuted. Malaligned or overriding multiple fragments can jam against each other and prevent anatomical reduction. In some cases, it is necessary to surgically expose fracture lines, appose them individually, and stabilize them with orthopedic wire or stainless steel pins. Accurate reduction is necessary for good occlusion and cosmetic appearance. Severe maxillary or facial fractures in puppies can disturb normal growth and result in facial deformities in the adult (see Fig. 7–3). Compromise of normal sinus drainage can result in subsequent blockage and infection. Displaced fragments with excessive callus formation may also cause obstruction of the nasal passages.

Sequestration of bone fragments within the nasal cavity is infrequent, and generally there is no reasonable indication for exploring each fracture specifically for the purpose of removing potential sequestered bone. However, this should be considered as a potential complication and investigated if rhinitis follows the healing of a maxillary fracture.

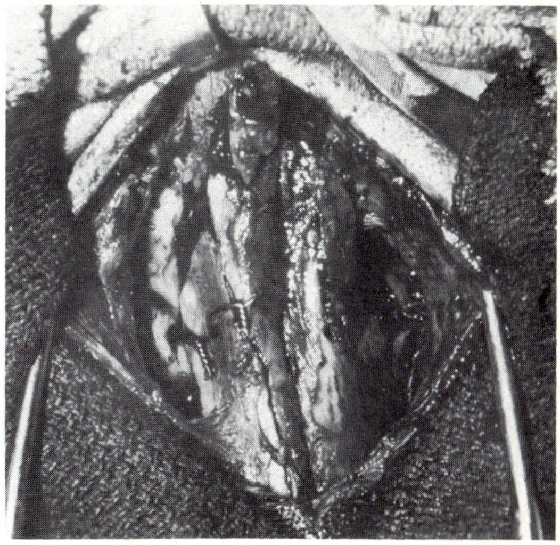

Figure 9–1. The fracture fragments in this nasomaxillary multiple fracture are lifted into position through a dorsal midline approach and are stabilized with wire placed through the bone.

Methods of Repair

Surgery. Fixation of maxillary fractures is accomplished by internal surgical techniques through midline skin incisions that are carried directly to the bone when possible. Subcutaneous tissues, facial muscles, and periosteum should be lifted from the bone and retracted as a unit. This preserves the myoperiosteal covering of the bone, which is important for normal healing. Bone fragments are lifted, positioned, and fixed by placing wire through the bone or by placing a pin and wire combination (Fig. 9–1).[2] Since the force acting on these facial bones is small, light fixation is adequate. If fracture lines extend through the hard palate, occlusive alignment must be maintained and the fixation must be supported by intraoral appliances or muzzling with tape.

Bone Pins and Acrylic Resin. There are several methods for the external fixation of maxillary fractures. The first method involves the application of bone pins that protrude through the skin and are stabilized by external acrylic resin.[3,4] The acrylic method is versatile because pin placement can be random. If occlusive forces are reduced by keeping the animal on a semiliquid diet, there is little stress on the fracture lines. The abundant blood supply will enhance healing.

Intraoral Acrylic Splint. The second method of external fixation involves the application of an intraoral acrylic splint or appliance that is wired to the teeth.[5] In this case, the fracture first must be reduced and an alginate impression of the palate and dentition must be made. A plaster cast is then prepared from the impression. The acrylic splint is constructed on the cast, which is described in Chapter Seven. Wires are incorporated into the acrylic splint for its fixation to the maxilla and the surrounding teeth (Fig. 9–2).

It is sometimes difficult to prepare the intraoral acrylic splint so that it allows the carnassial teeth to interlock properly. An additional problem is the accumulation of food debris between the splint and the oral tissues. Generally, intraoral acrylic splints may be kept in place for as long as 6 to 8 weeks without serious secondary problems developing.

Interdental Wiring. Other methods of maxillary fracture fixation involve interdental wiring. The Stout multiple loop technique can be applied to both the upper and lower arcades. Both arcades are wired together, maintaining occlusive alignment; however, a pharyngostomy tube must be placed.[6] The jaw remains shut until sufficient callus has formed to allow removal of the wire without loss of occlusive alignment. This takes about 3 weeks. The fracture is then treated conservatively by allowing only a gruel diet until it has completely healed. Most maxillary fractures heal well without surgical intervention. The most critical factor in deciding on the choice of treatment modality is occlusive alignment.

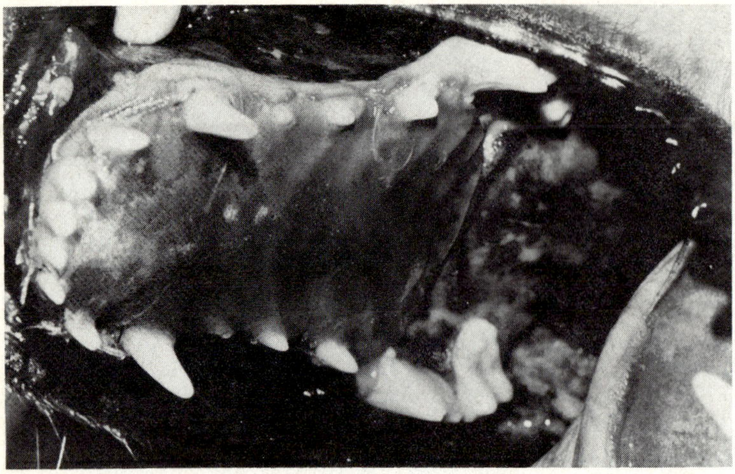

Figure 9–2. This acrylic plate was formed from a cast model and was then wired to the teeth.

MANDIBULAR FRACTURES

Fractures of the mandible in small animals present several unique problems. The mandible withstands a different set of forces than do the weight-bearing limb bones. As a result, fixation of mandibular fractures must take into consideration the forces of occlusion. The proper positioning of orthopedic implants such as wire, Steinmann pins, and plates may be difficult in the mandible because of its curved contour and its unique mechanical requirements. The presence of teeth within fracture lines is another special consideration. The secondary effects of oral trauma and the loss of function affect the intake of fluids and food. Dehydration and inanition may result within a few days in a dog with an unstable mandibular fracture.

The basic principles of mandibular fracture repair include (1) a perfect anatomical or occlusive alignment, (2) neutralization of distracting forces by proper fixation placement, (3) prevention of soft tissue entrapment within fixation implants, (4) prevention of unnecessary damage to tooth roots or developing tooth buds, (5) removal of broken or loose teeth within the fracture line, (6) treatment of open and contaminated fractures, (7) good quality radiographic evaluation, (8) consideration of previous occlusal defects, and (9) an associated program of nutritive maintenance. One must also remember that physiological function is more important than union of individual fracture lines.

Methods of Repair

In the treatment of any mandibular fracture, correct alignment of occlusive surfaces is critical. Small malalignments that are well tolerated in limb bone fractures are not well tolerated in the mandible when complete closure of the mouth cannot take place. Malalignments of 2 mm to 3 mm can result in the jaw failing to close to the extent of 0.5 cm to 1 cm. The condition becomes more complicated when multiple fractures are present or when fractures are complicated by temporomandibular joint subluxations or fractures. Therefore, the surgeon should concentrate primarily on occlusive alignment and consider the fracture fragment alignment secondarily.

Intraoral Screws and Elastic Bands. Dental interlock is a convenient way of achieving proper alignment and fixation. Certain fractures, such as those occurring caudal to the dentition, are very difficult to repair by conventional orthopedic methods. The intraoral application of screws into the maxilla and mandible and the placement of dental bands or elastics to maintain dental interlock are useful in small dogs and cats[7] (Fig. 9–3). The placement of these screws and bands is determined preoperatively by noting the direction of malalignment. The bands are placed on the opposing side in order to pull the mandible into proper alignment. Screws should avoid tooth roots. Bands must be checked periodically and must be replaced when broken. Fractures in large dogs are hard to stabilize by this method, since frequent adjustment and replacement is required. When the mandible is held in occlusion forcibly, two possible complications must be considered: (1) heat prostration from inadequate ventilation and (2) aspiration pneumonia if the animal vomits. The owner should be instructed how to remove the bands if an emergency occurs.

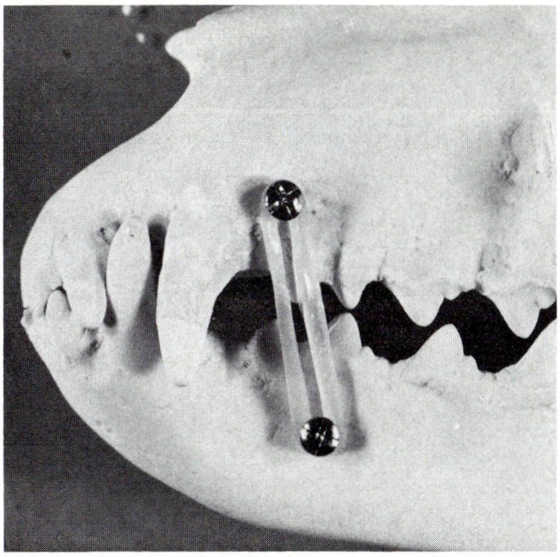

Figure 9–3. Elastic bands stretched around bone screws will maintain occlusive alignment. The screws are placed through the gingivae and into the bone, allowing the screw head to protrude into the buccal space. The screws and bands should be strategically positioned to resist displacement of the fractured mandible.

Interdental Wiring. Orthopedic wire may also be used to secure dental interlock or proper alignment of individual dental arcades. Wiring of the upper fourth premolar to the lower first molar ensures stability and alignment[8] (Fig. 9–4). However, in this technique, the fixation is difficult to release if vomiting occurs. The long-term effects on the periodontium from wire placed in periodontal pockets and perigingival spaces is unclear.

Wiring of an individual dental arcade does not require locking the jaw shut, but it may require specific additional fixation at the fracture site for adequate stability. Techniques such as the Ivy loop, Stout procedure, Risdon, and Essig wiring patterns have been described for use in the dog[5] (Figs. 9–5 through 9–7). Small-gauge wire is usually advised, and in some cases the enamel surfaces of the teeth may have to be grooved to hold the wire in place.

Acrylic Splints. Intraoral acrylic splints

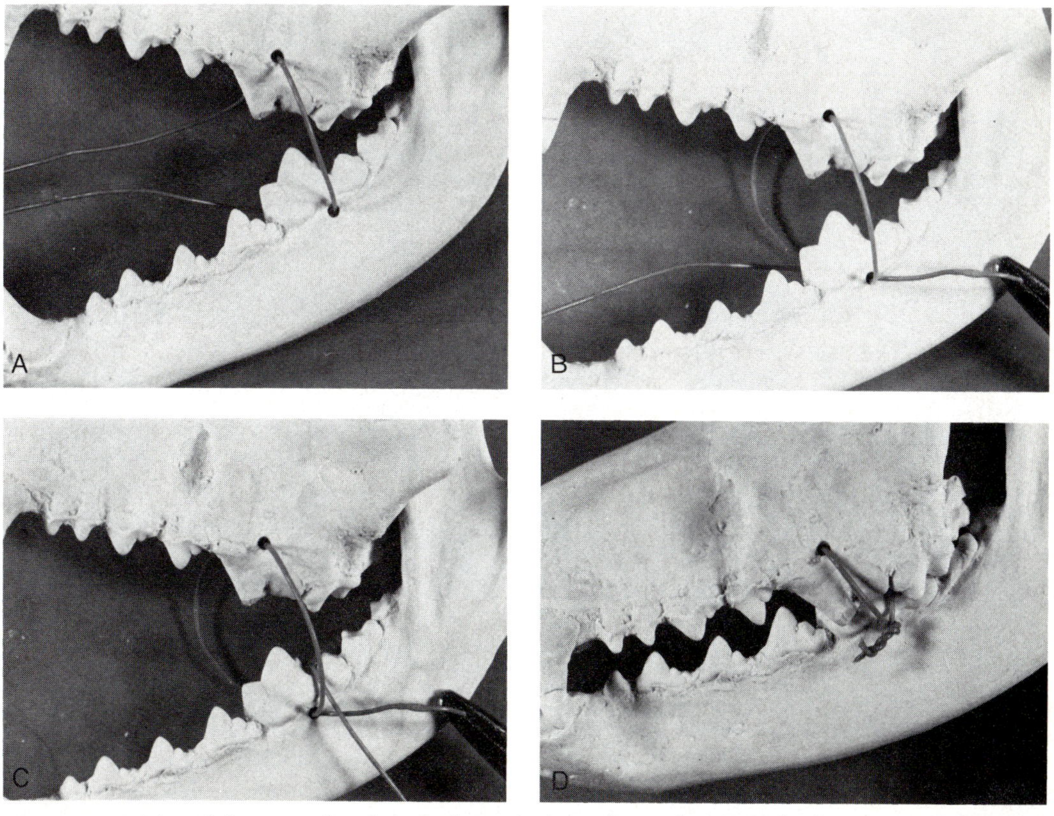

Figure 9–4. Wiring of the upper fourth premolar to the lower first molar. *A*, A wire loop is passed through the interradicular space of the upper fourth premolar and the lower first molar from the buccal to the lingual side. *B*, The upper arm of the loop is brought down and is passed through the interradicular space of the lower first molar to exit into the buccal space. *C*, The lower arm of the loop is brought caudad and over the caudal notch of the lower first molar. *D*, The wire loop is tightened with the twisted end on the buccal side.

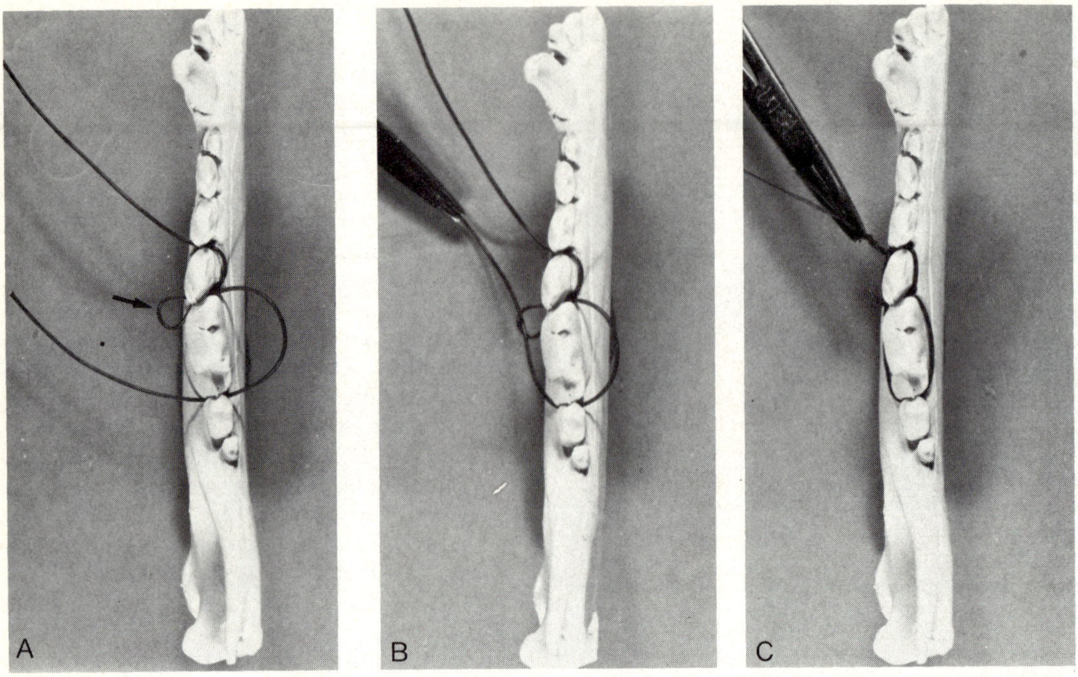

Figure 9–5. The Ivy loop technique. *A*, A single wire is passed through the interproximal space of two adjacent teeth. A portion of this wire is twisted forming a secondary loop *(arrow)*. *B*, One arm of the primary loop is passed through the secondary loop. *C*, The primary loop is pulled tightly and twisted. The secondary loop is also pulled tightly and twisted.

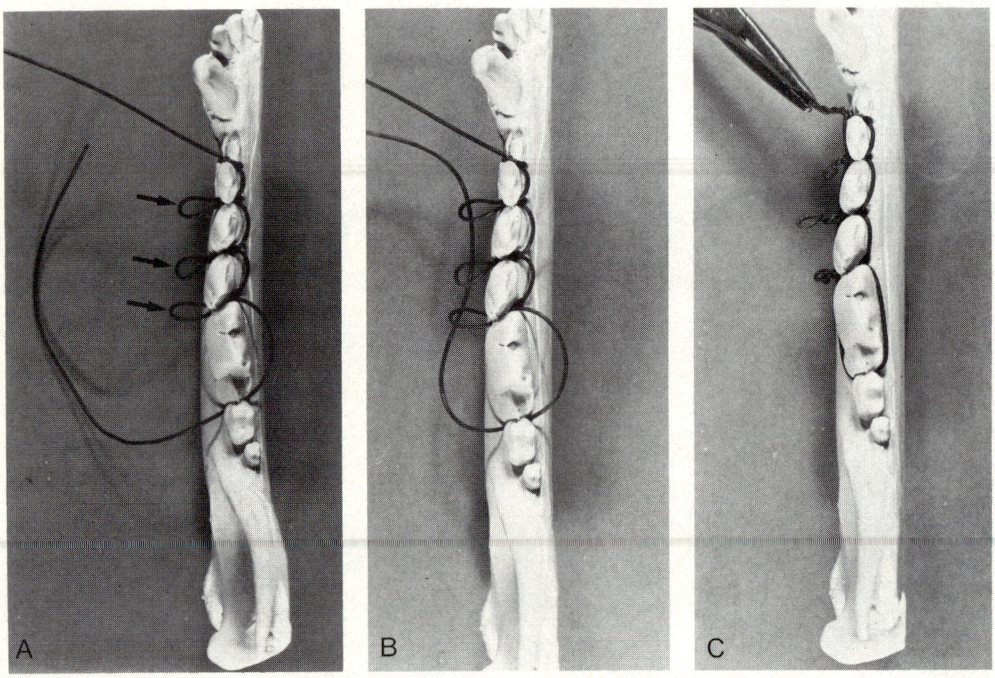

Figure 9–6. A modified Stout loop technique. *A*, A single wire can be passed through the interproximal space of as many as four adjacent teeth. Secondary loops *(arrows)* are then formed. *B*, One arm of the primary loop is passed through the secondary loops. *C*, The primary loop is pulled tightly and twisted. Each of the secondary loops are pulled tightly and twisted.

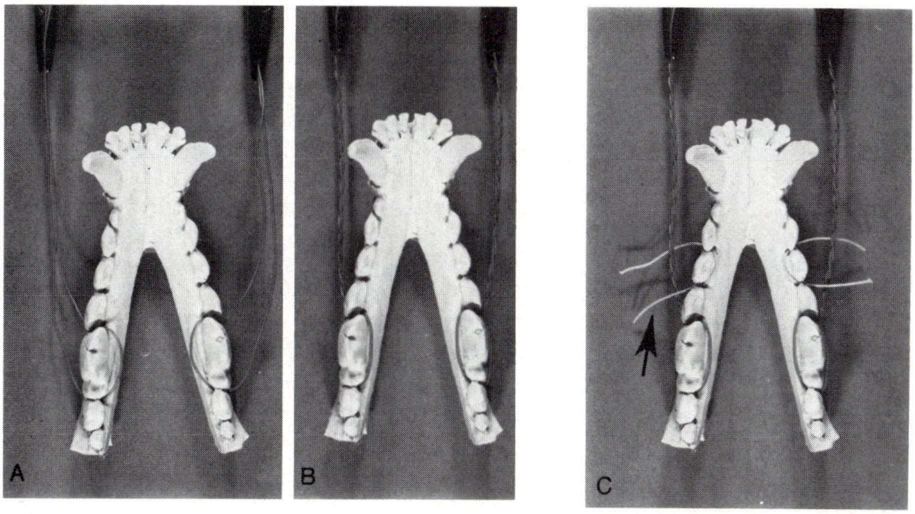

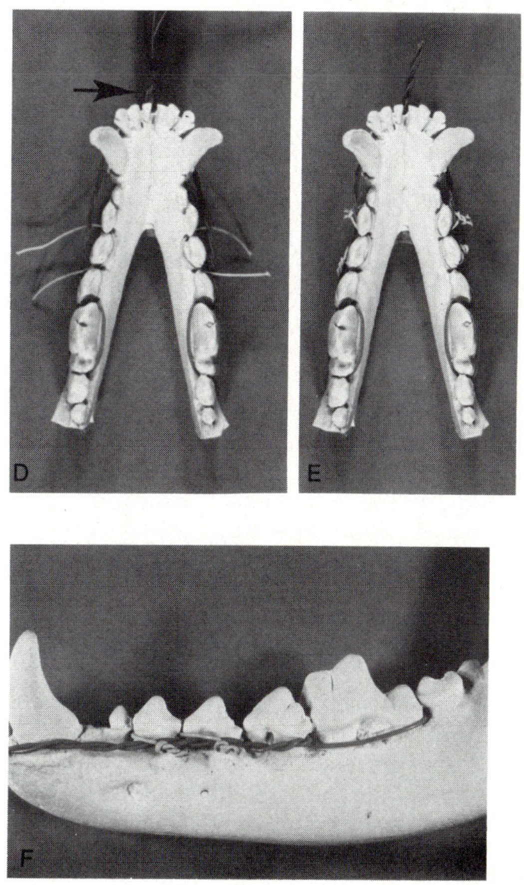

Figure 9–7. The Risdon technique. *A*, A single loop of wire is passed around the base of each lower first molar tooth forming two primary loops. *B*, The long arms of each primary loop are pulled tightly and are twisted throughout their length. *C*, Shorter secondary loops of wire (*arrow*) are passed around the base of individual premolars. *D*, The twisted arms of the primary loops are pulled tightly and are twisted together (*arrow*). *E*, Each secondary loop is pulled tightly and twisted over the twisted arms of the primary loop. *F*, A lateral view of the Risdon technique. This technique can augment stability for fixation of symphyseal fractures.

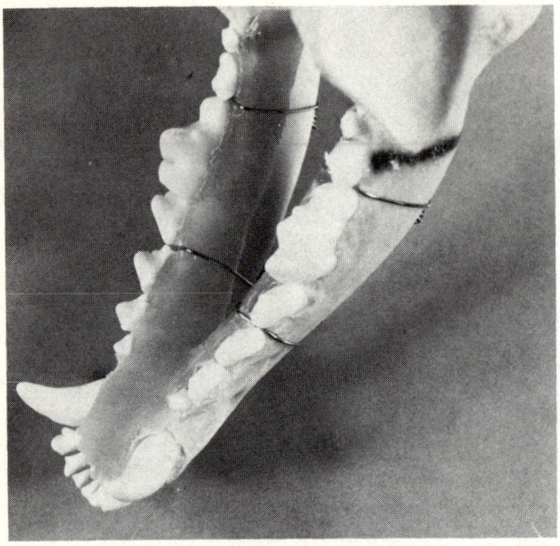

Figure 9–8. The acrylic plate is first formed from a cast model and is then wired to the mandible with multiple circummandibular wires. These wires are positioned flat against the bone. Soft tissue should not be trapped between the wire and the bone.

can also be applied to the mandible.[9] The principle difficulty with this technique is the need to reduce the fracture and hold it in reduction while the initial impression is made. However, the fracture can be approached surgically and can be wired before the impression is made. The acrylic splint will support the inner fragment fixation and is capable of withstanding the magnitude of occlusive forces. It is wired directly to the teeth or is positioned on the mandible and stabilized with circummandibular wires (Fig. 9–8). Washing the oral cavity helps prevent the accumulation of debris during the convalescent period. Pressure necrosis of oral mucosae and gingivae has not been observed.

Tape Muzzle. Tape muzzling affords a very practical means of aligning and stabilizing mandibular fractures by maintaining dental interlock. Muzzling that allows a 0.5-cm to 1-cm gap for tongue protrusion lets the patient lap liquid diets. In the adult dog with normal premolar and canine dentition, adequate alignment can be maintained. Rigid stability is not present, but this will not impede healing of the fracture. Tape muzzles that avoid sticking tape directly to the skin and hair have been described;[10] the tape is applied with the adhesive surface away from the skin and hair. A single strip is initially placed along one side of the face and is brought around the back of the head caudal to the ears and over the neck to the other side of the face. This tape strip should extend for several inches beyond the rostral end of the muzzle. A second strip is placed completely around the muzzle, again with the adhesive surface away from the skin. The rostral portions of the initial strip are folded back and are applied to the tape that extends alongside the face (Fig. 9–9). The owner can remove these muzzles by simply lifting them over the head and ears. A variety of muzzles can be fashioned and applied, but rigid materials must be adequately padded. Ulcerative dermatitis can be prevented with good muzzling techniques and home care, and these muzzles can usually be removed in 4 to 8 weeks.

Use of Pharyngostomy Tubes. When stabilizing mandibular fractures by complete restriction of jaw movement, a pharyngostomy tube must be placed to permit nutritive maintenance. It is not advisable to have the end of the tube pass through the gastroesophageal sphincter, since such placement predisposes to reflux esophagitis and megaesophagus. Liquid diets should be administered through the tube slowly and in small amounts to prevent regurgitation and vomiting. Prolonged use of a pharyngostomy tube is not advisable because of the complication of esophagitis.

Surgery. Surgical repair of mandibular fractures in the dog is infrequent. In a nationwide survey, only 639 of 2178 mandibular fractures in dogs were surgically repaired,* indicating that most are handled by non-surgical methods.

Indications for surgical invasion and correction of a mandibular fracture include (1) bilateral or multiple fractures, (2) a symphyseal separation or fracture, (3) severe instability, (4) a delayed or non-union mandibular fracture with impaired function, and (5) the inability to apply conservative measures.

Orthopedic Wire. Many techniques that are used in the treatment of limb bone fractures have also been used for mandible repair in the dog and cat. Orthopedic wire fixation is economical and popular. The guidelines for its use include (1) a ventral surgical approach, (2) the use of the tension band principle, (3) the avoidance of soft alveolar bone, (4) the use of solid teeth in some fixation patterns, (5) the secure fastening of all orthopedic wire, (6) the use of additional sup-

*Data obtained from the Veterinary Medical Data Program, 1983.

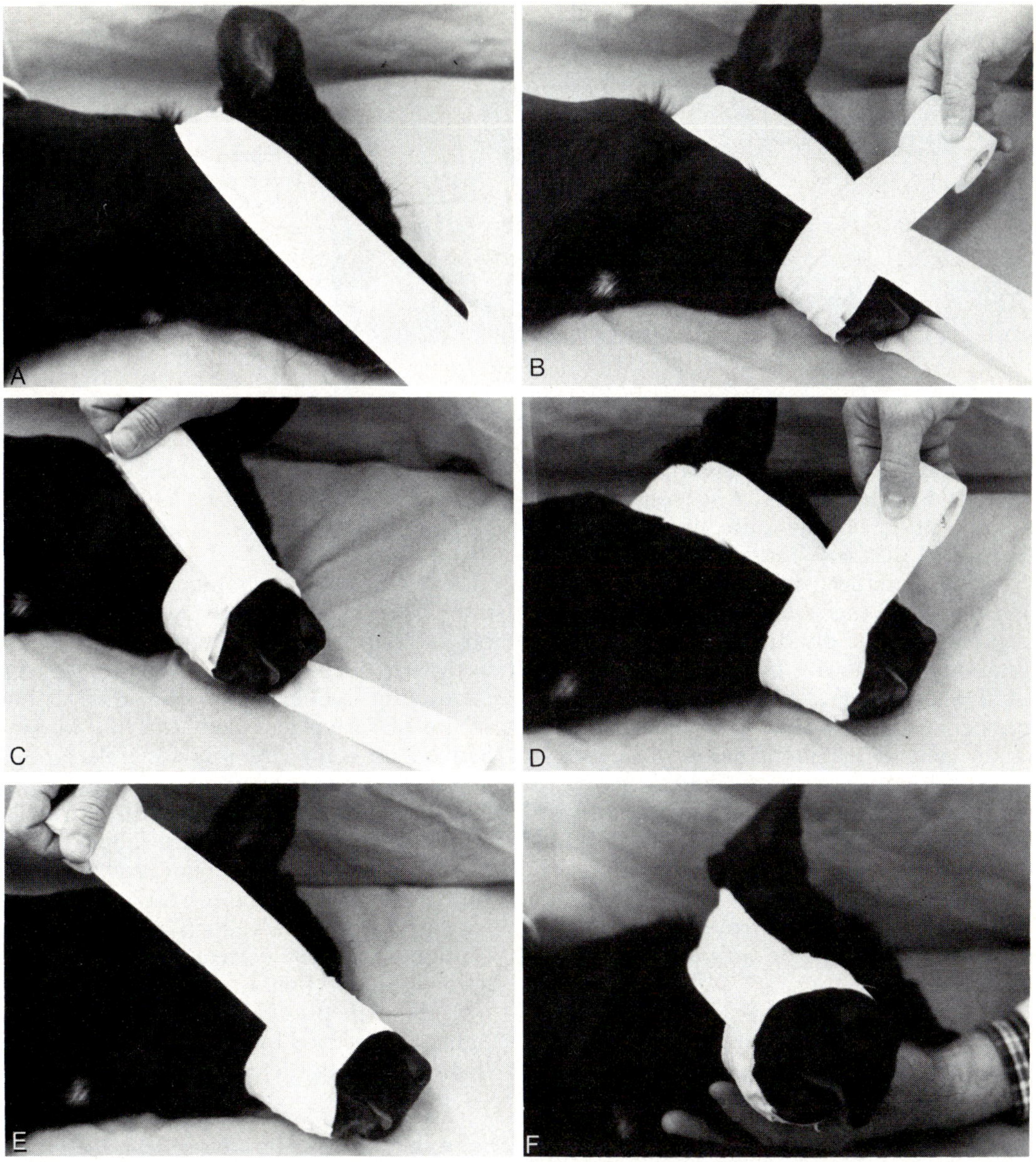

Figure 9–9. Application of a tape muzzle. *A*, A single strip of tape is passed around the back of the head with the adhesive surface away from the skin. *B*, Tape is now passed around the muzzle with the adhesive surface away from the skin. *C*, The rostral extension of the initial strip is now folded back. *D* and *E*, The tape muzzle can be reinforced with additional tape. *F*, A gap of 0.5 cm to 1 cm will allow for tongue protrusion.

port, (7) the use of multiple wires, and (8) the avoidance of reactive or infected bone in the fixation.

The oral approach is generally not appropriate when applying orthopedic wire to the mandible. The level of contamination is high, and one cannot effectively reach the ventral cortex of the mandible to apply the wire. The alveolar portion of the mandible is easily accessible from the oral approach, but it is not sufficiently dense to support orthopedic implants.

The muscular and occlusive forces in the oral cavity create tension and compression sides to a fracture (Fig. 9–10). Shear forces are accentuated in oblique fracture lines. Occlusive forces create tension on the alveolar border of the mandibular body. Interdental wiring, as previously discussed, has been proposed by dentists and veterinary surgeons

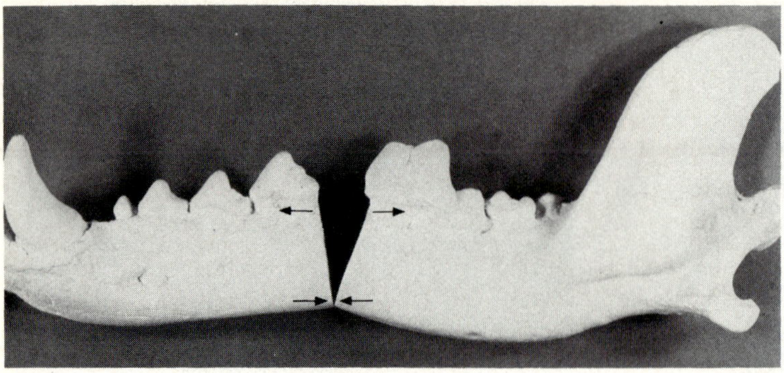

Figure 9–10. Occlusive forces create tension and compression sides to the mandible *(arrows).*

for use in animals. It shows promise in neutralizing the distraction force of tension; however, the teeth of the carnivore are conical in profile and elliptical in cross section, making the application of wire difficult. It must be emphasized that wire must be tight in order to ensure fracture stability. Grooving the teeth facilitates the stability of such wire application. Another disadvantage concerns the limitations of the wire gauge in these interdental techniques. Twenty six–gauge wire has been suggested, but it is generally too thin to control fragment mobility. If interdental techniques are used, additional fixation at the fracture site is necessary to ensure adequate stability. Heavier wire, which is not used in interdental wiring, can be applied directly to the mandible.

There have been many proposals for the placement of orthopedic wire directly across a mandibular fracture.[2, 5, 9, 11–13] It is essential to apply at least two wires across any single fracture line. Additional support should be applied, especially when dealing with bilateral mandibular fractures. This support may be applied directly to the fracture, for example, an intramedullary pin, or it may be applied to the mandible, for example, an intraoral acrylic splint or some other form of external fixation.

When applying orthopedic wire to bone, it must be secured as tightly as possible. This is best accomplished by first applying tension to the wire, then twisting or bending it while continuing to hold the tension. Using a long strand of wire is less likely to cause kinking. Kinked or bent wire will not pull through holes or around corners, thus preventing the application of even tension on the wire. The tightening of orthopedic wire should be performed with an instrument that pulls the wire in tension before twisting. Orthopedic wire with a small "eye-loop" at one end can be tightened very effectively with a simple wire tightener that is designed to be used with this type of wire. After pulling the wire tight, it is secured by bending it in the direction opposite to the pull (Fig. 9–11).

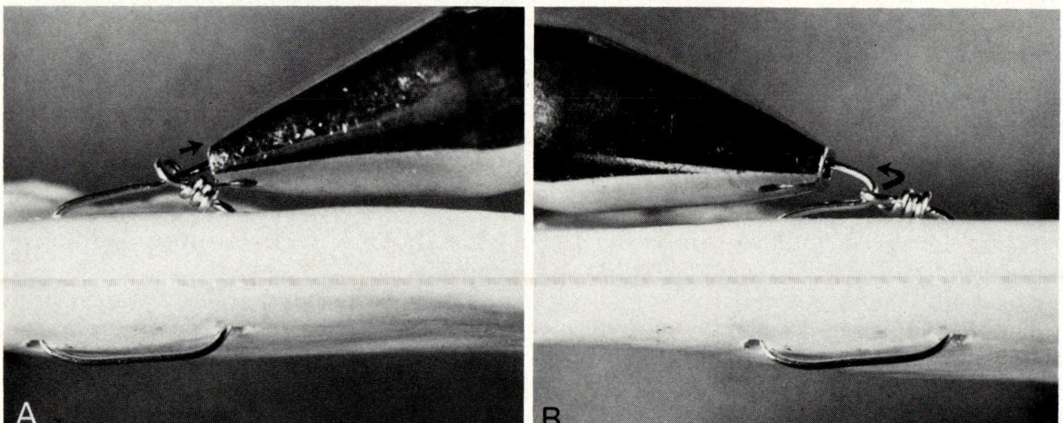

Figure 9–11. Tightening of orthopedic wire. *A*, The wire is tightened in tension. *B*, Once fully tightened, the wire is secured by a single bend created by swinging the tightener (while the wire is still held in tension) 180 degrees opposite the direction of pull.

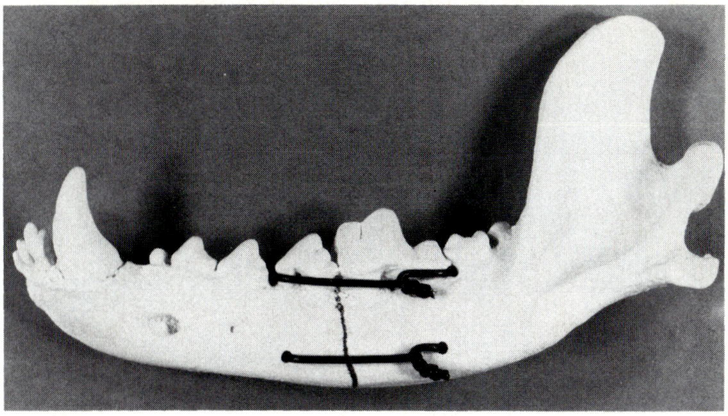

Figure 9–12. In this example, two orthopedic wires have been properly placed for good stabilization.

Dense cortical bone is necessary for good stability of any orthopedic wire. The ventral border of the body of the mandible is the most ideal location. The alveolar bone around the roots of the teeth is less dense and compact and is therefore less likely to hold wire for a prolonged time. If there is an indication for wire placement in this region of the mandible, the teeth should be considered as a base of support for the wire (Fig. 9–12). The surgeon should avoid diseased bone, especially areas of osteolysis from chronic periodontal disease.

The gauge of wire is an important consideration. Thick heavy wire cannot be applied effectively in tiny mandibles. Thick wire is difficult to place in a small area, as it tends to bind and kink. While applying tension, heavy wire can overpower the bone and fracture it. A loose wire across a fracture line inhibits healing. Recommended sizes for toy breeds are 24 gauge wire, and for large or giant breeds, 18 gauge wire.

In summary, two wires per fracture line is a good "rule of thumb." Less than two wires increases the risk of fragment movement, whereas too many wires can weaken the bone and inhibit vascularity and the development of adequate callus. In my experience, orthopedic wiring of mandibular fractures has not been as successful in general as have other fixation methods, except in the case of a separated mandibular symphysis.

Intramedullary Pinning. Intramedullary pinning has been used for mandibular fracture fixation.[11, 13, 14] Pinning techniques require a small investment in equipment and can be applied quickly; however, there are many disadvantages for their use in the mandible. Stability in all planes, and especially in rotation, is difficult to obtain with round, smooth-shafted pins. The demand for stability is further accentuated in bilateral fractures. The roots of the teeth should be avoided, and the pin should not follow the caudal mandibular aveolar canal, since the pin will resist bending and will cause fragment displacement[14] (Fig. 9–13). Because the canine tooth has a long root, the rostral placement of a pin is restricted. The only indication for mandibular pinning is in unilateral fractures of its body in the area from the second premolar to the first molar teeth.[14] The pin is most easily applied by retrograde

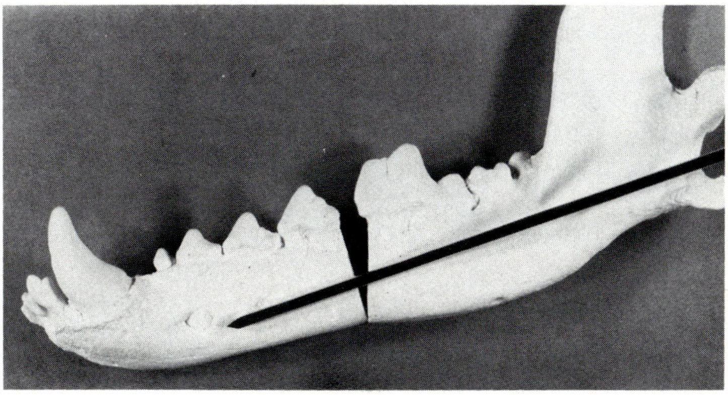

Figure 9–13. A pin placed within the mandibuloalveolar canal will cause distraction of a transverse fracture.

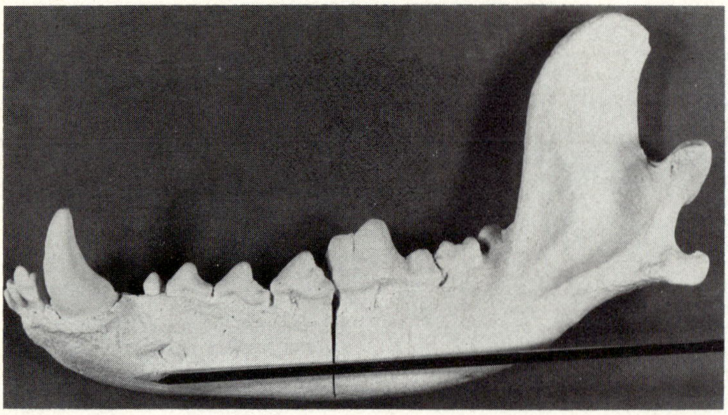

Figure 9–14. A properly placed pin will penetrate the cortex of the ventral border of mandible.

application into the caudal fragment. Again, note that the pin should exit the cortex of the mandible caudally, just as the mandibular canal begins to curve dorsally. The pin needs to extend rostrally to the level of the canine root, but must not penetrate it (Fig. 9–14). Fractures in other areas of the mandible are sometimes repaired by using pins, but application is more difficult, and additional fixation may be necessary to achieve adequate stability.

Intramedullary pins in the body of the mandible may damage the mandibuloalveolar nerves and vessels that supply the dentition, though the effects of damage to the neurovascular structures are unknown. In conclusion, the use of intramedullary pins in the mandible is limited, and when used additional support should be considered.

Bone Plating. This procedure is a very effective means of treating mandibular fractures[11, 13, 15, 16] (Fig. 9–15). Its most desirable advantage is the early return of function and the reduced postoperative care and maintenance. The primary disadvantages are expense and the increased surgical time required for application. Expense is a factor when one considers the need for specialized equipment such as miniplates and miniscrews and their respective installation tools, such as special drills, guides, and screwdrivers.

Compression plating is ideal, but maintaining occlusive alignment takes precedence in mandibular fractures. If there is missing bone or a slight malalignment in the fracture line, compression can further distort fragment alignment, causing malocclusion. Compression with minor malalignment may be acceptable in the limb bones, but if proper occlusion is obstructed by malalignment in the mandible, compression should be avoided.

The plate must conform to the bone for a proper fit. During the application of the plate, the bone fragments will line up along the plate; therefore, if the plate does not conform to the anatomical shape of the bone, the fragments will not reduce anatomically, and the occlusion will be distorted. Intubation through a pharyngostomy or tracheostomy incision allows the surgeon to examine for proper occlusion during the surgery.[17]

Surgical exposure for plating should be made through a ventral approach. Screw

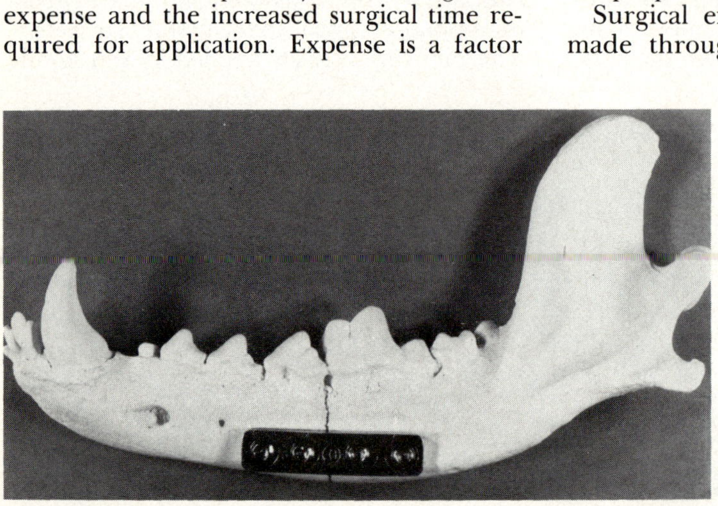

Figure 9–15. A properly applied and well-contoured bone plate provides an excellent means of fixation for certain mandibular fractures.

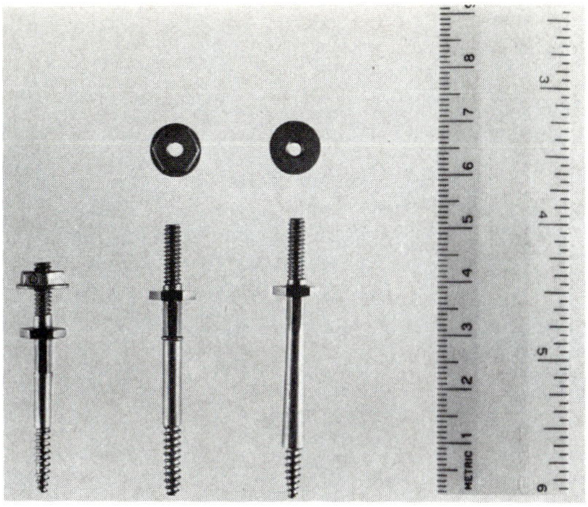

Figure 9–16. Biphase fixation bolts with washer-faced nuts come in three sizes as shown here. (From Weigel JP, Dorn AS, Chase DC, Jaffrey B: The use of the biphase external fixation splint for repair of canine mandibular fractures. *J Am Anim Hosp Assoc* 17:550, 1981.)

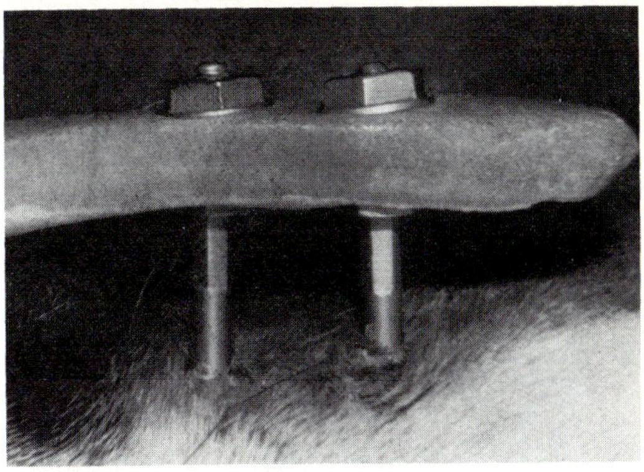

Figure 9–17. The external acrylic fixaton bar, while still soft, is placed over the protruding ends of the bolts. As the acrylic hardens the washer-faced nuts are applied and tightened.

placement should avoid dental roots and the neurovascular structures of the mandibular canal. A minimum of four screws, two on each side of a plated fracture, is necessary for stability in the mandible.

External Fixation. This method of repair is very useful and is preferred in certain types of mandibular fractures, such as complex fractures involving comminution or loss of bone and multiple fractures that are difficult to stabilize internally. The Kirschner-Ehmer system is good for limb fractures, but is cumbersome and heavy, and difficult to apply in the mandible. Obtaining good occlusive alignment with multiple pins and straight external rods is a technical challenge. External fixation systems with more versatility and lighter composition are better suited for use in the mandible.

Biphase Splint. The Morris biphase external mandibular splint is the most appropriate external splint.[18–20] The apparatus is fixed to the mandible by means of specially designed bolts (Fig. 9–16). These bolts are stabilized externally by an acrylic bar (Fig. 9–17). The splint is most useful in large-breed dogs, since the mandibles of dogs weighing less than 20 kg are too small to hold the bolts, which are applied to the bone through small stab incisions and predrilled holes. The first phase in using the biphase splint is the application of the bolts, reduction of the fracture, and temporary stabilization with a single stainless steel rod and two clamps (Fig. 9–18). The second phase consists of preparing the acrylic by mixing powder and fluid resins until a soft, doughy consistency is obtained, placing the mix in a metal form for 1 to 2 minutes, and applying the soft acrylic to the bolts. The acrylic is then allowed to polymerize to a rigid state. The nuts are applied but are not tightened until the acrylic hardens After 10

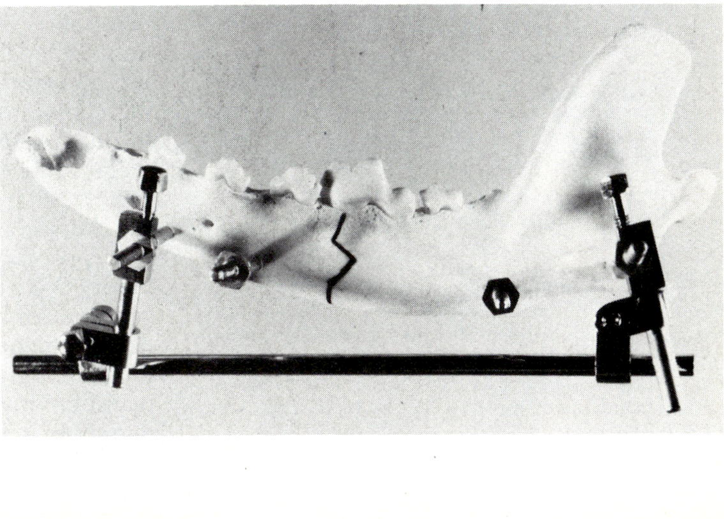

Figure 9–18. Phase I of the biphase splint temporarily holds reduction while the acrylic is mixed and applied to the bolts.

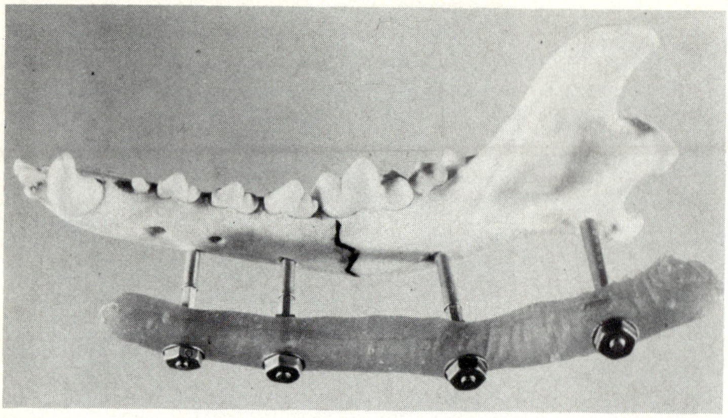

Figure 9–19. Once the acrylic bar has fully polymerized, the steel rod and clamps are removed. The acrylic bar of phase II maintains fixation throughout the healing period.

minutes, the acrylic polmerizes, and the nuts are tightened. The temporary fixation (the steel rod and clamps) is removed, completing the second phase (Fig. 9–19).

To achieve adequate stabilization, two bolts should be applied on either side of the fracture line. The splint can be applied unilaterally or bilaterally by spanning across the midline (Fig. 9–20). Generally, the patient accepts the splint well. If the splint is stable, it can remain on the mandible for as long as 6 months. Drainage around the bolts does occur, and the risk of drainage will increase if the bolts are applied to thin or diseased bone. Instability of the splint or of the fracture, or of both, will also enhance infection and drainage. However, in most cases, this type of local infection does not interfere with fracture healing.

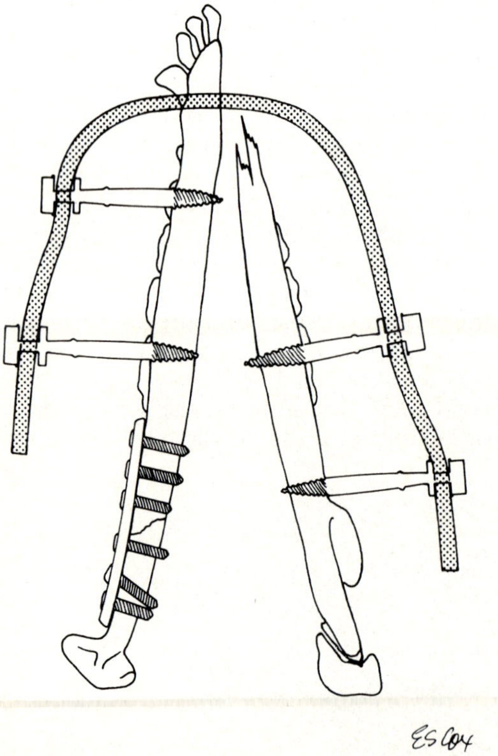

Figure 9–20. In multiple fractures, the biphase splint can be applied to both sides in the same patient and can be used in conjunction with other forms of fixation. (From Weigel JP, Dorn AS, Chase DC, Jaffrey B: The use of the biphase external fixation splint for repair of canine mandibular fractures. *J Am Anim Hosp Assoc* 17:550, 1981.)

The primary disadvantage of the biphase splint is expense. Each bolt costs about $50. The acrylic is inexpensive, versatile, and strong. The bolt is a critical part of the splint, and modifications that use a substitute for the bolt, such as bone screws, threaded pins, or smooth pins, are not as stable or durable and are more difficult to apply.

Indications for Particular Mandibular Fracture Fixation Techniques

There are certain regions of the mandible that are fractured frequently; some lend themselves well to fixation whereas others do not. The mandible can be considered to consist of seven regions: (A) the symphysis to the canine teeth, (B) the canine teeth to the second premolar teeth, (C) the second premolar teeth to the first molar teeth, (D) the first molar teeth to the angle of the mandible, (E) the angle of the mandible, (F) the coronoid process, and (G) the condyloid process. Figure 9–21 indicates the relative occurrence of fractures by region in the mandible of the dog. A major determining factor in choosing the method of fixation is the region of the mandible involved, since the contour of the mandible is so variable.

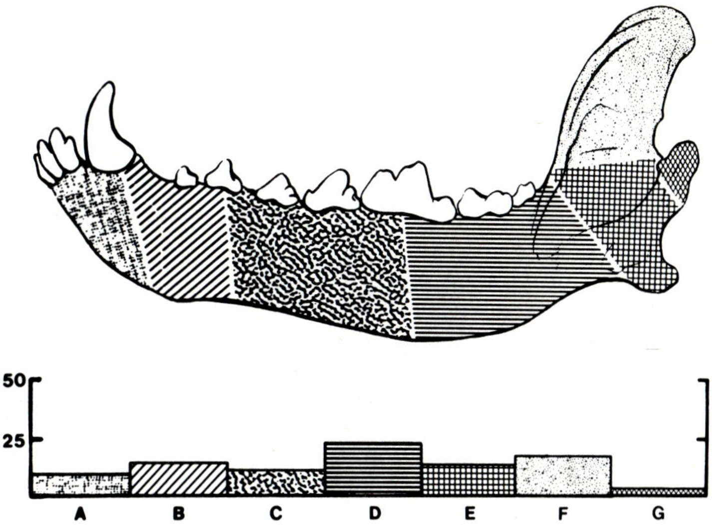

Figure 9–21. This diagram and graph represent a survey of 87 fractures in 41 dogs. The values on the vertical axis represent a percentage of the total fractures surveyed, whereas the horizontal axis represents the regions of the mandible that were involved.

Region A includes all symphyseal separations and fractures of the chin. Symphyseal separations are easily wired, and if bone is missing, a combination of pin and wire is adequate. These fractures are described on page 154. If there is a major loss of bone, external fixation, tape muzzling, or transmandibular screws can be used. If the bone loss is unilateral and surgery is not an option, conservative therapy may be used. If healing does not occur with this approach, a nonunion may be functionally acceptable in isolated cases.

Region B can be difficult to repair by internal methods, since the root of the canine tooth occupies most of the mandible in this area. Orthopedic wiring is best suited for this area unless there is a bilateral fracture. External fixation or wiring the jaws closed would be suitable in the case of a bilateral fracture through region B.

Region C is the straightest part of the horizontal ramus and has the fewest tooth roots. Intramedullary pinning, bone plating, orthopedic wiring, intraoral acrylic resin, and external fixation can all be conveniently applied for fractures in this area. Tape muzzling is not ideal in this area, since the tape would act as a fulcrum against the fracture, especially if it is bilateral.

Region D has a relatively high incidence of fracture compared with the other areas. The mandible begins to change contour in this region, and the density of the bone varies greatly. Internal fixation can be applied but with more difficulty than in region C. Plates are best suited for region D. Conservative measures such as tape muzzling can also be applied. Wiring the jaw shut or using the screw and band technique is also applicable.

Fractures in region E are extremely difficult to stabilize internally. These fractures are best supported by maintaining occlusion with a tape muzzle or by wiring the teeth.

Fractures in region F heal without surgical intervention. Maintaining occlusive alignment is all that is required.

Fractures in region G involve the condyloid process of the mandible. If left alone, these fractures do not generally cause a problem

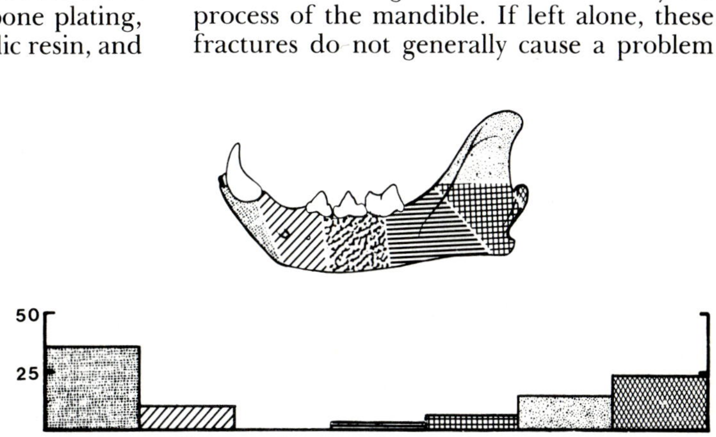

Figure 9–22. This diagram and graph represent a survey of 29 fractures in 15 cats. The values on the vertical axis represent a percentage of the total fractures surveyed, whereas the horizontal axis represents the regions of the mandible that were involved.

in the dog, and the joint is not immobilized. Severe comminuted fractures of the condyloid process may require condylectomy (Chapter Seven, page 113) if callus formation or arthritis interfere with joint function following healing.

The pattern of fracture incidence in the cat differs from that in the dog (Fig. 9–22). Symphyseal separations account for the majority of fractures in the feline mandible. They can easily be repaired with orthopedic wire. There is also a high incidence of fractures in region G. In these cases, the fracture is allowed to heal without repair, and the patient is monitored. Severe fractures and secondary joint abnormalities are treated by condylectomy.

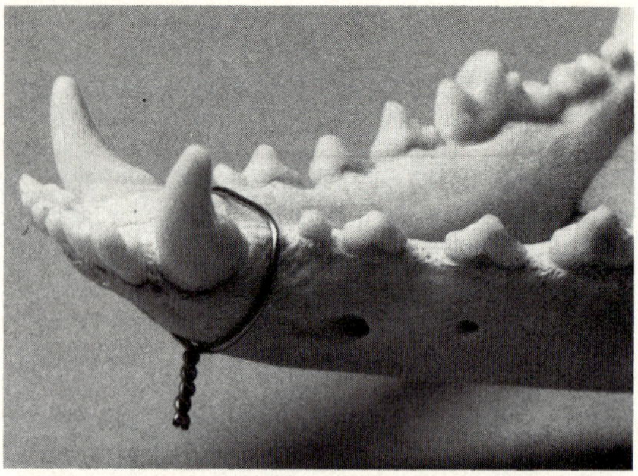

Figure 9–23. Symphyseal separations are quickly and effectively stabilized by passing a single strand of orthopedic wire around both bodies of the mandible just caudal to the canine teeth.

SYMPHYSEAL FRACTURES

Symphyseal fractures are a special type of fracture that merits separate discussion. Although they occur in dogs, symphyseal fractures are most common in cats. Of 15,432 fractures in cats, 809 involved the mandible, and 702 were symphyseal fractures or separations. Of 87,655 fractures in dogs, 2178 were mandibular and only 216 were symphyseal fractures or separations.*

There are three types of symphyseal fractures. Type I is a separation at the symphysis with no break in the intraoral or extraoral soft tissue and no comminution of bone or fracture of teeth. Type II involves tearing of the intraoral soft tissue and exposure of the symphysis. Type III is the complex symphyseal fracture with torn intraoral soft tissue and comminution of bone and fracture of teeth. There is a high incidence of type I symphyseal fractures in the cat.

Generally type I separation does not require surgical fixation in the cat. Types II and III require surgical stabilization, especially if the temporomandibular joint is also involved. Stabilizing the mandibular symphysis will help to control instability and dislocation within the temporomandibular joint.

The most practical method of fixation for the mandibular symphyseal separation is to pass a loop of orthopedic wire around both mandibular bodies caudal to the canine teeth[2,21] (Fig. 9–23). Direct wiring of the canine teeth is difficult because of the conical shape of the crowns. Most dental wiring techniques are borrowed from the human literature. In humans, the mandibular symphysis is parallel to the vertical axis of the teeth. In the dog and cat, the symphysis is oblique to the long axis of the teeth. Therefore, wiring of the teeth alone is insufficient for controlling stability.

When symphyseal fractures are comminuted, additional techniques, such as a combination of pin and wire placement, can be used. The pins may migrate after a short time; however, they will provide enough stability for a fibrous union or early callus formation. Pins must be placed to avoid damage to tooth roots.

FRACTURE COMPLICATIONS

Teeth in the line of fracture can be an impediment to healing. This is especially true if the tooth is unstable. Teeth can act as foreign bodies, making it difficult for granulation tissue to bridge the fracture gap. This problem is accentuated if the fracture is open to contamination, fluid, and debris from the oral cavity. In this situation, the teeth in the line of fracture should be extracted.

Delayed and non-union complications can occur with mandibular fractures. Complications of this type occur most frequently with unstable fractures that have been invaded surgically. The same principles that are used for similar problems in limb fractures are used for the treatment of these complications and include securing rigid stability and graft-

*Data obtained from the Veterinary Medical Data Program, 1983.

ing with autogenous cancellous bone. Not all non-union fractures of the mandible need to be corrected. Some animals with unilateral non-union fractures will function well if pain and infection are not present.

Complications are not limited to the healing process. They can also be present after the fracture has healed. Malocclusions can result in abnormal tooth wear or excessive plaque and tartar build-up, resulting in periodontal erosion and premature loss of affected teeth. In such patients, prophylactic teeth scaling (page 66) may be required on a more frequent basis than it was prior to the fracture. Extraction of teeth because of the previous trauma leaves bare gingival bridges that can be traumatized by hard food trapped between the edentulous gingivae and the teeth from the opposing arcade. If secondary damage to the gingiva is seen, the crowns of the opposing teeth should be cut down or the entire tooth should be extracted. Following mandibular and maxillary fractures in humans, additional periodontal and orthodontic therapy is occasionally necessary to ensure normal occlusion. As the practice of veterinary orthodontics and periodontics develops, these techniques will be available to correct the occlusal problems following fracture repair in patients with healed maxillary and mandibular fractures. Satisfactory fracture repair is often a multistaged procedure requiring considerable time and patience and periodic re-evaluation of the patient.

References

1. Shafer WG, Hine MK, Levy BM: Healing of oral wounds. *In* A Textbook of Oral Pathology, Vol. II, 3rd ed. Philadelphia, WB Saunders Co., 1974, pp. 542–563.
2. Rudy, RL: Fracture of the maxilla and mandible. *In* Bojrab MJ (ed): Current Techniques in Small Animal Surgery. Philadelphia, Lea & Febiger, 1975, pp. 364–375.
3. Charnock M: Surgical correction of severe bilateral fractures of the maxilla in the dog. *Vet Rec* 108:123–124, 1981.
4. Stambaugh JE, Nunamaker DM: External skeletal fixation of comminuted maxillary fractures in dogs. *Vet Surg* 11:72–76, 1982.
5. Tholen MA: Dental orthopedics. *In* Concepts in Veterinary Dentistry. Edwardsville, Kansas, Veterinary Medicine Publishing Co., 1983, pp. 135–156.
6. Merkley DE, Brinker WO: Facial reconstruction following massive bilateral maxillary fracture in the dog. *J Am Anim Hosp Assoc* 12:831–833, 1976.
7. Nibley, W: Treatment of caudal mandibular fractures: A preliminary report. *J Am Anim Hosp Assoc* 17:555–562, 1981.
8. Lantz GC: Interarcade wiring as a method of fixation for selected mandibular injuries. *J Am Anim Hosp Assoc* 17:599–603, 1981.
9. Ross DL: Anterior mandibular fracture fixation. *In* Bojrab MJ (ed): Current Techniques in Small Animal Surgery. Philadelphia, Lea & Febiger, 1975, pp. 363–364.
10. Withrow SJ: Taping of the mandible in treatment of mandibular fractures. *J Am Anim Hosp Assoc* 17:27–31, 1981.
11. Chambers JN: Principles of management of mandibular fractures in the dog and cat. *J Vet Orthop* 2:26–36, 1981.
12. Chaffee VW: A technique for fixation of bilateral mandibular fractures caudal to the canine teeth in the dog. *Vet Med Small Anim Clin* 73:907–909, 1978.
13. Brinker WO, Piermattei DL, Flo GL: Handbook of Small Animal Orthopedics and Fracture Treatment. Philadelphia, WB Saunders Co., 1983, pp. 184–192.
14. Cechner PE: Malocclusion in dogs caused by intramedullary pin fixation of mandibular fractures: Two case reports. *J Am Anim Hosp Assoc* 16:79–85, 1980.
15. Leach JB: Stabilization plating of the canine mandible. *Vet Med Small Anim Clin* 68:985–988, 1973.
16. Sumner-Smith G: Fractures of the mandible. *In* Brinker WO, Hohn RB, Prieur WB (eds): Manual of Internal Fixation in Small Animals. New York, Springer-Verlag, 1984, pp. 210–218.
17. Hartsfield SM, Gendreau CL, Smith CW, Rouse GP, Thurmon JC: Endotracheal intubation by pharyngotomy. *J Am Anim Hosp Assoc* 13:71–74, 1977.
18. Morris JH: Blind application of biphase external skeletal fixation. *In* Archer WH (ed): Oral and Maxillofacial Surgery, Vol. II, 5th ed. Philadelphia, WB Saunders Co., 1975, pp. 1129–1136.
19. Greenwood KM, Creagh GB: Bi-phase external skeletal splint fixation of mandibular fractures in dogs. *Vet Surg* 9:128–134, 1980.
20. Weigel JP, Dorn AS, Chase DC, Jaffrey B: The use of the biphase external fixation splint for repair of canine mandibular fracture. *J Am Anim Hosp Assoc* 17:547–554, 1981.
21. Hinko PJ: A method for reduction and fixation of symphyseal fracture of the mandible. *J Am Anim Hosp Assoc* 12:98–100, 1976.

Chapter Ten

Oral Surgery

CE Harvey

INTRODUCTION

Oral surgical procedures on cats and dogs are almost always performed with the animal under deep sedation or general anesthesia. Injection sites for local analgesia have been described;[1] however, lack of patient cooperation makes them impractical for most purposes. When bone is to be incised or vital teeth are to be invaded, the following anesthetic technique is recommended: a narcotic and atropine preanesthetic, thiobarbiturate induction, and oxygen-methoxyflurane maintenance.

The oral surgeon is blessed by working with tissues having abundant blood supply and an epithelial surface that is constantly bathed with saliva—a fluid rich in antimicrobial protection systems. The result is that healing of incisional wounds in oral mucosa is more rapid than it is in skin. Phagocytic activity is greater, it occurs earlier, and it is mostly due to monocytes rather than to polymorphonuclear leukocytes; epithelial migration occurs earlier; and epithelialization is completed earlier. The higher metabolic activity and higher mitotic rate of oral mucosa are believed to be responsible for these differences and may be due to the richer blood supply and higher temperature of oral mucosa.[2] Infections following oral surgical procedures are very rare, even though the surgical preparation for oral surfaces cannot permit the same attention to detail as that for skin, and isolating the affected area for postoperative cleanliness is impractical.

In a study of sutures used in the oral tissues of normal dogs, monofilament nylon was found to cause the least reaction, polyglycolic acid and surgical gut was found to cause a mild to moderate reaction, and silk was found to cause the most severe tissue response.[3] However, in another study, silk and Mersilene (Dacron) sutures caused a similar moderate leukocytic infiltration, and surgical gut caused a significantly greater cellular response.[4] Most sutures with knots on the mucosal surface, whether absorbable or non-absorbable, are sloughed within 2 to 4 weeks. Based on my own clinical observations, synthetic absorbable sutures appear to last somewhat longer than surgical gut, they do not interfere with healing when compared with non-absorbable sutures, and they do not require removal: I recommend them for routine use during oral surgical procedures. A vertical mattress pattern ensures some contact between connective tissue surfaces as well as epithelial apposition; this technique is particularly recommended for use when the suture line will not be supported by underlying tissue, as in many palate procedures.

Wire is not recommended for use in the mouth because the small diameter of wire, when compared with other suture materials, causes the sutures to saw through the tissue more readily: in addition, wire will not prevent tongue movements, and it will cause lacerations in the tongue from licking. Preventing damage to oral suture lines is best achieved by attention to suture technique in order to provide apposition of tissues without suture tension or excessive tightness. In the occasional case in which glossal or pharyngeal muscle activity is particularly likely to cause a breakdown of the suture line, a temporary acrylic obturator can be cemented or wired to the teeth to protect the healing tissues. Pharyngostomy tubes have been recommended as a means of reducing tension on oral or pharyngeal suture lines; documentation of a beneficial or protective effect is not available, and esophagitis may result.[5] In my experience, pharyngostomy is not necessary.

Temporary occlusion of both carotid arteries through an incision in the neck should be considered if extensive surgery is likely,[6] particularly in an animal who is in poor condition or who is anemic because of blood loss from an ulcerated lesion.

PERIODONTAL SURGERY

Periodontal techniques are described in Chapter Five.

DENTAL SURGICAL TECHNIQUES

Endodontic, restorative, and extraction techniques are described in Chapter Six.

JAW AND OCCLUSIVE SURGERY

The correction of jaw, occlusal, and temporomandibular joint abnormalities is described in Chapter Seven. Techniques for repair of oral trauma are described in Chapter Nine. Resection of tumors involving the jaws is described further on in the section on Resection of Mass Lesions.

ORAL SOFT TISSUES

The Tongue

Congenital Anomalies. It is rare for congenital anomalies of the tongue to be amenable to surgical repair. Lateral protrusion of the tongue without hypoglossal nerve damage has been described (Fig. 10–1), and repair by plication has been attempted with limited success.[7] Macroglossia has been treated by resection of the rostral section of the tongue, with good clinical results.[8] Many brachycephalic dogs have tongues that seem grossly long when compared with their jaw length, though they have good control of function, and the tongue does not become traumatized from exposure. A short frenulum in a dog, which caused difficulty in eating and drinking, was treated successfully by incising the frenulum for 2 cm.[9]

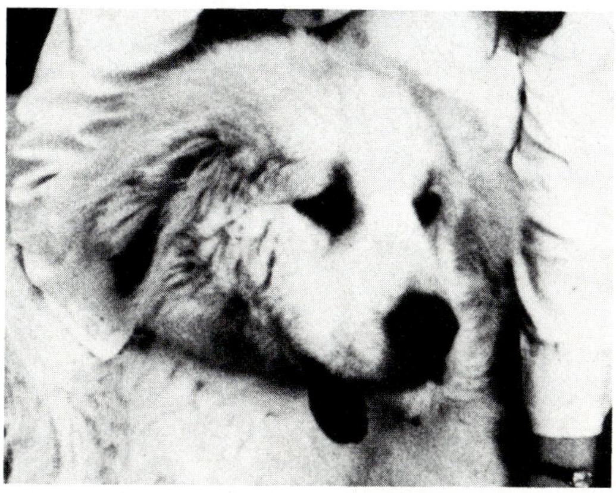

Figure 10–1. Lateral drooping of the tongue in a dog. The tongue was not paralyzed. Lateral plication partially corrected the condition.

The injuries most frequently observed are lacerations, which are caused by the animal licking sharp surfaces, by penetrating foreign bodies such as chicken bones or wood splinters, by the animal chewing electric cords (Fig. 10–2 *A*), and by ingestion of caustics. Clinical signs include bleeding, drooling, an inability or unwillingness to eat, and pawing at the mouth. Diagnosis is by inspection of the mouth, which may require sedation in an animal who is in pain. It is particularly important to inspect the sublingual area to ensure that no foreign bodies are embedded in the tongue or are wrapped around its root.

Surgical incisions or clean lacerations are sutured with absorbable material, both to control hemorrhage and to appose the epithelial edges. Jagged lacerations require débridement prior to suturing. Barbed foreign bodies, such as fish hooks and some bone chips or wood splinters, require incision of overlying tissue to prevent more severe damage by blunt removal.

Tongue injury from electric cords rarely requires much by way of definitive management; the injured tissues are best left to necrose so that the maximum amount of tongue tissue is retained (Fig. 10–2 *B*). Use of a pharyngostomy or gastrostomy tube for several days may be necessary for feeding. Once the necrotic portion of the tongue has sloughed, the remaining stump is rapidly covered by epithelium.

Mass lesions on the tongue can be resected with good results if the resection can be confined to the free rostral portion. Protuberant, ulcerated lesions on the tongue should be biopsied prior to resection (or before euthanizing the animal if the lesion appears to be too extensive for surgery or radiation therapy) because eosinophilic granuloma of the tongue, which is treated medically (see page 49, Chapter Four), appears similar to an invading neoplasm in some cats and dogs. Surgical resection of part of the tongue is likely to be a bloody procedure; therefore, electrosurgery is useful. Ideally, tongue tissue is removed as a wedge so that the mucosa can be apposed with synthetic absorbable sutures (Fig. 10–3). The wedge technique can be used to remove lesions from the dorsal part of the root of the tongue. Neoplastic lesions that are deep in the root of the tongue or that cause the tongue to be

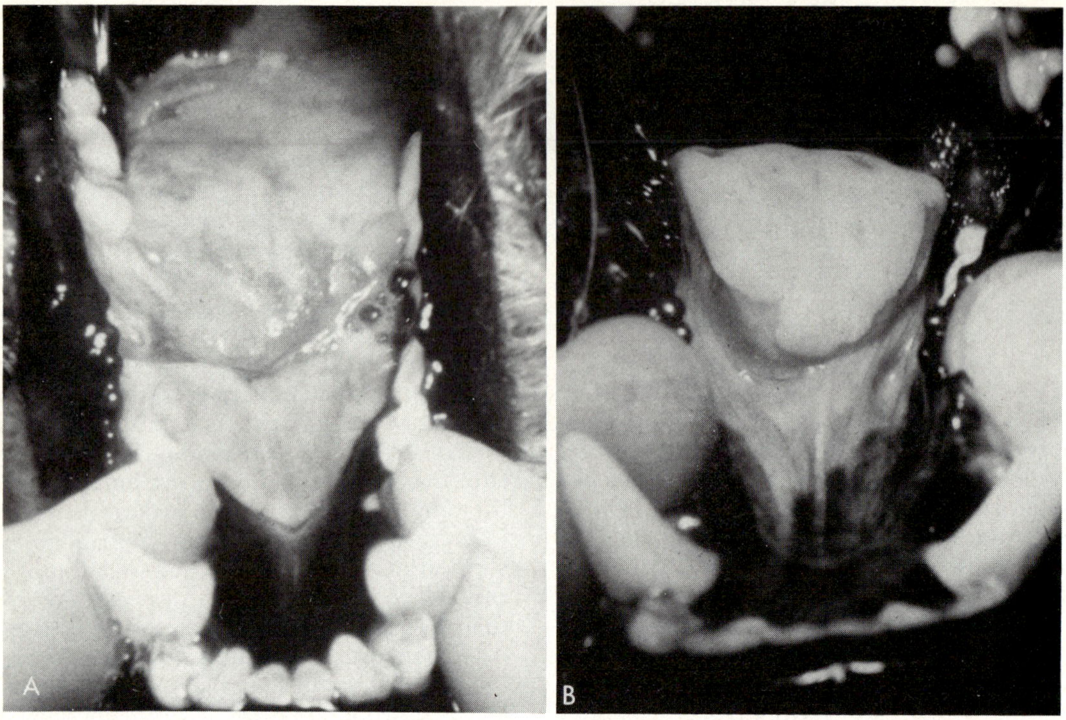

Figure 10–2. Necrosis of the tongue in a dog caused by chewing on an electric cord 1 day after injury *(A)*, and 18 days after injury *(B)*. (From Harvey CE, O'Brien JA. *In* Ettinger SJ (ed): Textbook of Veterinary Internal Medicine, Ch. 39. Philadelphia, WB Saunders Co., 1975.)

tied down to the adjacent soft tissues are not amenable to resection in veterinary patients.

Dogs and cats that have lost the entire free portion and some of the root of the tongue often manage well by sucking in food and water or by tossing chunks of food to the back of the tongue. Cats, who are more fastidious groomers than dogs, may develop a poor hair coat if the length of tongue available for grooming is insufficient.[10]

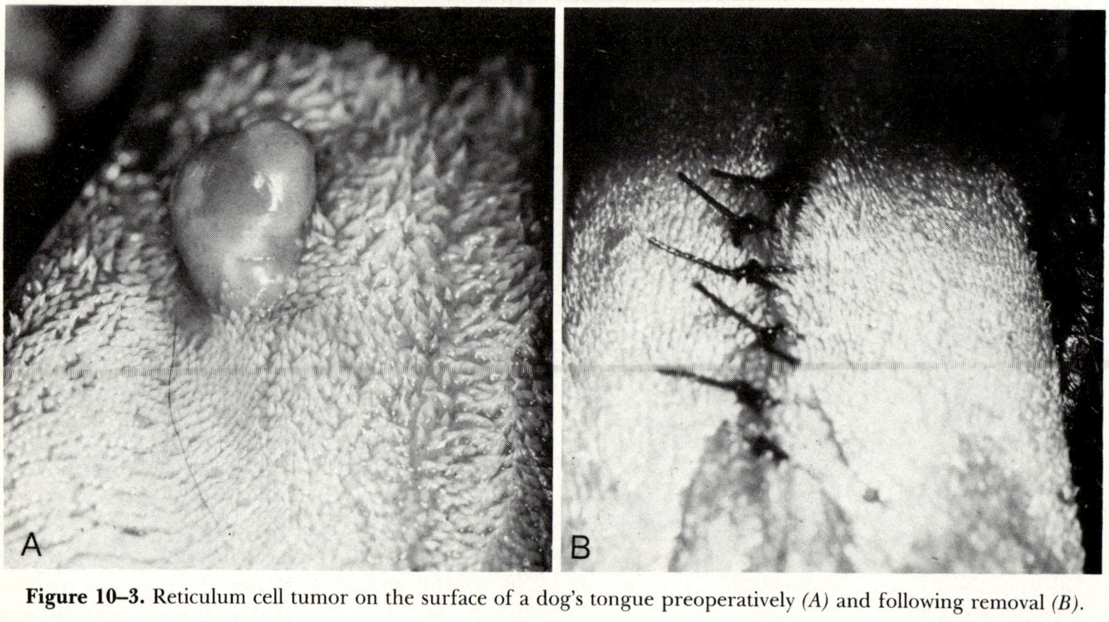

Figure 10–3. Reticulum cell tumor on the surface of a dog's tongue preoperatively *(A)* and following removal *(B)*.

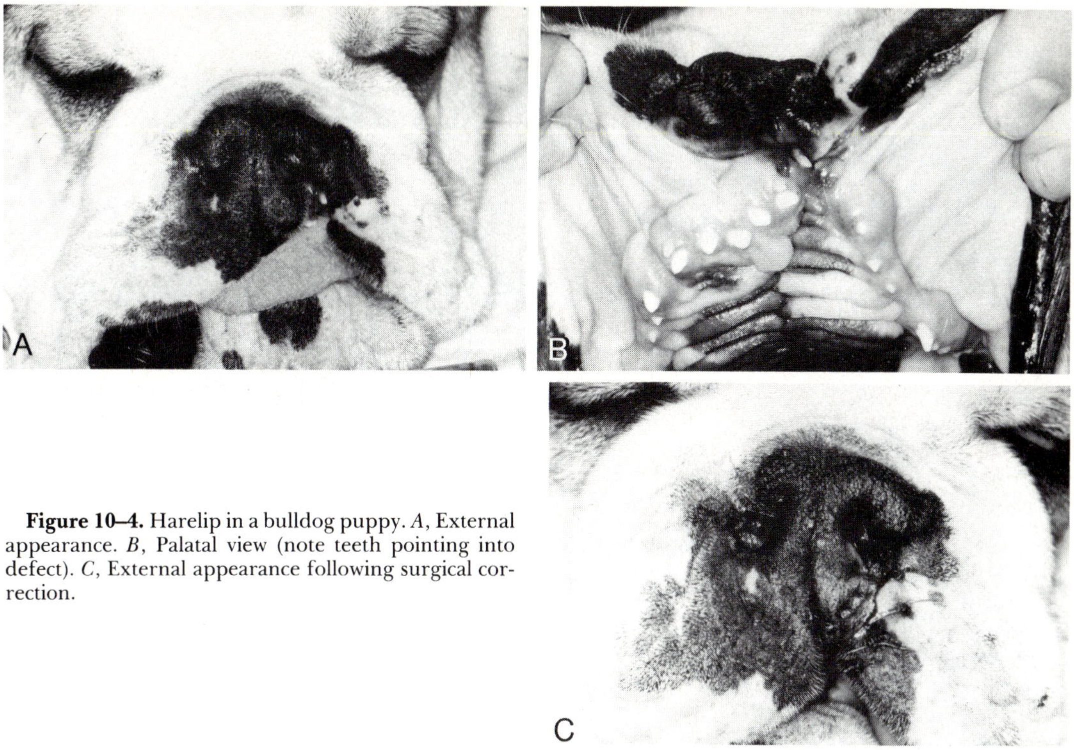

Figure 10–4. Harelip in a bulldog puppy. *A*, External appearance. *B*, Palatal view (note teeth pointing into defect). *C*, External appearance following surgical correction.

LIPS AND CHEEKS

Congenital abnormalities

Hare Lip. The most obvious abnormality affecting the lips is hare lip, in which the two sides of the primary palate fail to fuse normally. This condition is sporadically seen in a wide variety of breeds and is probably caused by intrauterine trauma or stress rather than by a genetic defect, though affected puppies have been born to affected parents.[11, 12] When the hare lip is unilateral in dogs, it is almost always on the left side, as is also the case in affected children.[12]

Treatment is by reconstruction of the lip (Fig. 10–4). Attempts to close the defect by simple sliding skin procedures are rarely successful, because there is no connective tissue bed to support the flap.[13] The floor of the nasal vestibule must be re-formed by creating flaps of oral or nasal tissue that are sutured with synthetic absorbable sutures. It is often necessary to remove one or more incisor teeth that would otherwise erupt into or through the repair (Fig. 10–4 *B*). The skin is closed over the defect by forming overlapping flaps on either side; absorbable subcutaneous sutures and monofilament skin sutures are then placed (Fig. 10–4 *C*). The philtrum (the midline crease between the lips) should be preserved or re-formed as symmetrically as possible.

Results depend on the care that is taken to form the flaps with minimal tension and accurate apposition of epithelial edges, resulting in minimal distortion of the lip edge.[13] Surgery of this type can be performed at any age, though the anesthetic risk suggests delaying the procedure until the animal is several months old; delayed surgery for hare lip without secondary cleft palate is not a problem, since airway aspiration is rarely a complication.

Lip-Fold Dermatitis. The most frequent congenital abnormality affecting the lips and cheeks is the abnormal lip fold conformation seen in some spaniels, and occasionally in some other breeds. The lips form a channel that causes saliva to flow onto the skin of the lip. The result is chronic moist dermatitis that is very foul-smelling. Diagnosis is by inspection of the lips (Fig. 10–5). The major differential diagnosis is halitosis caused by periodontal disease, which often coexists. Treatment is by resection of the folds, making a V-shaped incision through the skin and mucosa (Fig. 10–5 *B*). The two layers are sutured separately (Fig. 10–5 *C*). Results are usually excellent. Both sides usually require treatment in affected dogs.

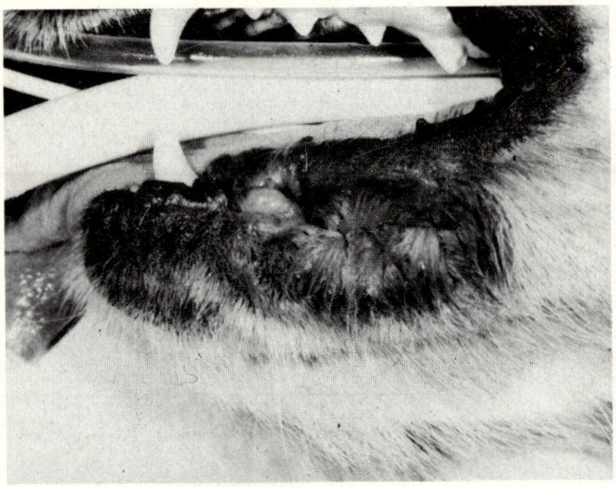

A

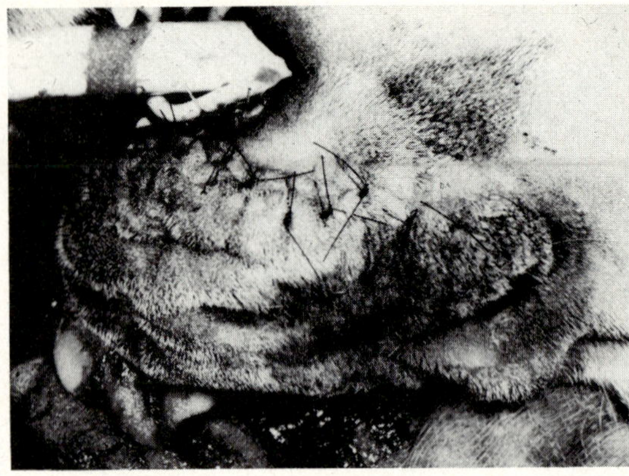

C

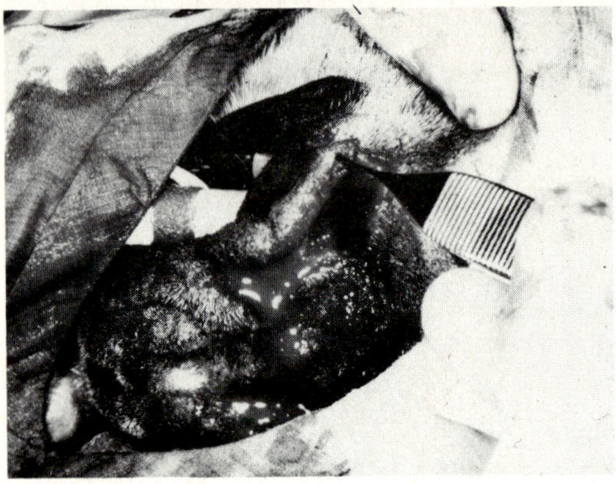

B

Figure 10–5. Lip-fold pyoderma in a dog. *A*, Preoperative appearance. *B*, Resection of tissue completed. *C*, Closure of incisions.

Giant-breed dogs with conformational drooling can be treated by bilateral mandibulosublingual gland ligation or resection (page 191); resection of the lip folds as already described, combined with salivary duct ligation, is a simple and effective technique. A more involved form of cheiloplasty has been described for this condition; a flap of the lower lip is isolated and is sutured to a defect created in the upper lip, forming a sling that channels the saliva back into the oral cavity.[14]

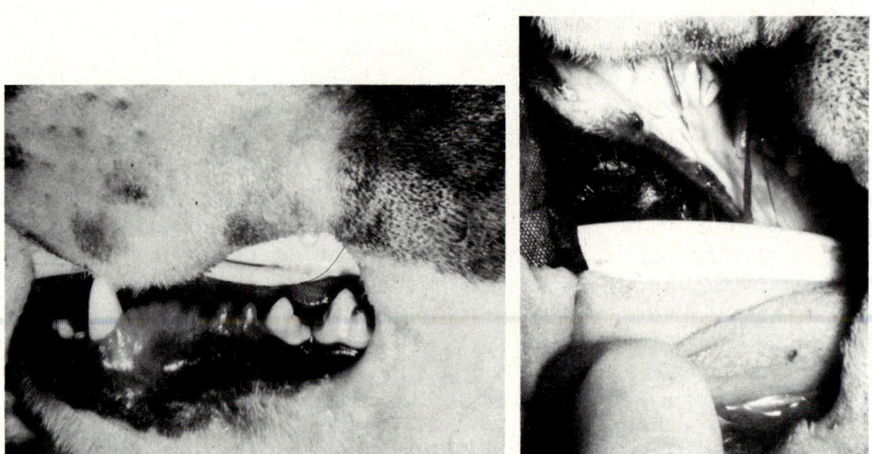

A B

Figure 10–6. Scarring of the commissure of the lip following an electric cord injury in a dog. *A*, Preoperative view. *B*, The commissure has been enlarged by incision and closure of epithelial surfaces.

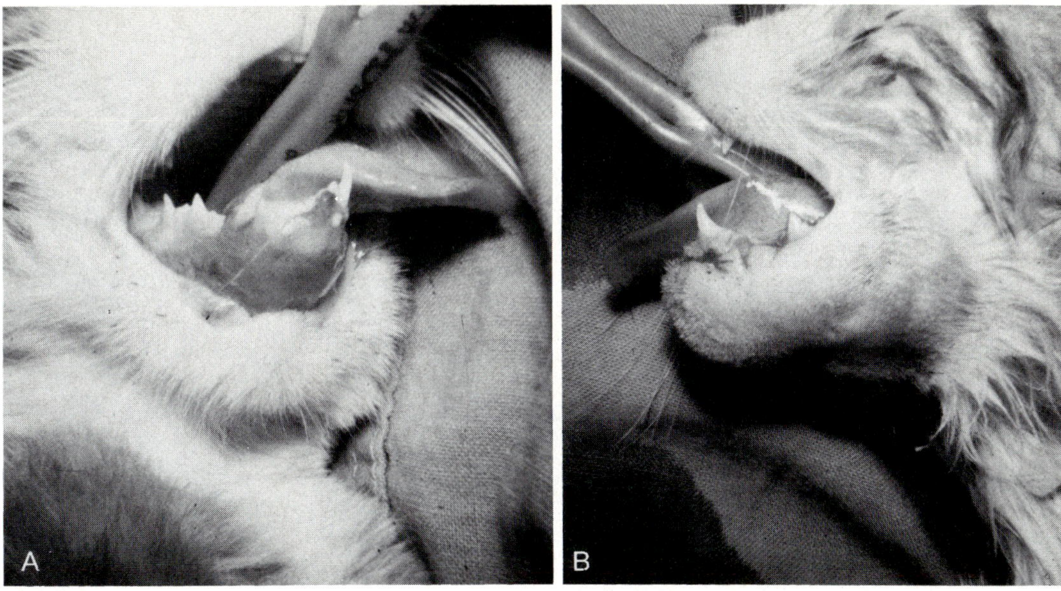

Figure 10–7. *A*, Avulsion of the lower lip in a cat. *B*, Following reattachment of the lip in its normal position. Sutures were placed around the canine teeth.

Trauma

Simple lacerations are sutured with separate layers on the mucosal and skin surfaces. Abscesses are lanced and drained, avoiding the parotid duct as it courses over the side of the face.[15]

Necrosis of part of the lip can be caused by electric cord injury or abscess and may result in stricture of the oral commissure and an inability of the animal to open the mouth (Fig. 10–6). This can be corrected by incising the scar at the commissure and closing the mucosa and skin as two layers to lengthen the commissure (Fig. 10–6 *B*); this procedure can be improved by performing a Z-plasty so that the healing incision is not located at the new commissure.

Avulsion injuries may cause severe skin loss. Because the mandible is an exposed prominence with not enough available skin for covering bare areas, every effort should be made to retain skin at the rostral end. This can be done by reattaching the avulsed skin to the gingival attachment if the skin is healthy (Fig. 10–7) or by rotating a flap of skin from the intermandibular area, with the subsequent repair of the defect created. Lip skin can be held in place at its rostral end by placing sutures through the skin and around

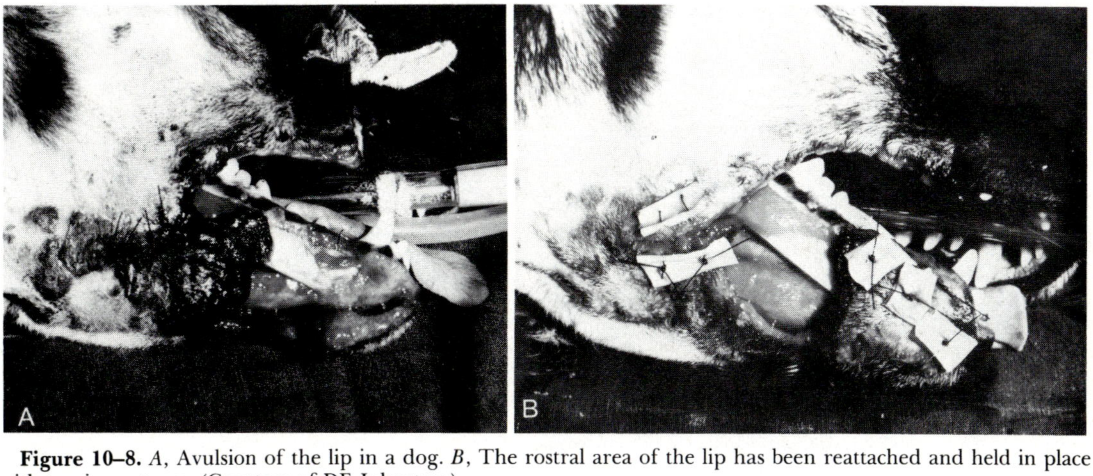

Figure 10–8. *A*, Avulsion of the lip in a dog. *B*, The rostral area of the lip has been reattached and held in place with tension sutures. (Courtesy of DE Johnston.)

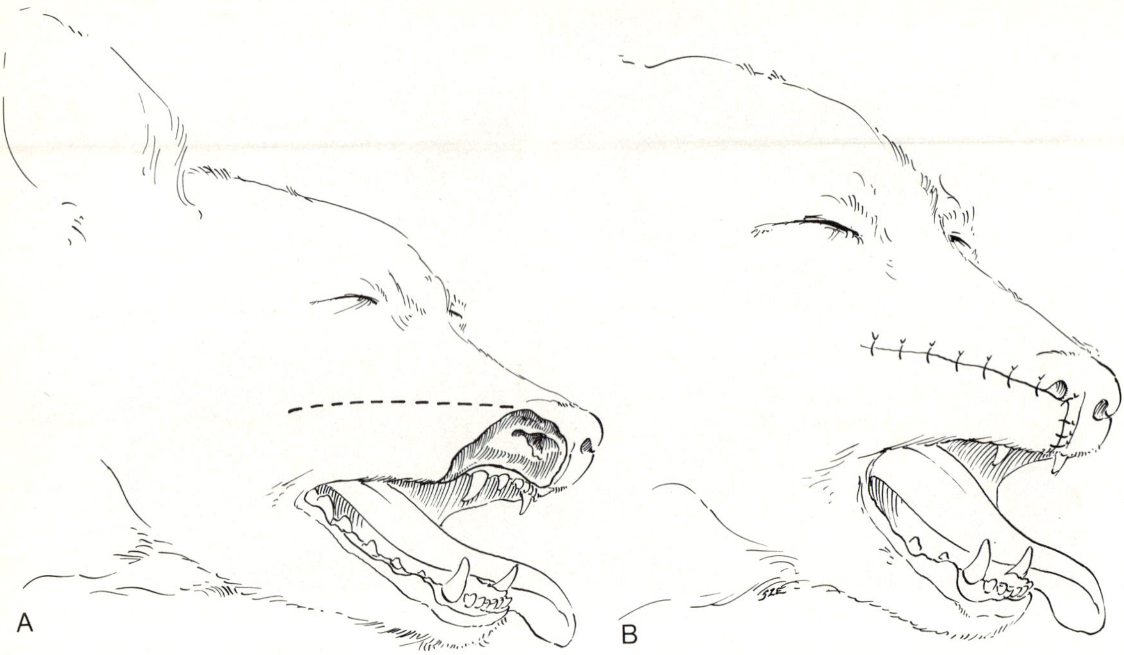

Figure 10–9. *A*, Loss of part of the upper lip and rhinarium in a dog. Incision for lip flap is shown *(dotted line)*. *B*, The flap has been sutured in place.

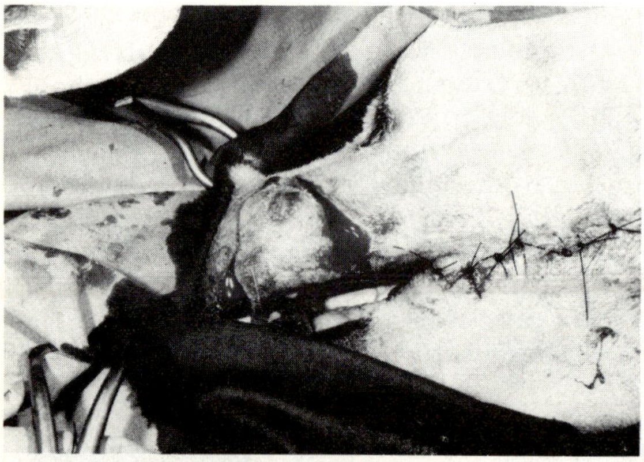

A

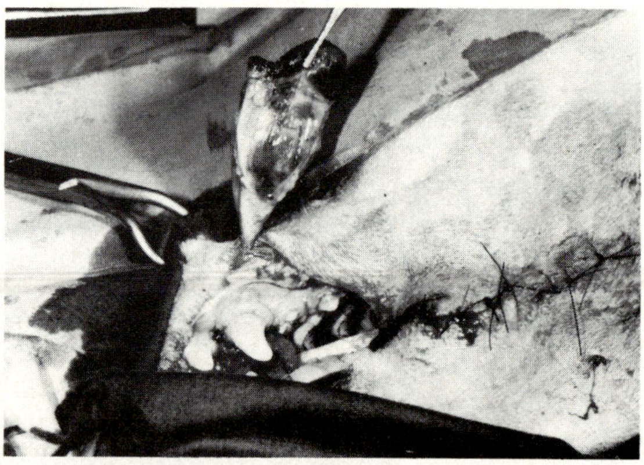

B

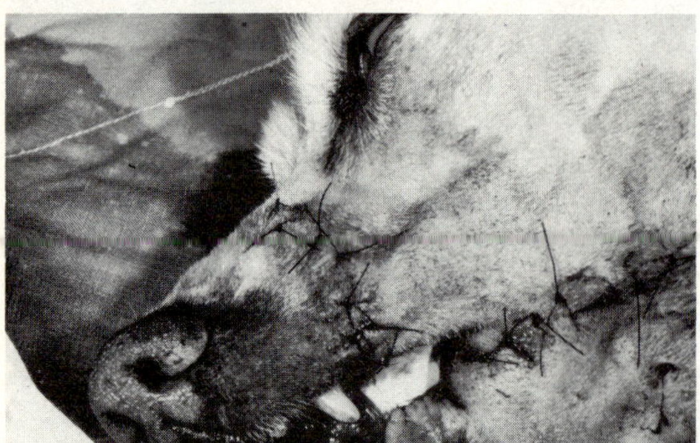

C

Figure 10–10. *A*, Basal cell tumor on the lip of a dog. *B*, The full thickness of the lip has been excised. *C*, The wound has been closed in two layers.

adjacent teeth (Fig. 10–7 *B*);[16] a soft rubber drain or plastic tubing can be used to form tension-relieving sutures (Fig. 10–8).[17]

Avulsion of the upper lip is less common but more spectacular if the nasal cavity is exposed. Disrupted tissues are débrided, are kept in normal apposition by sutures that are placed through the avulsed lip, and are anchored to one or more incisor or canine teeth.[18] A full-thickness upper lip pedicle flap can be formed and sutured in place to cover avulsion defects of the area around the philtrum; the buccinator muscle may have to be severed to obtain sufficient freedom of movement for the flap (Fig. 10–9).[19] The effect is to bring the lip commissure forward on that side, which does not interfere with the animal's ability to fully open the mouth.

Neoplastic and Hyperplastic Lesions

The principles of surgical management for lip and cheek lesions include biopsy of all lesions suspected of being malignant, wide excision of known malignant lesions, maintenance of a functional commissure so that the mouth can open (which may require lengthening of the commissure or use of rotation flaps), separate closure of the incisions in the mucosa and the skin when the resection is full thickness (Fig. 10–10), avoidance of the parotid salivary duct when possible, or ligation or transposition when avoidance is not possible.

Lesions that may appear to be neoplastic, but are in fact hyperplastic, include lip (eosinophilic) granuloma of cats and occasional single or multiple masses in the lip skin, which are probably chronic granulomata from foreign body penetration. Eosinophilic granulomata of cats should be managed medically when possible[20] (page 49, Chapter Four). Surgical resection and cryosurgical destruction[21] provide the least cosmetically acceptable results. Recurrence is possible with all treatment methods.

PALATE DEFECTS

Etiology

Formation defects of the palatal structures may be inherited, or they may result from an insult during the critical stage of fetal development when the two palatine shelves fuse to separate the oral and nasal cavities. A wide variety of dog and cat breeds are known to be affected. The sporadic nature of these conditions and the wide range of dog and cat breeds that are affected suggest that in most cases the cause is an intrauterine insult. Breeding studies have shown evidence of an inherited pattern with incomplete penetrance in the Shih Tzu breed, and possibly in pointers, bulldogs, and Swiss sheep dogs.[22] Other congenital defects, such as meningocele, may also be present occasionally.[23]

Primary palate (incisive bone) congenital abnormalities of formation appear as hare lip. They may be associated with abnormalities of the secondary palate (hard and soft palate), but they rarely result in clinical signs in and of themselves. Repair is made for esthetic reasons and is described on page 159.

Clefts of the secondary palate or acquired defects of the palate or maxilla are more serious, though they are rarely obvious externally. Affected animals are usually presented to the veterinarian because of nasal discharge. The prognosis without surgical repair is guarded because of the risk of lower airway aspiration.

Surgical correction of congenital cleft palate in dogs is usually possible if the animal can survive and grow to a suitable size for anesthesia and surgery. Milk substitute or puppy food fed by tube several times daily is necessary in most dogs and cats to avoid recurrent, and eventually fatal, aspiration pneumonia. The larger the animal is at the time of surgery the better; most procedures of this sort are performed on animals who are 2 to 4 months of age.

Congenital cleft hard palate is almost always in the midline and is usually associated with a midline soft palate abnormality (Fig. 10–11). Soft palate defects without hard palate defects may occur in the midline or may be unilateral.

Repair

The principles for the surgical treatment of palate defects follow:

1. The covering flaps should be large in comparison to the size of the defect. This ensures that tension on the suture line will be minimized, and it may permit overlapping of tissues to provide support for the suture line.
2. Tissues should be sutured so as to appose cleanly incised epithelial edges. A flap sutured to an intact epithelial surface will not heal.

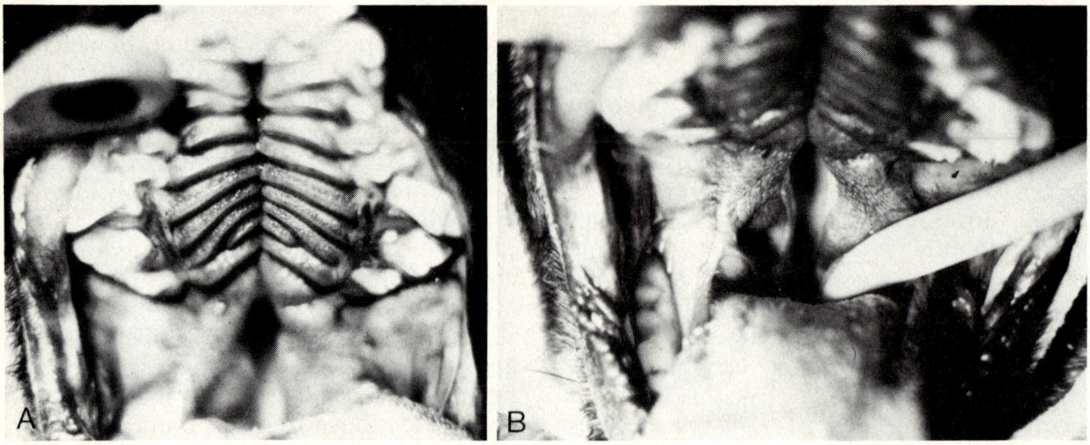

Figure 10–11. Hard *(A)* and soft *(B)* cleft palate in a dog.

3. When possible, suture lines should be arranged so that they lie over connective tissue rather than over the defect. This will prevent drying and contamination of the connective tissue side of the flap and will increase the likelihood that the repair will remain intact during the healing process.

4. Tissues should be sutured gently, using large bites of tissue to minimize tension and interference with the blood supply at the wound edges.

The surgical area is limited by the presence of the mandible and the tongue, particularly when repairing soft palate defects. Mandibular symphysiotomy provides additional exposure[24, 25] (page 179); however, it has rarely been necessary in my experience.

Types

Midline Palate Defects

When correcting midline congenital defects, the foregoing principles are best met by using the overlapping flap technique (Fig.

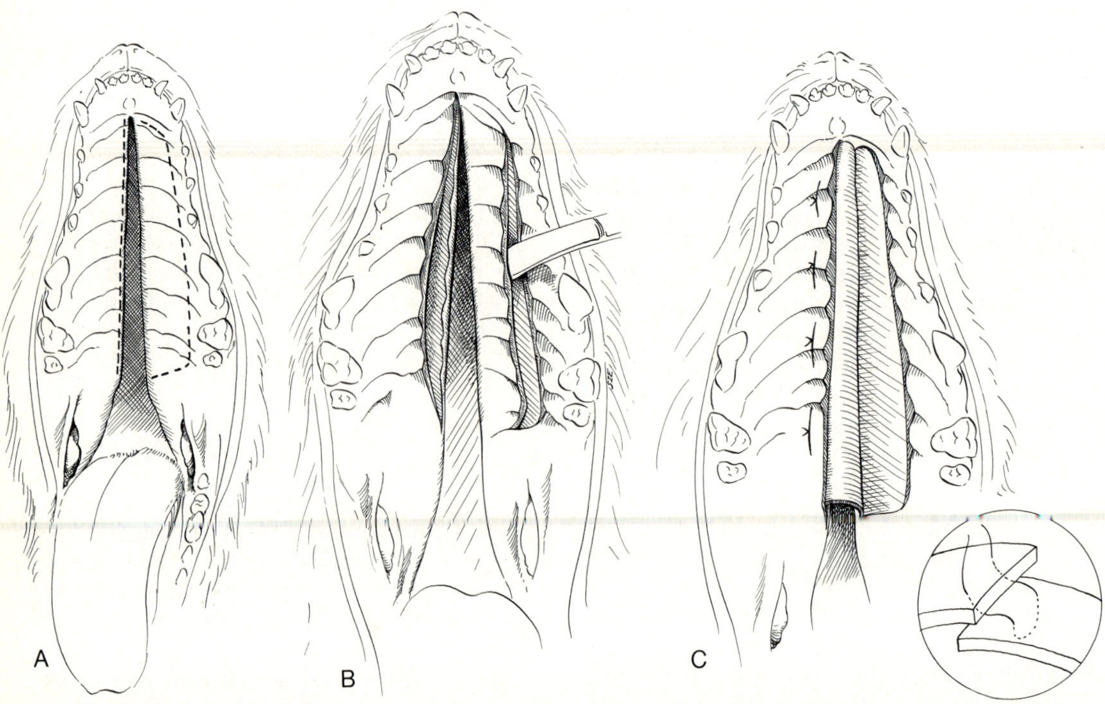

Figure 10–12. Overlapping flap technique for closure of midline hard palate defects. *A*, Incisions to create flaps. *B*, A periosteal elevator is used to raise the flaps. *C*, One flap is turned and laid under the other, and the flaps are sutured to each other.

10–12).[26] Incisions in the palate mucosa are made down to bone, and a periosteal elevator is used to separate the mucoperiosteum from the bone to form two flaps. One flap is hinged at the edge of the cleft, and the other is attached at the lateral aspect of the palate (Fig. 10–12 *A*, and *B*). Hemorrhage is usually brisk and is controlled with pressure. The incisions extend to the junction of the hard and soft palates. The flap that is hinged at the defect margin is turned under the other flap, and the connective tissue surfaces of the two flaps are kept in apposition by horizontal mattress sutures of synthetic absorbable material (Figs. 10–12 *C* and 10–13). This technique does not result in apposition of epithelial cut edges, but it does provide a wide area of connective tissue contact without tension. The epithelial defect fills in by epithelialization. It is rare for repairs that use this technique to break down if the formed flaps retain sufficient vascularity.

The alternative technique is to form two symmetrical flaps by making incisions at the edges of the defect, then suturing the flaps over it (Fig. 10–14).[27] It is usually necessary to make relieving incisions on one or both sides so that the mucoperiosteal flaps can be slid over to appose each other.[25, 28] In my hands, this technique usually results in tension at the suture line, which is located directly over the defect, and is followed by partial breakdown of the repair. The relieving incision gapes, and a lateral oronasal defect may result, particularly in narrow-nosed dogs (Fig. 10–15). For these reasons, I recommend the overlapping flap technique previously described.

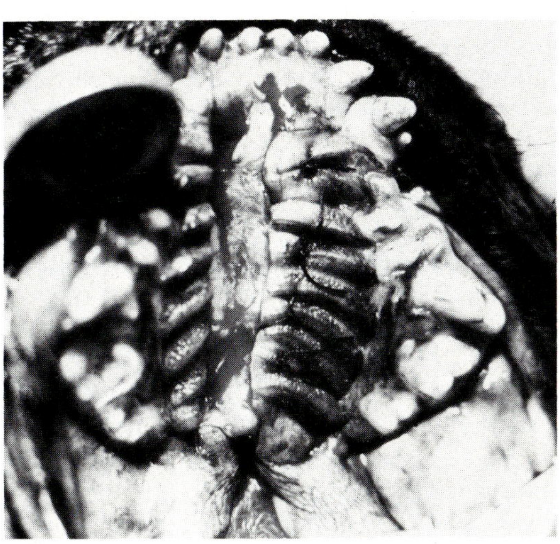

Figure 10–13. Correction of the cleft palate shown in Figure 10–11.

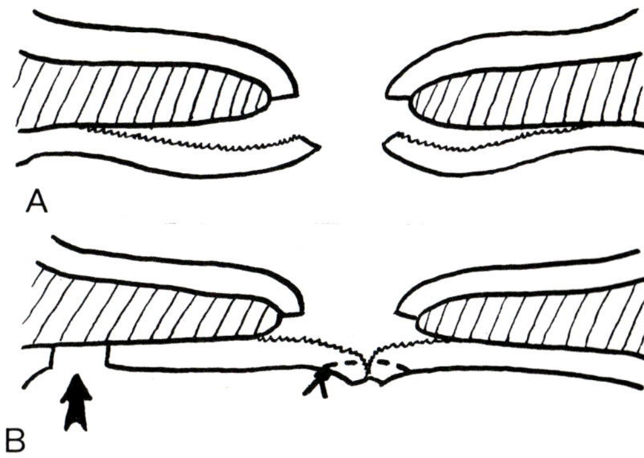

Figure 10–14. Alternative technique for cleft palate repair. *A*, Incisions are made along the cleft, and flaps are raised. *B*, A relieving incision or incisions *(arrow)* are made as necessary to join the edges of the flaps, and the flaps are sutured in the midline.

With either technique, closure of the soft palate defect is performed in the same manner (Fig. 10–16). Incisions at the end of the hard palate are continued onto the soft palate at the junction of the oronasal epithelium to the level of the middle of the tonsils. These incisions are deepened by gentle blunt dissection to form a dorsal and a ventral flap on each side. The dorsal flaps are sutured to appose the nasal epithelial edges, and the suture knots are placed on the epithelial surface to minimize scar tissue formation

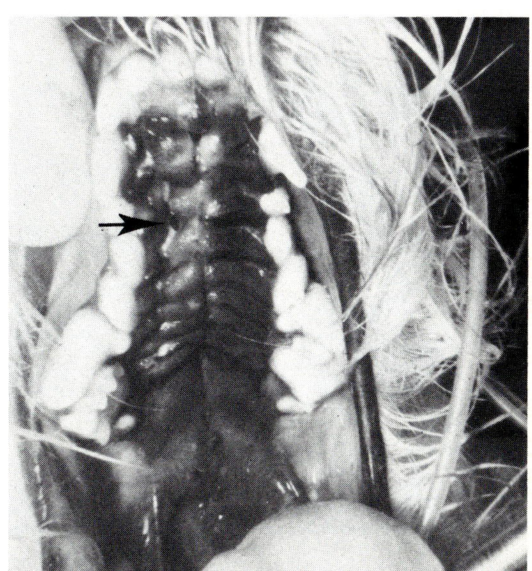

Figure 10–15. Result of the use of the technique shown in Figure 10–14. The midline defect has healed, but a lateral defect *(arrow)* has formed through one of the relieving incisions in this narrow-nosed dog.

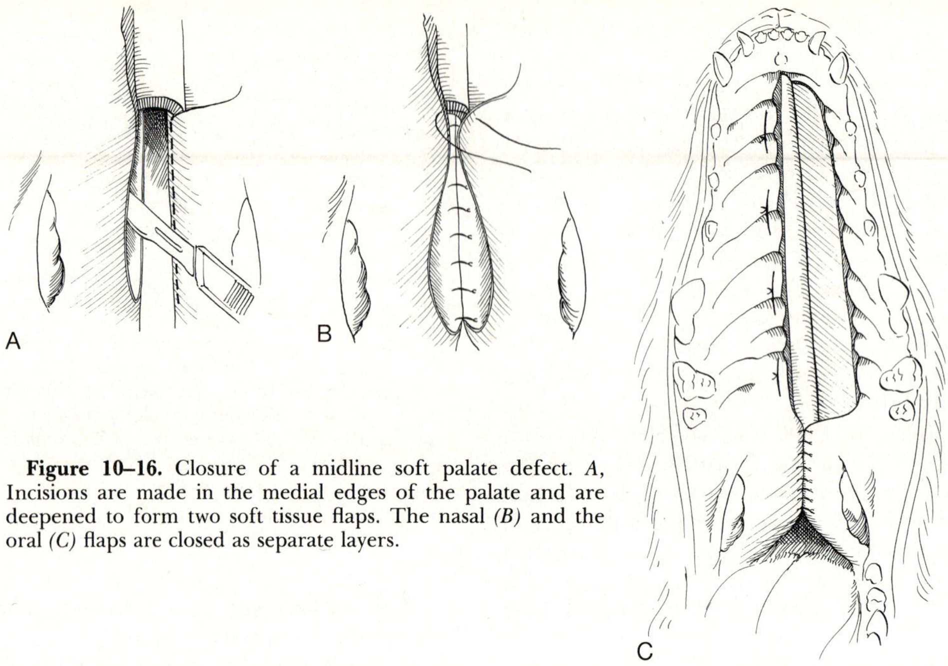

Figure 10–16. Closure of a midline soft palate defect. *A*, Incisions are made in the medial edges of the palate and are deepened to form two soft tissue flaps. The nasal *(B)* and the oral *(C)* flaps are closed as separate layers.

within the muscle tissue of the palate. The ventral flaps are then sutured together to appose the oral epithelium (Fig. 10–17). This technique works well for closing the rare midline cleft of the soft palate, or for closing incisions in the soft palate that were made for access to the nasopharynx.

Closure of palate defects in cats is similar (Fig. 10–18): the tissues in these animals are thinner and must be handled gently.

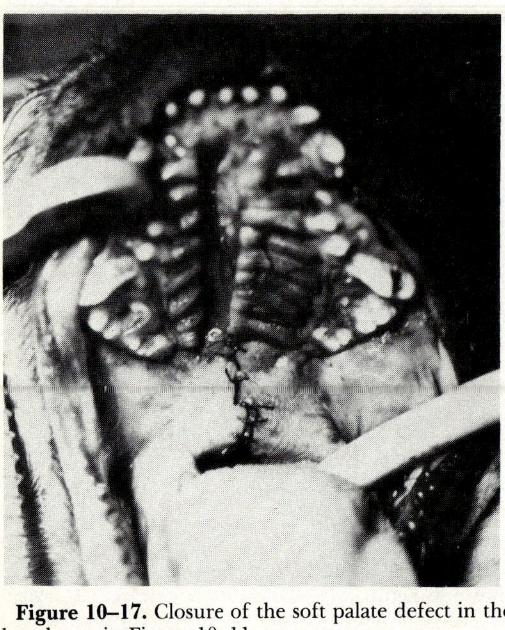

Figure 10–17. Closure of the soft palate defect in the dog shown in Figure 10–11.

Unilateral Soft Palate Defects.

Unilateral hypoplasia, or failure of fusion of the soft palate on one side, occurs sporadically in a number of breeds (Fig. 10–19). This condition is seen less commonly than midline cleft of the hard and soft palates. Often, the simple flap technique for closing midline soft palate defects is not successful on unilateral soft palate defects, perhaps because the tension produced by muscle activity during swallowing is more disruptive when the repair is not symmetrical.[29] More elaborate flap techniques are necessary. The tonsil on the affected side can be removed, providing tissue for dorsal and ventral flaps that can be sutured to flaps made by incising the palatal edge on the "normal" side (Fig. 10–19 *B* through *F*).[30, 31] If this repair breaks down, the entire lateral pharyngeal wall is available for the creation of flaps.[31] A flap that is formed entirely from nasopharyngeal mucosa and submucosa was used successfully in one dog.[29]

Bilateral Absence of Part of the Soft Palate

There is a rare, but severe, deformity that is seen as a very short soft palate and is referred to as bilateral absence of part of the short palate. A midline "uvula" may represent the only soft palate tissue present (Fig. 10–20). Presenting signs include nasal dis-

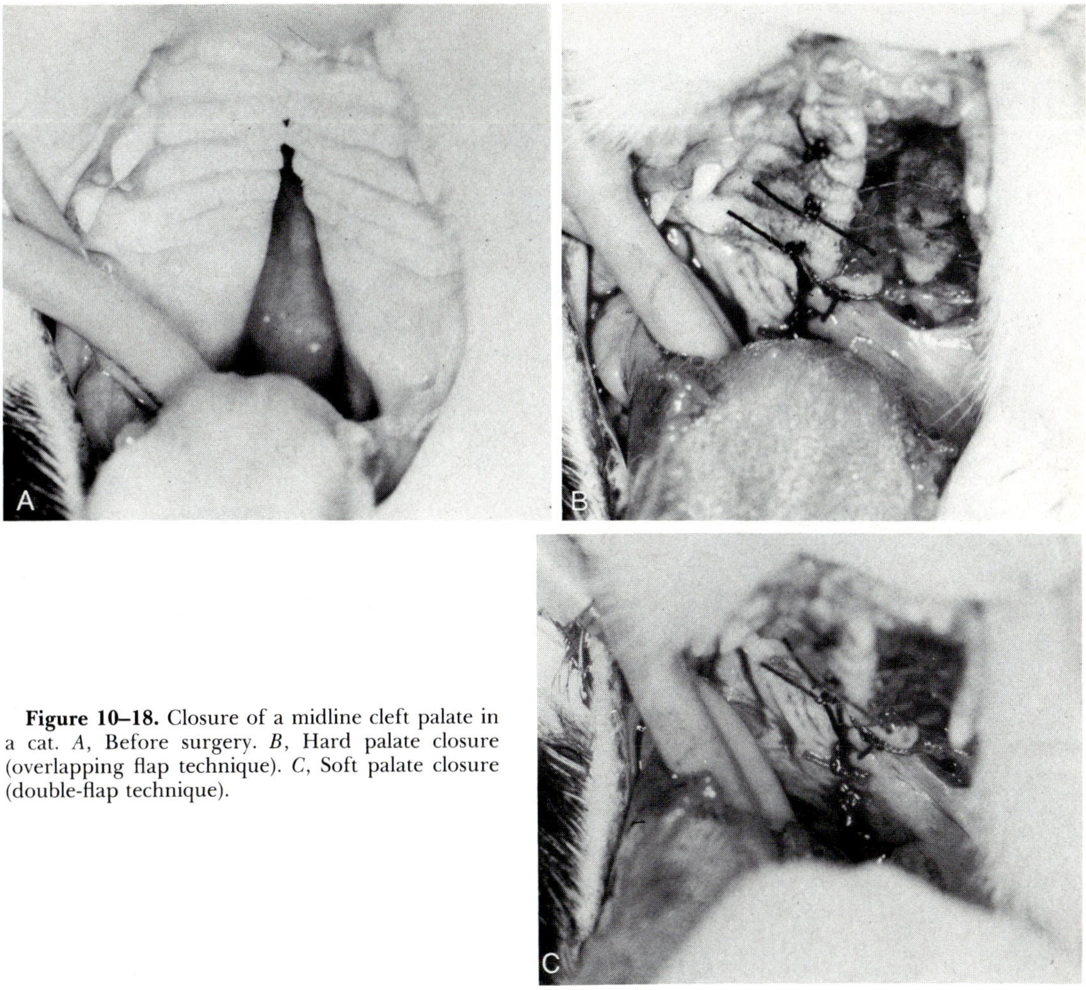

Figure 10–18. Closure of a midline cleft palate in a cat. *A*, Before surgery. *B*, Hard palate closure (overlapping flap technique). *C*, Soft palate closure (double-flap technique).

charge and cough or respiratory distress resulting from pneumonia. Because the palate is symmetrical, and is intact in the midline, this abnormality may be missed on casual inspection of the pharynx. Attempts to correct this defect by sliding hard palate mucoperiosteum caudally have not been successful.[31]

Acquired Palate Defects

The most common cause of acquired defects between the nasal and oral cavities is the loss of maxillary bone associated with severe periodontal disease or tooth extraction; this defect is usually referred to as an oronasal fistula. Trauma (dog bites, electric cord injury), severe chronic infections, surgery, and radiation therapy of palatal tumors are other causes.

Oronasal Fistula. This defect most commonly occurs following loss of the canine tooth. If an abnormality is obvious at the time of tooth extraction (as evidenced by bleeding from the nose during the procedure or the appearance of fluid from the external nares when the socket is gently flushed), absorbable sutures can be placed in an attempt to collapse the sides of the alveolus and prevent formation of a fistula. An established fistula is repaired by creating a buccal flap (Fig. 10–21), advancing it over the defect, and suturing it to cleanly incised epithelium on the palatal margin.[32, 33] Results are excellent with this technique if the flap is large enough and includes some connective tissue to retain vascularity.

Hard Palate. Most defects in the hard palate can be closed by some form of mucoperiosteal flap. Because the mucoperiosteum has so little elasticity, it cannot be stretched to cover a large area. Therefore, it is essential to plan the position of the flap in advance so that a large enough area of tissue can be obtained to ensure healing. Rotation and advancement flaps can be created. In general, one should use the technique that will pro-

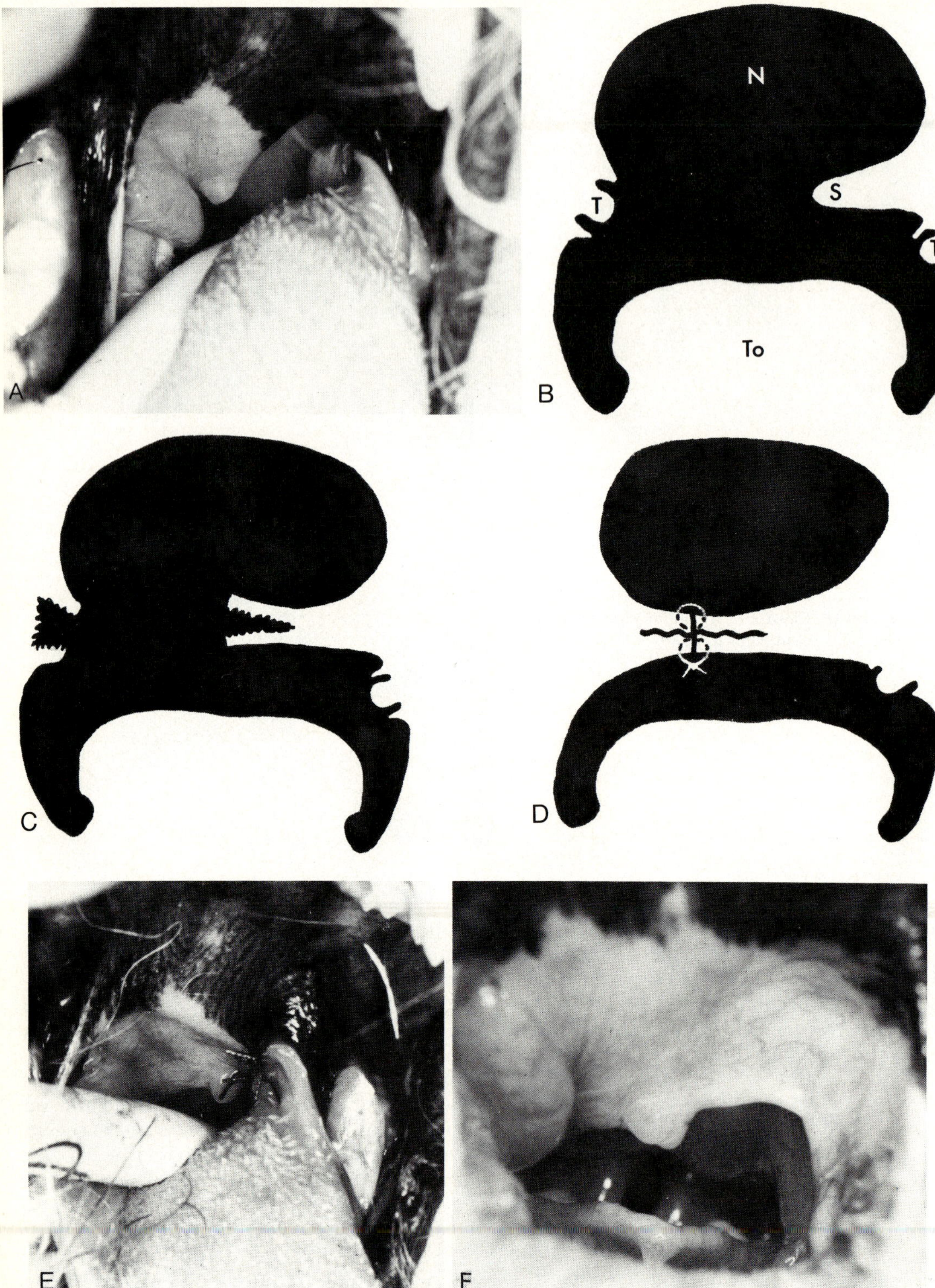

Figure 10–19. *A*, Unilateral soft palate defect in a dog. The tonsil is attached to a "common" pharynx on the abnormal side. *B–D*, Diagram of cross section of the head to show the closure technique. The tonsil is removed and flaps are formed from the tonsillar crypt and from the soft palate on the "normal" side *(C)*, and the four flaps are sutured *(D)*. (N = nasopharynx, S = soft palate, T = tonsil, To = tongue.) *E*, Immediate postoperative appearance. *F*, Appearance 6 months later.

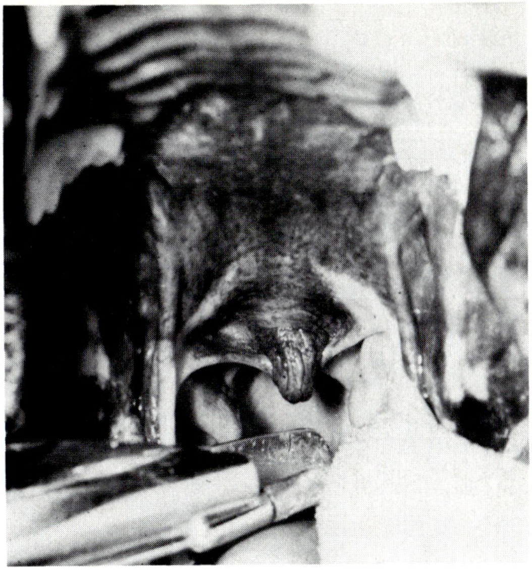

Figure 10–20. Bilateral soft palate defect in a dog. Both tonsils are attached to an enlarged common pharynx.

vide the largest flap. The area of the palate that is left devoid of mucosa will heal readily by epithelialization, and necrosis of the bare palatine bone is almost unknown. For small, circular defects, rotation flaps usually are best (Fig. 10–22). For long midline or paramidline defects (such as those resulting from midline palatal separation in cats who have fallen from a height or who have been hit by a car), the overlapping technique described previously for congenital defects can be used if the epithelium at the defect has matured. Alternatively, relieving incisions can be made to allow two lateral flaps to be apposed.

Fresh midline lacerations in palates of cats may not need surgical repair if there is no bubbling through the defect from the nose, because the stump of the vomer bone or nasal septum plugs the defect until a blood clot forms and healing commences. Fresh defects with obvious communication into the nasal cavity can be closed successfully by simply placing sutures to join the tissue edges, as for a clean skin wound.[34]

Large defects that cross the midline require the use of an advancement flap,[35] which necessitates the elevation of the mucoperiosteum caudally to include part of the soft palate so that sufficient tissue can be pulled forward to prevent tension on the suture line (Fig. 10–23). With flaps of any shape, it is essential that the epithelium around the defect be removed to provide a surface for healing. For very large defects (covering more than half the width of the palate), a buccal-based flap can be formed and sutured across the defect, though the teeth and remaining palatal mucosa adjacent to the defect must first be removed. An alternative method is to create a permanent or removable acrylic or metal obturator (Fig. 10–24).[36,37] Tech-

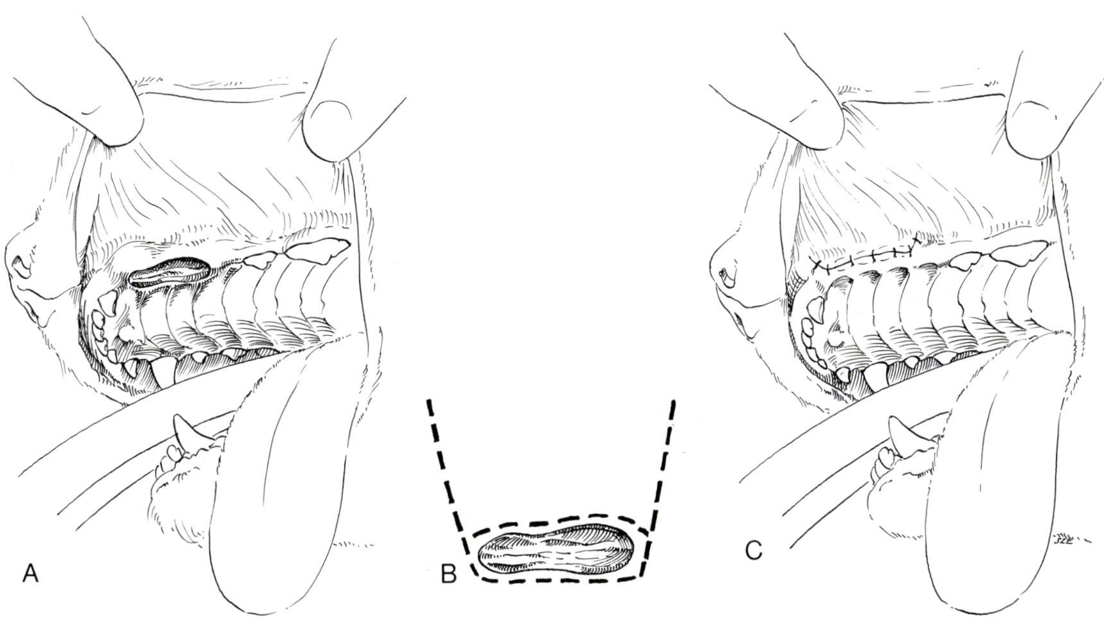

Figure 10–21. *A*, Oronasal fistula following extraction of a canine tooth. *B*, Planned incisions to form a buccal flap and a bed to receive it. *C*, Following closure.

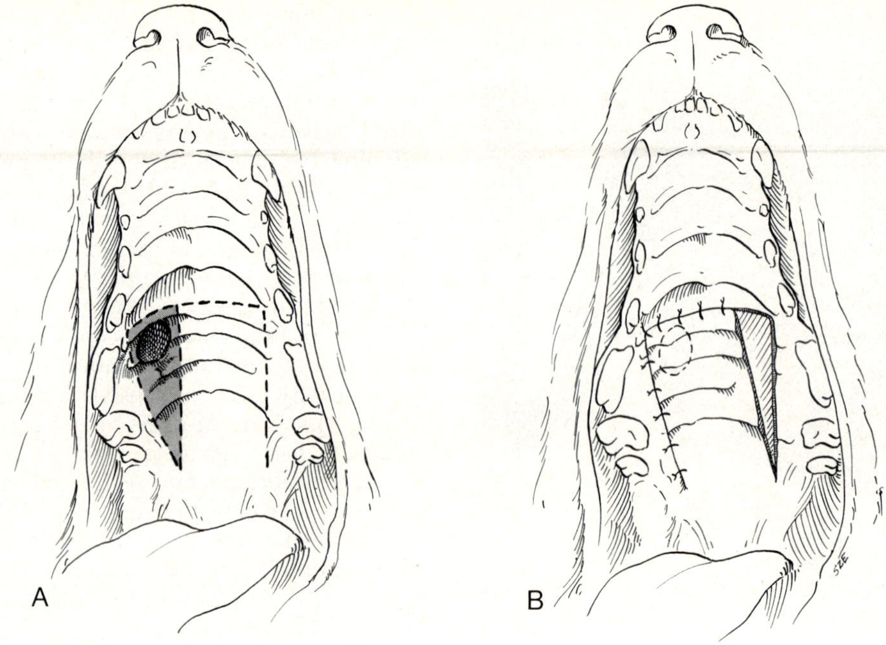

Figure 10–22. *A*, Defect in the hard palate with planned incisions. *B*, Closure with a rotation flap.

niques and materials for making dental impressions and acrylic obturators are described in Chapter Seven.

ORAL MASS LESIONS

Diagnosis and treatment planning for oral neoplasms is described in Chapter Eight. Cystic lesions and chronic infection are also indications for en bloc resection of oral structures.

Cystic lesions may be congenital[38, 39] or neoplastic.[40] Other lesions arising from the tooth-forming structures in young dogs may consist of multiple, odd-shaped dental structures or bony proliferation.[41, 42]

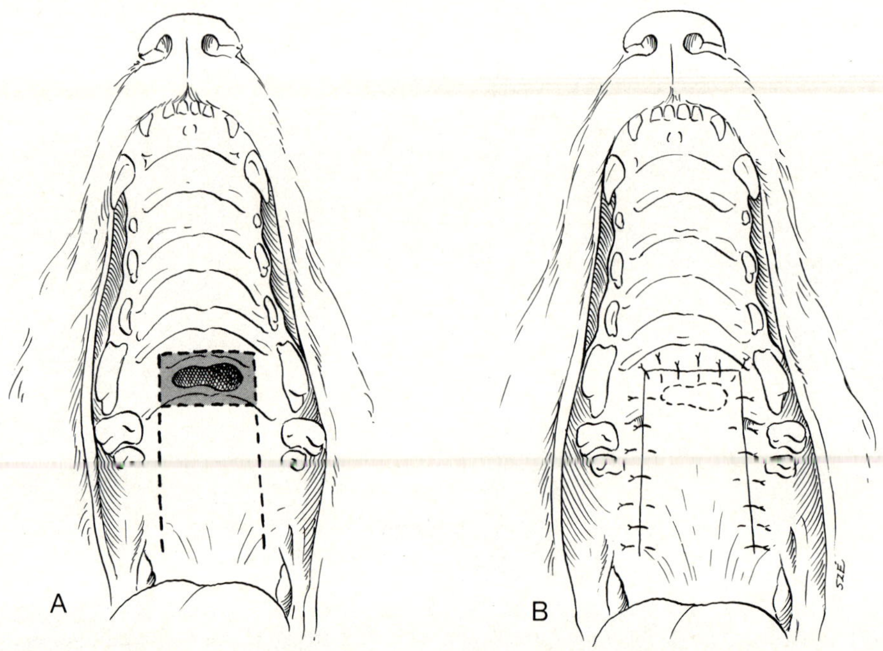

Figure 10–23. *A*, Midline defect in the hard palate and planned incisions, which extend onto the soft palate. *B*, Closure with an advancement flap.

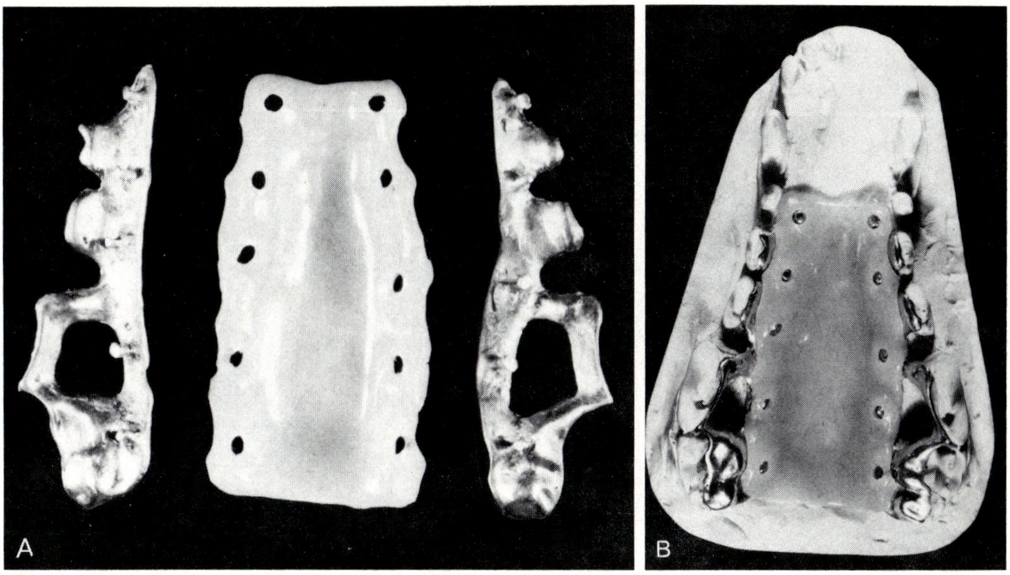

Figure 10–24. Acrylic obturator to close a large defect in the hard palate. *A*, Metal retention devices that can be bonded to teeth and acrylic obturator. *B*, Obturator snapped into place on posts in retention devices on a model. (Courtesy of Dr. A Thomas.)

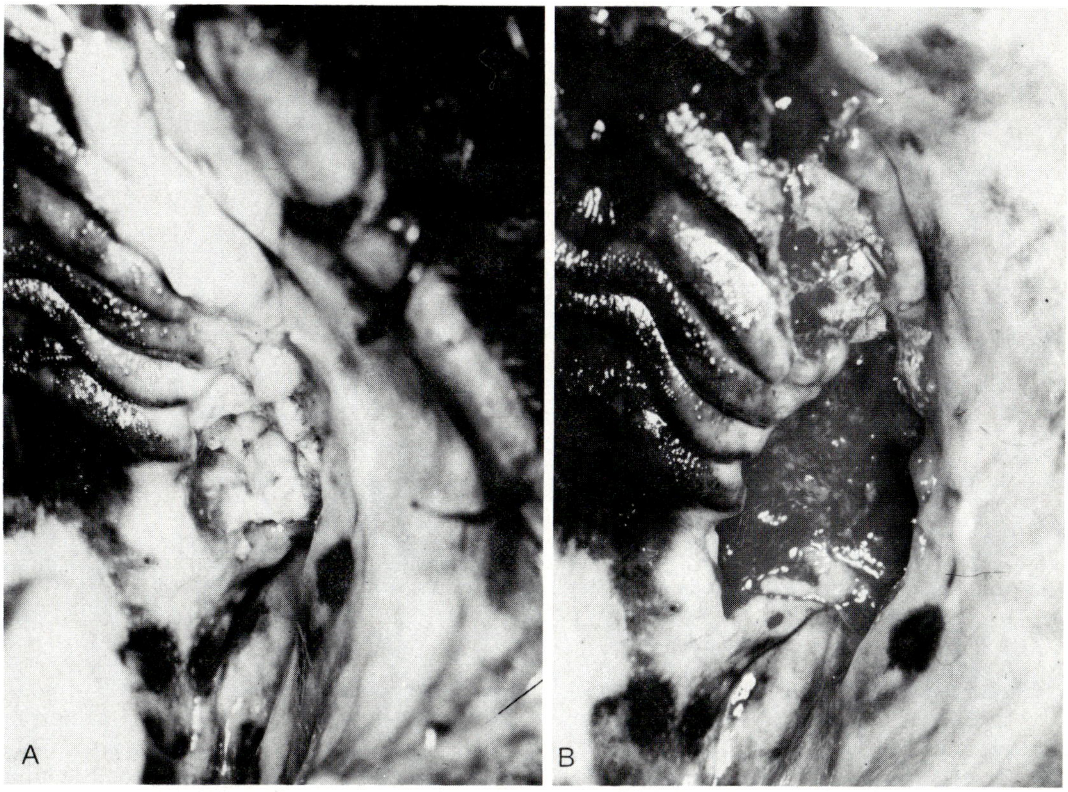

Figure 10–25. *A*, Longstanding osteomyelitis of the maxilla in a dog secondary to periodontal disease and extraction. *B*, Following curettage.

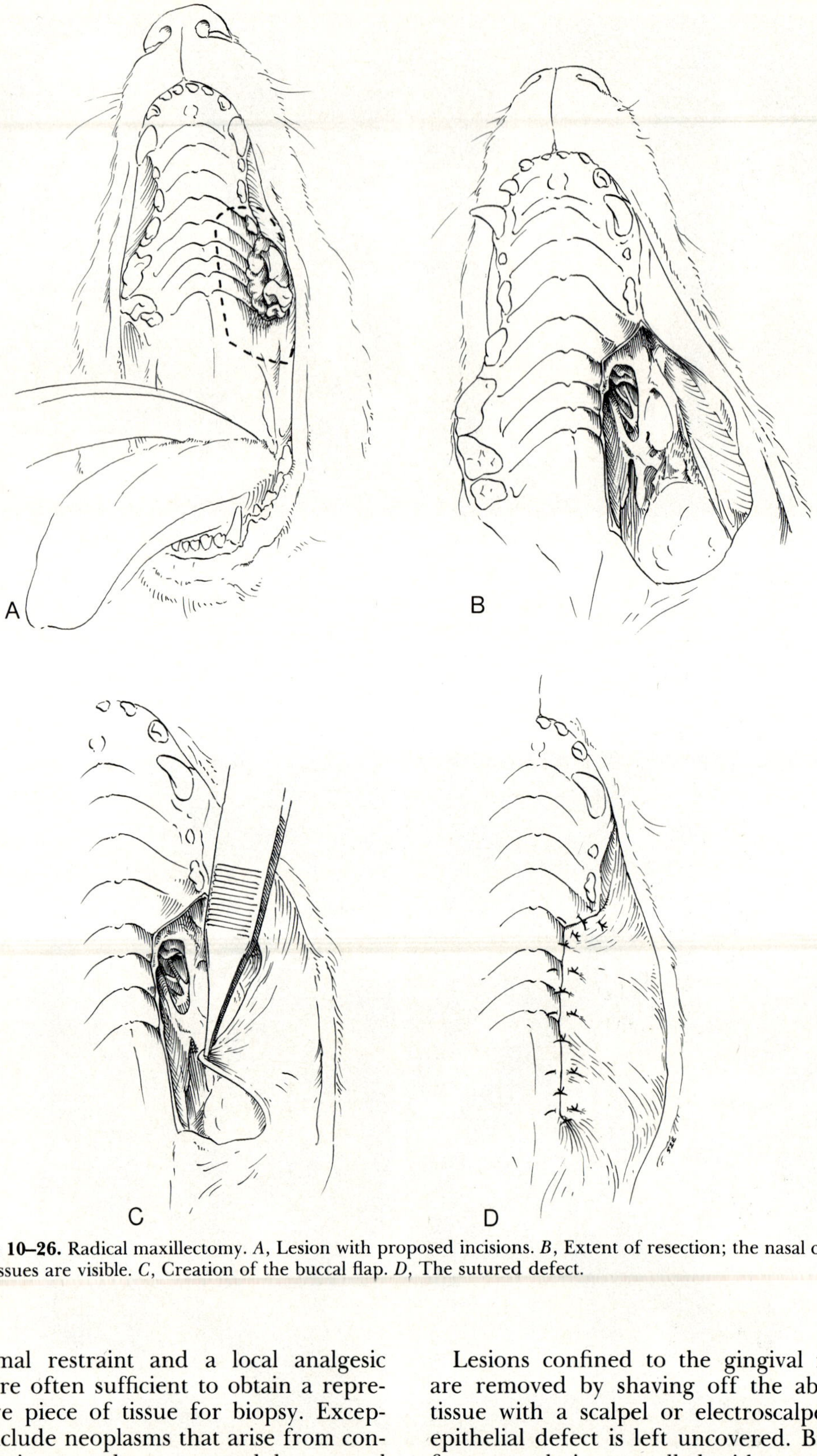

Figure 10–26. Radical maxillectomy. *A*, Lesion with proposed incisions. *B*, Extent of resection; the nasal cavity and orbital tissues are visible. *C*, Creation of the buccal flap. *D*, The sutured defect.

Minimal restraint and a local analgesic spray are often sufficient to obtain a representative piece of tissue for biopsy. Exceptions include neoplasms that arise from connective tissue and are covered by normal mucosa.

Lesions confined to the gingival mucosa are removed by shaving off the abnormal tissue with a scalpel or electroscalpel. The epithelial defect is left uncovered. Bleeding from vessels is controlled with pressure or electrocoagulation. Lesions on the mucosa of the hard palate can be removed in a similar fashion. This superficial method of excision is applicable only to hyperplastic or benign lesions that have not penetrated the basement membrane. Often, it is not even sufficient for benign lesions such as fibromatous epulis. When there has been recurrence of a benign lesion following conservative resection, consideration should be given to radiation therapy or radical surgery, though intermittent conservative resection is also possible.

Fortunately, generalized maxillary or mandibular osteomyelitis is uncommon. This condition usually results from chronic periodontitis. As the periodontitis progresses, most or all of the teeth on the affected jaw will fall out or will be removed. Large areas of necrotic bone, with reactive new bone surrounding it, are seen on examination of the mouth (Fig. 10–25). The maxilla or mandible may be grossly swollen. Nasal discharge is not common. Medical treatment of osteomyelitis in this location is often unavailing, though drugs that are particularly effective against the spectrum of bacteria associated with severe periodontitis, such as tetracycline (20 mg/kg TID PO for a minimum of 4 weeks) or metronidazole (50 mg/kg daily PO, 5 days on and 5 days off, repeated twice) should be tried before resorting to radical surgery. Conservative surgical treatment, such as limited curettage of obviously necrotic bone, followed by a prolonged course of antibiotics, usually is only successful temporarily. Radical resection of affected tissue back to normal bone (Fig. 10–25 *B*) is much more likely to cure the condition.

Maxillectomy

Invasive or recurrent lesions of the maxilla or palate can only be cured surgically by radical resection. Radical partial maxillectomy and palatectomy are practical and cause little or no long-term problem for the animal. Since the mucosa of the cheek is not resected, it is available to cover the lesion. The cosmetic defect is a sunken-in appearance to one side of the face, and even this is not noticeable in long-haired dogs. Partial maxillectomy is easier to perform on lesions located in the middle third of the hard palate because of the desirability of maintaining a bony platform for the nasal cartilage at the rostral end of the nose. A 1-cm margin of grossly normal tissue is removed with the tumor when possible.

The procedure commences with an incision in the palatal, gingival, and buccal mucosae to outline the extent of resection, staying at least 1 cm away from the gross margins of the lesion (Fig. 10–26). The epithelium is reflected to expose the underlying bone. Hemorrhage is often profuse, particularly when the palate is incised, but can usually be controlled with pressure until the resected tissue is lifted out, at which time the vessels themselves can be located and ligated or electrocoagulated. Temporary occlusion of one or both carotid arteries through an incision in the neck should be considered in animals having a low hematocrit prior to surgery. The maxilla and palate are fractured along the incision lines with a bur driven by a high speed dental or orthopedic handpiece,

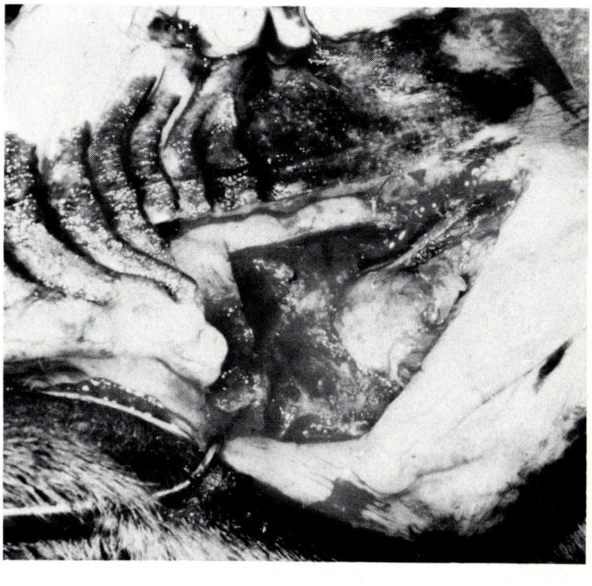

Figure 10–27. Maxillectomy. A shelf of bone has been left to form a support for the buccal flap.

an osteotome or oscillating bone saw (Fig. 10–26 *B*). Ideally, a shelf of bone is left so that closure of the mucosal incision is supported (Fig. 10–27); however, this is not generally possible given the size of most oral malignancies at the time of surgery. The line of incision may include the infraorbital canal; if this is the case, the infraorbital artery must be picked up and ligated. The tissue to be resected is levered up; remaining attachments are separated; and the section, which usually includes several teeth *in situ,* is removed en bloc (Figs. 10–26 *B* and 10–28).

Normally, the nasal passage will be exposed at this point if the resection is adequate. If the nasal cavity is not exposed, the resection is unlikely to be adequate as primary treatment of an oral malignancy. Hemorrhage is controlled, blood clots are removed, and the remaining tissues are examined. If there are areas of turbinate that were partially severed or traumatized during the resection, they are cut with scissors to leave a clean edge. Hemorrhage that cannot be controlled by ligation or pressure may respond to surface application of a 5 per cent cocaine solution. The use of diluted epinephrine is to be avoided, particularly when the anesthetic agent used is halothane.

The defect between the nose and the mouth is covered with a buccal flap that is created by incising the buccal mucosa and undermining it until sufficient tissue is formed to cover the defect without tension (Fig. 10–26 *C*). Most of the connective tissue layer is left attached to the buccal mucosa to ensure viability of the flap in its new position.

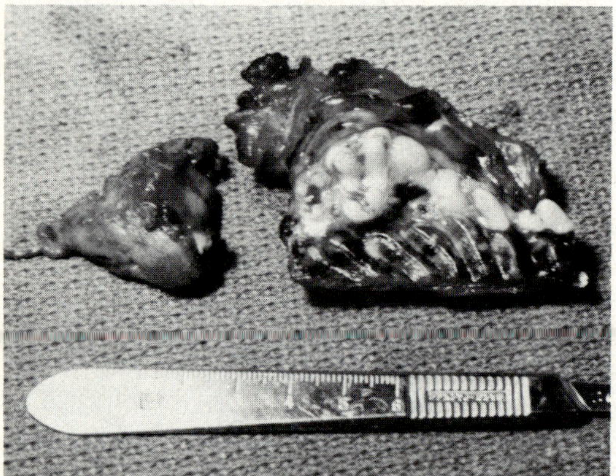

Figure 10–28. Maxillectomy and orbital resection for fibrosarcoma in a dog. Surgical specimen showing the maxilla and palate tissue *(right side)* and the zygomatic salivary gland and infraorbital nerve tissue *(left side)*.

The flap is sutured into position with a combination of vertical mattress and simple interrupted synthetic absorbable sutures (Fig. 10–26 *D*). Drains are not necessary. The connective tissue surface of the flap that faces the nasal cavity heals by granulation and epithelialization of the nasal mucosa.

Radical maxillectomy may result in the loss of most of the lateral external skeleton of the nose; a soft tissue flap closed across the defect may cause obstruction of nasal airflow. If this appears likely at the time that the flap is created, sections of nasal conchae can be resected with scissors to create free air space in the re-formed nasal cavity. The bone forming the conchae is very delicate; tissue that is to be retained should not be retracted or crushed by sponges.

The animal may experience pain during recovery from anesthesia, but eating usually takes place without difficulty the following day. Breakdown of the sutures holding the flap in place may occur 2 to 3 days following surgery; in this case the animal is reanesthetized, and the flap is resutured. Feeding the animal through a pharyngostomy or gastrostomy tube is of doubtful value in preventing dehiscence. Antibiotics are not necessary. The animal should be fed a soft diet and should be prevented from chewing hard objects for the next several weeks to protect the flap while it heals.

This procedure can be adapted for lesions that penetrate into the orbit by extending the resection to include the entire infraorbital canal and adjacent bone. The zygomatic salivary gland can be resected through this approach (see Fig. 10–28), and the tissues forming the medial wall of the orbit are available for resection if necessary. Perhaps surprizingly, the eye remains in a normal position and retains its ability to rotate following this extensive resection.

Unilateral or bilateral radical premaxillectomy can also be performed on dogs with good results (Fig. 10–29).[43] The lesion is outlined by incision into the oral mucosa, and the palate and premaxilla are removed en bloc with an osteotome or bone saw, exposing the nasal vestibule (Fig. 10–29 *B*). Hemorrhage is then controlled. The defect between the oral and nasal cavities is covered by creating unilateral or bilateral buccomucosal advancement or rotation flaps (Fig. 10–29 *C*). If bilateral surgery is performed, the flaps are placed so that they both cover the oronasal defect when sutured together, one with the epithelial surface facing dorsally to form

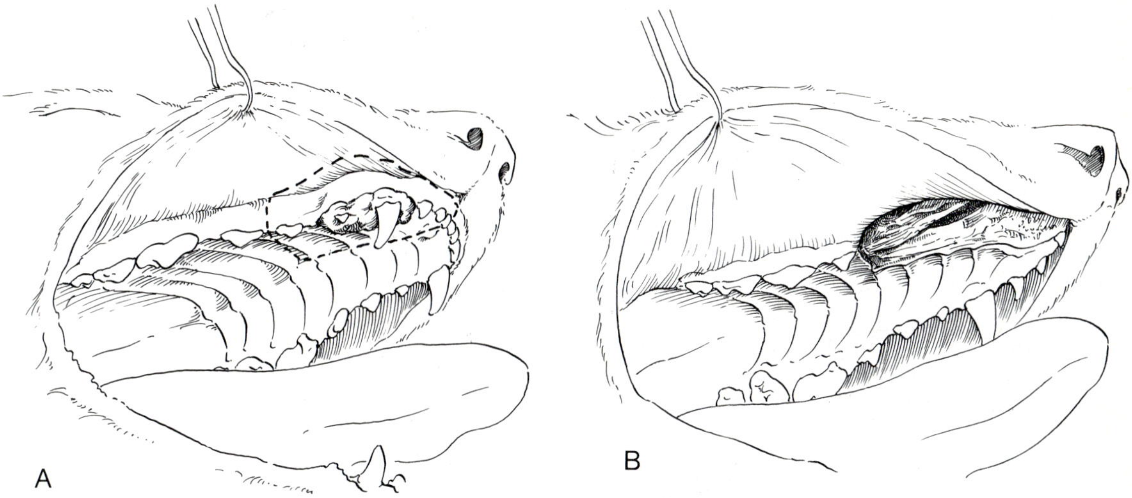

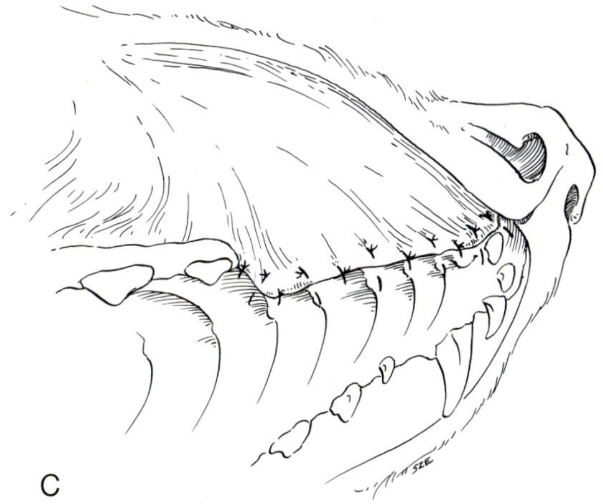

Figure 10–29. Premaxillectomy. *A*, Lesion and planned incisions. *B*, Defect following resection. *C*, Closure with a unilateral buccal flap.

the floor of the nasal vestibule, and the other with the epithelium facing ventrally to form the new palate surface. As for maxillectomy, part of the ventral nasal concha may need to be resected to retain space for air movement in the nasal cavity following closure.

Lesions on the lateral aspect of the upper canine tooth can be removed by resecting the lateral alveolar plate and the canine tooth only (Fig. 10–30). Suturing is not necessary if the nasal cavity is not penetrated (Fig. 10–30 *B*).

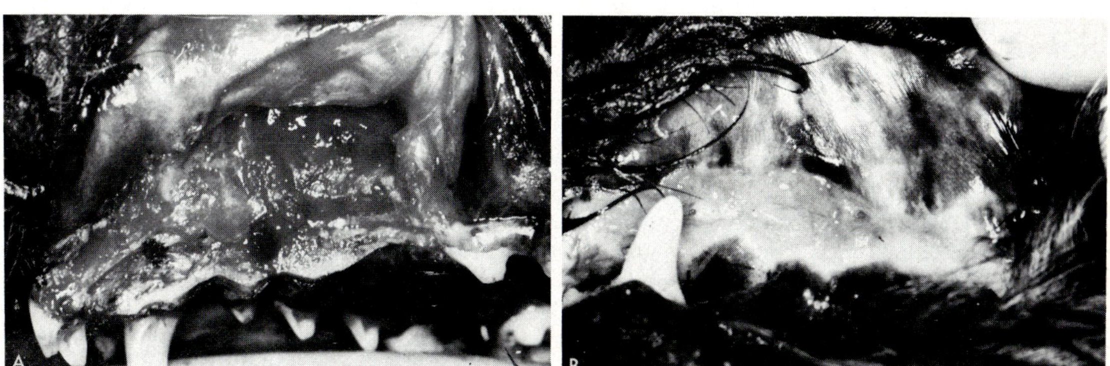

Figure 10–30. Acanthomatous epulis arising from the lateral alveolar plate of an upper canine tooth. *A*, Following resection of the lateral alveolar plate and tooth. The defect was not sutured. *B*, Three weeks later.

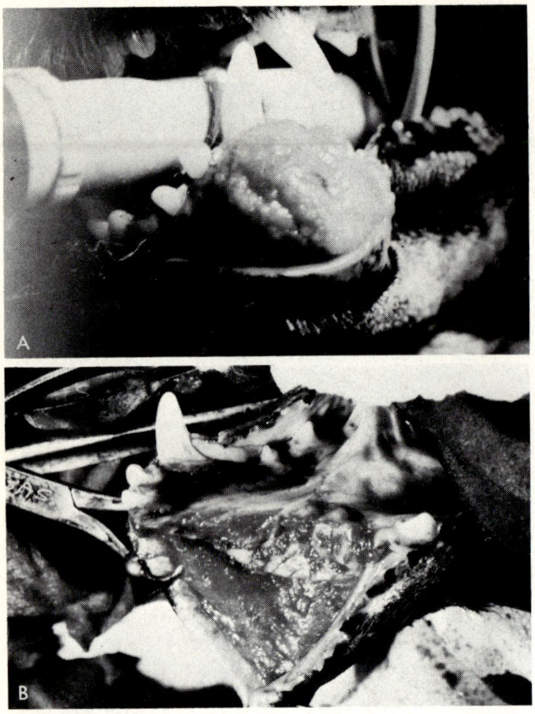

Figure 10–31. Rostral mandibulectomy. *A*, Acanthomatous epulis of the mandible. *B*, The lesion and surrounding mandible, including canine and incisor teeth, have been resected.

Mandibulectomy

Rostral mandibulectomy has been performed for many years, with excellent functional results. If the procedure is confined to the incisor and canine teeth area, and the mandibular symphysis is not completely separated, no supportive procedures are necessary (Fig. 10–31). The skin can be retracted following the initial incision through the free gingivae and can be reattached to the shortened mandible. If necessary, excess skin can be resected. For more extensive lesions caudal to the canine teeth, the symphysis must be resected. The line of resection should be at least 1 cm away from grossly or radiographically visible lesional tissue. The horizontal rami of the mandible are stabilized with cross pins prior to cutting bone. The mucosa around the lesion is incised, the bone is transected with a dental bur or an oscillating saw, and bleeding vessels are ligated. Excess skin is resected, leaving the mucocutaneous junction intact if possible, and a flap of skin is created to cover the re-formed point of the jaw.[44]

Recovery from the effects of surgery is rapid, and most animals learn to drink and eat normally within a few days. Because the canine teeth have been removed, the tongue may tend to hang out of that side of the mouth when relaxed, but this does not interfere with normal prehension and swallowing.

For lesions located in the premolar or molar area, hemimandibulectomy can be performed.[45, 46] This is particularly well-tolerated by cats. Incisions are made well away from the lesional tissue in the free gingivae (Fig. 10–32), and the mandible is undermined by blunt dissection. The symphysis is separated by bone cutters or scissors (Fig. 10–32 *B*), and the lateral attachments of the tongue are separated, leaving the mandibular and sublingual gland ducts intact if they can be identified. This frees the mandible to swing independently, which facilitates dissection of the masseter and pterygoid muscles from their attachments (Fig. 10–32 *C*). These muscles are reflected laterally and medially, respectively, exposing the vertical ramus of the mandible. Exposed or incised vessels are ligated. The mandible is cut with a bone cutter, and the digastric muscle is transected, allowing the jaw to be removed from the surgical site.

Alternatively, the entire hemimandible can be removed by continuing blunt and sharp dissection to separate muscular and tendinous attachments from the mandible; the temporomandibular ligaments are exposed by rotating the mandible (Fig. 10–32 *D*) and are incised.

A drain can be placed in the cavity beneath the suture line, exiting through the skin. The incision is closed by absorbable sutures aposing the incised oral mucosal edges (Fig. 10–32 *E*). The opposite mandible will swing over toward the midline, which may result in the remaining mandibular canine tooth impinging on the palate when the mouth is closed; to prevent this occurrence, 2 to 3 mm of the crown can be filed down without exposing the pulp cavity. A soft diet will probably be necessary for the duration of the animal's life.

Other than persistent protrusion of the tongue in some animals, there is little externally visible evidence of the surgery in cats. In dogs, the commissure of the lip on that side can be shortened (by excising the mucocutaneous junction, then suturing skin to skin and mucosa to mucosa until the new commissure is reached) to form a sling to keep the tongue in the mouth.[46]

Lesions of the coronoid process of the vertical ramus of the mandible can be re-

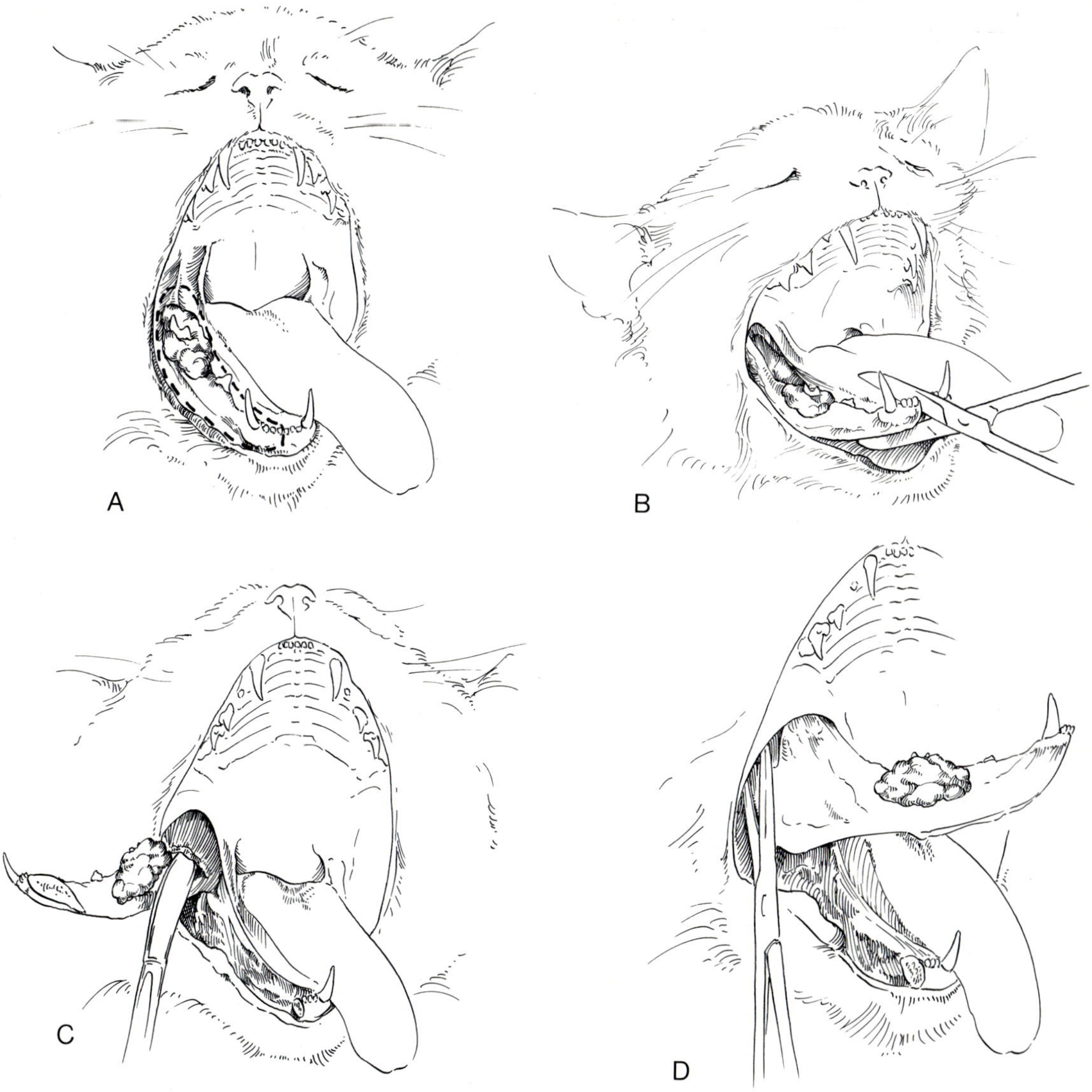

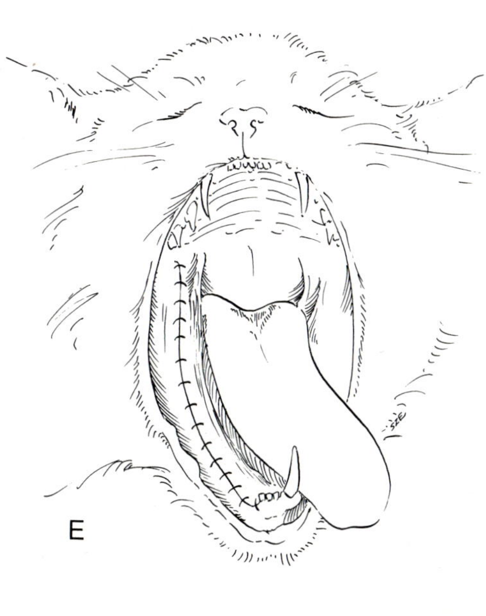

Figure 10–32. Total hemimandibulectomy in a cat. *A*, Lesion and proposed incisions in the mucosa *(dashed lines)*. *B*, The mandibular symphysis is split. *C*, The mandible is rotated to facilitate muscle dissection. *D*, The lateral ligament and condylar attachments are separated. *E*, The mucosal incisions are sutured.

sected by an approach through the zygomatic arch and the masseter muscle. The periosteum of the zygoma is incised and reflected (Fig. 10–33 *A* and *B*); the zygoma is resected full thickness with an osteotome or rongeur (Fig. 10–33 *C*); and the temporal, massetter, and pterygoid muscles are reflected from the coronoid process (Fig. 10–33 *D*), which can then be partially or completely removed with a rongeur or osteotome (Fig. 10–33 *E*). The incision is closed by apposing the periosteum of the zygomatic arch and the orbital fascia (Fig. 10–33 *F*). If muscle dissection was extensive, soft rubber drains can be placed through the masseter muscle, avoiding the parotid duct.

Dogs and cats can usually eat and swallow adequately, or even normally, following the radical maxillary and mandibular procedures just described, though some animals require a period of 10 to 14 days to adapt to the changes in their mouths. Short-term complications consist mainly of mucosal wound breakdown. This is less likely to occur if there is minimal tension on the flap and if the flap incision is located over some supporting tissue. If the flap becomes necrotic, one should wait until the epithelium has healed to form an oronasal fistula, then another flap should be created and sutured in place (page 167). Long-term complications are most often due to recurrence of disease. Management and

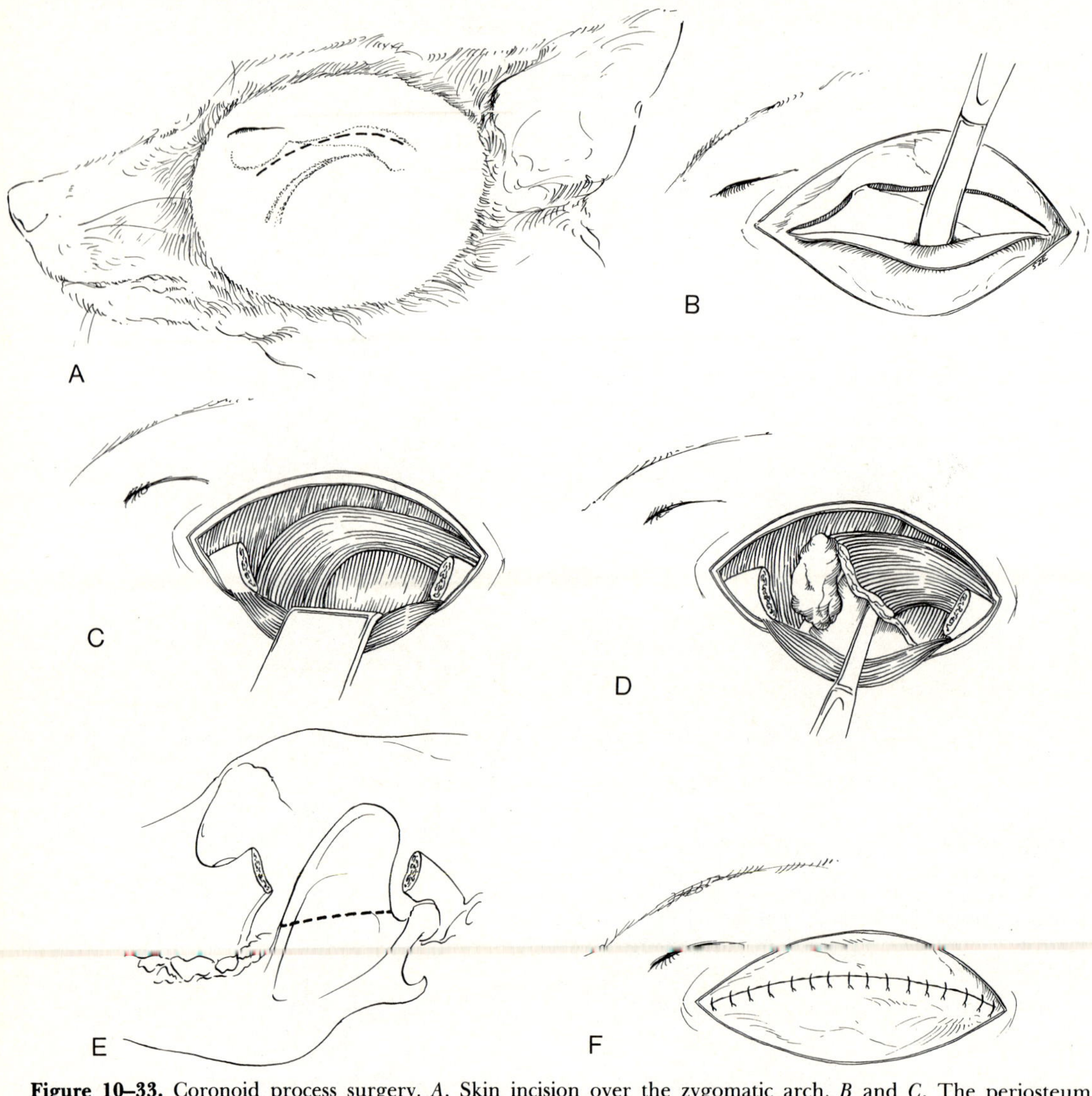

Figure 10–33. Coronoid process surgery. *A*, Skin incision over the zygomatic arch. *B* and *C*, The periosteum covering the zygoma is reflected and the zygoma is resected, revealing the temporal muscle. *D*, Temporal and pterygoid muscles are dissected from the coronoid process. *E*, The dorsal half of the zygoma can be resected. *F*, The fascial incision is sutured.

prognosis for particular tumor types are described in Chapter Eight. Cryosurgical and hyperthermic treatment of oral tumors are also described in Chapter Eight.

Mandibular Symphysiotomy

Access to the caudal oral cavity and pharynx can be enhanced by mandibular symphysiotomy.[24, 25]

The mandible and cranial neck area is prepared for surgery. A midventral skin incision is made from the basihyoid bone to the tip of the mandible. The mylohyoid muscle is incised, separated, and reflected. The mandible is exposed, and the symphysis is split with a scalpel. The mandibles are spread to tense the genioglossus muscle as it is incised about 1 cm from the midline. The sublingual mucosa is incised lateral to the salivary ducts. The mandibles can then be spread maximally, and the tongue is retracted caudally to expose the pharynx.

Closure is made by suturing the oral mucosa and the genioglossus and mylohyoid muscles with absorbable suture material. The mandibular symphysis is closed with cross pins or encircling wires. There is little postoperative discomfort or interference with prehension or swallowing.[24]

References

1. Wright JG, Hall LW: Regional analgesia of the dog's head. *In* Veterinary Anesthesia and Analgesia, 5th ed. London, Balliere Tindall & Cox, 1961, pp. 55–58.
2. Sciubba JJ, Waterhouse JP, Meyer J: A fine structural comparison of the healing of incisional wounds of mucosa and skin. *J Oral Pathol* 7:214–227, 1978.
3. Lilly GE, Cutcher JL, Jones JC, Armstrong JH: Reaction of oral tissues to suture materials. IV. *Oral Surg Oral Med Oral Pathol* 33:152–157, 1972.
4. Bergenholtz A, Isaksson B: Tissue reaction in the oral mucosa to catgut, silk, and Mersilene sutures. *Odontol Rev* 18:237–250, 1967.
5. Lantz GC, Cantwell HD, Van Fleet JF, Blakemore JC, Newman S: Pharyngostomy tube induced esophagitis in the dog: an experimental study. *J Am Anim Hosp Assoc* 19:207–212, 1983.
6. Hedlund CS, Tangner CH, Elkins AD, Hobson HP: Temporary bilateral carotid artery occlusion during surgical exploration of the nasal cavity of the dog. *Vet Surg* 12:83–85, 1983.
7. Dent RSC: Operation for correction of lateral protrusion of the tongue in the dog. *Vet Rec* 64:276, 1952.
8. Greene RW: Personal communication, 1982.
9. Wolff A: Tongue-tie in a dog? *Canine Pract* 7:6, 1980.
10. Stauffer VD: Loss of the tongue in a cat and the resulting skin problem. *Vet Med Small Anim Clin* 68:1266–1267, 1973.
11. Jurkiewicz MJ: Cleft lip and palate in dogs. *Surg Forum* 15:457–458, 1964.
12. Jurkiewcz MJ: A genetic study of cleft lip and palate in dogs. *Surg Forum* 16:472–473, 1965.
13. Howard DR, Merkley DF, Lammerding JJ, Ford RB, Bloomberg MS, Davis DG: Primary cleft palate (harelip) and closure repair in puppies. *J Am Anim Hosp Assoc* 12:636–640, 1976.
14. Stoll SG: Cheiloplasty. *In* Bojrab MJ (ed): Current Techniques In Small Animal Surgery, Philadelphia, Lea & Febiger, 1975 pp. 286–292.
15. Harvey CE: Parotid salivary duct rupture and fistula in the dog and cat. *J Small Anim Pract* 18:163–168, 1977.
16. Bartels P: Kurzbericht zur naht von skalpierwunden am unterkiefer. *Kleinter Prax* 22:171–172, 1977.
17. Farrow CS: Surgical treatment of lower lip avulsion in the cat. *Vet Med Small Anim Pract* 68:1418–1419, 1973.
18. Olmstead ML, Stoloff DR, O'Keefe CM: Correction of traumatic avulsion of the upper lip in two dogs. *Vet Med Small Anim Clin* 71:1228–1229, 1976.
19. Pavletic MM: Nasal and rostral labial reconstruction in the dog. *J Am Anim Hosp Assoc* 19:595–600, 1983.
20. Scott DW: Observations on the eosinophilic granuloma complex in cats. *J Am Anim Hosp Assoc* 11:261–270, 1975.
21. Willemse A, Lubberink AAME: Eosinophilic ulcers in cats. *Tijdschr Diergeneesk* 103:1052–1056, 1978.
22. Cooper HK, Mattern GW: Genetic studies of cleft lip and palate in dogs. *Carnivore Genet Newsletter* 9:204–209, 1970.
23. Samuelson ML, Dennis SM: Cleft palate associated with meningocele in a pup. *Vet Rec* 104:436, 1979.
24. Curley BM, Nelson AW, Kainer RA: Mandibular symphysiotomy in the dog and cat: a surgical approach to the nasopharynx. *J Am Vet Med Assoc* 160:981–987, 1972.
25. Sinibaldi KR: Cleft palate. *Vet Clin North Am* 9:245–257, 1979.
26. Howard DR, Davis DG, Merkley DF, Krahwinkel DJ, Schirmer RG, Brinker WO: Mucoperiosteal flap technique for cleft palate repair in dogs. *J Am Vet Med Assoc* 165:352–354, 1974.
27. Knight G: Surgical closure of the cleft palate. *Vet Rec* 70:680–681, 1958.
28. Long DA: Surgical repair of cleft palate. *Vet Med Small Anim Clin 70*:434–436, 1975.
29. Hammer DL, Sacks M: Surgical closure of cleft soft palate in a dog. *J Am Vet Med Assoc* 158:342–345, 1971.
30. Archibald J, Reed JH, Johnston DE: Soft palate defect. p349 *In* Archibald J (ed): Canine Surgery. Wheaton Illinois, American Veterinary Publications, 1965.
31. Baker GJ: Surgery of the canine pharynx and larynx. *J Small Anim Pract* 13:505–513, 1972.
32. Harvey CE: Oronasal fistula. *Am Vet Dent Soc Newsletter*, Nov. 1980.
33. Slocum B: Oronasal fistula repair in a dog. *Mod Vet Pract* 61:769–771, 1980.
34. Rickards DA: Disjunction of the upper jaw and traumatic cleft palate. *Feline Pract* 5:51–52, 1975.
35. Lammerding JJ, Howard DR, Bloomberg MS: Repair of an acquired oral-nasal fistula in a dog. *J Am Anim Hosp Assoc* 12:64–69, 1976.
36. Hobson HP, Heller RA, Wilson JB: Use of a removable maxillary appliance to correct a palatal defect in a dog. *Vet Med Small Anim Clin* 66:1085–1087, 1971.

37. Thoday KL, Charlton DA, Graham-Jones O, Frost PL, Pullen-Warner E: Successful use of a prosthesis in the correction of a palatal defect in a dog. *J Small Anim Pract* 16:487–494, 1975.
38. Arenzo AR, Glauser GFJO: Quiste dentigero en un perro. *Rev Med Vet Brazil* 44:349–355, 1963.
39. Field EA, Speechley JA, Jones DE: The removal of an impacted maxillary canine and associated dentigerous cyst in a Chow. *J Small Anim Pract* 23:159–163, 1982.
40. Langham RF, Mostosky UV, Schirmer RG: Ameloblastic odontoma in the dog. *Am J Vet Res* 30:1873–1876, 1969.
41. Brodey RS, Morris AL: Odontoma associated with an undifferentiated carcinoma in the maxilla of a dog. *J Am Vet Med Assoc* 137:553–559, 1960.
42. Figueiredo C, Barros HM, Alvares LC, Damante JH: Composed complex odontoma in a dog. *Vet Med Small Anim Pract* 69:268–270, 1974.
43. Withrow SJ: Premaxillectomy in the dog. Annual Meeting of the American College of Veterinary Surgeons, 1983.
44. Vernon FF, Helphrey M: Rostral mandibulectomy; three case reports in dogs. *Vet Surg* 12:26–29, 1983.
45. Bradley RL, MacEwen EG, Loar AS: Mandibular resection for removal of oral tumors in 30 dogs and 6 cats. *J Am Vet Med Assoc* 184:460–463, 1984.
46. Withrow SJ, Holmberg DL: Mandibulectomy in the treatment of oral cancer. *J Am Anim Hosp Assoc* 19:273–286, 1983.

Chapter Eleven

Diseases of the Pharynx

CE Harvey

The pharynx is a crossroads. During ventilation, air traverses between the nasal and laryngeal airways. During swallowing, the food or fluid bolus passes from the mouth to the esophagus. These pathways cross at the common pharynx. Animals having conditions that affect the pharynx are likely to present because of respiratory signs, such as cough or respiratory distress, or because of swallowing abnormalities, indicated by drooling, awkward gulping motions, or the inability to swallow after picking up food. Often, both sets of signs are present, particularly when the abnormality results in nasal regurgitation of food or fluids.

Discussion in this chapter is confined to conditions affecting the oral cavity and the oropharynx.

CONGENITAL ABNORMALITIES

The most common congenital abnormality of the pharynx in the dog is over long soft palate, which is usually seen in brachycephalic dogs. This condition rarely causes oropharyngeal disease; diagnosis and management have been described in detail elsewhere.[1,2] Brachycephalic dogs that are sedated or anesthetized for diagnosis or treatment of oral disease must be kept under observation until recovery from the sedation or anesthesia is complete to avoid airway obstruction by the relaxed soft palate.

Cleft soft palate occurs sporadically in dogs and cats, usually in association with cleft hard palate; variations and management are described on page 163. Other congenital abnormalities of the oropharynx, such as branchial cleft cysts and lymphoepithelial cysts, are extremely rare as causes of pharyngeal or neck masses in dogs and cats.

Congenital abnormalities of the tonsil are noticed only if they interfere with swallowing. They are also seen as incidental findings. Dogs and cats manage well without tonsils; therefore, hypoplastic or absent tonsils will not be noticed. Occasionally, the shape of the tonsil will cause it to protrude abnormally from the tonsillar crypt and may cause chronic retching or pain on swallowing (Fig. 11–1).[3] Diagnosis is by inspection of the abnormal tonsil in an otherwise normal pharynx. Treatment is tonsillectomy, which is described further on.

PHARYNGITIS

Primary pharyngitis (inflammation of the pharyngeal mucosa) is uncommon in dogs and cats, though signs resulting from pharyngeal pain may cause the owner to seek veterinary attention. Pharyngitis can be caused by local disease (such as ingestion of

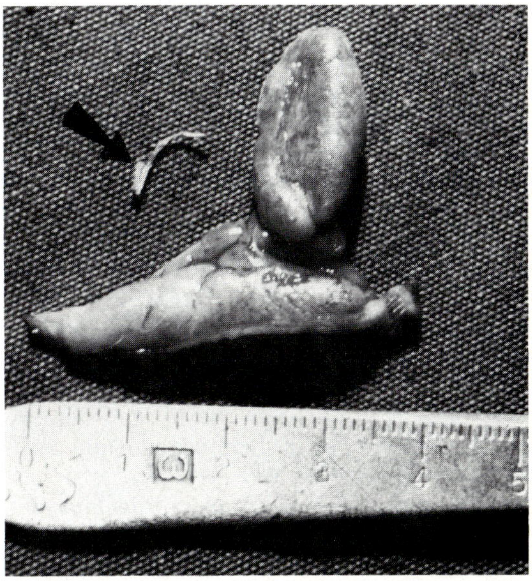

Figure 11–1. Abnormally shaped tonsil from a dog showing pharyngeal irritation. There is a protuberance extending medially. Cause not known. There was also a grass awn caught in the tonsillar crypt *(arrow)*.

caustic chemicals; local viral infections, such as canine distemper, feline viral rhinotracheitis or calicivirus infection; or spread of infection from the periodontal tissues in cats) or by local irritation from disease in other areas (such as nasal disease causing chronic nasopharyngeal discharge or chronic vomiting or coughing causing the pharynx to be showered intermittently by gastric secretions or lower airway discharges). Foreign bodies often penetrate the pharyngeal oral mucosa, and they may become lodged in the soft tissues of the pharynx to cause an acute abscess, or they may lacerate the pharynx, exposing the submucosal tissues.

Signs of pharyngitis, whether the cause is local or systemic, include gagging or retching. The fluid or mucus freed during gagging is rarely expectorated, though coughing is frequent because gagging often results in minor lower airway aspiration. Because of the discomfort produced during swallowing, anorexia is common, and occasionally it may progress to drooling if the discomfort is severe enough to limit the ability to swallow. Pharyngeal abscessation causes depression and fever.

Pharyngeal swellings, such as neoplasms or mucoceles, interfere with swallowing or respiration because of the space they occupy, and they commonly result in secondary pharyngitis.

TONSILLAR DISEASE

The tonsils form part of a ring of lymphatic tissue that encircles the naso- and oropharynx. Tonsils are not essential for life, but they probably play an important part in recognizing and processing antigenic materials that enter the body through the nose or mouth. Large numbers of a wide variety of microorganisms are present in the tonsillar crypts and epithelial folds of the tonsillar surface (see Table 3–1, page 29), but few penetrate into the deeper lymphatic tissue to stimulate antigen production. When large numbers of organisms successfully penetrate the tonsillar epithelium, the normal defense mechanisms are overwhelmed, allowing pathogens to proliferate and spread or to persist as a chronic infection.[4] Primary tonsillitis may represent an overloading of this antigenic filter mechanism in immature animals.[5] Based on their observations of the microscopic changes seen in excised tonsils from young dogs with primary tonsillitis, Kutschmann and Schafer suggest that routine tonsillectomy is not indicated, since the inflammation will recede when the animal reaches maturity.[5] The tonsils may act as a reservoir of infection in dogs with endocarditis and other chronic infections.[6, 7]

Tonsillitis is often diagnosed but is rarely a primary disease except in young small-breed dogs. As the most obvious feature in the pharynx and the most prone to react to irritants because of the lymphatic tissues, the tonsils are more readily noted to be inflamed than is the surrounding pharyngeal epithelium. Causes and clinical signs of tonsillitis are the same as described for pharyngitis. A complete history should be taken and a thorough physical examination should be made for all animals that appear to have tonsillitis on initial examination. Other causes of chronic pharyngitis, such as chronic vomiting or coughing or nasal disease, should be investigated before a definitive diagnosis of chronic tonsillitis is made. It is necessary to use sedation or anesthesia in some animals so that the pharynx can be examined to rule out foreign body, abscess, tumor, or mucocele.

The value of bacterial culture from an inflamed tonsil is questionable. The most common organisms associated with tonsillitis in the dog are *Escherichia coli, Staphylococcus aureus* and *S. albus,* hemolytic *Streptococci, Diplococci,* and *Proteus* and *Pseudomonas* spp., all of which can be found in the throat of normal dogs. If the sample is taken from an area of obvious purulent exudate on the surface of the tonsil or from material squeezed from deep within an inflamed tonsil, the culture probably will represent the organisms causing local infection. "Tonsil" cultures taken by the uncontrolled thrust of a swab into the pharynx of an uncomfortable, uncooperative dog are as likely to capture normal pharyngeal flora as organisms causing infection.

The medical management of tonsillitis consists of antibiotics given orally, or by injection initially if the animal is too uncomfortable to swallow (see Table 4–3, page 54). Clinical improvement is seen with almost any antibiotic, culture and sensitivity results are rarely available except in chronic or severe recurrent cases. Treatment for 5 to 7 days is usually sufficient. Prolonged antibiotic therapy, or frequent changes of antibiotic, should be avoided to prevent the establishment of resistant organisms. The purpose of antibiotic therapy is to allow the normal defense mechanisms to re-establish control. Tonsillectomy is indicated in the occasional animal in whom chronic or recurrent pharyngitis may cause failure to thrive because of the animal's reluctance to eat.[8]

Trauma from a sharp ingested object may cause the tonsil to protrude abnormally, either because of a retrotonsillar abscess or as a result of laceration of tonsillar tissue. Foreign bodies, such as grass awns or fox tails, occasionally become lodged within the tonsillar crypt (see Fig. 11–1), and they cause a severe unilateral tonsillitis. Treatment consists of draining the abscess, if present, inspecting the tonsillar crypt, and removing the foreign body, if present. Tonsillectomy is an alternative treatment.

Pharyngeal Neoplasia

Most tumors in the pharynx arise from the tonsil (see Figs. 8–6 and 8–7), but occasional tumors invade the pharyngeal tissues from the nasal cavity or the base of the skull. The incidence, presenting signs, methods of diagnosis, management, and prognosis for tonsillar tumors are discussed in Chapter Eight. Tonsillectomy combined with partial pharyngeal wall and soft palate resection will occasionally result in cure in dogs with squamous cell carcinoma with no lymph node or lung metastasis. Neoplastic pharyngeal tissue is best resected with an electroscalpel to reduce hemorrhage. If soft palate tissue is to be removed, one should avoid penetrating through the full thickness of the palate so that the nasopharyngeal closure mechanism will be retained during swallowing. Involved nodes can be resected, though this is of little value unless adjuvant therapy is to be used. Resection is complicated if the retropharyngeal node is enlarged, because of its protected position deep to the mandibular salivary gland, and the adjacent neurovascular structures.

Tonsillectomy

Tonsillectomy is indicated for the treatment of chronic or recurrent tonsillitis, or as one step in the treatment of tonsillar neoplasia.

The animal's mouth is held open with a mouth retractor. To prevent aspiration of blood, an endotracheal tube is placed, the cuff is inflated, and a moist sponge is wrapped around the tube in the pharynx. The tonsil is everted from its crypt and is held at its rostral margin with a hemostat. With a scissors or electroscalpel, the tonsil is incised at the junction of the lymphoid tissue and pharyngeal epithelium both dorsally and ventrally (Fig. 11–2 *A*). Blunt scissors can be used instead of a scalpel to cause shearing of tissues, and thus reduce hemorrhage.[10] Medial retraction on the partially resected tonsil will cause the hidden lateral lobe to appear, which is resected with the main tonsillar lobe. Because the surgery is done through the mouth, the caudal end of the tonsil cannot be seen clearly; therefore, care is taken to prevent unnecessary caudal extension of the epithelial incision. Bleeding vessels are picked up with hemostats and are ligated (Fig. 11–2 *B*). The incised edges of the tonsillar crypt epithelium are sutured with 000 absorbable sutures to allow healing by first intention (Fig. 11–2 *C* and *D*).

Complications of tonsillectomy include postoperative hemorrhage and pharyngeal muscle or nervous tissue injury with resultant dysphagia. These conditions are unlikely to develop if the resection is limited to the lymphoid tissue and if the surgical site is thoroughly inspected for hemorrhage before the animal is allowed to recover from anesthesia. Another possible complication is airway obstruction that may result from pharyngeal swelling, particularly in brachycephalic dogs or in other animals predisposed to airway obstruction. Careful monitoring is essential for 12 hours following surgery. Retching is frequent during this period because of the irritation caused by pharyngeal manipulation; therefore, food is withheld for 24 hours. Moistened food is fed for 7 to 10 days following surgery. Antibiotic administration is not necessary.

Alternatives to the electroscalpel or scissors-suture technique include simple excision with scissors after injection of 1:5000 epinephrine solution into the tissues lateral to the tonsils;[11] excision with an electrocautery snare;[12] and retraction of the tonsil from its crypt, placement of a forceps lateral to the tonsil, and excision distal to the forceps.[8]

When techniques are used in which the tonsillar crypt epithelium is not sutured, healing takes place by granulation and contraction. This prolongs the duration of pharyngeal irritation and dysphagia and increases the risk of aspiration.

Cryotonsillectomy in dogs has been shown to result in considerable pharyngeal edema 12 to 24 hours later,[13] which could result in

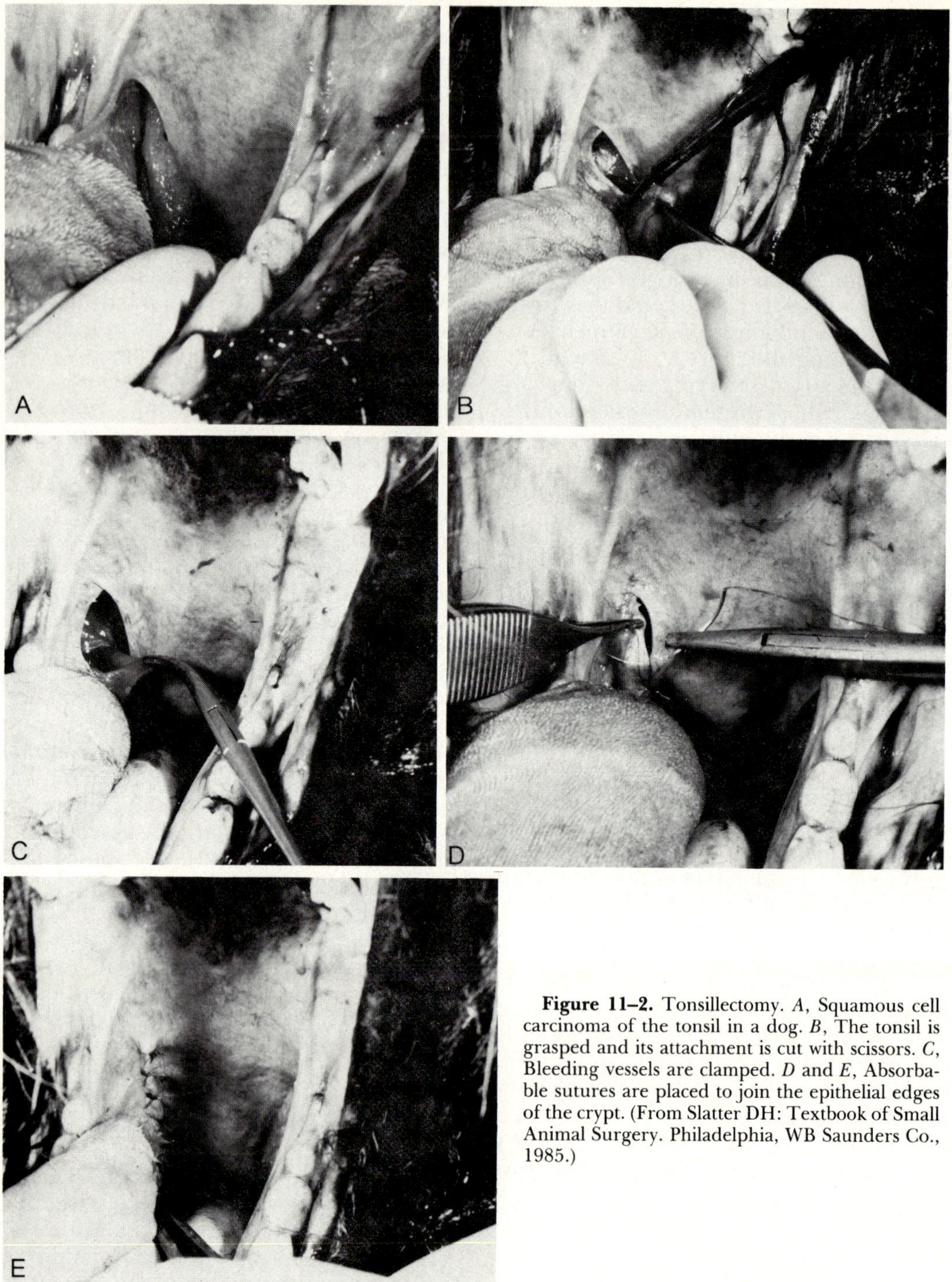

Figure 11–2. Tonsillectomy. *A*, Squamous cell carcinoma of the tonsil in a dog. *B*, The tonsil is grasped and its attachment is cut with scissors. *C*, Bleeding vessels are clamped. *D* and *E*, Absorbable sutures are placed to join the epithelial edges of the crypt. (From Slatter DH: Textbook of Small Animal Surgery. Philadelphia, WB Saunders Co., 1985.)

airway obstruction. The risk of hemorrhage at the time of surgery is minimal; however, the possibility of airway obstruction, or hemorrhage during sloughing of the tonsillar tissue several days later, plus the protracted healing, suggests that this technique is not suitable for clinical use.

SWELLINGS IN THE RETROPHARYNGEAL AREA

The most common causes of retropharyngeal swellings are abscesses caused by pharyngeal foreign bodies (see further on), sali-

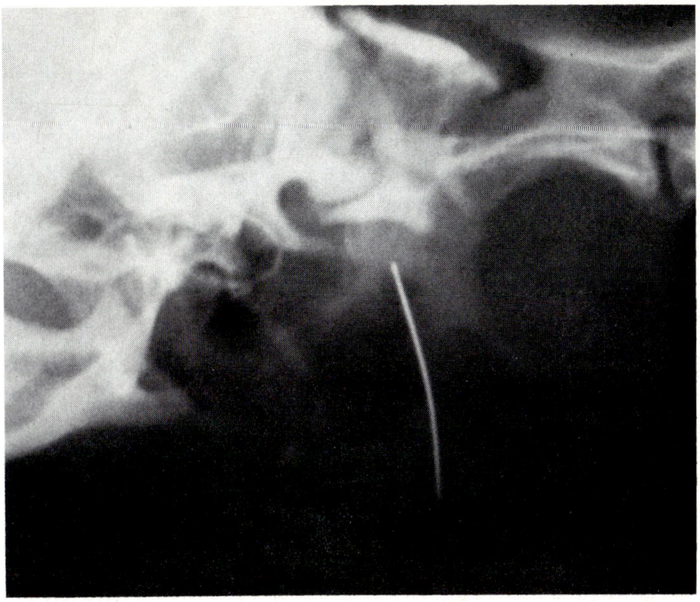

Figure 11–3. Radiograph showing a sewing needle caught in the pharynx of a cat.

vary mucoceles (Chapter 12, page 193), and metastatic tumors in mandibular and retropharyngeal lymph nodes (Chapter Eight). Plain radiographs will confirm the presence of a mass and will demonstrate a radiopaque foreign body or bony invasion by a tumor, but they are of little value in differentiating the cause of soft tissue masses.[14] Palpation and aspiration of the mass, thorough examination of the oropharynx, and biopsy of solid neoplastic masses usually result in a diagnosis. The diagnosis of the rare congenital causes of fluid-containing neck swellings such as branchial cleft cyst[15–17] is made by microscopic examination of the lining of the swelling.

Retropharyngeal Abscess

The mouth or pharynx in the dog and cat is frequently lacerated or penetrated by objects such as chicken bones, fish hooks, sewing needles (Fig. 11–3), grass awns, or wooden sticks.[8, 9] These objects may be retained within the sublingual, retrobulbar, or pharyngeal soft tissues, in which they cause a localized infection or acute abscess. When the animal is presented because of acute disease, there is usually pyrexia, and the pharyngeal tissues are hot, firm, and painful. The swelling is usually surrounded (particularly rostrally) by edema, and it may have a soft central area that is undergoing necrosis. The sublingual tissues may be swollen and edematous because of interference with venous return, and they may appear as a ranula grossly (Fig. 11–4). Acute pharyngeal abscess is treated by lancing, flushing, and draining the abscess with the animal under sedation (Fig. 11–5); the abscess cavity is explored digitally to break down loculations and is palpated for a foreign body. The pharynx should be examined through the mouth for evidence of foreign body penetration. An antibiotic is often given, but it is unnecessary if drainage is thorough. The causative foreign body often is not found.

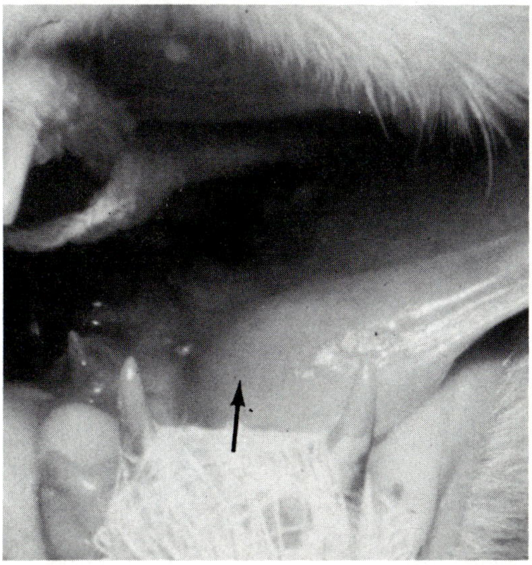

Figure 11–4. Sublingual edema in a cat resulting from a pharyngeal abscess. (From Harvey CE, O'Brien JA: *In* Ettinger SJ (ed): Textbook of Veterinary Internal Medicine, Ch. 39. Philadelphia, WB Saunders Co., 1975.)

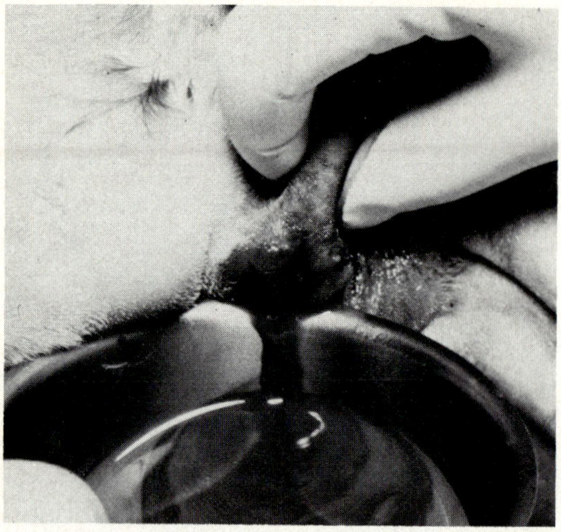

Figure 11–5. Draining a retropharyngeal abscess in a dog.

Chronic pharyngeal abscesses develop when antibiotic therapy or local defense mechanisms effectively sterilize a foreign body in the connective tissues. The tissues continue to react to the foreign substance, and a serosanguineous effusion collects in the area. As with a salivary mucocele, this fluid takes the path of least resistance and is seen as a firm or soft, usually non-painful swelling in the neck.

It is possible to confuse an acute or chronic pharyngeal abscess with a salivary mucocele,[18] though aspiration is usually sufficient to differentiate the two conditions; if doubt exists, some of the aspirate can be stained with a mucopolysaccharide-specific stain such as periodic acid–Schiff (PAS) to identify the mucous strands found in a mucocele. Radiographs are made of the neck to check for the presence of a radiodense foreign body, and the pharynx is examined. The swelling is incised, loculations are broken down, and the walls are thoroughly scraped. If a foreign body is not found, the incision is left open, and the cavity is packed with antiseptic-soaked sponges to encourage granulation but to prevent the skin edges from sealing. The packing is replaced daily until the swelling has been obliterated by granulation and contraction; this usually takes 2 to 3 weeks.

Retro-orbital abscess arises from an oral foreign body penetrating through the soft tissues medial to the vertical ramus of the mandible. Animals with retro-orbital abscess are usually presented to the veterinarian because of exophthalmos of rapid onset or because of an inability to open the jaw resulting from pressure that causes pain in the orbital area. Differential diagnoses are orbital or invasive frontal sinus or nasal tumors. Radiographs may disclose a foreign body. Treatment consists of draining the abscess into the mouth through an incision in the oral mucosa just caudad to the last upper molar tooth (Fig. 11–6); a soft rubber drain can be placed, extending through the oral incision and exiting the orbit through a skin incision caudal to the globe. A systemic antibiotic is given for several days. Recovery is usually complete, even when no foreign body is found.

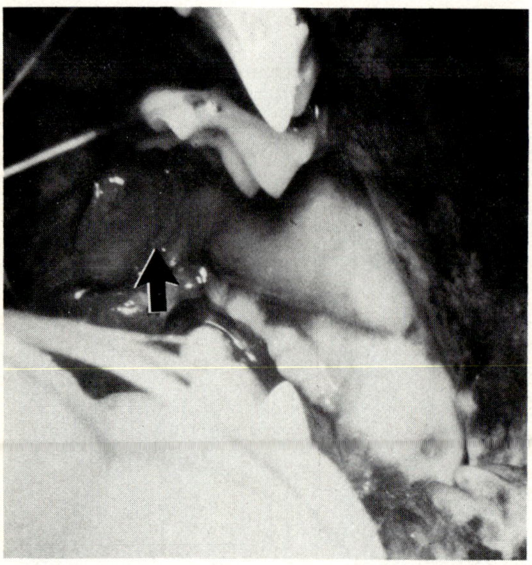

Figure 11–6. Drainage site for a retro-orbital abscess into the mouth. (From Harvey CE, O'Brien JA: *In* Ettinger SJ (ed): Textbook of Veterinary Internal Medicine, Ch. 39. Philadelphia, WB Saunders Co., 1975).

References

1. O'Brien JA, Harvey CE: Diseases of the upper airway. *In* Ettinger SJ: Textbook of Veterinary Internal Medicine, 2nd ed. Philadelphia, WB Saunders Co., 1983.
2. Harvey CE: Upper airway obstruction surgery: 2. Soft palate resection in brachycephalic dogs. *J Am Anim Hosp Assoc* 18:538–544, 1982.
3. Petrick SW: Ectopic tonsil in a dog. *J South Africa Vet Med Assoc* 49:378, 1978.
4. Anon: The tonsils in the pathogenesis of disease. *Vet Rec* 95:234, 1974.
5. Kutschmann K, Schafer R: Zur Tonsillitis und Tonsillektomie beim Hund. *Monat Veterinarmed* 30:381–383, 1975.
6. Dimic J, Andric R, Milivojevic J: Zur Frage der Pathologie und Therapie der Tonsillenerkrankungen der Hunde. *Kleinter Prax* 17:77–81, 1972.

7. Von Scupin E: Tonsillitis-Endocarditis Syndrom beim Hund. *Deutsche Tierarzt Wschr* 85:313–317, 1978.
8. Hallstrom M: Surgery of the canine mouth and pharynx. *J Small Anim Pract* 11:105–111, 1970.
9. Brennan KE, Ihrke PJ: Grass awn migration in dogs and cats: A retrospective study of 182 cases. *J Am Vet Med Assoc* 182:1201–1204, 1983.
10. Hofmyer CFB: Indications for and technique of tonsillectomy in the dog. *J South Africa Vet Med Assoc* 26:9–14, 1955.
11. Kaplan B: A technic for tonsillectomy in the dog. *Vet Med Small Anim Clin* 64:805–810, 1969.
12. Rickards DA: Tonsillectomy and soft palate resection. *Canine Pract* 1:29–33, 1974.
13. Kataura A, Doi Y, Narimatsu E: Histological research concerning cryotonsillectomy in dogs. *Arch Otorhinolaryngol* 209:33–45, 1975.
14. Lee R: Radiographic examination of localized and diffuse tissue swellings in the mandibular and pharyngeal area. *Vet Clin North Am* 4:723–740, 1974.
15. Karbe E, Schieffer B: Branchial cyst in a dog. *J Am Vet Med Assoc* 147:637–640, 1965.
16. Karbe E: Lateral neck cysts in the dog. *Am J Vet Res* 26:717–722, 1965.
17. Miskowiec JF, Hankes GH, Engel HN, Bartels JE: Internal branchial fistula in a kitten. *Vet Med Small Anim Clin* 69:259–263, 1974.
18. Scott WA: Treatment of sub-mucus cysts. *Vet Rec* 72:133–134, 1960.

Chapter Twelve

Salivary Gland Diseases

CE Harvey

The anatomy of the salivary glands in the dog and cat is described on page 19. The major functions of saliva in dogs and cats are lubrication of food in its passage from the mouth to the stomach and protection of the oropharyngeal mucosa. Saliva contains a rich assortment of antimicrobial and buffering agents. Evaporative heat loss during panting is a secondary function in dogs.

There is very little digestive enzyme activity in carnivore saliva. The mandibular and sublingual glands produce a tryptic inhibitor—anti-insulin factor.[1] Salivary flow is reduced in some diabetic humans,[2,3] which may, in part, account for the increased severity of periodontal disease in these patients.

CLINICAL SIGNS AND METHODS OF EXAMINATION

Swelling is the most common sign of salivary gland disease, and is caused by swelling of the gland itself or by accumulation of salivary secretions in an abnormal area. The swelling may be on the side of the face, in the intermandibular area, or in the sublingual tissues, or it may present as exophthalmos. The swelling may be soft (extravasation) or firm (neoplasia). With the exception of mandibular gland necrosis, swellings caused by salivary gland disease are rarely painful. Fluid-containing swellings in the head and

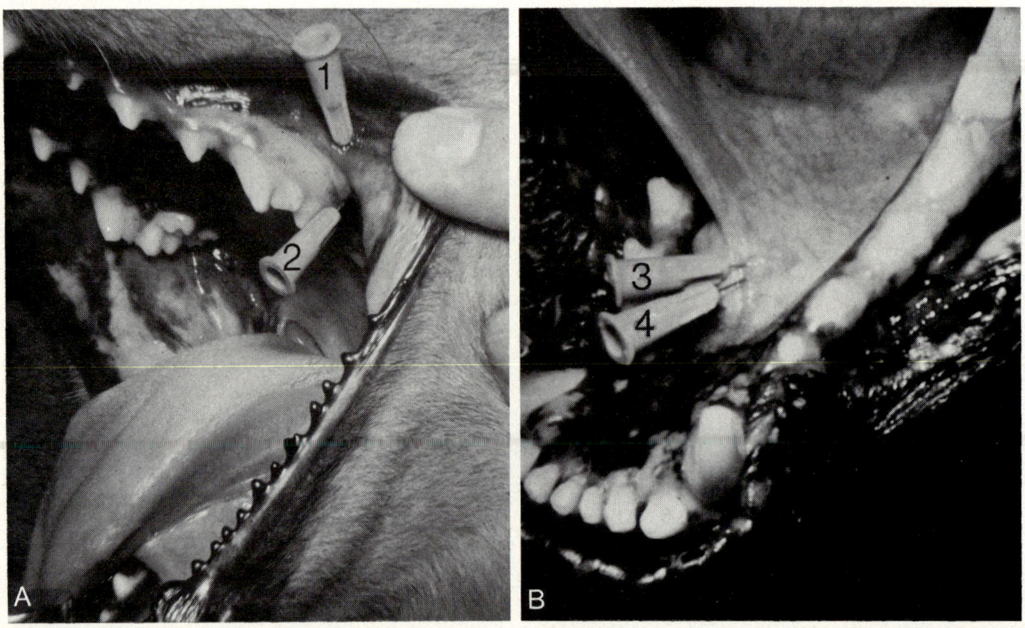

Figure 12–1. Cannulae in openings of the salivary ducts. *A*, Parotid *(1)* and zygomatic *(2)*. *B*, Sublingual *(3)* and mandibular *(4)*. (From Harvey CE: Sialography in the dog. *Vet Radiol* 10:18–27, 1969.)

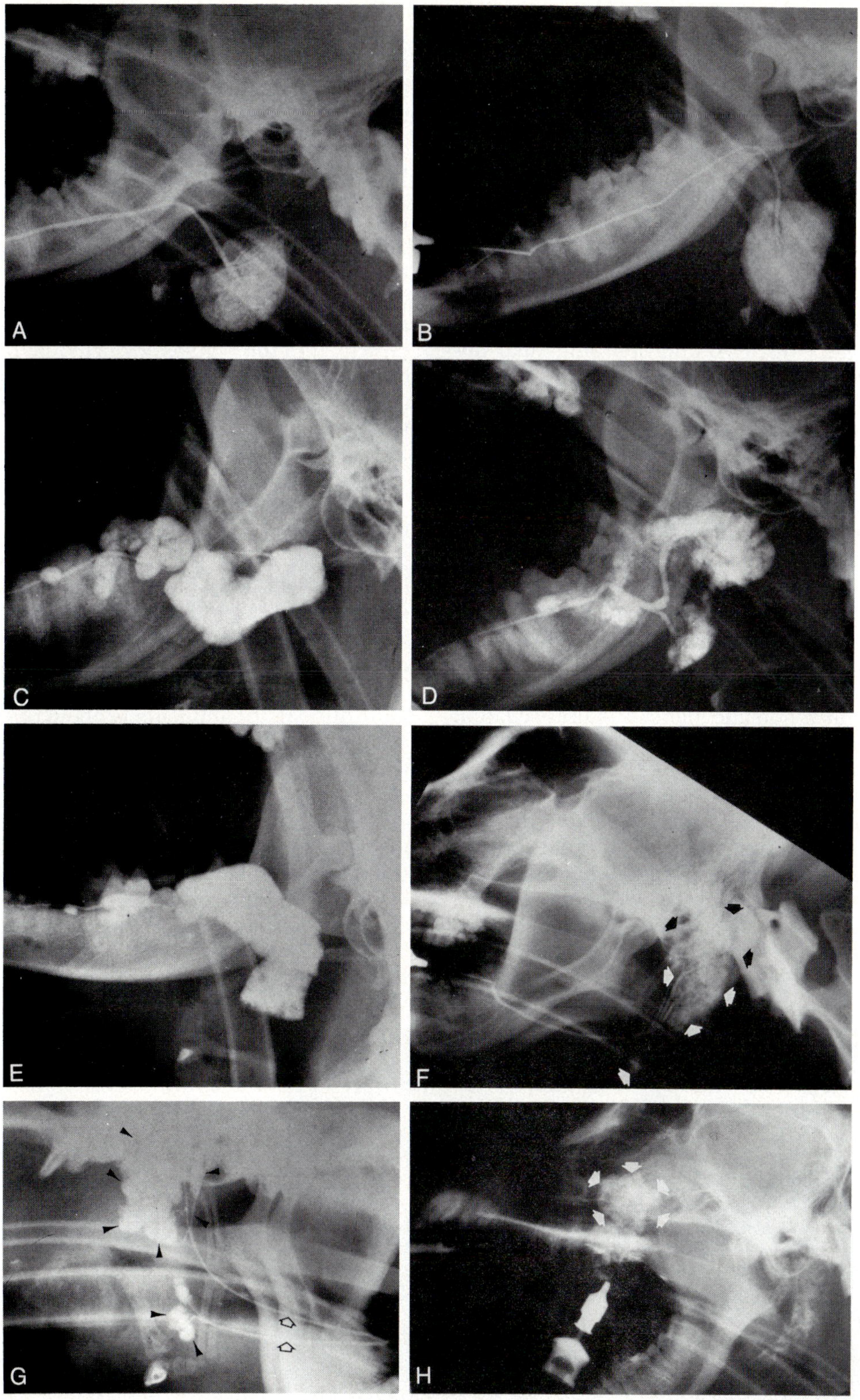

Figure 12–2. Normal sialograms of dogs. *A* and *B*, Mandibular gland. *C, D,* and *E*, Sublingual gland (see also Figure 12–8). *F* and *G*, Parotid gland *(arrows)*: Note double duct in *G (open arrows)*. *H*, Zygomatic gland *(arrows)*.

neck area are almost always of salivary origin or the result of foreign body penetration. Congenital abnormalities, such as branchial cleft or lymphoepithelial cysts, are extremely rare in the dog and cat.[4–6] The differential diagnosis of retropharyngeal swellings is described in Chapter Eleven.

Drooling is usually the result of oral or pharyngeal pain or swelling that restricts or prevents swallowing. Other causes of drooling include poisons, such as organophosphate insecticides, lead, and cyclonite; viral diseases, such as canine distemper or feline respiratory diseases; and neuromuscular abnormalities that interfere with the normal swallowing reflex. The mouth and pharynx should be examined carefully in drooling dogs, and the examination should include watching the animal eat and drink.

Cervical pain or reluctance to open the mouth is a prominent sign in dogs with mandibular gland necrosis; more common causes of these signs include pharyngeal or retrobulbar abscess, masticatory muscle disease, cervical disc disease, and trauma.

The parotid and mandibular glands are readily palpable. Examination of the sublingual and zygomatic glands requires sedation or anesthesia. Gland and duct function can be evaluated by placing a drop of topical ophthalmic atropine solution on the tongue; in a normal dog or cat, a copious flow of saliva occurs, though usually it is not possible to distinguish from which ducts the flow originates. Parotid saliva is aqueous when compared with the mixed mucoaqueous saliva from the other salivary glands in dogs and cats.

Plain film radiography is rarely useful in investigating salivary gland disease, though a sialolith may be radiopaque. Contrast radiography (sialography) is performed under anesthesia. A water-soluble radiopaque dye, such as that used for intravenous urography, is injected into a salivary duct through a blunt small-gauge needle at a dose of 1 ml/10 kg/injection.[7–9] The parotid and zygomatic duct openings are usually easy to find on the buccal mucosa opposite the upper fourth premolar tooth and the first molar tooth, respectively (Fig. 12–1 *A*). The cannula slides directly into the zygomatic duct. The parotid duct bends medially just before opening onto the mucosal surface at the papilla. Cannulation is made easier by grasping the mucosa just caudal to the duct opening and pulling it rostrally to straighten the bend.

The mandibular and sublingual duct openings are recognized as slits on the lateroventral surface of the lingual caruncles, which lie at the ventral end of the frenulum of the tongue (Fig. 12–1 *B*). The mandibular duct is the larger and more rostral of the two and is usually easy to cannulate once identified. The sublingual duct is sometimes frustratingly difficult to cannulate; in about one third of dogs, there is no separate opening, because the sublingual duct joins the mandibular duct along its course.[10–12]

Typical sialographic patterns of normal glands are shown in Figure 12–2 *A–H*. Radiographically visible abnormalities include a loss of continuity of the duct, extravasation of dye from the gland or duct, dilatation of the duct, or failure of the dye to penetrate fully into the duct and gland.[8]

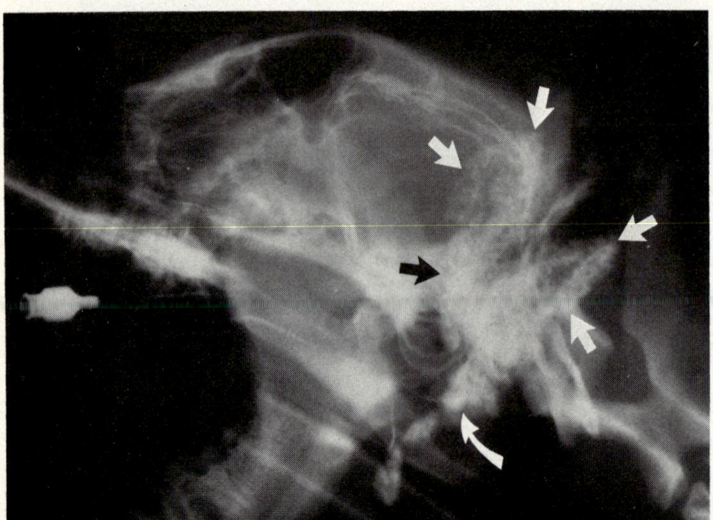

Figure 12–3. Sialogram of a dog with an enlarged parotid gland *(arrows)*. The dog's face was constantly moist. (From Harvey CE: Hypersialosis and parotid gland enlargement in a dog. *J Small Anim Pract* 22:19–25, 1981.)

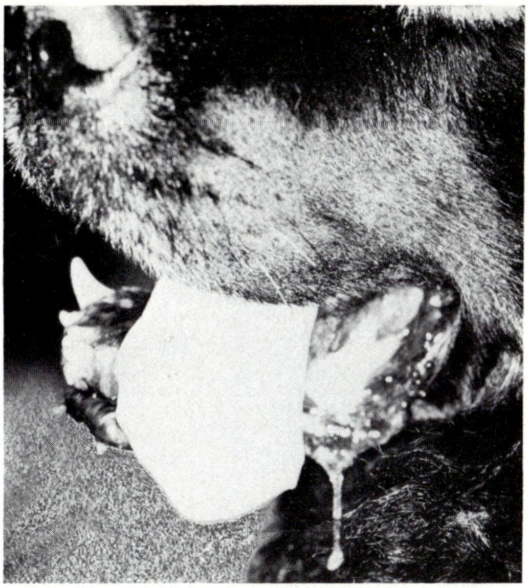

Figure 12–4. Drooling of mucoid saliva from the pendulous lip fold of a Newfoundland dog.

CONGENITAL ANOMALIES

Because there is such an abundance of functional salivary tissue, congenital atresia of salivary ducts or absence of one more salivary glands is not likely to be noted.

It is very rare to see hypersialism (drooling) as a primary salivary gland abnormality in dogs and cats. Drooling of a clear, serous secretion was the clinical sign noted in two dogs with congenital enlargement of the parotid salivary glands (Fig. 12–3).[13, 14] Treatment by parotid duct ligation (see further on) was successful in both dogs, as well as in a third dog seen recently by the author.

Drooling that starts at a young age in giant-breed dogs is usually due to an abnormal conformation of the lips (Fig. 12–4). The saliva hangs in mucoid ropes from the lower lip furrows and is sent flying in all directions when the dog shakes its head. Treatment consists of bilateral mandibular and sublingual gland ligation (Fig. 12–5) or resection, lip fold resection (Chapter Ten, page 159), or cheiloplasty, or by a combination of these procedures.

INFECTIOUS, INFLAMMATORY, AND IMMUNE-MEDIATED DISEASES

Many non-traumatic and non-neoplastic conditions are known to affect the salivary glands of humans.[15] Few of them are recognized in veterinary species. Xerostomia (dry mouth) is seen in some dogs with keratoconjunctivitis sicca.[16] Dogs with this combination of reduced ocular and oral secretions may be suffering from a condition equivalent to Sjögren's syndrome in humans, which is a chronic inflammatory disease presenting as keratoconjunctivitis sicca and xerostomia, associated with rheumatoid arthritis, systemic lupus erythematosus, scleroderma, polymyositis, or polyarteritis.[17]

The paramyxovirus that causes mumps in humans can cause parotid, and less often mandibular, gland infections in dogs.[18, 19] Clinically obvious disease is uncommon and

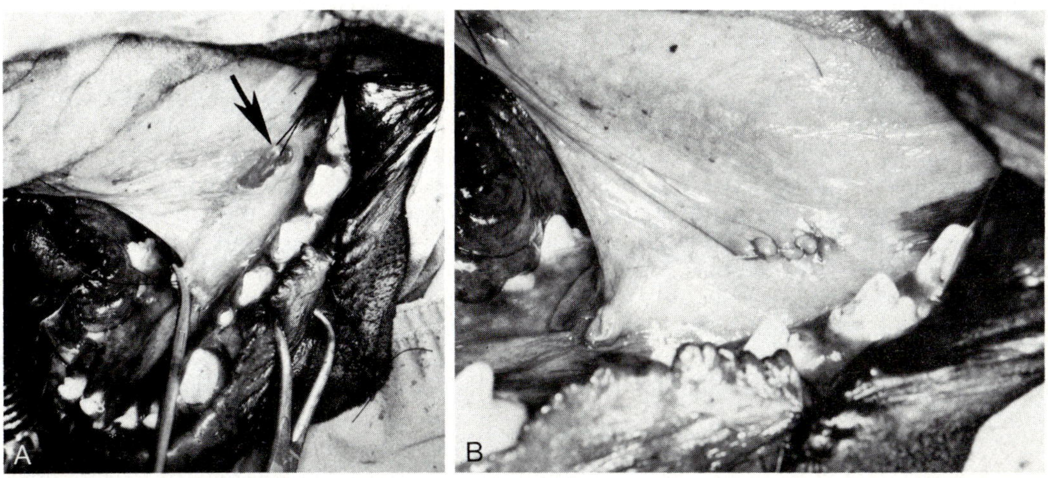

Figure 12–5. Ligation of the mandibular and sublingual ducts. *A*, The ducts have been identified through an incision in the sublingual mucosa, and suture material has been passed around the ducts *(arrow)*. Lengths of monofilament nylon are present in the ducts. *B*, The mucosal incision has been sutured following duct ligation.

is usually seen in households in which a human occupant has mumps. Clinical signs include pyrexia, depression, and swollen, tender salivary glands; recovery is rapid and treatment is not necessary.

Mandibular Gland Necrosis

Mandibular gland necrosis is a more serious, but also uncommon, inflammatory disease of the salivary glands.[20, 21] Because the mandibular gland is enclosed within a tight and strong capsule, any rapid increase in the size of the gland can lead to vascular compromise and necrosis. The cause of the inflammation in this syndrome is not known, though viral infection is a likely possibility.

Dogs are presented to the veterinarian because of exquisite pain on swallowing or on palpation of the mouth and neck. There may be little obvious swelling of the mandibular gland, though the mandibular lymph nodes are usually swollen to some extent. Radiographic and laboratory examinations provide no useful diagnostic information. Conservative treatment with antibiotics and corticosteroids has no beneficial effects. Surgical resection of the mandibular glands may provide relief for some dogs, though the pain often persists following surgery[21] and the dog is euthanized. Pathological examination of the resected gland shows acute inflammation and necrosis.[20]

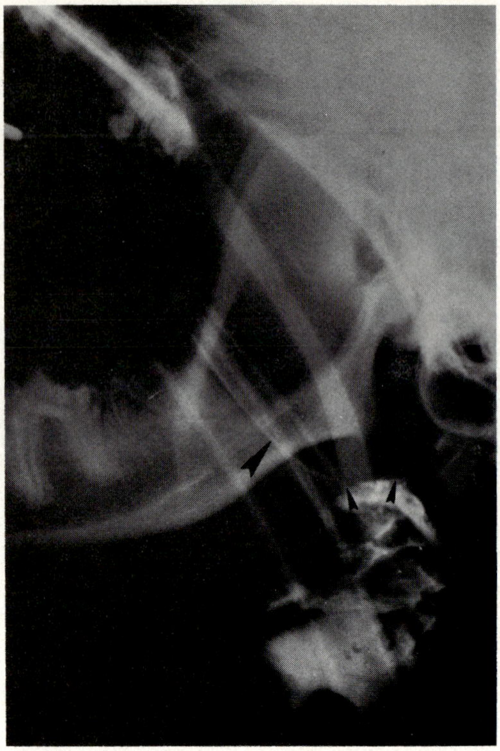

Figure 12–6. Sialogram from a dog with a parotid duct fistula. The contrast medium passes from the duct *(large arrow)* through the area of damage *(small arrows)* to the skin. (From Harvey CE: Parotid salivary duct rupture and fistula in the dog and cat. *Sm An Pract* 18:163, 1977.)

INJURY TO THE SALIVARY GLANDS AND DUCTS

If a salivary gland or duct is injured, and stenosis of the duct or diversion of salivary flow to a new opening into the mouth results, there will be no long-term clinical consequences of note. For this reason, facial trauma that may involve the salivary glands does not require that any initial management be directed at the salivary glands. Long-term consequences of salivary gland or duct injury include sialocele or fistula formation. Ligation of salivary ducts results in an initial increase in size, then in atrophy,[22] though some secretory activity can be stimulated for at least several months following ligation.[23]

The Parotid Gland

The parotid gland or duct may be injured by bites or blunt trauma during surgery on the side of the face or as a result of adjacent disease, such as carnassial abscess. If the duct is severed, and saliva establishes a route of escape through the subcutaneous tissues to the skin, a fistula will result.[24] The fistula typically leaks a clear, thin fluid, which may be more noticeable or even copious during eating. The fluid accumulates in a soft, nonpainful pocket on the side of the face if the skin is not damaged.[8, 25] Sialography is diagnostic, though the pattern varies (Fig. 12–6); the distal duct may be completely obstructed, in which case dye is injected into the fistulous opening. Treatment may be to divert[25] or reconstruct the duct,[24] though simple ligation is quick and effective.[24]

Parotid Duct Ligation. Monofilament nylon 00 suture material is inserted into the duct opening in the mouth or into the fistula if the openings are not connected. A skin incision on the side of the face is used to locate the duct between the buccal nerves, lying on the surface of the masseter muscle aponeurosis. The proximal duct is undermined, the suture material in the duct is removed, and two or three ligatures are placed. The caudal (proximal) ligature is tied less tightly to distribute the back pressure that follows ligation.[24]

The Zygomatic Gland

Trauma to the face may cause saliva to leak from a damaged zygomatic salivary gland.[26, 27] Dogs with zygomatic mucocele are presented to the veterinarian because of exophthalmos. Diagnosis is by aspiration of mucoid material from the ventral aspect of the orbit, and it is confirmed by sialography. Treatment is by surgical resection of the gland[26, 27] (page 200) or by marsupialization (see description further on) of the swelling into the mouth.[28] The gland should be examined microscopically following resection, because zygomatic gland carcinoma may cause a large mucocele.[29]

The Mandibular Gland

The mandibular gland is contained within a firm, fibrous capsule, so clinically obvious, long-term effects of trauma to this gland in the dog are uncommon.[30, 31] The mandibular gland has been shown to be the cause of a salivary mucocele in rare cases;[32] treatment consists of mandibular gland resection (page 197).

The Sublingual Gland

Salivary Mucocele

The most common condition of the salivary glands in the dog and cat is salivary mucocele, which is collection of mucoid saliva that has leaked from a damaged salivary gland. It has been suggested from small sample populations that toy or miniature poodles and German shepherd dogs have an abnormally high

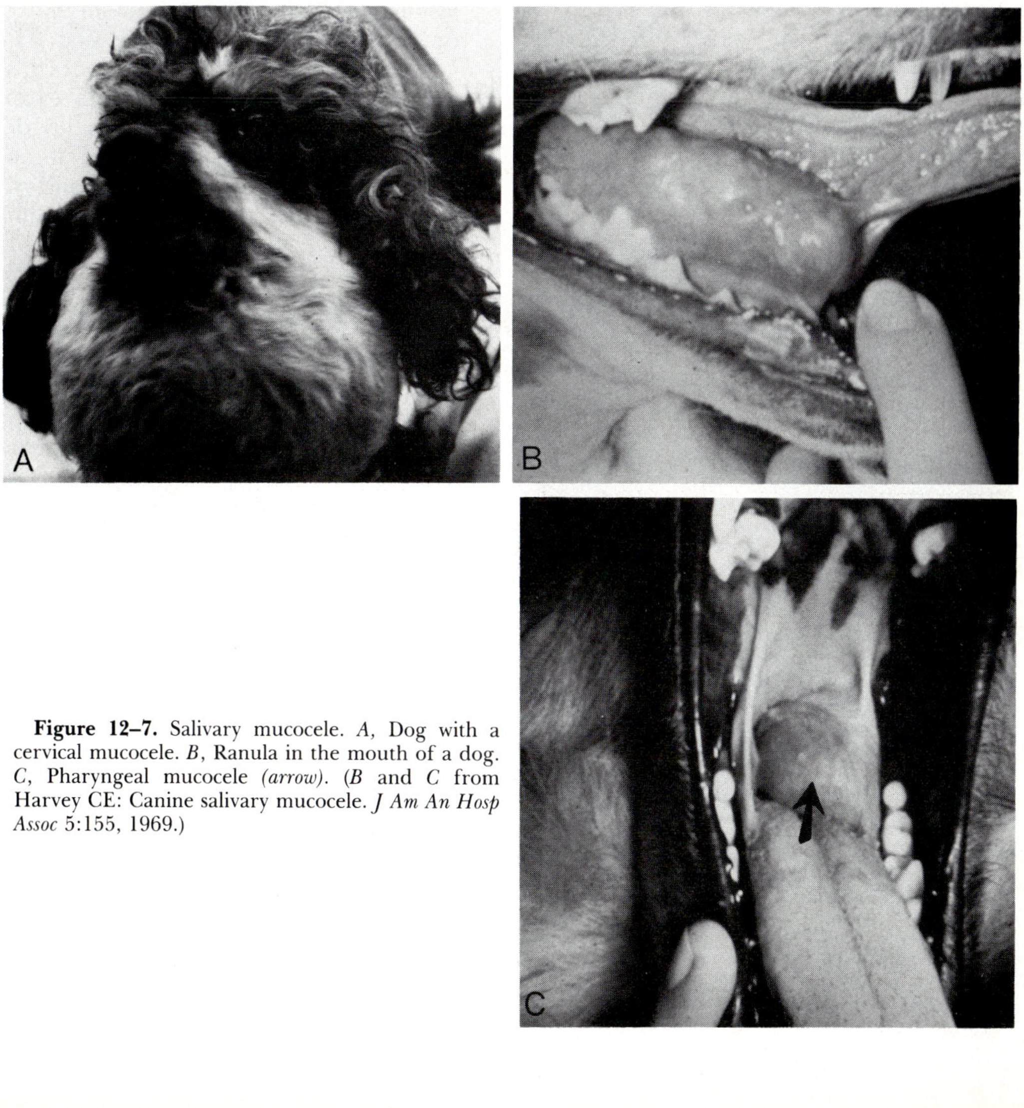

Figure 12–7. Salivary mucocele. *A*, Dog with a cervical mucocele. *B*, Ranula in the mouth of a dog. *C*, Pharyngeal mucocele *(arrow)*. (*B* and *C* from Harvey CE: Canine salivary mucocele. *J Am An Hosp Assoc* 5:155, 1969.)

incidence of this disease;[33,34] other studies showed no breed predisposition.[10,35] The sublingual gland is most frequently affected.[7,11,35–37] As with any fluid in body tissues, saliva takes the path of least resistance. The most common sites for the extravasated saliva to collect are the subcutaneous tissues of the intermandibular or cranial cervical area ("cervical mucocele," Fig. 12–7 *A*) and sublingual tissues on the floor of the mouth ("ranula," Fig. 12–7 *B*). A less common site is the pharyngeal wall (Fig. 12–7 *C*).[38]

The cause of the damage, which can occur anywhere in the gland or duct,[10] is rarely known, though occasionally a foreign body penetrating the sublingual gland is found (Fig. 12–8).[8,39] Blunt trauma caused by bones or sticks that the animal chews is a likely cause, since they may crush the sublingual gland against the mandible. Grass seeds may penetrate the oral mucosa and cause disruption of the duct system and mucus accumulation.[40] Cervical mucoceles and ranulas occasionally occur in cats.[41–43] Mucoceles formed in 44 percent of 27 experimental cats following ligation of the sublingual duct rostral to the lingual nerve.[44]

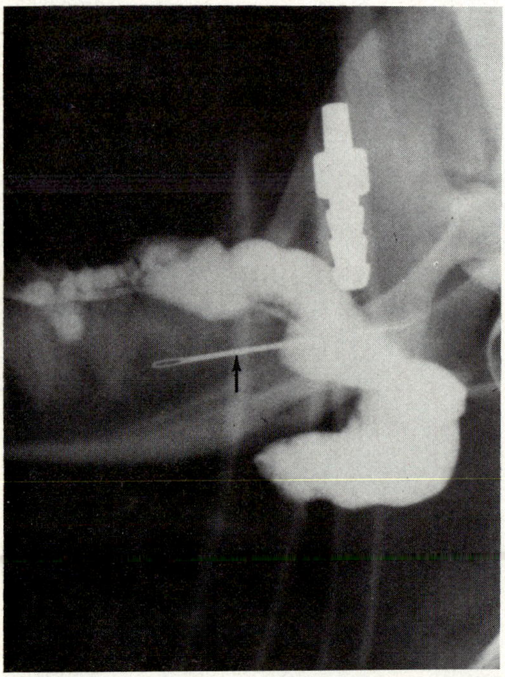

Figure 12–8. Sialogram of a dog with a mucocele caused by a needle that penetrated the sublingual gland. The sialogram shown is from the opposite, normal side. (From Harvey CE: Sialography in the dog. *Vet Radiol* 10:18–27, 1969.)

Clinical Signs. These depend on the position of the mucocele. A cervical mucocele may commence with an acute phase when the swelling is firm and somewhat painful, followed by a reduction in the swelling as the initial inflammatory response to the saliva[31] subsides; however, this initial period is often not observed by the owner, and the usual presenting complaint is of gradual enlargement of a soft, non-painful mass. A ranula may be seen by the owner or may become noticeable when it is damaged by the teeth, causing bleeding around the mouth or into the animal's water bowl. A pharyngeal mucocele can cause more significant disease by obstructing the pharyngeal airway; emergency treatment by lancing the mucocele may be necessary in occasional animals to relieve respiratory distress.

Diagnosis of Salivary Mucocele. Diagnosis is made by palpation and aspiration of the swelling. Sedation may be required if the lesion is oral or pharyngeal. Golden colored or blood-stained mucus is obtained. The mucus is invariably viscid enough to form strings when exuded from the syringe through a needle (Fig. 12–9). It is occasionally difficult to distinguish between a mucocele and the serosanguineous fluid that is found in association with a foreign body. Examining smears of the cells in the fluid is not likely to be helpful; however, staining a smear of the fluid with a mucus-specific stain, such as periodic acid–Schiff (PAS), will effectively confirm the diagnosis. Although sialography can be used to confirm the diagnosis (Fig. 12–10), it is time-consuming and may be unrewarding because the mandibular and sublingual ducts are conjoined, often preventing cannulation of the sublingual duct. A mucocele can be differentiated from the very rare congenital branchial cleft cyst by microscopic examination of the wall of the swelling, which, in the case of a mucocele, is composed of inflammatory or connective tissue cells, with occasional areas of epithelium at the junction with the gland or duct.[31] Occasionally, a mucocele contains hard, round objects that initially appear as calculi of some sort; they are mineralized folds of the inflammatory lining that have sloughed into the lumen.[45]

Definitive Treatment of Salivary Mucocele. Treatment consists of removing the damaged salivary gland, to prevent further accumulation of mucus, and draining the mucocele. However, in many cases (particularly when the animal may be a severe anes-

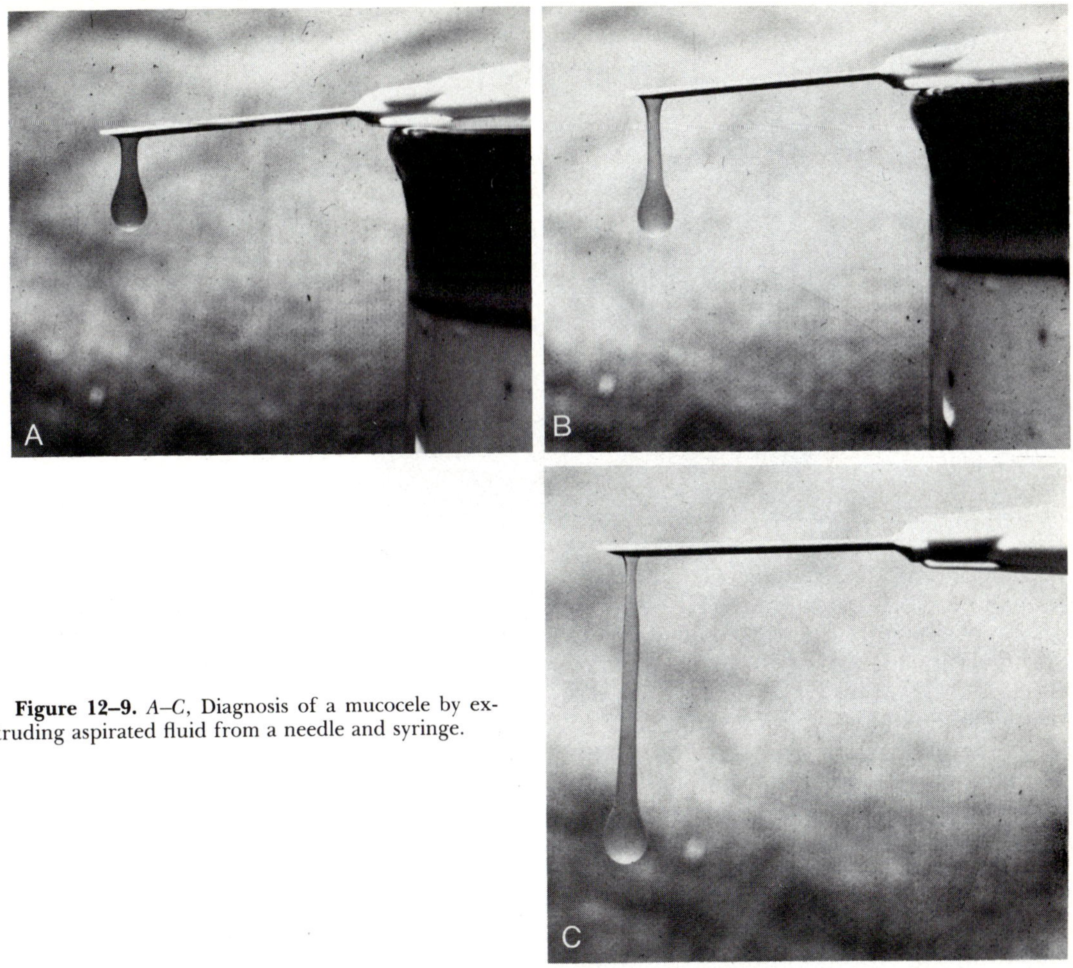

Figure 12–9. *A–C*, Diagnosis of a mucocele by extruding aspirated fluid from a needle and syringe.

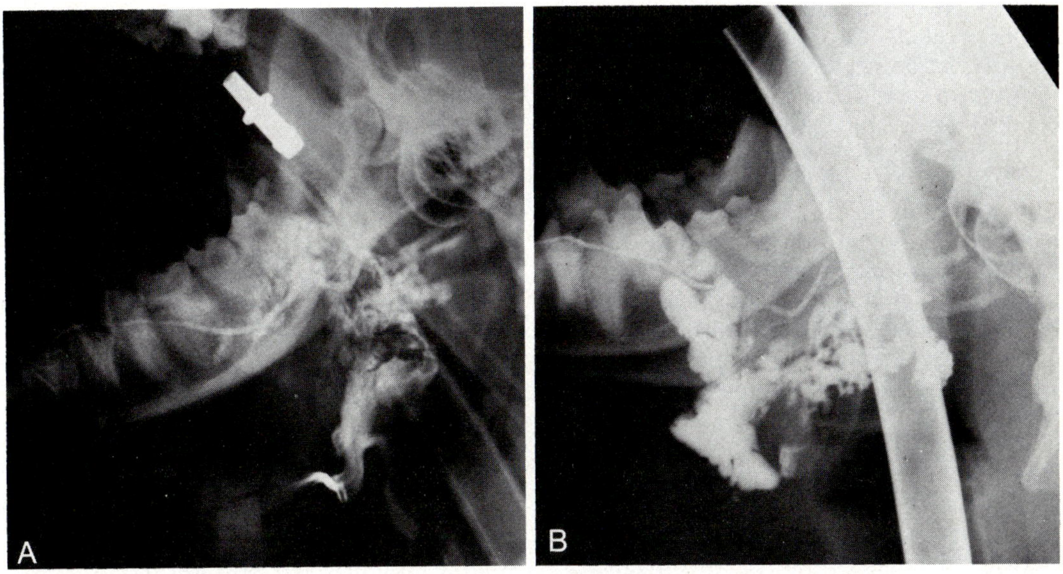

Figure 12–10. *A* and *B*, Sialograms showing leakage from sublingual glands.

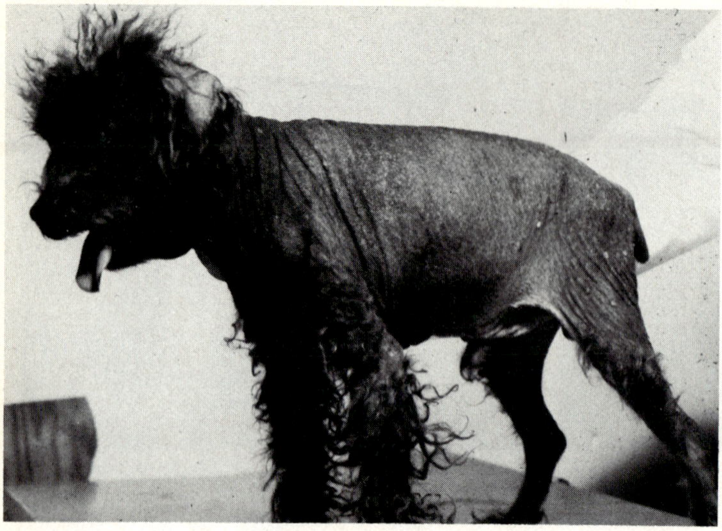

Figure 12–11. An aged poodle presented because of a cervical salivary mucocele. The dog also had severe cardiac disease and was cushingoid. The mucocele was treated by periodic aspiration.

thetic risk), periodic drainage of the mucocele may be more appropriate (Fig. 12–11). Periodic drainage is not recommended for pharyngeal mucoceles, or for some ranulas, if the mucocele is causing respiratory distress or difficulty in eating or swallowing.

If conservative treatment is selected, drainage, using a 20-gauge needle and a 10-ml to 50-ml syringe, can usually be accomplished without anesthesia. In most cases, the mucocele will have recurred and will have grown to its former size in 6 to 12 weeks, though in a few dogs scar tissue will seal the area of leakage, and no further saliva will accumulate.

Redirection of salivary flow has been suggested as an alternative to salivary gland resection, particularly for a ranula or pharyngeal mucocele.[46] This process is known as marsupialization. A section of the mucocele wall is removed with a scalpel or scissors, and the lining of the mucocele is sutured to the oral or pharyngeal mucosa. This is not likely to provide satisfactory long-term results, because the lining of the mucocele consists of fibrous or inflammatory tissue. Stainless steel sutures have been suggested as a means of maintaining the patency of the fistula.[47] Since anesthesia is necessary to perform marsupialization, it seems more appropriate to perform salivary gland resection, since it will provide a much greater chance for preventing recurrence.

When an animal is presented to the veterinarian in respiratory distress because of a pharyngeal mucocele, immediate relief of the distress and confirmation of the diagnosis can be obtained by aspirating or lancing the swelling. When in doubt, a diagnostic tap should be performed first. Definitive treatment can be performed during the same anesthetic episode.

Resection of a cervical salivary mucocele is possible, but it is tedious and may result in damage to vascular or neural structures in the area. More important, it will not prevent recurrence,[48] since the cause of the mucocele has not been dealt with. Therefore, resection of a mucocele is not recommended. In an exceptional case in which the mucocele is very large, the dependent skin can be resected following salivary gland resection and drainage of the mucocele.[49]

Resection of the sublingual gland without resection of the mandibular gland is not practical because of the close apposition of the two glands. Thus, even though the sublingual gland is almost always the gland affected, treatment consists of removing the mandibular-sublingual gland complex. Removing both of these glands does not affect the animal adversely, even if the procedure is performed bilaterally.[11] Generally, it is obvious which side is affected from the clinical history or physical examination. When this is not the case, palpation and observation with the animal under anesthesia and in dorsal recumbency are helpful. Sialography may determine which side is affected, but it is time-consuming and may not be successful because of the frequency of combined mandibular-sublingual duct openings. A practical alternative is to incise the mucocele and palpate the wall from the lumen; the unaffected side will usually be rounded and smooth, whereas the affected side will have a tunnel or tract that descends dorsally into the deeper tissues of the intermandibular area. When the affected side cannot be determined by one of these methods, the mandibular-sublingual gland complex can be removed from both sides.

Mandibular-Sublingual Gland Resection for Salivary Mucocele. This is accomplished with the animal in dorsolateral recumbency under general anesthesia. The intermandibular and cranial neck area is clipped and prepared for aseptic surgery. A skin incision is made over the mandibular salivary gland, which can be palpated caudal to the mandible (Fig. 12–12). The maxillary and linguofacial veins should be avoided; they can be identified by digitally occluding the jugular vein. The thin platysma muscle is penetrated, and the incision is continued more deeply until the fibrous capsule covering the mandibular gland is reached and penetrated. The incision is extended, and the gland is separated from the capsule by blunt dissection, commencing at the caudoventral edge. The gland is grasped with Allis tissue forceps and is prolapsed from the capsule (Fig. 12–12 *B*). Blunt dissection is continued to further free the gland. An artery and vein are often seen entering the medial aspect of the gland; they are clamped and ligated. The attachment of the capsule to the cranial end of the gland must be penetrated without damaging the ongoing sublingual gland; this is achieved by directing the dissection parallel to the long axis of the mandibular duct and sublingual gland as they disappear beneath the digastric muscle. A branch of the lingual artery that curves backward to supply the salivary glands is often visible at this point; it is dissected free, clamped, and ligated.

Blunt dissection is continued rostrally with scissors or a finger (Fig. 12–12 *C*). By tunneling the sublingual gland and duct underneath the digastric muscle, or by transecting

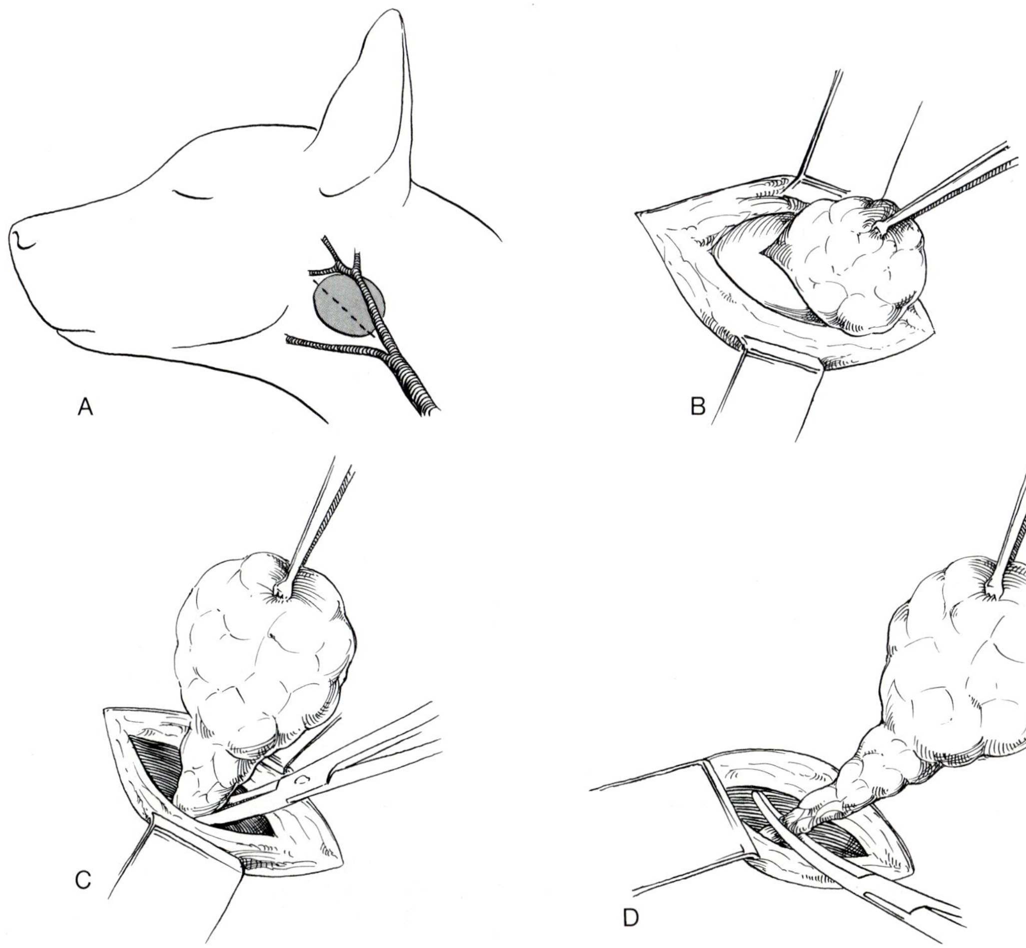

Figure 12–12. *A*, Mandibulosublingual salivary gland resection. *A*, Lateral view of the head and neck showing the position of the jugular vein, mandibular salivary gland *(shaded area)*, and skin incision *(dashed line)*. *B*, The mandibular gland is prolapsed through an incision in its capsule. *C*, The sublingual gland is dissected deep to the digastric muscle. *D*, The sublingual gland is retracted caudally with a hemostat.

the muscle, more complete removal of the rostral, polystomatic part of the sublingual gland can be achieved;[50] however, this is very rarely necessary clinically. Particular care is required to prevent separation of the lobules of the sublingual gland, because the sublingual duct is small, and the lobules of the gland are loosely connected. Dissection of the sublingual gland is continued as far rostrally as possible, then a hemostat is placed across the most rostral part of the dissected gland and is pulled caudally (Fig. 12–12 *D*). Another hemostat is placed across the newly exposed gland. This process is continued until the sublingual gland and duct finally tear. No ligatures are needed when this retraction technique is used. The incision is closed by apposing the capsule edges and subcutaneous tissues with absorbable sutures, followed by skin sutures.

The mucocele is drained following resection of the glands; a stab incision is made into the lumen and the contents are milked out. A soft rubber drain is placed in a cervical mucocele to encourage the elimination of remaining fluid; ranulas and pharyngeal mucoceles are allowed to drain into the oral or pharyngeal cavities. Antibiotics are not necessary following salivary gland surgery.

Prognosis and Management of Recurrence. Occasional dogs show slight swallowing abnormalities following surgery.[11, 36]

Recurrence following mandibular-sublingual gland resection is less than 5 percent in reported series of cases.[11, 35, 36, 51] In the occasional case in which recurrence is obvious, there are two possible causes: (1) failure to resect all of the affected gland (or resection of the wrong gland) or (2) damage to the sublingual gland on the opposite side. When salivary gland resection has been performed previously, sialography is particularly useful to determine the amount of glandular tissue remaining, thus allowing a more exact treatment plan to be made.

When part of the sublingual gland remains in place and is known or suspected of being the site of leakage, treatment consists of resecting the remaining glandular tissue. Location and removal are facilitated if some methylene blue dye is injected through a blunt cannula into the sublingual duct immediately prior to dissection. An incision is made in the oral mucosa between the tongue and the vertical ramus of the mandible (Fig. 12–13). The gland is identified by its salmon-pink coloration and lobular structure or by the blue coloration if dye has been injected. The gland lies beneath the oral mucosa, between the styloglossus and mylohyoid muscles. The gland is freed by blunt and sharp dissection, which proceeds caudally as far as necessary to remove it completely (Fig. 12–13 *B*). The oral mucosa is sutured with absorbable material.

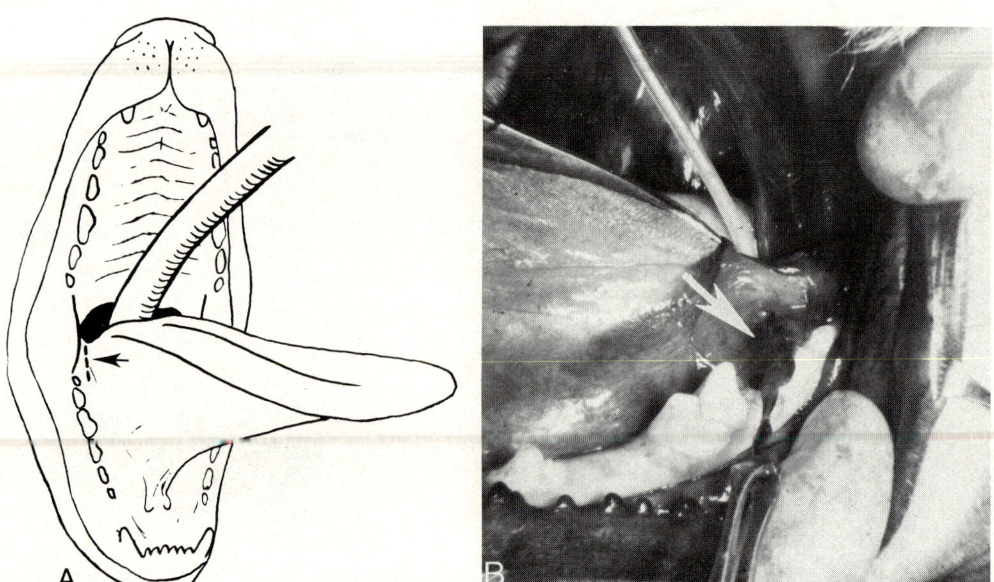

Figure 12–13. Resection of the rostral part of the sublingual gland. *A*, Incision (*dashed line, arrow*) in the oral mucosa lateral to the root of the tongue. *B*, The sublingual gland (*arrow* stained dark by methylene blue) is dissected free.

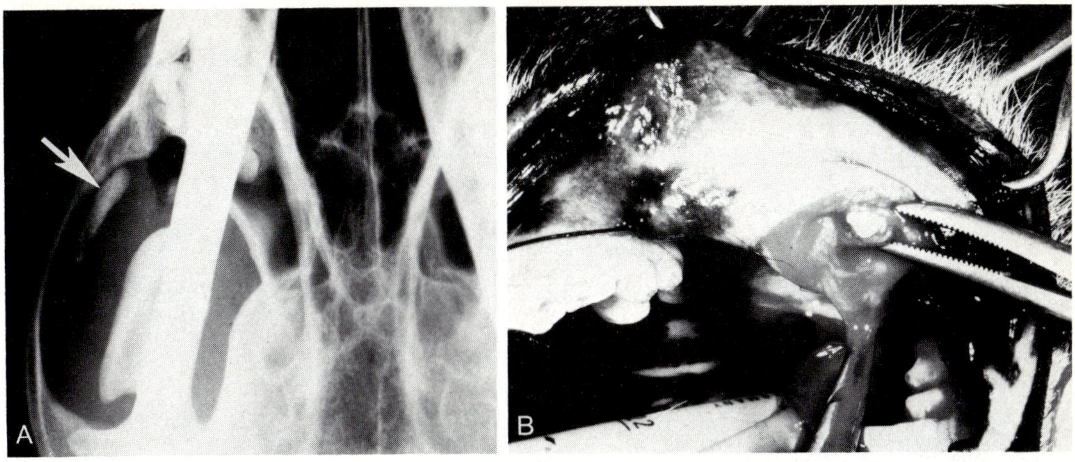

Figure 12–14. *A*, Radiograph of the head of a dog showing a sialolith *(arrow)*. *B*, A sialolith (the white structure held in the jaws of the hemostat) in the parotid duct seen through an incision in the oral mucosa.

SIALOLITHS

Sialoliths are stones in a salivary duct. They are seen occasionally in the parotid salivary ducts of dogs.[52, 53] They may cause obstruction of the duct, and the animal is presented to the veterinarian because of the resultant painful swelling. Foreign bodies are possible causes.[54] Sialoliths do not cause salivary mucoceles. The sialolith may be palpable, or it may be visible on survey radiographs (Fig. 12–14) or sialograms. Treatment consists of incising the duct over the sialolith through the oral mucosa and expressing the sialolith (Fig. 12–14 *B*). The duct is flushed to ensure that the obstruction has been cleared. Because the incision is made into the mouth, there is no need to suture the incision.

SALIVARY GLAND NEOPLASIA

Neoplasms of the salivary glands occur occasionally. The animal is usually presented to the veterinarian because of a palpable mass. Adenocarcinomata of the parotid and mandibular glands are most common and occur in dogs and cats with a mean age of 10 years.[55–57] Occasionally, very aggressive lesions may invade the skull and cause behavioral or endocrinopathic signs.[58] Oncocytomas arising from the parotid gland have been reported in a dog and cat.[59] Unilateral firm masses in a salivary gland should be biopsied. Distant metastasis may occur. Thoracic radiographs should be examined prior to definitive treatment. Lesions confined to the salivary gland itself may be amenable to surgical treatment.

The mandibular gland is particularly easy to resect because of the firm, easily recognizable capsule and the compact shape of the gland. The gland is dissected rostrally until normal sublingual gland is reached. A ligature is placed at that point, and the mandibular and caudal sublingual glands caudal to the ligature are resected.

The other salivary glands are more difficult to resect.

Parotid Gland Resection. This requires tedious dissection of the poorly defined gland, with identification and preservation of the facial nerve branches and blood vessels that traverse under and through the gland. Because of the diffuse nature of the parotid gland, complete resection of an infiltrating mass arising from this gland is rarely possible. Because of the surgical difficulties and superficial position of the parotid gland, orthovoltage radiotherapy was used to treat parotid adenocarcinomata in three dogs; all were alive with no evidence of recurrence or metastasis a minimum of 1 year later.[60] The staging system proposed for parotid carcinoma in dogs follows:

T: Primary tumor
- T1: Tumor 0 cm to 3 cm; solitary, freely movable; facial nerve intact
- T2: Tumor 3.1 cm to 6 cm; solitary, freely movable or reduced mobility or skin fixation; facial nerve intact
- T3: Tumor more than 6 cm with multiple nodules, ulceration, deep fixation, or facial nerve dysfunction

N: Regional lymph node
- N0: Regional lymph nodes not palpable

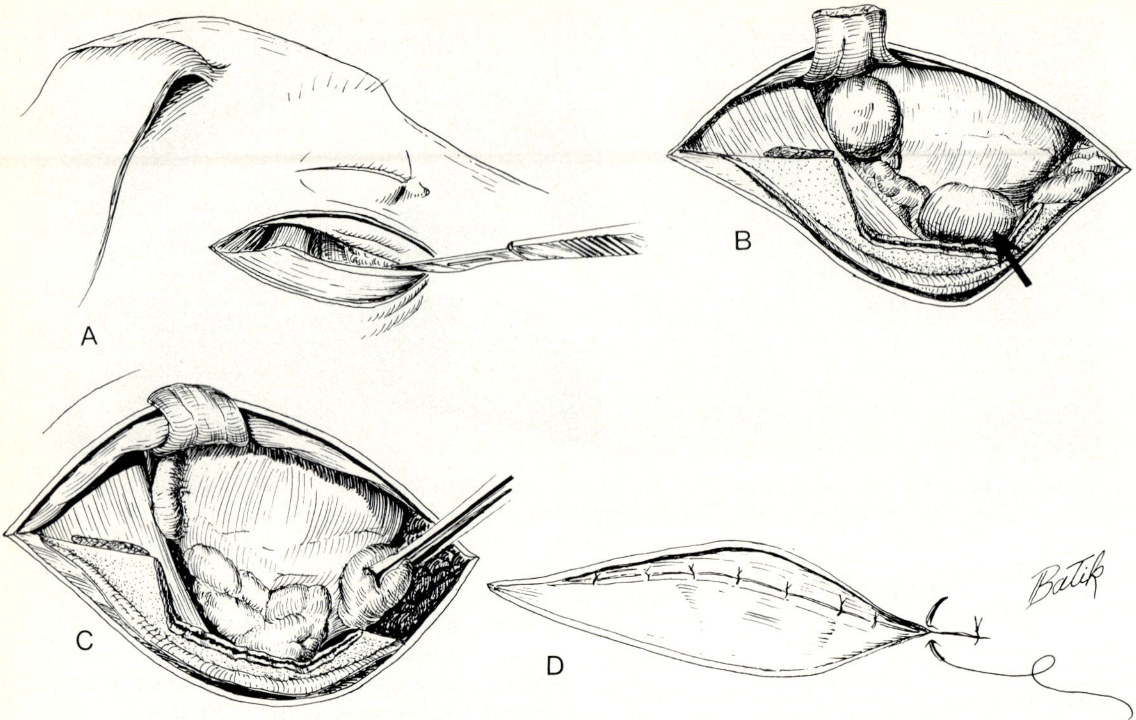

Figure 12–15. Zygomatic salivary gland resection. *A*, Incision over the zygomatic arch through the skin and periosteum. *B*, The dorsal section of the zygomatic arch has been resected, revealing the zygomatic salivary gland *(arrow)* beneath the orbital fat. *C*, The gland is retracted dorsally and is dissected free. *D*, The masseter aponeurosis and orbital fascia are sutured. (From Harvey CE: *In* Bistner SI, Aguirre GD, Batik G: Atlas of Veterinary Ophthalmic Surgery. Philadelphia, WB Saunders Co., 1977.)

N1: Movable homolateral nodes considered to contain growth
N2: Movable contralateral or bilateral nodes considered to contain growth
N3: Fixed nodes
M: Distant metastasis
M0: No evidence of distant metastasis
M1: Distant metastasis present

Stage 1 = T1N0M0
Stage 2 = T2N0M0
Stage 3 = T3N0M0
Stage 4 = any T1N2 or N3, M0; any T, N1, 2 or 3, any N, M

Zygomatic Gland Resection. This resection is complicated by the protected position of the gland behind the zygomatic arch. The skin is incised directly over the dorsal rim of the zygomatic arch, and the periosteum is incised and reflected, taking with it the orbital fascia dorsally and the masseter muscle aponeurosis ventrally (Fig. 12–15 *A*).[61] The dorsal half of the zygomatic arch is removed with a rongeur or bone saw (Fig. 12–15 *B*), or a bone flap is created by rostral and caudal incisions in the zygoma,[27] exposing the orbital fat. The zygomatic gland is found beneath the orbital fat, which is removed by gentle blunt dissection. The gland is lifted out, is dissected free from the loose connective tissue surrounding it (Fig. 12–15 *C*), and is removed. The incision is closed with interrupted absorbable sutures in the periosteum and orbital fascia (Fig. 12–15 *D*). For a large mass in the orbital area, the entire zygoma can be resected to facilitate dissection; closure is as described previously.

References

1. Godlowski Z, Gaza M, Withers BT: Ablation of salivary glands as initial step in the management of selected forms of diabetes mellitus. *Laryngoscope* 81:1337–1358, 1971.
2. Conner S, Iranpour B, Mills J: Alteration in parotid salivary flow in diabetes mellitus. *Oral Surg Oral Med Oral Pathol* 30:55–59, 1970.
3. Marder MZ, Abelson DC, Mandel ID: Salivary alterations in diabetes mellitus. *J Periodontol* 46:567–569, 1975.
4. Karbe E: Lateral neck cysts in the dog. *Am J Vet Res* 26:717–722, 1965.
5. Karbe E, Nielson SE: Branchial cyst in a dog. *J Am Vet Med Assoc* 147:637–640, 1965.
6. Miskowiec JF, Hankes GH, Engel HN, Bartels JE:

Internal branchial fistula in a kitten. *Vet Med Small Anim Clin* 69:259–263, 1974.
7. Christoph HJ: Zur Erkrankung der Speicheldrusen und deren Ausfuhrungsgange beim Hund. *Berl Munch Tierartz Wschr* 69:227–231, 1956.
8. Harvey CE: Sialography in the dog. *Vet Radiol* 10:18–27, 1969.
9. Leonardi L: La scialografia nel cane. *Gaz Vet* 18:20–24, 1965.
10. Gill MA: Diseases of the salivary glands of the dog. Thesis, Glasgow University, 1980.
11. Glen JB: Canine salivary mucoceles: results of sialographic examination and surgical treatment of fifty cases. *J Small Anim Pract* 13:515–526, 1972.
12. Michel G: Beitrag zur Topographie der Ausfuhrungsgange der gl. mandibularis und der gl. sublingualis major des Hundes. *Berl Munch Teirartz Wschr* 69:132–134, 1956.
13. Bedford PGC: Unilateral parotid hypersialism in a dachshund. *Vet Rec* 107:557–558, 1980.
14. Harvey CE: Hypersialosis and parotid gland enlargement in a dog. *J Small Anim Pract* 22:19–25, 1981.
15. Epker BN: Obstructive and inflammatory diseases of the major salivary glands. *Oral Surg Oral Med Oral Pathol* 33:2–27, 1972.
16. Kaswan MD: Rheumatoid factor determinations in dogs with keratoconjunctivitis sicca. *J Am Vet Med Assoc* 183:1073–1075, 1983.
17. Daniels TE, Silverman S, Michalski JP, Greenspan JS, Sylvester RA, Talal N: The oral component of Sjogren's syndrome. *Oral Surg Oral Med Oral Pathol* 39:875–885, 1975.
18. Chandler EA: Mumps in the dog. *Vet Rec* 96:365–366, 1975.
19. Smith RE: Mumps in the dog. *Vet Rec* 96:296, 1975.
20. Kelly DF, Lucke VM, Denny HR, Lane JG: Histology of salivary gland infarction in the dog. *Vet Pathol* 16:438–443, 1979.
21. Kelly DF, Lucke VM, Lane JG, Denny HR, Longstaffe JA: Salivary gland necrosis in dogs. *Vet Rec* 104:268, 1979.
22. Harrison JD, Garett JR: Histological effects of ductal ligation of salivary glands of the cat. *J Pathol* 118:245–254, 1975.
23. Emmelin N, Garrett JR, Ohlin P: Secretory activity and the myoepithelial cells of salivary glands after duct ligation in cats. *Arch Oral Biol* 19:275–283, 1974.
24. Harvey CE: Parotid salivary duct rupture and fistula in the dog and cat. *J Small Anim Pract* 18:163–168, 1977.
25. Hurov L: Surgical correction of blocked parotid duct. *Can Vet J* 2:348–349, 1961.
26. Knecht CD, Slusher R, Guibor EC: Zygomatic salivary cyst in a dog. *J Am Vet Med Assoc* 155:625–626, 1969.
27. Schmidt GM, Betts CW: Zygomatic salivary mucoceles in the dog. *J Am Vet Med Assoc* 172:940–942, 1978.
28. Martin CL: Orbital salivary mucocele in a dog. *Vet Med Small Anim Clin* 66:36–38, 1971.
29. Buyukmihci N, Rubin LF, Harvey CE: Exophthalmos secondary to zygomatic adenocarcinoma in the dog. *J Am Vet Med Assoc* 167:152–155, 1975.
30. DeYoung DW, Kealy JK, Kluge JP: Attempts to produce salivary cysts in the dog. *Am J Vet Res* 39:185–186, 1978.
31. Hulland TJ, Archibald J: Salivary mucoceles in dogs. *Can Vet J* 5:109–117, 1964.
32. Beaumont PB: Atypical cervical sialocele in a dog. *Canine Pract* 7:56–58, 1980.
33. Harvey CE: Letter to the editor. *J Am Vet Med Assoc* 158:1454, 1971.
34. Knecht CD, Phares J: Characterization of dogs with salivary cyst. *J Am Vet Med Assoc* 158:612, 1971.
35. Spreull JSA, Head KW: Cervical salivary cysts in the dog. *J Small Anim Pract* 8:17–35, 1967.
36. Harvey CE: Canine salivary mucocele. *J Am Anim Hosp Assoc* 5:155–165, 1969.
37. Glen JB: Salivary cysts in the dog: identification of sublingual duct defects by sialography. *Vet Rec* 78:488–492, 1966.
38. Harvey HJ: Pharyngeal mucoceles in dogs. *J Am Vet Med Assoc* 178:1282–1283, 1981.
39. Battershell D: What is your diagnosis? *J Am Vet Med Assoc* 158:256–258, 1971.
40. Durtnell RE: Salivary mucocele in the dog. *Vet Rec* 101:273, 1977.
41. Harrison JD, Garrett JR: Ultrastructural and histochemical study of a naturally occurring salivary mucocele in a cat. *J Comp Pathol* 85:411–416, 1975.
42. Pantel M, Wissdorf H: Anatomische und klinische Aspekte zur Ranula bei einer Katze. *Kleinter Prax* 277–280, 1976.
43. Wallace LJ, Guffy MM, Gray AP, Clifford JH: Anterior cervical sialocele (salivary cyst) in a domestic cat. *J Am Anim Hosp Assoc* 8:74–78, 1972.
44. Harrison JD, Garrett JR: Experimental salivary mucoceles in the cat: a histochemical study. *J Oral Pathol* 4:297–306, 1975.
45. Preibisch J: Kamienie slinowe u psa. *Med Wet* 16:277–279, 1960.
46. Bennett D: Canine salivary mucoceles. *J Small Anim Pract* 13:669–670, 1972.
47. Prescott CW: Ranula in the dog—a surgical treatment. *Aust Vet J* 44:382–383, 1968.
48. Denis D: Kistes salivaires et des kistes branchiaux chez le chien. Thesis. Alfort, 1973.
49. Teague HD: Surgical correction of a large sialocele in a dog. *Canine Pract* 6:11–14, 1979.
50. Hoffer RE: Surgical treatment of salivary mucocele. *Vet Clin North Am* 5:333–341, 1975.
51. Kealy JK: Salivary cyst in the dog. *Vet Rec* 76:119–120, 1964.
52. Chastain CB: What is your diagnosis? *J Am Vet Med Assoc* 164:415–416, 1974.
53. Mulkey OC, Knecht CD: Parotid salivary gland cyst and calculus in a dog. *J Am Vet Med Assoc* 159:1774, 1971.
54. Bell DA: Grass seed in the parotid duct of a dog. *Vet Rec* 102:340, 1978.
55. Koestner A, Buerger L: Primary neoplasms of the salivary glands in animals compared to similar tumors in man. *Vet Pathol* 2:201–226, 1965.
56. Head KW: Tumors of the upper alimentary tract. *Bull World Health Org* 53:3427, 1976.
57. Karbe E, Schiefer B: Primary salivary gland tumors in carnivores. *Can Vet J* 8:212–215, 1967.
58. Bright JM, Bright RM, Mays MC: Parotid carcinoma with multiple endocrinopathies in a dog. *Compend Cont Ed Pract Vet* 5:728–734, 1983.
59. Case MT, Simon J: Oncocytomas in a dog and a cat. *Vet Med Small Anim Clin* 61:41–43, 1966.
60. Evans SM, Thrall DE: Postoperative orthovoltage radiation therapy of parotid salivary gland adenocarcinoma in three dogs. *J Am Vet Med Assoc* 182:993–994, 1983.
61. Knecht CD: Treatment of diseases of the zygomatic salivary gland. *J Am Anim Hosp Assoc* 6:13–19, 1970.

Section Two

Oral Diseases of the Horse

Chapter Thirteen

Oral Anatomy of the Horse

GJ Baker

The study of the cheek teeth in the horse is a well-documented feature of horse evolution.[1-3] The teeth of the modern horse (*Equus caballus*) have evolved into the structure and form that they now have as a result of the change from a browsing habitat to a grazing habitat. The Eocene ancestor of the family Equidae (*Hyracotherium* or *Eohippus*) was a small (65-cm) three-toed animal with low-crowned (brachydont) cheek teeth and an arcade made up of four premolar and three molar teeth. All the teeth had simple crown patterns, and chewing depended mainly on the three molar teeth. Subsequent changes in the environment during the later Miocene period brought about a rapid evolution of the tooth, resulting from the survival of favorable mutations. These changes included a modification of the crown pattern, an increase in the height of the crown, and the development of crown cementum. What had been two open valleys on the teeth now became deep closed pits, and numerous wrinkles and spurs appeared on the sides of the main crest. These changes were similar in both jaws, but they were less extreme in the lower teeth.

The process by which the premolar teeth became anatomically similar to the molar teeth has been described as molarization. The formation of the high-crowned cheek teeth of *Merychippus* in the late Miocene period was accompanied by the development of cementum. This cementum appeared on the outside of the enamel crown and developed to fill all its valleys, thereby protecting the brittle enamel. In this way a permanently erupting cheek tooth was formed, with a crown having a height at least twice its width. The rate of eruption of such a tooth was equal to that of the crown's rate of wear by attrition.

DENTAL FORMULA OF EQUUS CABALLUS

Deciduous: $i\frac{3}{3}$, $c\frac{0}{0}$, $p\frac{3}{3} \times 2 = 24$
Permanent:
$I\frac{3}{3}$, $C\frac{1}{1}$, $P\frac{3}{3}$ or $P\frac{4}{3}$, $M\frac{3}{3} \times 2 = 40$ or 42

Eruption Times[4]

A. Deciduous. First incisor: birth or first week of life. Second incisor: fourth to sixth weeks of life. Third incisor: 6 to 9 months of age. First and second premolar, third premolar: birth to first 2 weeks of life.
B. Permanent. First incisor: 2½ years of age. Second incisor: 3½ years of age. Third incisor: 4½ years of age. Canine: 4 to 5 years of age. First premolar (wolf tooth): 5 to 6 months of age. Second

premolar: 2½ years of age. Third premolar: 3 years of age. Fourth premolar: 4 years of age. First molar: 10 to 12 months of age. Second molar: 2 years of age. Third molar: 3½ to 4 years of age.

A number of standard variations in the dental formula are recognized. The canine teeth are absent or rudimentary in the mare, thus reducing the total number of teeth found in mares by four. It is usual to include the vestigial first premolar in the upper jaw in the dental formula, but it can also be found in the lower jaw, thus increasing the total number of teeth here by two. In a study of Thoroughbred fetuses and neonates, the first premolar was found in the upper jaw in 20 percent of those studied. Figures are not available for other horse types.[5]

GROSS MORPHOLOGICAL CHARACTERISTICS
(Figs. 13–1 and 13–2)

Incisor Teeth

There are six teeth in each jaw, and they are placed close together so that their labial edges almost form a semicircle. The occlusal surface has a deep enamel invagination, the infundibulum, which is only partially filled with cementum. As the teeth are worn, a characteristic pattern forms in which the infundibulum is surrounded by rings of enamel, dentin, enamel, and crown cementum in a concentric pattern. Each incisor tooth tapers evenly from a broad crown to a narrow root so that as the midportion of the incisor is exposed with wear, the two cross section diameters are about equal. Observations of the state of eruption, the table pattern and shape, and the angle of incidence are used as guides for aging horses. With age, the infundibulum becomes smaller, approaches the lingual border, and finally disappears. It persists for a longer period in the upper incisors than in the lower ones because of its greater depth in this location. The rate of its disappearance should not be relied upon too closely when aging horses. As the size of the infundibulum diminishes, a mark appears on the labial aspect of the table of the incisor tooth. This mark represents the arch of secondary dentin that is formed to protect the pulp cavity from exposure by attrition of the crown. The average length of the crown of an incisor tooth in a 6 year old Thoroughbred is 7 cm.

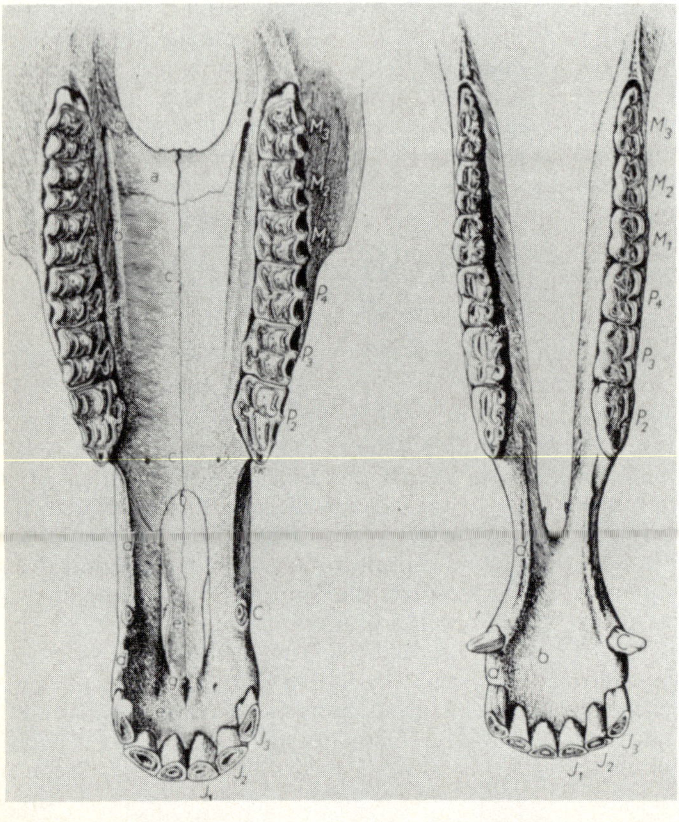

Figure 13–1. Upper and lower arcades of 7 year old Thoroughbred gelding. P2 = second premolar tooth. (From Schummer A, Nickel R, Sack WO: Viscera of the Domestic Mammals. Berlin, Paul Parey, 1979.)

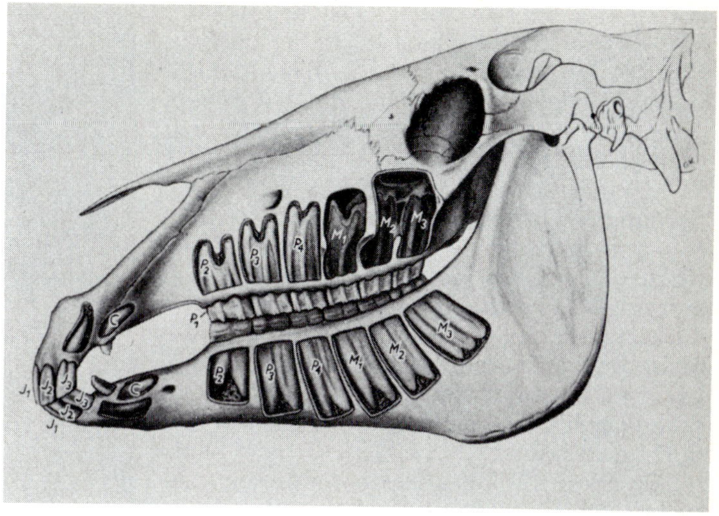

Figure 13–2. Sculpted skull to show reserve crowns and root structures. (From Schummer A, Nickel R, Sack WO: Viscera of the Domestic Mammals. Berlin, Paul Parey, 1979.)

The deciduous teeth are smaller than are permanent incisors, and they have a distinct neck at the junction of the root and crown when viewed from the front. The crown is shell-shaped rather than rectangular, and the infundibulum is shallow.

Canine Teeth

The canine teeth are simple (i.e., without complex crown and cementum) and curved. The crown is compressed and is smooth on its labial aspect, but it carries two ridges on its lingual aspect. The upper canine is situated at the junction of the premaxilla (incisive bone) and maxilla, whereas the lower canine is nearer the corner incisor. No occlusal contact is made between the upper and lower canine teeth.

Cheek Teeth

It is common in veterinary work to call all the cheek teeth of the horse molar teeth, since the premolars (with the exception of the wolf [1 PM] tooth) do not differ materially from true molars in size or form. In this chapter, the term "cheek teeth" will be used to include both premolars and molars and they will be numbered 1 through 6 (i.e., cheek tooth 1 = PM 2 and cheek tooth 4 = M1).

The constant number of cheek teeth is 24, composing four dental arcades with six teeth in each arcade. In addition, the persistent wolf teeth are commonly found in the upper jaw. At their maximum development, the crowns of these teeth are small and irregularly conical, giving some indication of the enamel folding that is so characteristic of the other cheek teeth in the horse. When less developed, these crowns are generally small and simple cones. It is this latter pattern that is seen with the greatest frequency (Fig. 13–3).

Upper Cheek Teeth. Each tooth, with the exception of the first one, has the shape of a slightly bent four-sided prism. The first tooth is three-sided because its rostral border does

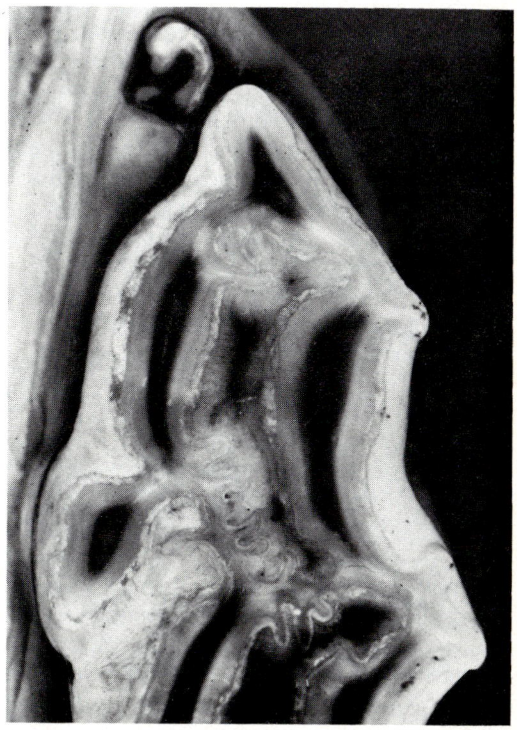

Figure 13–3. Occlusal surface of wolf tooth (PM1) and first cheek tooth (PM2). (From Mansmann RA, McCallister ES: Equine Medicine and Surgery, 3rd ed, Santa Barbara, American Veterinary Publications Inc, 1982.)

not contact another tooth. The first tooth also differs in the character of its buccal surfaces. In the second to the sixth teeth, this surface carries a longitudinal rounded ridge (cingulum) that separates two grooves. However, in the first tooth there are two such ridges, the rostral one being somewhat less prominent. The lingual surface of each tooth crown is marked by a longitudinal ridge whose position corresponds to the groove and ridge of the chewing surface. The occlusal surface is not positioned at right angles to the longitudinal vertical plane of the tooth, but is set somewhat obliquely, the labial side of the maxillary cheek tooth being taller than the lingual side.

The unworn upper cheek tooth presents a surface on which there are two undulating and narrow ridges (styles), one of which is lateral, whereas the other is medial. On the rostral and lingual side of the medial style there is an extra hillock. The central portion of the surface is indented by two depressions that are comparable to, but much deeper than, the infundibulum of the incisor teeth. When the teeth have been subjected to wear, the enamel that clothes the ridges is worn through and the underlying dentin appears on the surface. The result is that after a time, the chewing surface displays a complicated pattern that may be likened to the outline of an ornate letter B, the upright stroke of the B being on the lingual aspect. Dentin supports the enamel internally, cementum supports the enamel lakes, and the peripheral cementum fills in the spaces between the teeth so that all six teeth function as a single unit, that is, the dental arcade (Fig. 13–4). Each tooth is crossed by transverse ridges so that the whole maxillary arcade seems to consist of a serrated edge. The serrations are formed so that a valley is present at the area of contact with adjacent teeth.

The true roots of the cheek teeth are short when compared with the total length of the teeth. There are three roots, two small lateral roots and one large medial root. If the term "crown" is held to include all that part of the tooth on which enamel is present, the teeth of the horse must be described as having a considerable amount of crown buried beneath the gum. It is customary to refer to this portion of the crown as the reserve crown and to confine the term "root" to that area of the tooth that is comparatively short and enamel free. As the tooth wears away, the reserve crown is gradually exposed, and the roots lengthen.

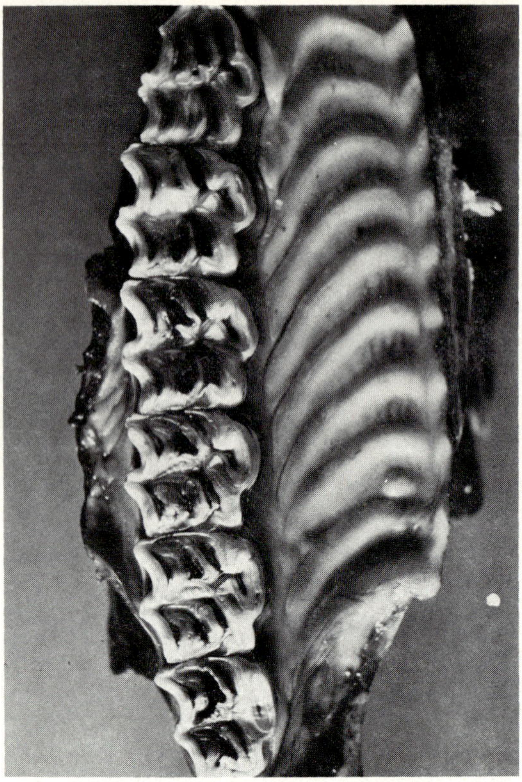

Figure 13–4. Right upper arcade.

The exposed crowns are in close contact, forming a slightly curved continuous row with the convexity on the buccal aspect. The embedded crowns vary in length and lie at a slight angle to each other so that emerging crowns fit close together to form a compact arcade mass. In the adult horse, the first upper cheek tooth is directed upward and slightly forward and is 6.8 cm long. The second upper cheek tooth is vertical and is 8.3 cm long. The third and subsequent upper cheek teeth incline backward to an increasing degree and are 9 cm, 7.8 cm, 8.7 cm, and 7.6 cm long, respectively. The tooth measurements given are an average of the root apex to crown measurements taken from the rostral and caudal roots in adult Thoroughbred horses. The embedded portions of the third to sixth cheek teeth occupy part of the paranasal maxillary sinuses (see Fig. 13–2). In younger horses, the position of the teeth in relation to the sinuses changes because of the extent of the reserve crown and the caudorostral angle of the erupting teeth. This effectively reduces the size of the rostral maxillary sinus.

Growth changes can be illustrated by considering the position of a perpendicular line drawn from the front of the orbit. In a 180 day old fetus this line bisects the molar arcade between the last two deciduous cheek teeth. At birth it is caudal to the third cheek tooth. At 2 years it is caudal to the fifth cheek tooth. Subsequent to this, the teeth move rostrally in the mouth so that at 19 years of age, this line crosses the arcade caudal to the last cheek tooth.

Lower Cheek Teeth. These teeth are generally as long as the upper teeth, but their transverse measurement is much less; consequently, they have an oblong instead of an approximately square occlusal surface. There is a longitudinal groove on the labial aspect of the first five teeth. The sixth tooth has two longitudinal grooves on its labial aspect. The lingual aspect is irregularly grooved longitudinally. The exposed part of the crown is taller on the inner, or lingual, side, resulting in a chewing surface that is oblique to the longitudinal plane of the mouth, as is also true for the upper teeth. The pattern assumed by the worn occlusal surface on the lower teeth is simpler than that of the upper teeth (Figs. 13–5 and 13–6). Although there are two infundibula, they are not closed on the lingual side until cementum has been extensively developed. Consequently, in the worn tooth the enamel fold lingual to each infundibulum is incomplete. The occlusal surface is serrated in a manner that presents a mirror image of the serrations of the upper arcade. Each of the lower cheek teeth has two relatively short roots, with the exception of the last tooth, which usually has three roots.

Each lower dental arcade is straighter than its upper partner. In general, the lower arcades are 30 percent narrower than the upper arcades (anisognathism), so the lingual margins of the lower cheek teeth lie medial to the lingual aspect of the upper cheek teeth (see Fig. 13–1). Therefore, the horse is equipped with an efficient dental apparatus for grazing and grinding food. The hypsodont and reserve crown nature of its cheek teeth ensures that the arcades are maintained throughout life. The deposition of crown cementum and the close apposition of individual teeth in each arcade give a grinding surface that presents essentially one complex occlusal surface.

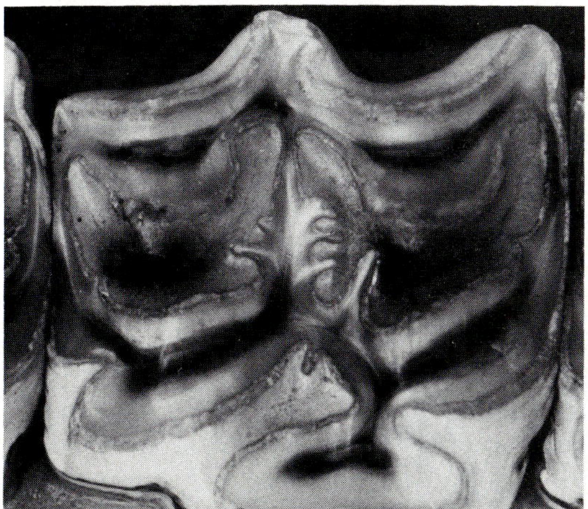

Figure 13–5. Fourth upper cheek tooth. Occlusal surface. (From Baker GJ: Dental disorders in the horse. *Compend Contin Educ Pract Vet* 4:S507–515, 1982.)

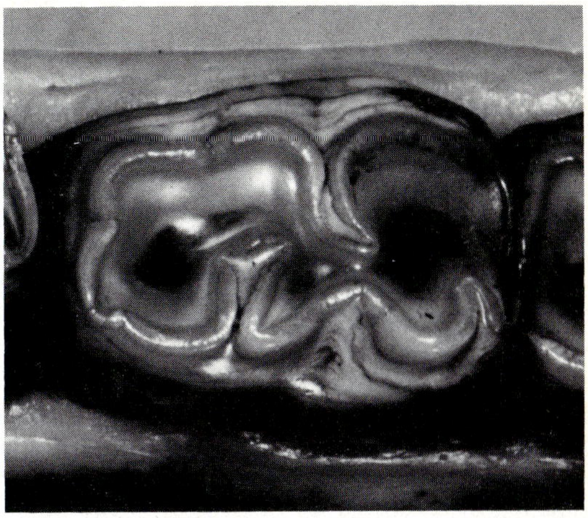

Figure 13–6. Fourth lower cheek tooth. Occlusal surface.

DENTAL HISTOLOGICAL CHARACTERISTICS

Dentin

Dentin is the major component of the tooth. It consists of 72 percent inorganic material and 28 percent organic material. It is harder than compact bone, and in section it is seen to be formed of a mass of fine canals or tubules—the dentinal tubules. Dentin formation is cyclical so that growth lines (Owen's lines) can be seen in sections of a fully developed tooth. Each tubule may be up to 4 μ in diameter, with the tubules of greater diameter forming peripheral rings that conform to the intricate shape of the tooth within the peripheral enamel. In the peripheral layers of dentin, the tubules may branch or fuse together. There are no nerve fibers or blood vessels in the dentin. Sensations of touch, cold, and pH changes are conducted by Tome's dentinal fibers. Odontoblasts covering the pulp cavity remain viable throughout life and respond to irritation (e.g., attrition of the crown) by producing layers of secondary dentin. In this manner, the pulp is protected from exposure.

Enamel

The enamel pattern of the horse's tooth and its unique gross structure have been described. Its chemical composition is predominantly inorganic, 90 percent of which is calcium phosphate. Enamel consists of myriad uniformly wide crystals of hydroxyapatite packed into an organic matrix. A repetitive pattern of change in the orientation of its constituent elements is responsible for its division into so-called prisms and interprismatic areas. The crystals of hydroxyapatite are formed as an extracellular secretion from the ameloblast cell layer. Each prism of enamel formed is perpendicular to the surface of the dentin. Confirmation of the pattern of crystallite orientation resulted from scanning electron microscopy of the developing teeth. Enamel formation is completed prior to the eruption of the tooth, and at this stage the enamel anlage has a series of integuments. These integuments are lost after eruption. As the tooth remnants and integuments of embryological origin are worn away in the horse, the enamel acquires secondary cuticles, as happens in other species. In animals with brachydont teeth, these cuticles are formed from salivary mucins to which bacterial plaque, food debris, and calculus become attached. In animals with hypsodont teeth, the major structure surrounding the exposed enamel is peripheral crown cementum.

Cementum

Cementum is very similar to bone in chemical composition, being two-thirds inorganic and one-third organic material. Its microscopic structure is also similar to compact bone, having an intracellular matrix, or ground substance, canaliculi, and cell lacunae that contain cementocytes that are structured to resemble a haversian system. The matrix is eosinophilic in nature. The peripheral cementum is formed continuously from modified odontoblasts (cementoblasts) within the alveolar periodontal membrane. This cementum is nourished by blood vessels and lymphatics within the periodontal membrane. As the tooth erupts, carrying the peripheral cementum with it, nutrition to the peripheral crown cementum is lost and compact cementum is acellular. The cementum within the enamel invagination of the upper cheek teeth is also deprived of its blood supply at eruption and cannot receive material from the pulp or dentin because of the impervious, avascular nature of the formed enamel and dentin. Sections of this cementum, therefore, show empty cell lacunae and canaliculi that can become packed with cellular material from the animal's feed, particularly along the infundibulum (Fig. 13–7).

Tooth Attachment

Each tooth is independently and firmly attached to the alveolar process of the mandible or maxilla within an alveolus that is formed from the connective tissue of the dental sac and the surrounding bone of the jaw. The teeth are suspended and attached by bundles of connective tissue fibers making

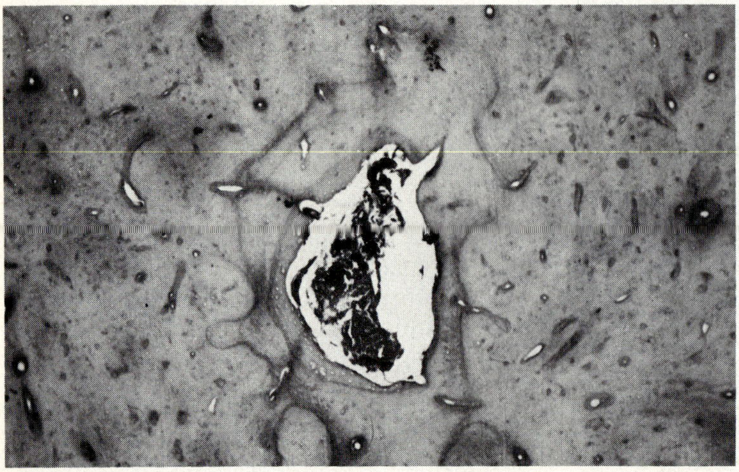

Figure 13–7. Upper tooth lake cementum. Acellular cementum and debris filled infundibulum (decalcified hematoxylin-eosin, magnification × 35).

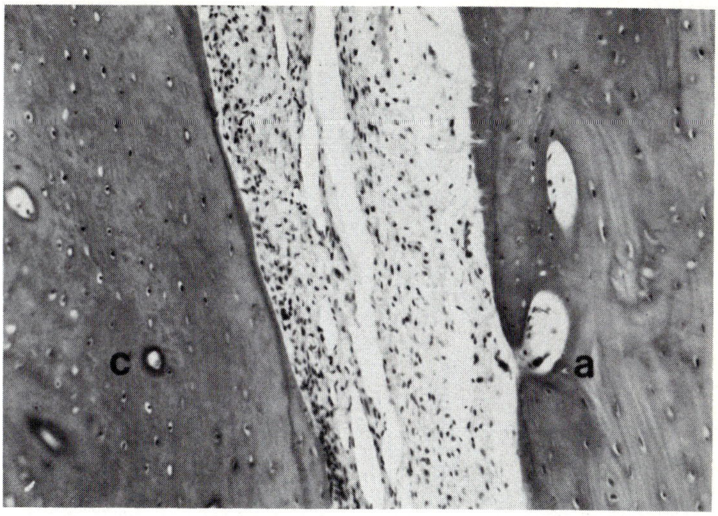

Figure 13–8. Vertical section of periodontal ligament. c = cementum; a = alveolar bone (decalcified hematoxylin-eosin, magnification × 110).

up the periodontal ligament. The arrangement of fibers in this periodontal ligament is complex, and dense bundles of collagen run in various directions from the bone of the socket wall to the cementum covering the roots and reserve crowns. The embedded portions of these fibers are called Sharpey's fibers. The periodontal ligament contains blood vessels and nerves; the collagen bundles are arranged so that these vessels and the pulp vessels are protected from ischemia that may result from occlusal pressure. In this way the tooth is suspended firmly within the bone, and at the same time it is permitted some slight movement within its own alveolus (Fig. 13–8).

Because of the relative sizes of the teeth, there is only a thin plate of bone covering the lateral aspects of the roots and reserved crowns. This thin covering is subject to erosion and lysis during eruption of the permanent teeth, and it may appear as porous areas of thin bone in skulls of young horses.

The mucous membranes of the mouth cover the alveolar processes externally. The gums are composed of dense, fibrous tissue intimately connected with the periosteum. The gums are covered by a smooth, stratified squamous cell epithelium and have few glands. In addition, they are relatively insensitive and do not bleed easily. A free margin of gum extends from the epithelial attachment of the gum to the crown of the tooth and encloses the gingival crevice. This crevice is continuous between adjacent teeth of the arcade, but it is reduced by the intimate contact of teeth at the interdental areas. These arrangements are modified during eruption of the teeth. It is assumed that in the continually erupting teeth of the horse, movement of the reserve crown is accommodated by a rearrangement of collagen bundles within the periodontal ligament and the formation of new attachments between root cementum and the alveolar margin.

An efficient food grinding apparatus that is adapted to a life of almost continuous grazing has evolved in the horse. The lips are prehensile, and the horse is selective in grazing. The incisor teeth form an efficient cutting apparatus, and the arrangement of the cheek teeth into a single functional arcade in each jaw results in an elegant food processing apparatus. The rate of increase in food intake may be determined by cubing the rate of increase in body size; thus a doubling of height requires eight times the food intake. Evolutionary changes in the cheek teeth accommodated such an increase in food uptake during the development from *Eohippus* to *Equus caballus.*

Continuous grazing and mastication result in dental attrition from wear; the development of hypsodont teeth, with the continuous eruption of reserve crowns, maintains the functional integrity of each arcade. Peripheral crown cementum is important in forming a supporting structure to maintain the integrity of each arcade.

Effective mastication in the horse has also been enhanced by the structure and function of the temporomandibular joint and the size of the masticatory muscles. Although the horse follows the general herbivore adaptation pattern, there is limited side-to-side movement when compared with ruminant herbivores. The multilayered masseter muscle and the medial pterygoid muscle form

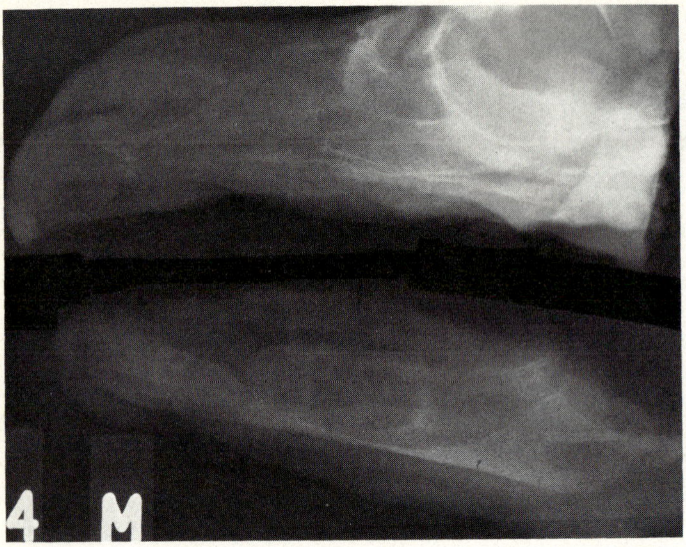

Figure 13–9. Radiograph of 120 day Thoroughbred fetal maxilla and mandible showing developing tooth buds.

the main masticatory muscle mass. The temporal muscle is relatively weak.

The mandibular articular condyle has a thick meniscus. Its dorsal position, above the occlusal plane of the cheek teeth, gives great mechanical advantage to the masseter and medial pterygoid muscle action. The articular condyle fits a flat facet on the temporal bone.

DEVELOPMENTAL ANATOMY

Examination of fetal mandibles and maxillas shows that the dental lamella is enveloped by the gums; three distinct cyst-like structures are visible in a 120 day fetus (Fig. 13–9). The relative sizes indicate that the bud of the second premolar tooth leads the development sequence. A cupped enamel organ overlies the dental papilla within each tooth bud (Figs. 13–10 and 13–11). The folding of the maxillary and mandibular enamel organs of the horse was first studied by Kupfer in 1937;[6] his fundamental pioneer studies are

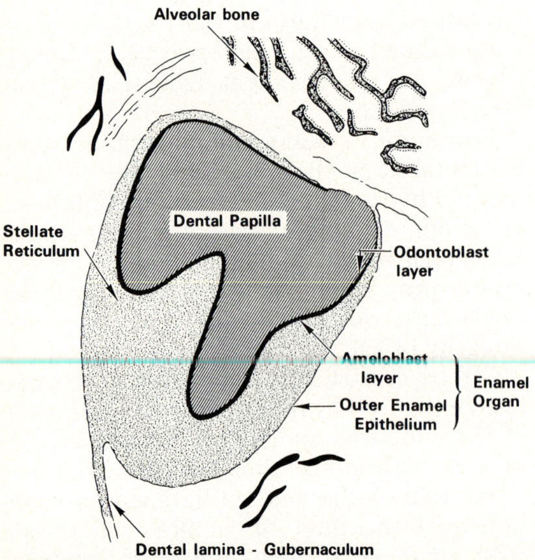

Figure 13–10. Diagram of developing equine cheek tooth. (From Baker GJ: Dental disorders in the horse. *Compend Contin Educ Pract Vet* 4:S507–515, 1982.)

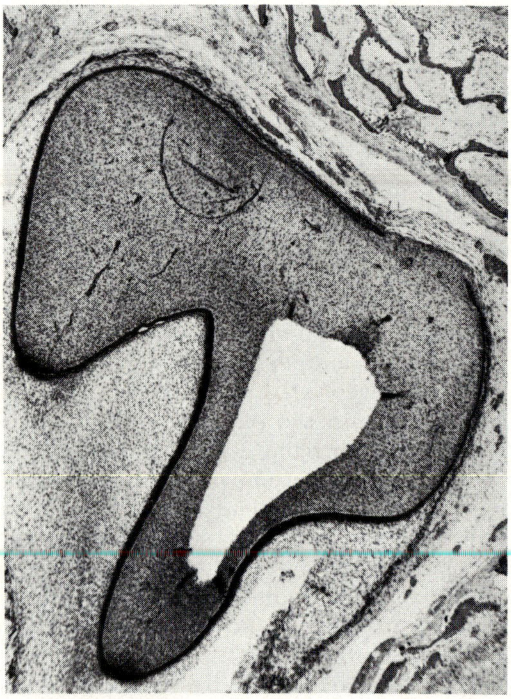

Figure 13–11. Cryostat section of upper tooth bud from 120 day Thoroughbred fetus (hematoxylin-eosin, magnification × 25). (From Baker GJ: Dental disorders in the horse. *Compend Contin Educ Pract Vet* 4:S507–515, 1982.)

recommended for further reading. The differences in development between the upper and lower teeth can be summarized by describing the enamel organ changes that take place during maturation. In principle, both upper and lower jaw enamel organs fold in the same manner. There are, however, important distinctions that lead to the morphological differences in the teeth of the upper and lower jaw (see Figs. 13–5 and 13–6). A double cup forms within the enamel organ, but the rate of growth is less on the lingual edges of the lower teeth, and consequently the cup becomes split by infolds on the lingual surface. As a result of invaginations on the buccal surface, double enamel folds are produced (Figs. 13–12 and 13–13). Odontogenesis and amelogenesis are seen as the maturation of individual ameloblasts into tall columnar cells with oval nuclei close to the basement membranes. At their interface with the inner enamel layer, the cells of the dental papilla develop into the odontoblast and secrete dentin tubules (Fig. 13–14). Each odontoblast has a long cell body extending through a terminal web into the odontoblast process within the dentin itself. Odontoblasts

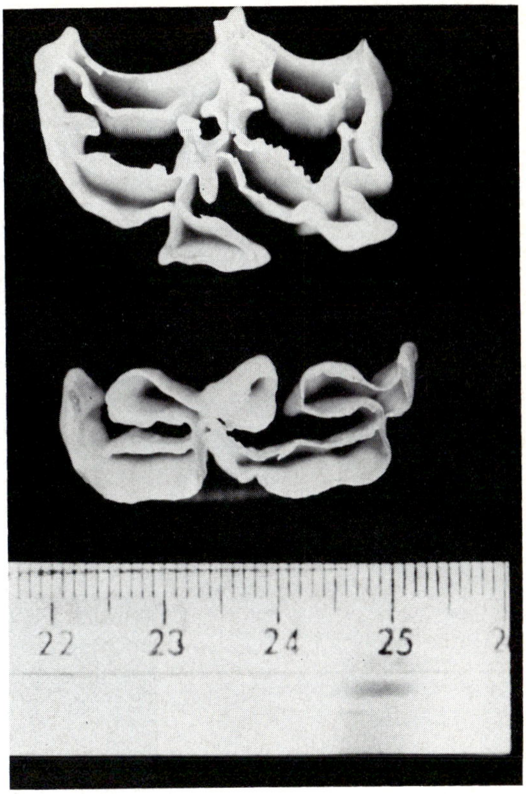

Figure 13–13. Horizontal sections of upper and lower tooth germs from fetus shown in Figure 13–12.

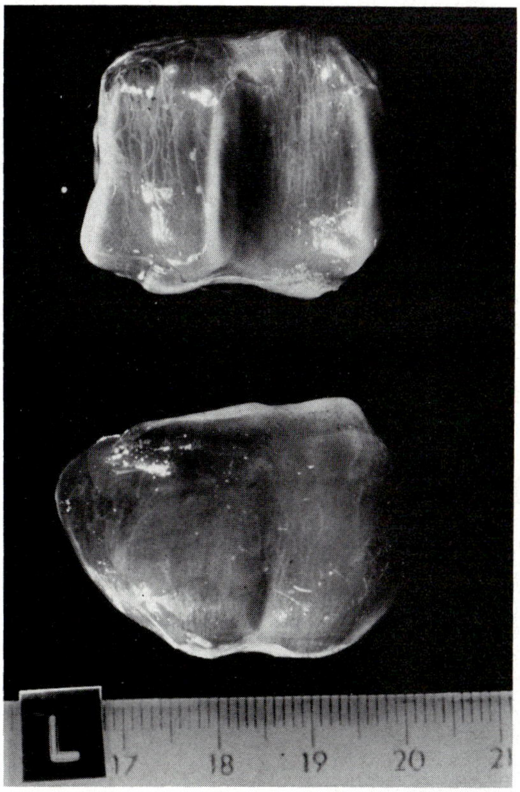

Figure 13–12. Lateral view of upper and lower tooth germs from 270 day Thoroughbred fetus.

may be separated from each other by clefts containing collagen fibers and later capillaries. Initially, odontoblasts are separated from the ameloblasts by the basement membrane only. The odontoblasts deposit a collagen-rich material, composing fibrils that become oriented perpendicular to the basement membrane. The dentin formed is produced as a matrix (predentin) and is calcified within 24 hours of its secretion. It is produced in layers; the cytoplasmic processes of the odontoblasts become trapped within the calcified matrix and canals known as dentinal tubules. As further layers of dentin are secreted, the odontoblasts are removed from their original position but maintain their contact with the basement membrane by elongation of the odontoblastic processes.[5]

The first thin layer of dentin that is produced is thought to be the stimulus for the ameloblasts to produce enamel. It forms a poorly calcified matrix that later becomes almost totally calcified. Enamel forms in rods that retain the shape of the cells, so they are therefore prismatic. The first radiographic signs of calcification within the tooth bud can

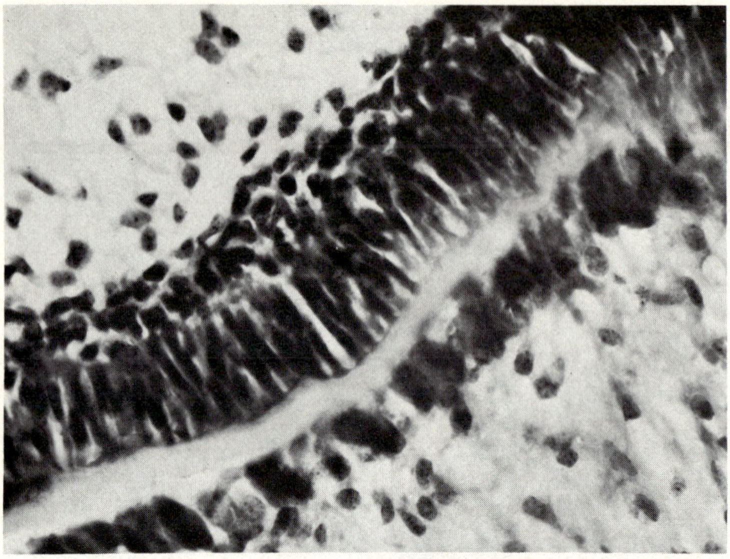

Figure 13–14. Predentin separating odontoblasts and ameloblast layers (hematoxylin-eosin, magnification × 950).

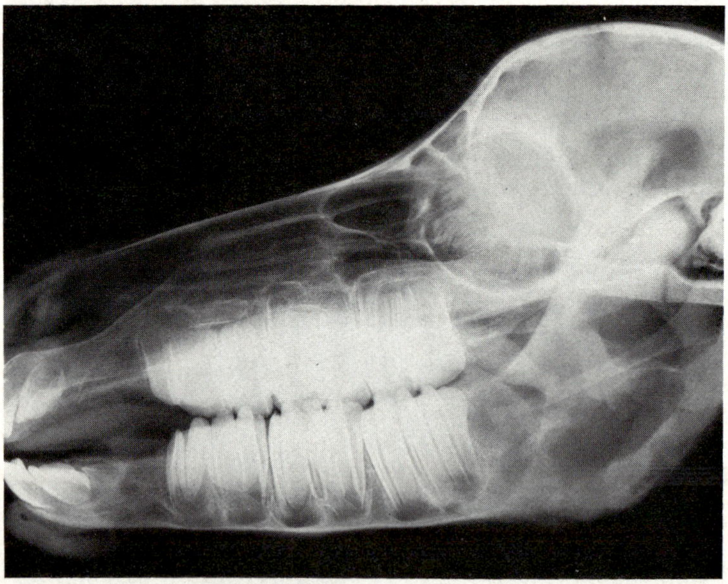

Figure 13–15. Radiograph of 3 week Thoroughbred, showing developing teeth.

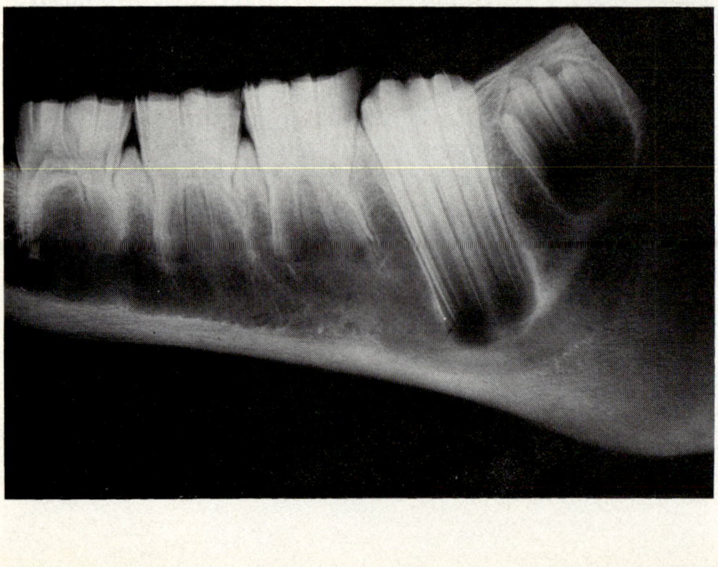

Figure 13–16. Radiograph of the mandible of 10 month Thoroughbred. Note maturation of M1 and development of M2 when compared with Figure 13–15.

be seen at 120 days, and it takes a total of 240 days for the complete enamel anlage to form.[7,8] The wave of formation and maturation of the permanent teeth tooth buds is first seen at 9½ months of fetal life. Calcification within the bud of the fourth cheek tooth (M1) is seen starting at 10 months of fetal age. The upper tooth bud precedes the lower tooth bud by up to 3 weeks. Subsequent enamel anlages form in sequence, each taking 360 days to develop from bud to eruption (Figs. 13–15 and 13–16).

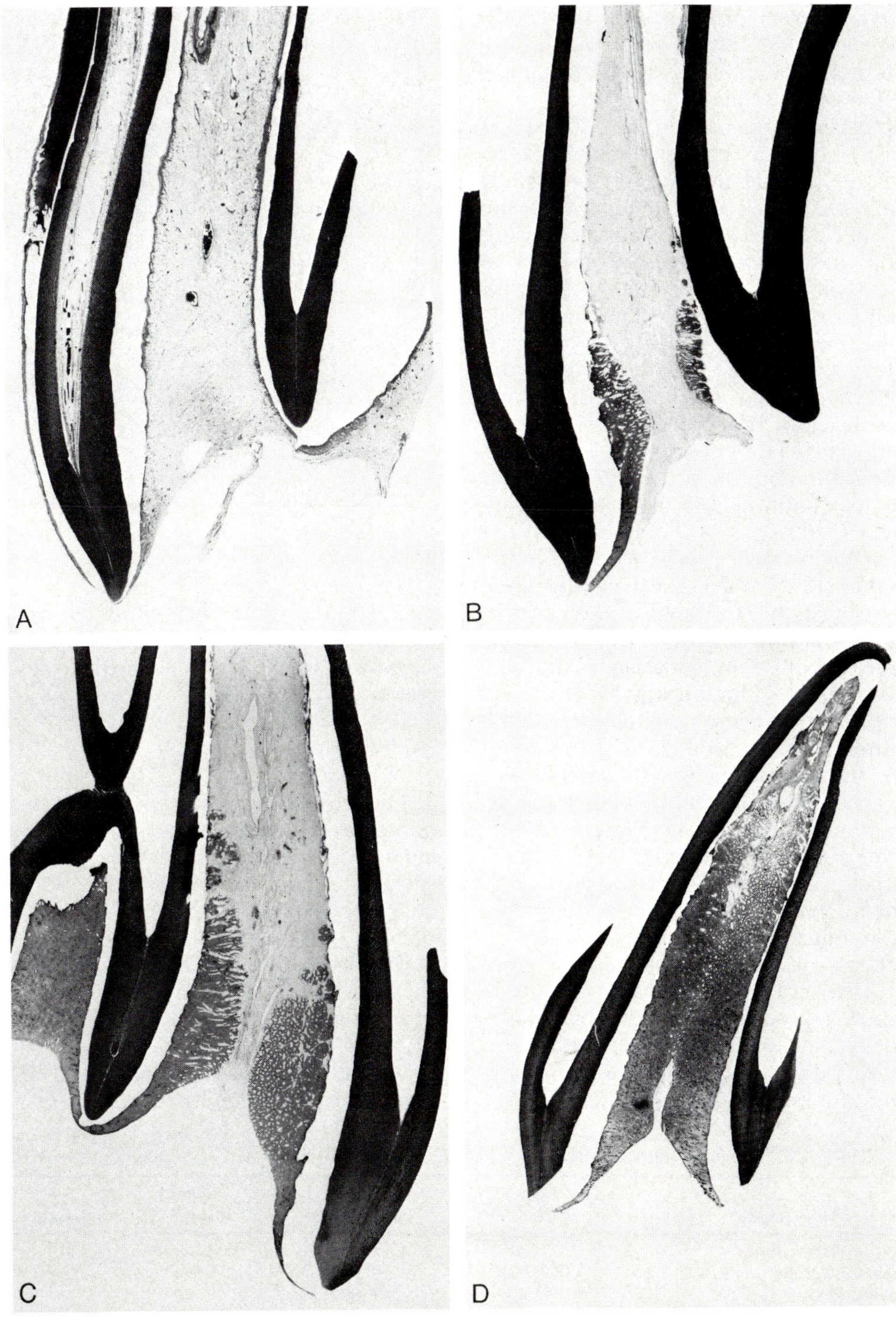

Figure 13–17. Cementogenesis in enamel lake. *A, A* 240 day fetus (magnification × 8.25). *B, A* 270 day fetus (magnification × 8.25). *C, A* 300 day fetus (magnification × 8.25). *D, A* 49 day neonate (magnification × 4.25).

The mesenchymal tissue that surrounds the developing tooth is continuous with that of the dental papilla, and it differentiates into connective tissue that makes up the dental sac. In the area of the future root, its inner cells differentiate into cementoblasts, and as the enamel epithelial sheath (outer enamel cell layer) disintegrates, these cells deposit root cementum. These changes can be seen in the deciduous cheek teeth starting at 280 days of fetal life.

At an earlier stage (starting at 210 days of fetal age), cellular changes can be seen around the occlusal margins of the central invaginations in the enamel anlage of the upper cheek teeth. Cementoblasts arising from the mesenchymal cells of the dental papilla break through the epithelial sheath and come to rest beneath the ameloblast layer. In this manner, a collar of cementoblasts forms within the enamel invagination. These cells are nourished from the dental sac that develops capillaries within the stratum reticulare. The gubernacular cord, and later the infundibulum, are the remnants of this vascular pathway into the enamel invagination. By 280 days (a 9-month fetus) the discrete cement collar can be seen within the anlage (Fig. 13–17 *A–D*). Subsequently, these areas expand to fill the depth of each enamel invagination with cementum. At first the cementum is sponge- or coral-like in appearance, but in the 7-day neonatal foal the occlusal collar is formed of mature dense cementum. In the central third of the invagination, the cementum retains its coral-like appearance, and at the apex of the enamel invagination it is hypoplastic; that is, eruption cementogenesis appears to be incomplete in most upper cheek teeth (Fig. 13–18).

Cementogenesis in the lower teeth is initiated by a similar differentiation of mesenchymal cells to form cementoblasts. They come to rest beneath the ameloblast layer so that cementum is produced to fill the buccal and lingual invaginations of the lower teeth. Starting at 210 days of fetal life, cementum is produced so that at eruption the occlusal, buccal, and lingual surfaces are covered with mature cementum. This process is mimicked as peripheral crown is formed around the teeth.

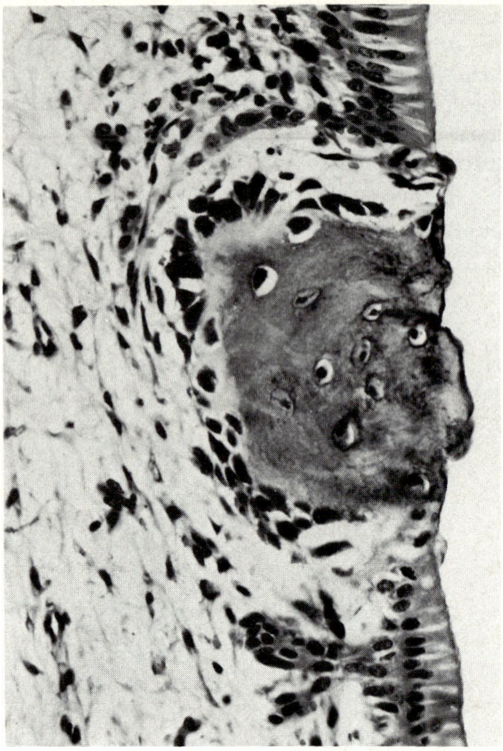

Figure 13–18. Cementoblast activity in the ameloblast layer.

AGING

The age of horses up to 8 years is determined by examining the state of eruption and the degree of attrition in the occlusal surfaces of the incisor teeth. An estimate of later age is gained by examining the incisor occlusal surface, its shape, and the changes in the incisor profile. Table 13–1 summarizes the changes that occur in the occlusal surfaces of the lower incisors in horses up to 15 years of age. Variations in the occlusal surface occur in horses with malocclusion, for example, in parrot-mouthed horses, in horses

Table 13–1. Changes in Occlusal Surfaces of the Mandibular Incisors as Guide to Aging in Horses

Stage	Central Incisor (1)	Lateral Incisor (2)	Corner Incisor (3)	Canine
Deciduous eruption	1 wk	1 mo	6 mo	
Permanent eruption	2½ yr	3½ yr	4½ yr	4½–5 yr
Loss of enamel cup	6 yr	7 yr	8 yr	
Dental star	8 yr	9 yr	10 yr	
Change from oval to triangular	11 yr	12 yr	14 yr	
Loss of enamel star	12 yr	12 yr	15 yr	

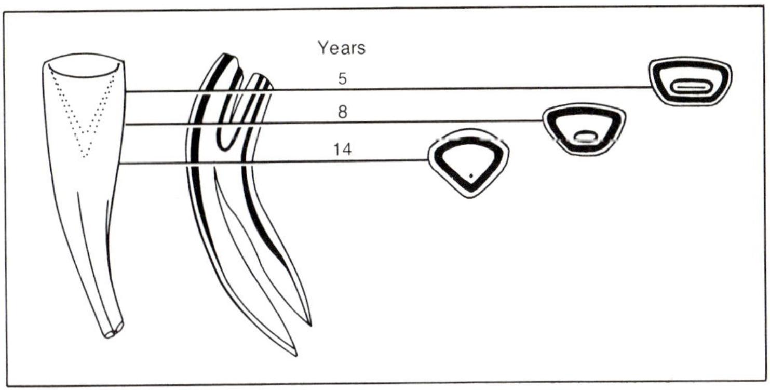

Figure 13–19. Diagram of incisor wear as guide to aging of the horse.

that habitually crib bite, or in horses having an abnormal diet, such as those who eat sand. Cementogenesis within the base of the enamel invagination ceases when the incisor erupts. Consequently, the depth of the enamel cup (infundibulum) within the invagination and its subsequent erosion depend on the rate of erosion and the amount of cementum that persists (Fig. 13–19).[9, 10]

In principle, the rate of tooth eruption in the horse follows that of the general mammalian pattern; the wave of eruption is from a rostral to a caudal position, with eruption of the deciduous cheek teeth preceding that of the molar cheek teeth (the fourth, fifth, and sixth cheek teeth) being succeeded by the eruption of the permanent premolars (the first, second, and third cheek teeth). The vascular forces associated with eruption consistently cause mandibular and maxillary swellings at this time. Such swellings and their radiographic appearance have been described and denoted as eruption cysts (Fig. 13–20). Impactions of the erupting permanent premolar dentition (the second and third cheek teeth) may be caused by adjacent teeth. Such impactions may lead to the development of apical osteitis and fistula formation. As the crowns are worn away, the cheek teeth continually erupt so that the dental arcades maintain functional occlusion. In this process, the reserve crown is reduced and the true roots are lengthened (Fig. 13–21 *A* and *B*). In extreme old age the teeth are finally lost. Under normal circumstances, dental attrition from wear occurs at a rate of 3 mm/year. Consequently, with an effective

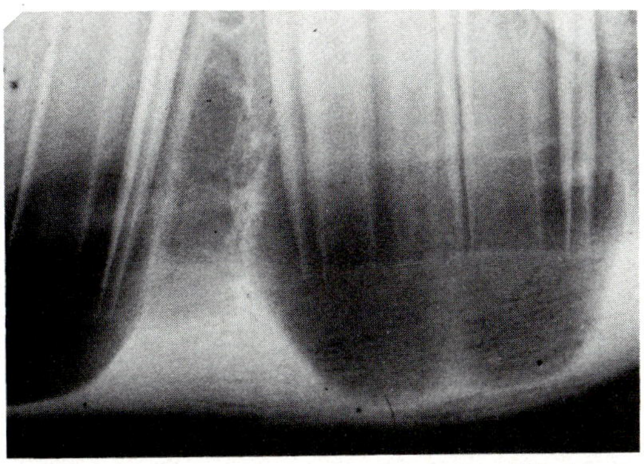

Figure 13–20. Radiograph of erupting third lower cheek tooth showing cystic distension of lamina dura (eruption cyst). (From Mansmann RA, McCallister ES: Equine Medicine and Surgery, 3rd ed. Santa Barbara, American Veterinary Publications, Inc., 1982.)

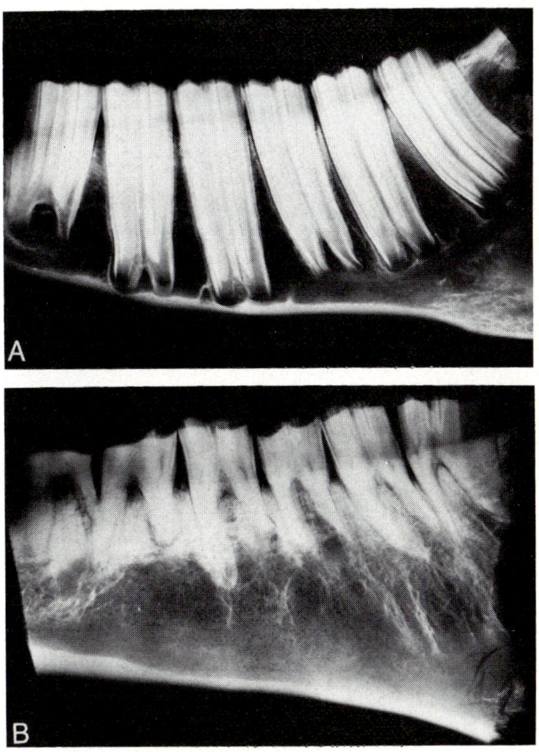

Figure 13–21. *A*, Radiograph of the mandible in a 4 year old Thoroughbred. *B*, Radiograph of the mandible in a 25 year old Thoroughbred. Note the increase in length of true roots and alveolar periostitis when compared with *A*. (From Mansmann RA, McCallister ES: Equine Medicine and Surgery, 3rd ed. Santa Barbara, American Veterinary Publications, Inc., 1982.)

tooth length of 80 mm to 90 mm and a deciduous arcade that lasts up to four years, it can be seen that after 30 to 34 years the domestic horse will be without teeth. Records show that with special diets, some horses may survive beyond this time. It has been suggested that the rate of attrition in donkeys may be less than that in horses, so that ages of up to 40 years may be reached.[5]

References

1. Clarke WH: Horses' Teeth. Oxford, Oxford University Press, 1880.
2. Simpson GG: Horses. Oxford, Oxford University Press, 1951.
3. Romer AS: The Vertebrate Story, 2nd ed. Chicago, University of Chicago Press, 1962.
4. Sisson S, Grossman JD: Anatomy of the Domestic Animals. WB Saunders, Philadelphia, 1910.
5. Baker GJ: A Study of Dental Disease in the Horse. PhD thesis. Glasgow, University of Glasgow, 1979.
6. Kupfer M: Tooth Structure in Donkeys and Horses. Jena, Gustav Fischer, 1937.
7. Baker GJ: Some aspects of equine dental disease. *Equine Vet J* 2:105–110, 1970.
8. Baker GJ: Some aspects of equine dental radiology. *Equine Vet J* 3:46–51, 1971.
9. Galvayne S: Horse Dentition: Showing How to Tell Exactly the Age of a Horse up to Thirty Years, 2nd ed. Glasgow, Thomas Murray, 1921.
10. American Association of Equine Practitioners: Official Guide for Determining the Age of the Horse. Golden, Colorado, 1966.

Chapter Fourteen

Oral Examination and Diagnosis: Management of Oral Diseases

GJ Baker

HISTORY AND CLINICAL SIGNS OF DENTAL DISEASE

A complete history should be taken, including an inquiry into the eating habits of the horse and the quality and quantity of the diet. The classic signs of dental disease in the horse include difficulty and slowness in feeding together with progressive unthriftiness and loss of body condition. In some instances, the horse may quid (drop poorly masticated food boluses from the mouth), and halitosis may be obvious. Additional problems reported by owners include biting and riding problems and head shaking or shyness. Facial or mandibular swelling and nasal discharge can result from dental disease associated with maxillary sinus empyema. Mandibular fistulae are frequently caused by lower cheek tooth apical infections (Figs. 14–1 and 14–2).

Although signs such as quidding are diffi-

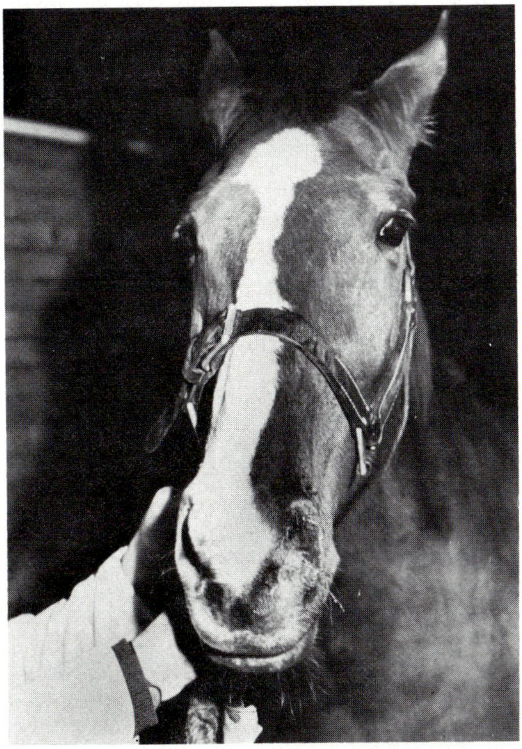

Figure 14–1. Nasal discharge in an 8 year old Thoroughbred mare. (From Baker GJ: Dental disorders in the horse. *Compend Contin Educ Pract Vet* 4:S507–515, 1982.)

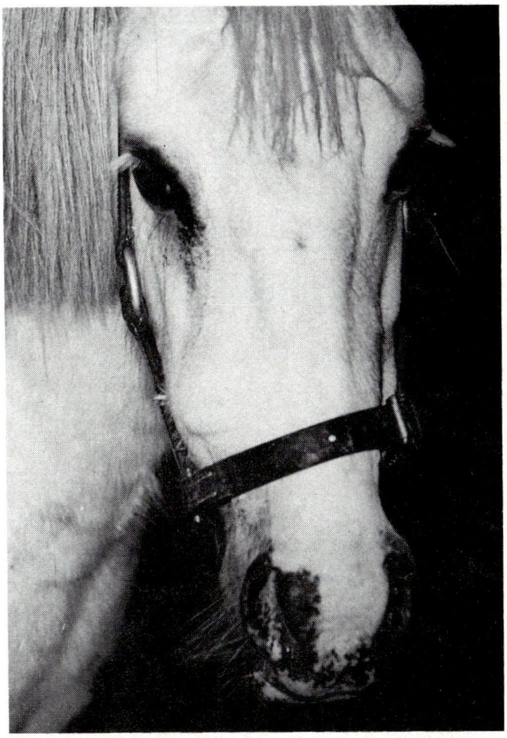

Figure 14–2. Apical infection of the upper third right cheek tooth. Note facial swelling and nasal discharge. (From Mansmann RA, McAllister ES: Equine Medicine and Surgery, 3rd ed. Santa Barbara, American Veterinary Publications Inc., 1982.)

cult to miss, owners often delay seeking veterinary attention. A horse with a chronic mandibular dental sinus may change ownership more than once and may be accompanied by a description that the horse "banged his chin in the trailer coming from the sale ring," emphasizing that dental sinuses or fistulae do not appear to inconvenience the horse to any great extent. Conversely, dental attention is commonly sought for young horses in early training or for horses that are thought to have sore mouths and do not accept the bit. The veterinarian should be aware that other factors may influence an apparently spectacular improvement following removal of a wolf tooth.[1]

DENTAL EXAMINATION

By correlating the history with the animal's age and the clinical signs, it is often possible to make a presumptive diagnosis (Table 14–1).

It is impossible to satisfactorily examine a nervous, frightened, or stubborn horse. Therefore, one must take every precaution not to increase the animal's natural suspicion and distrust of strangers. It is uncommon for horses to permit dental examinations without suitable preliminaries to convince them that the examiner means no harm. In some cases, an examination for painful disorders may be impossible without the aid of ataractics or anesthetics. When sedation is necessary, care should be taken to avoid the use of ataractics in entire horses because of the danger of priapism. Xylazine is an effective drug but has the disadvantage that the sedated horse lowers the head in a way that may inconvenience the examiner.

The examination should commence by an inspection of the incisors after the lips are rolled back so that the angle of bite and any external abnormalities can be noted. The deciduous incisors should be checked for looseness if evidence indicates they are about to be shed. The mouth is opened by reaching into the interdental space and withdrawing the tongue, or by applying apposing pressure on the upper and lower lips. The animal's age should be determined as previously indicated.

The buccal edges of the first three cheek teeth can be assessed for sharpness by external palpation. Examination of the cheek teeth without a speculum is not difficult when the technique is mastered. However, a speculum may be necessary under some circumstances. The operator is warned that the application of a heavy speculum may create a potentially lethal weapon with which the horse can hit the examiner. Two methods may be employed to examine the horse's cheek teeth. In one method, both hands are used, and in the other method only one hand is used (Figs. 14–3 and 14–4). Each method has advantages and disadvantages that should be carefully evaluated by the practitioner.

Table 14–1. Clinical Signs and Age in the Diagnosis of Dental Disease in the Horse

Age	Examination Sites	Necessary Dentistry
2–3 yr	1. First premolar vestige (wolf teeth)	1. Remove wolf teeth if present
	2. First deciduous premolar (upper and lower)	2. Remove deciduous teeth if ready; if not, file off corners and points of premolars
	3. Hard swelling on ventral surface of mandible beneath first premolar	3. Examine with x-ray; extract retained temporary premolar if present
	4. Cuts or abrasions on inside of cheek in region of the second premolars and molars	4. Lightly float or dress all molars and premolars if necessary
	5. Sharp protuberances on all premolars and molars	5. Rasp protuberances down to level of other teeth in the arcade
3–4 yr	1. 1, 2, 4, and 5 above	1. 1, 2, 4, and 5 above
	2. Second deciduous premolars (upper and lower)	2. Remove if present and ready
4–5 yr	1. 1, 4, and 5 above	1. 1, 4, and 5 above
	2. Third, deciduous premolar	2. Remove if present and ready
5 yr and older	1. 1, 4, and 5 above	1. 1, 4, and 5 above
	2. Uneven growth and "wavy" arcade	2. Straighten if interfering with mastication
	3. Unusually long molars and premolars	3. Unusually long molars and premolars may have to be cut if they cannot be filed down

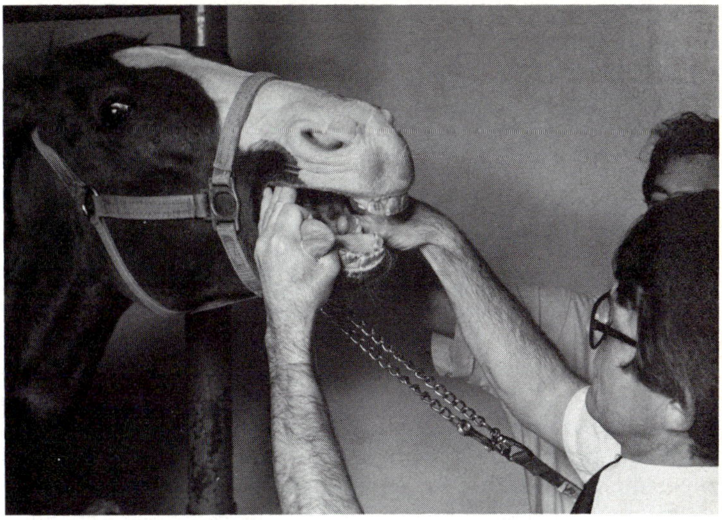

Figure 14–3. Dental examination. Two-handed technique.

In the two-handed method, the right side of the dental arcade is palpated by approaching the horse from the left-hand side. The left labial commissure is parted with the right hand, and the tongue is grasped and is pulled through the left interdental space. The cheek teeth of the right maxilla can then be examined by manipulating the right side of the lips with the left hand and by inserting the left hand into the horse's mouth. This process is then reversed to permit a similar inspection of the left arcades. A flashlight held by the clinician or by an assistant facilitates this examination. The examination must not be conducted in a leisurely fashion, because it annoys a horse to have its tongue clasped for long periods. If care is not taken, the tongue in males may be damaged by pressure from the canine teeth.

For experienced operators, the one-handed technique is recommended. The horse is approached from the front, and the right side of the mouth is palpated by inserting the right hand into the right interdental space with the palm facing laterad. The hand should be slightly flexed and the back of the hand should then be used to force the tongue between the left rows of the cheek teeth. This keeps the horse from completely closing the mouth and enables the examiner's fingers to run quickly along the arcades. The procedure is then repeated on the other side of the mouth using the left hand. As in the two-handed technique, it is best to carry out the procedure as quickly as possible. This method is not suitable for attempting to demonstrate specific lesions to owners or students.

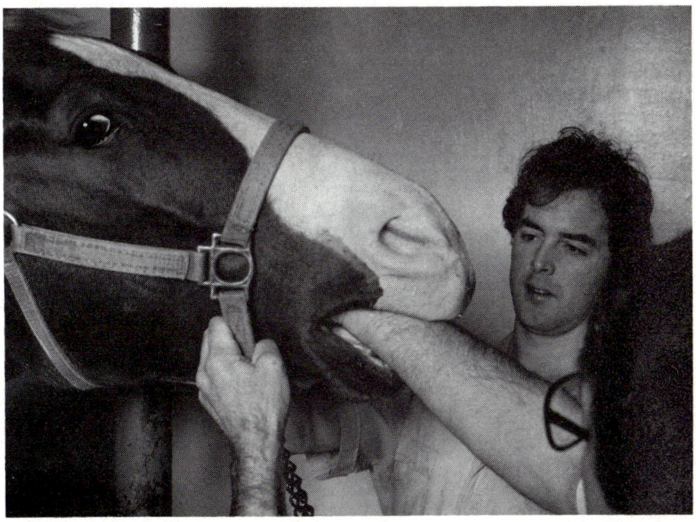

Figure 14–4. Dental examination. One-handed technique.

The cheek region around the labial commissure is readily palpated by placing the thumb in the commissure with the ball toward the buccal mucosa. Wolf teeth can be felt by inserting the thumb or forefinger into the interdental space and palpating the first upper and lower cheek teeth on both sides. At the same time that the arcades are examined for wolf teeth, the first cheek teeth should be palpated for protuberances and hooks; it is in this area that the bit draws the cheeks or tongue across the teeth, and sharp edges of the first premolars can cause painful lacerations.

In some cases, general anesthesia, oral lavage, and detailed arcade inspection (perhaps incorporating the use of endoscopic equipment) may be essential for a complete examination and an accurate diagnosis. Similarly, detailed inspections of gingival pockets and buccal ulcers, as well as probing infundibular pockets or mandibular fistulae with a dental pick, may be employed. General anesthesia is recommended for radiographic examination, thereby minimizing x-ray exposure to the attendant and lay personnel.

DENTAL RADIOGRAPHY IN THE HORSE

Satisfactory radiographs can be produced using standard veterinary equipment with exposures equivalent to 60 kvp to 70 kvp at 40 mas. Lateral and oblique films are taken using stationary grids, fast films, and screens. The mouth is held open with the anesthetized horse in lateral recumbency and the diseased side next to the cassette. In most cases, root and reserve crown detail rather than exposed crown detail are required. This can be achieved using a 30° to 45° oblique beam in a manner that projects the image of the normal arcade away from the diseased area.

Greater detail of individual upper and lower tooth roots can be obtained from intraoral dental films wedged 45° to the hard palate. The x-ray tube head needs to be angled correspondingly, with the affected side uppermost.[1–4]

EXAMINATION OF THE PARANASAL SINUSES

Fifty percent of paranasal sinus empyema cases in the horse are associated with dental disease.[5] A complete physical examination and a specific examination of the paranasal sinuses are indicated. The head is examined for the presence, color, and odor of any nasal discharge. It is more usual for the discharge to be unilateral, mucopurulent, and more copious after exercise. Hemorrhage and a bad odor may indicate conchal (turbinate) necrosis, dental infection, or neoplasia. Palpation may reveal heat, swelling, and pain. Percussion can confirm the presence of empyema, or a space-occupying granuloma or neoplasm by detecting areas of decreased or increased resonance when compared with the normal side. Endoscopic examination of the nasal chambers is used to detect the source of nasal discharge. The nasal drainage passages, conchae, auditory tube diverticula (guttural pouches), and pharyngeal tonsils should all be inspected. Erect lateral radiographs of the head using a horizontal beam should demonstrate paranasal sinus fluid lines in some cases or diffuse opacity when the sinus air spaces are obscured by exudate, granulation tissue, or new bone in other cases.

After applying a local anesthetic, an exploratory 3-mm trephine hole may be made into either the rostral or caudal maxillary sinus for the collection and culture of exudate or the biopsy of nasal granulomata or neoplasms. A short Steinmann pin or a drill bit may be used to create the hole.

CONGENITAL AND DEVELOPMENTAL ANOMALIES

The most common oral congenital deformity observed in the horse is "parrot mouth," in which the maxilla is relatively longer than the mandible (Fig. 14–5). The mirror-image condition in which the mandible appears longer than the maxilla is referred to as "monkey mouth" (or "sow mouth"). In apparent maxillary overgrowth, the defect is actually caused by mandibular shortening (brachygnathism) because the diastema in the mandible of a parrot-mouthed horse is shortened. The result is no occlusal contact between the upper and lower incisor teeth. An overbite of some 2 cm of the incisor arcade may be present in a horse with a mismatch of less than 1 cm when the first upper and lower cheek teeth are compared. Conversely, apparent mandibular overgrowth is caused by maxillary shortening (brachycephalism).

Both conditions are thought to be inherited. Some correction of incisor malocclusion

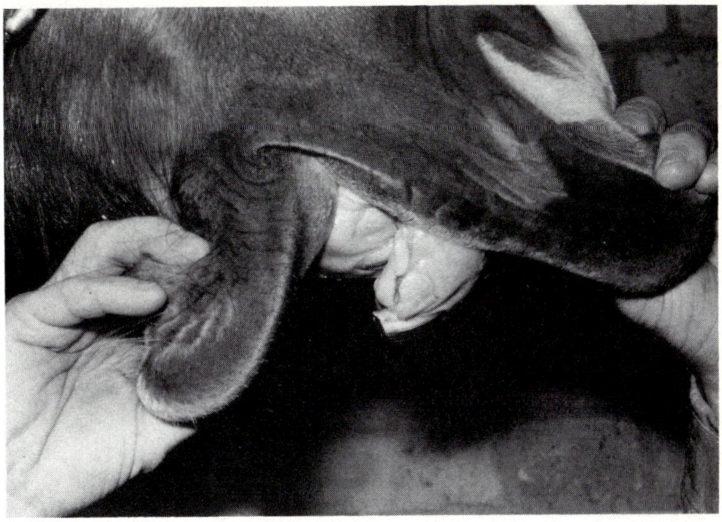

Figure 14–5. Parrot mouth (mandibular brachygnathia) in a 4 year old Thoroughbred. (From Mansmann RA, McAllister ES: Equine Medicine and Surgery, 3rd ed. Santa Barbara, American Veterinary Publications Inc., 1982.)

occurs up to 5 years of age. Definitions of parrot mouth and their recognition and detection are important in the examination of potential breeding stock.

SUPERNUMERARY TEETH

By definition supernumerary teeth exist in addition to the normal number of teeth (polyodontia). The wolf tooth should not be regarded as a supernumerary tooth, since it is part of the normal dentition. However, it has been shown that only 20 percent of foal and yearling Thoroughbreds have erupted wolf teeth. Extra incisors may arise as a result of the division of the permanent tooth germ. In some horses, it may be a complete double row, but often one finds only one or two extra teeth. Treatment depends on how the teeth develop. Those that wear more or less evenly and cause no apparent trouble should be left alone. However, if the extra teeth become elongated, they should be cut off or extracted to prevent damage to the occlusal surface. Owners frequently want supernumerary incisors removed for cosmetic reasons, and it may be necessary to accede to such a request when there are no other reasons for extraction. An extra cheek tooth may be present at the caudal end of the arcade or, less frequently, may appear displaced to the lingual or buccal aspect of the normal arcade. Extra cheek teeth should be extracted to prevent malocclusion.

DENTIGEROUS CYSTS

Dentigerous cysts are abnormal tooth developments of epithelial origin arising from Hertwig's sheath or its precursor, the enamel organ. Such cysts frequently contain tooth fragments and may distort the surrounding maxilla or mandible.

Dentigerous cysts that arise from the tooth germ of a branchial arch remnant appear as temporal cysts or teratomata and may drain into the ear (Fig. 14–6). The cysts are lined with stratified squamous epithelium and may on occasion contain one or more teeth. Clinical signs depend upon the site affected. In rare cases, cysts may form inside the cranial vault, but they more commonly occur as temporal cysts associated with oral fistulae and as maxillary or paranasal sinus cysts. Treatment consists of careful dissection and removal of the cyst followed by obliteration of the dead space and fistula (Fig. 14–7). Such lesions are usually seen in horses younger than 3 years of age.

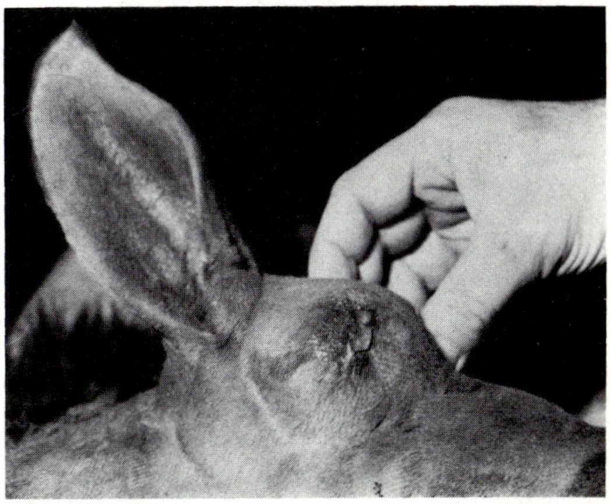

Figure 14–6. Dentigerous cyst (temporal teratoma) and aural fistula in an 8 month old Thoroughbred colt. (From Baker GJ: Dental disorders in the horse. *Compend Contin Educ Pract Vet* 4:S507–515, 1982.)

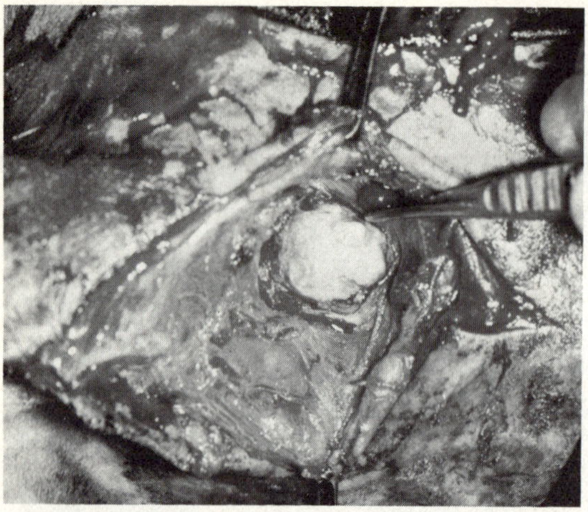

Figure 14–7. Exploration of dentigerous cyst to show developing tooth in the temporal bone. (From Mansmann RA, McAllister ES: Equine Medicine and Surgery, 3rd ed. Santa Barbara, American Veterinary Publications Inc., 1982.)

CYSTIC SINUSES

Cystic sinuses are also referred to as mucoid degeneration of the nasal conchae (turbinates), multiple mandibular cysts, or osteitis fibrosa cystica. It is typically seen in newborn or young horses. Affected animals may have facial or mandibular distortion, nasal obstruction, dyspnea, and nasal discharge from contact ulcers on the nasal mucosa. The differential diagnosis between multiple mandibular and maxillary cysts and dentigerous cysts may be difficult in mild cases. The lesions in these conditions are similar to those in classic hyperparathyroidism, with softening of bone caused by excessive resorption of calcium and fibrous tissue replacement. There is no evidence that the condition is influenced by dietary factors such as abnormal calcium or phosphorus ratios; it is more likely that genetic defects are involved. Another differential diagnosis in the young horse is ameloblastic odontoma. Confirmation of the diagnosis is by surgical biopsy.

Cystic sinusitis can be treated by surgical exploration and curettage through a frontomaxillary bone flap approach. Intraoperative hemorrhage should be controlled by irrigation with chilled saline and suture ligation when possible.

ABNORMAL TOOTH ERUPTION

Tooth eruption is a complex phenomenon involving the interplay of dental morphogenesis and the vascular forces responsible for creating the eruption pathway. The normal eruption times of the deciduous and permanent teeth have been listed in Chapter Thirteen. It should be noted that the third cheek tooth (fourth premolar) is the last permanent tooth to erupt, and it is the tooth that is most frequently found to be impacted, rotated, or misplaced.

Delayed Eruption or Impaction of Teeth

Wolf teeth may be displaced in a labial or rostral direction or may not be completely erupted. Such abnormalities may result in ulceration at the area of contact with the bit. Such teeth are easily extracted in sedated horses. Occasionally, there may be marked variation in canine tooth eruption in males, and one tooth may be impacted. In such cases, the gingivae should be split to allow the crowns to emerge.

Retention of Deciduous Teeth

The remnants of the deciduous cheek teeth (dental caps) may remain attached to the permanent teeth after these teeth have erupted. Caps should be removed once it has been determined that the permanent tooth has grown beyond the gingival line. It is best not to attempt to remove caps if it requires a great deal of effort to loosen them. Age and signs of pain generally dictate removal of offending caps. Occasionally, a dental cap may rotate following partial detachment and may cause buccal laceration and buccal deformity.

Perhaps the most significant abnormalities of tooth eruption are impaction and overcrowding. Under such circumstances, the vascular forces associated with the maturation of the enamel anlage and the eruption of the tooth result in the lysis of mandibular or maxillary bone, or of both. Such activity around the erupting permanent cheek teeth results in mandibular and maxillary swellings that are usually painless and symmetrical in young horses. However, if the erupting tooth is impacted (e.g., the third cheek tooth), contamination of the pulpal tissues results in mandibular or maxillary lysis and the formation of an external dental fistula.

ABNORMALITIES OF WEAR

The normal movement of the lower dental arcades across the upper arcades is accom-

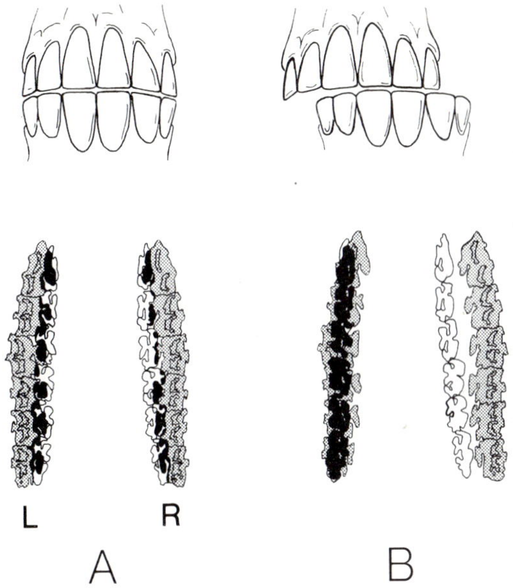

Figure 14–8. *A*, Incisor and arcade contact. *B*, Incisor and arcade contact illustrating effect of mandibular movement to the left side. Note upper teeth edges are not in occlusal contact.

panied by a slight retraction of the lower jaws. These movements, together with the way the lower arcades fit inside the upper cheek teeth, result in both the upper and lower arcades developing angled occlusal surfaces so that the outer (labial edges of the upper and the lingual edges of the lower) arcades are less worn (Figs. 14–8 and 14–9). The retraction of the lower arcade results in the formation of a small hook on the rostral point of the first upper cheek tooth and the

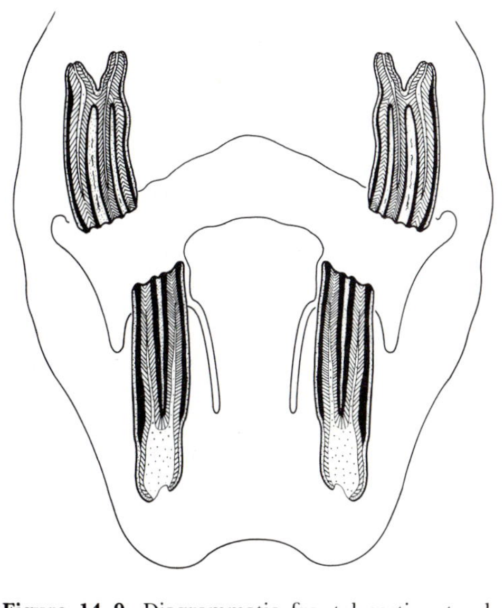

Figure 14–9. Diagrammatic frontal section to show inclination of occlusal surfaces.

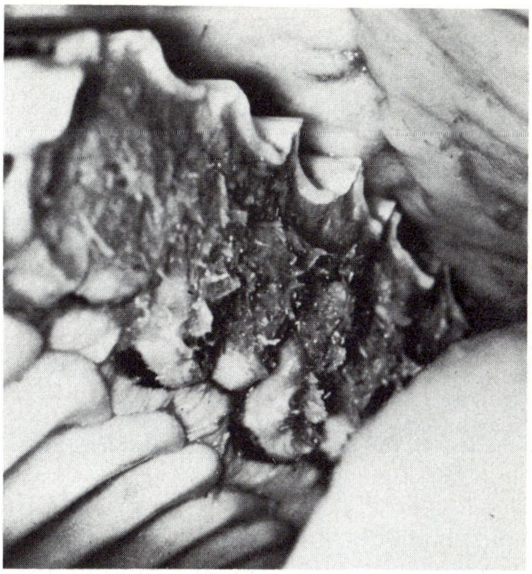

Figure 14–10. Enamel points and buccal ulceration. Note rostral hook on first cheek tooth. (From Mansmann RA, McAllister ES: Equine Medicine and Surgery, 3rd ed. Santa Barbara, American Veterinary Publications Inc., 1982.)

caudal point of the sixth lower cheek tooth. Exposed sharp enamel points develop along the unworn outer edges of the upper arcade and the inner edges of the lower arcade. The cheeks of the horse are closely applied to the teeth; consequently, the labial surfaces can be damaged and ulcerated by these points (Fig. 14–10). Areas of damaged buccal or lingual mucosa result in the horse changing the grinding pattern so that abnormal waves are formed along the dental arcade. Such changes in occlusal contact are always accompanied by gingivitis and periodontal infection. Without correction, severe periodontal pocketing and alveolar bone resorption and malocclusion will take place. Therefore, it is not surprising to find that the incidence of periodontal disease increases at the time of dental eruption and in old age. At these times, the shedding of the deciduous teeth and the long-term results of irregular wear, respectively, initiate the inflammatory changes of periodontal disease.[6]

When teeth are lost, broken, or displaced, enamel hooks and step deformities develop on the opposing arcade. These overgrowths may become so large that they make effective mastication impossible, and extensive dental work is required to restore normal occlusion and grinding action.

PERIODONTAL DISEASE

Periodontal disease in the horse is inflammatory and dystrophic in nature and can

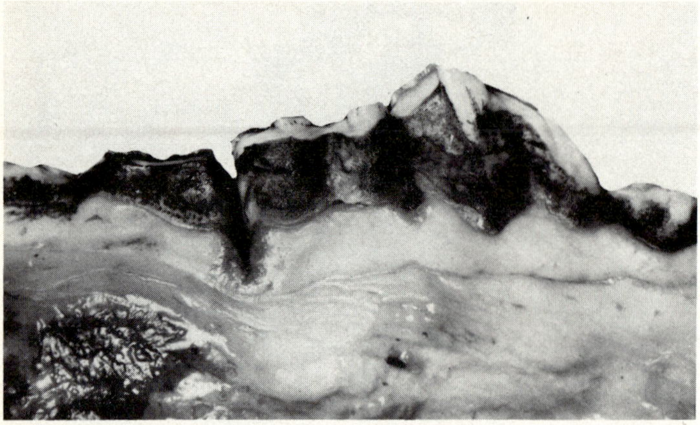

Figure 14–11. Periodontitis with gingival erosion. (From Mansmann RA, McAllister ES: Equine Medicine and Surgery, 3rd ed. Santa Barbara, American Veterinary Publications Inc., 1982.)

result in malnutrition, halitosis, maxillary and mandibular osteitis, paranasal sinusitis, quidding, nasal discharge, colic, and even death in severely affected animals. It has been described as the dental scourge of horses and is the most common dental disease in this animal.[7]

The initial lesion is marginal gingivitis with hyperemia and edema. The lateral gingival sulcus becomes eroded, and a triangular pocket is formed, usually on the buccal aspect (Fig. 14–11). This cavity harbors food, and a cycle of irritation, inflammation, and erosion is established that destroys gingival tissue deep into the periodontium. Ultimately, gross alveolar sepsis develops, and the tooth is lost.

In all species, the shearing forces produced by normal mastication are essential for the maintenance of a healthy periodontium. Gingivitis, which may lead to periodontitis, occurs in any situation in which there is abnormal occlusion and alteration in the shearing forces. The most severe form of periodontal disease, with gross pocketing, periodontal separation, and loosening of teeth, is associated with extreme abnormalities of wear. Such abnormalities include irregular arcades, hooks, the loss of teeth with corresponding overgrowth of the occluding arcade, displaced or split teeth, and mandibular or maxillary fractures.

Periodontal disease commonly occurs during the eruption of the permanent dentition. These lesions will heal once the normal grinding pattern is established. In severe cases, gross alveolar sepsis and unthriftiness may necessitate the animal's humane destruction. Treatment for periodontal disease is described in Chapter Fifteen.

DENTAL DECAY

Infection may be introduced into the pulp cavity of the tooth by a variety of routes. Hypoplasia of the upper cheek teeth enamel lake cementum may predispose to caries development at this site along with pulpitis (Fig. 14–12). Caries occurs through the fermentation of food within the infundibulum of

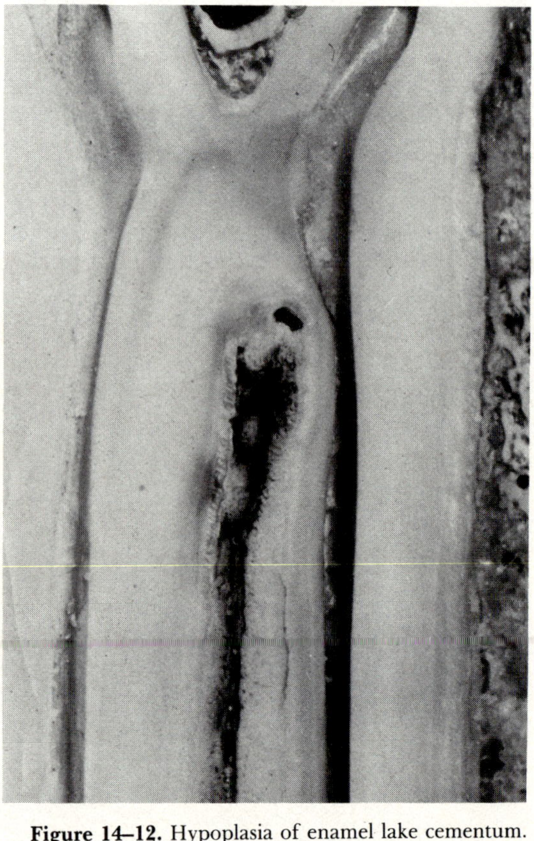

Figure 14–12. Hypoplasia of enamel lake cementum. Note position of pulp cavity.

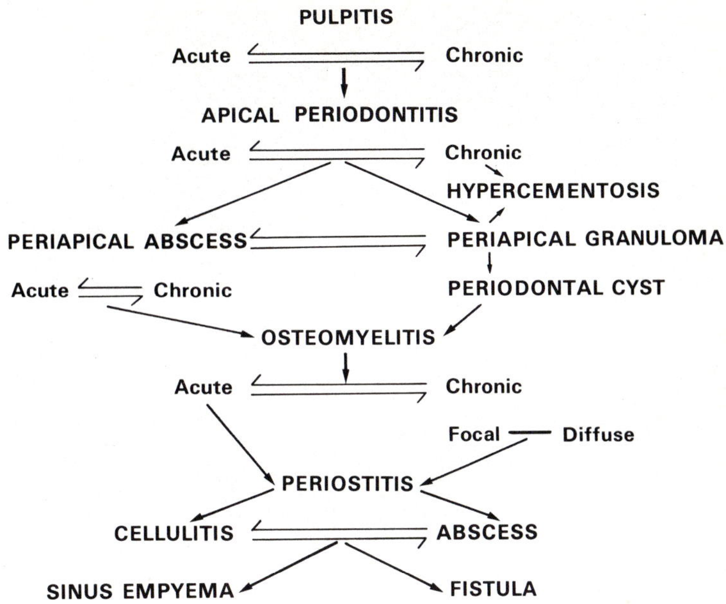

Figure 14–13. Potential sequelae and complications of apical osteitis-pulpitis in the horse.

the cement lakes and the subsequent dissolution of cementum by acid products. If these lesions expand to invade the surrounding enamel and dentin, infection will gain access to the pulp in spite of the production of secondary dentin by the pulp cavity. Pulpitis leads to periapical osteitis, and the subsequent clinical signs depend upon the site of the diseased tooth. There may be swelling, fistula formation, and infection (empyema) of the maxillary paranasal sinuses (Figs. 14–13 through 14–16).

The pathological features of decayed teeth are non-specific; consequently, the etiology of periapical infection in individual cases may be obscure. Many cases are not examined until the infection is advanced. Under such circumstances, tooth fractures may be pathological rather than primary. In both the upper and lower jaws, the majority of infected teeth are in a rostral position. Either the second or the third tooth is most commonly affected in the lower jaw, and the third tooth is more frequently diseased than

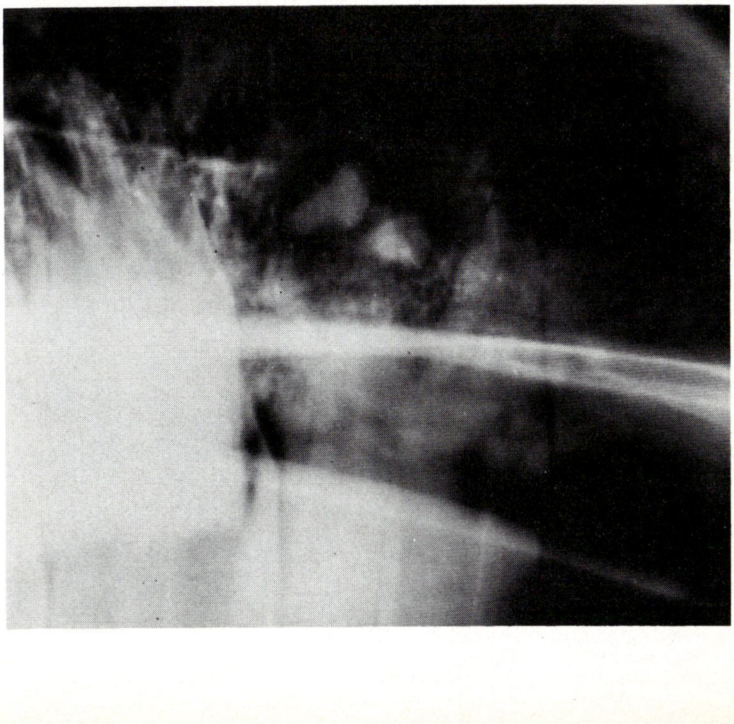

Figure 14–14. Apical infection of third cheek tooth, oblique projection. Eight year old Hunter gelding.

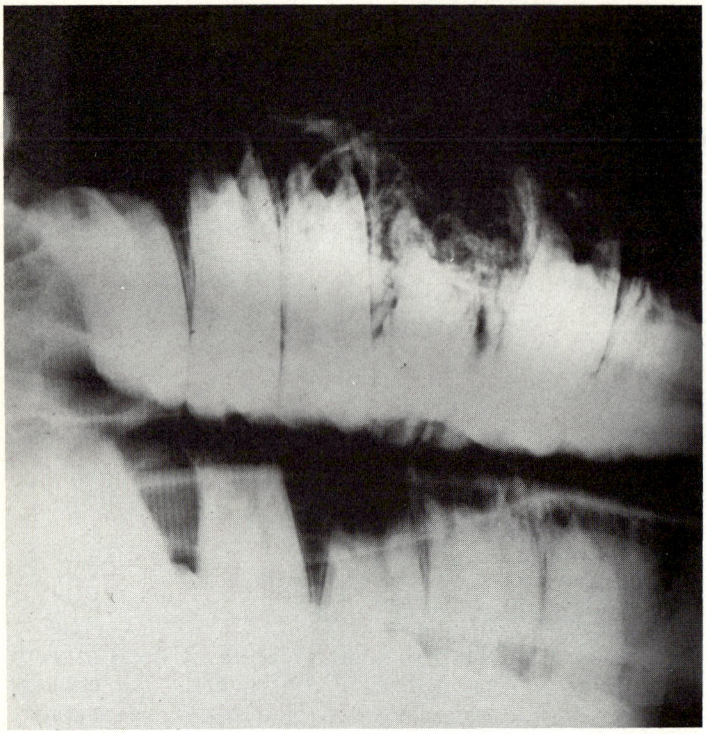

Figure 14–15. Apical osteitis with tooth fragments. Postextraction.

is the fourth tooth in the upper arcade. This observation led to the suggestion that in many cases delayed eruption and impaction are of primary etiological importance in the development of apical osteitis in the horse.[8–12]

DENTAL TUMORS

Dental tumors are classified as epithelial or mesenchymal according to their origin. An odontoma describes any tumor of odontogenic origin and refers to one in which both the epithelial and the mesenchymal cells produce functional ameloblasts and odontoblasts and, therefore, enamel and dentin within the tumor.

Most dental tumors occur in young animals and are congenital if they originate from a deciduous tooth germ or the first true molar tooth germ. They are usually benign but often defy treatment because of their size and the degree of facial, maxillary, or man-

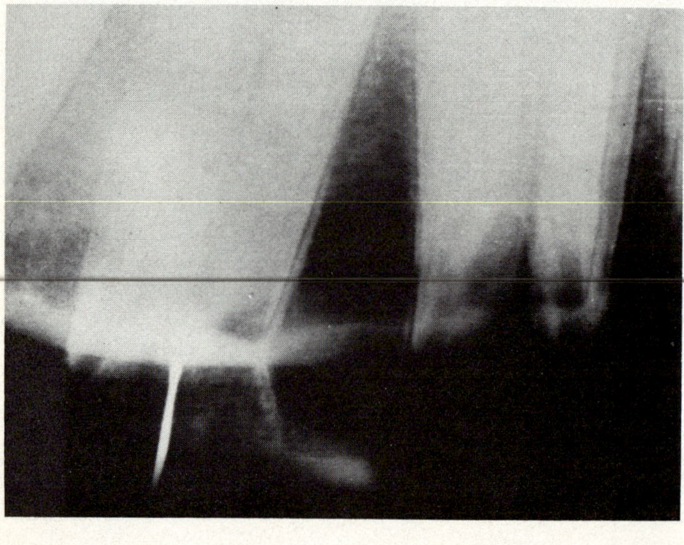

Figure 14–16. Mandibular dental fistulae.

dibular distortion that they cause. Affected animals may survive for several months or years before euthanasia is necessary.

Common dental tumors seen in the horse are ameloblastic odontomas (ameloblastoma) of the maxilla. Such tumors may be of epithelial and mesenchymal origin. The clinical signs may include facial swelling, nasal obstruction, dyspnea, dysplasia, quidding, and unthriftiness.[13]

DIFFERENTIAL DIAGNOSIS OF ORAL MUCOSAL LESIONS

Clinical signs and methods of diagnosis of oral disease are described at the beginning of this chapter.

Local lesions include oral trauma and foreign bodies (such as grass awns embedded in lips and gums).[14] Ulcers may appear on the lips, gums, and tongue from chemical irritants (such as from licking leg paints or blisters) as well as from viral infections (equine herpes viral infection [EHVI]) and from the prolonged use of phenylbutazone.[15] Epizootic diseases causing lesions in the oral cavity of the horse are described in Chapters Sixteen and Eighteen. In young horses, local hypertrophy of the palatine mucosa may result in a "tumor-like" swelling. The term "lampas" has been used to describe this condition. In the past, it was customary to excise, blister, or burn these sites—such treatment is no longer recommended, and it is very rare to associate any clinical disease with lampas. The hypertrophy regresses as permanent tooth eruption progresses. In order of decreasing frequency, oral papillomata (viral), fibromata, melanomata, fibrosarcomata and squamous cell carcinomata are seen.[16]

Masticatory myopathies as well as cranial nerve lesions (e.g., of the facial nerve) also interfere with prehension and mastication. Ingestion of yellow star thistle *(Centaurea solstitalis)* over an extended period (30 days) exposes horses to an unidentified toxic agent that causes negropallidal encephalomalacia. The disease is commonly called "chewing disease." The horse is unable to feed or drink because of paralysis of the muscles associated with prehension and swallowing. Recovery is very rare; diagnosis is confirmed by location of encephalomalacia of the substantia nigra of the brain.[17] A similar disease has been associated with the ingestion of Russian knapweed *(Centaurea repens).*

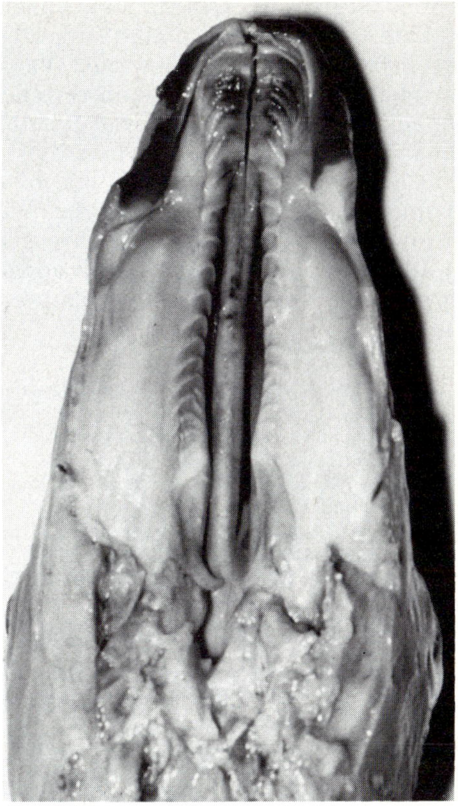

Figure 14–17. Palatine cleft in a 10 month Thoroughbred fetus.

Dysphagia may be seen with a number of systemic diseases that may cause local lesions of the mouth and throat, such as strangles *(Streptococcus equi),* tetanus, botulism, and a number of encephalitides, including rabies.

Clefts of the hard and soft palates are easily diagnosed in the neonatal foal (Fig. 14–17). The nasal return of milk when sucking is pathognomonic. Partial palatine clefts, palatine ulceration secondary to EHVI, and actinobacillosis infections may not be diagnosed until adulthood. Treatment is described in Chapter Fifteen.

Subepiglottic cysts are another uncommon cause of dysphagia and concomitant dyspnea in the young foal.

SALIVARY DISEASES

Wounds to the gland substance as well as lacerations of the ducts[18] are the most common salivary problem seen in the horse. Duct obstruction (congenital,[19] traumatic, or from calculus or foreign body obstruction-abscessation) will cause swelling and oral pain. Treatment is symptomatic and includes anti-inflammatory drugs, fomentation, dimethyl sulfoxide (DMSO) and specific surgical repair, debridement, and drainage. Parotid duct ligation[20] and parotid gland resection[21] have been used in horses for the treatment of benign parotid gland or duct disease.

The parotid salivary gland is one of the common sites for melanoma in the horse. Abscessation of the parotid salivary gland may follow retropharyngeal lymph adenopathy in strangles or guttural pouch empyema.

References

1. Baker GJ: Some aspects of dental radiology. *Equine Vet J* 3:46–51, 1971.
2. Baker GJ: The radiology of equine dental disease. *Acta Vet Radiol* (Suppl.) 67–69, 1972.
3. Baker GJ: Dental disease in the horse. In Practice. *Vet Rec* (Suppl.) 1:19–26, 1979.
4. Baker GJ: Dental disorders in the horse. *Compend Contin Educ* 4:S507–S515, 1982.
5. Mason BJE: Empyema of the equine paranasal sinuses. *J Am Vet Med Assoc* 167:727–732, 1975.
6. Baker GJ: Some aspects of equine dental disease. *Equine Vet J* 2:105–110, 1970.
7. Colyer F: Abnormal conditions of the teeth of animals and their relationships to similar conditions in man. *The Dental Board of the UK,* 1931.
8. Baker GJ: Some aspects of equine dental decay. *Equine Vet J* 6:127–130, 1974.
9. Baker GJ: Diseases of the teeth and paranasal sinuses. *In* Equine Medicine and Surgery, 3rd ed. Santa Barbara, California, American Veterinary Pub. Inc., 1982, pp. 437–458.
10. Hofmeyr CFB: Comparative dental pathology (with particular reference to caries and paradontal disease in the horse and the dog). *J South Afr Vet Med Assoc* 29:471–480, 1960.
11. Cook WR: Dental surgery in the horse. *Proc Br Equine Vet Assoc* 34–44, 1965.
12. Becker E: Joests' Handbook of Special Pathology of Domestic Animals. Berlin, Paul Parey, 1962.
13. Peter CP, Myers VS, Ramsey FK: Ameloblastic odontoma in a pony. *Am J Vet Res* 29:1495–1498, 1968.
14. Bankowski RA, Wichmann RW, Stuart EE: Stomatitis of cattle and horses due to yellow bristle grass *(Setaria lutescens). J Am Vet Med Assoc* 129:149–155, 1956.
15. Snow DH, Bogan JA, Douglas TA, Thompson H: Phenylbutazone toxicity in ponies. *Vet Rec* 105: 26–30, 1979.
16. Koch DB: The oral cavity, oropharynx and salivary glands. *In* Equine Medicine and Surgery, 3rd ed. Santa Barbara, California, American Veterinary Pub. Inc., 1982, pp. 458–475.
17. Cordy DR: Negropallidal encephalomalacia in horses, associated with ingestion of yellow star thistle. *J Neuropathol Exp Neurol* 13:330–341, 1956.
18. Cunningham, JA: A case of parotid fistula in a horse. *Vet Rec* 77:679–680, 1968.
19. Fowler ME: Congenital atresia of the parotid duct in a horse. *J Am Vet Med Assoc* 146:1403–1404, 1965.
20. Viborg E: Vorschlag zu einer verbesserten behandlung der speichelfisteln bey menschen und haustieren. *Sammlung Abhandlungen Tierarzte* 2:31–48, 1797.
21. Bracegirdle JR: Removal of the parotid and mandibular salivary glands from a pony mare. *Vet Rec* 98:507, 1976.

Chapter Fifteen

Oral Surgical Techniques

GJ Baker

DENTAL EQUIPMENT

A full set of dental instruments should include handles, molar cutters, extraction forceps, repellers or punches, bone chisels, mallets, a screwdriver, a dental pick, rasps, and a variety of floats, trephines, rongeurs, bone cutters, curettes, and splinter forceps (Fig. 15–1).

DENTAL PROCEDURES

Floating

It has been emphasized that the routine floating of horses' teeth to remove sharp enamel points and hooks is of value in ensuring that normal occlusal contact between the dental arcades is made and maintained.[1] In this way, many of the problems of irregular wear and periodontal disease may be prevented. It is recommended that teeth be checked and floated once a year in horses younger than 10 years of age and twice yearly in older animals. When horses are in training and during the erupting phase of their teeth (up to 4 years of age), they should also have biannual dental examinations and prophylactic work.

Floating is usually done without anesthesia and with minimum restraint. A speculum may be used or the tongue may be grasped and withdrawn to make the horse open the mouth. Usually, however, this is not necessary, because passage of the float causes the horse to open the mouth enough for the clinician to remove the sharp enamel points.

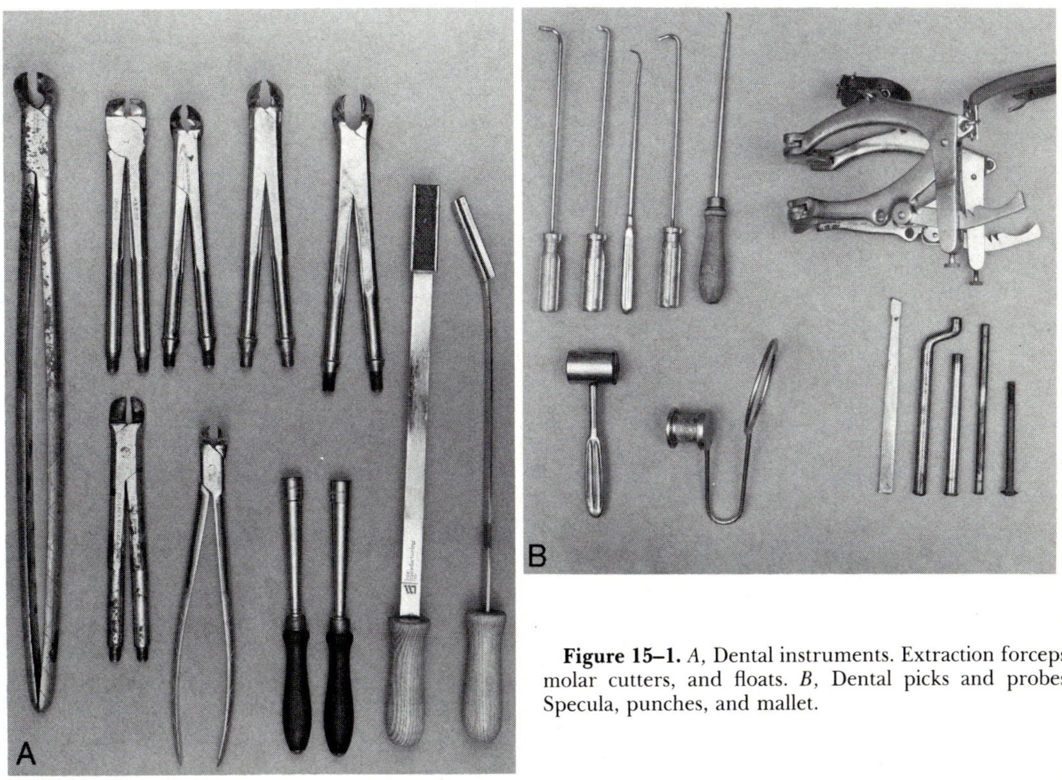

Figure 15–1. *A*, Dental instruments. Extraction forceps, molar cutters, and floats. *B*, Dental picks and probes. Specula, punches, and mallet.

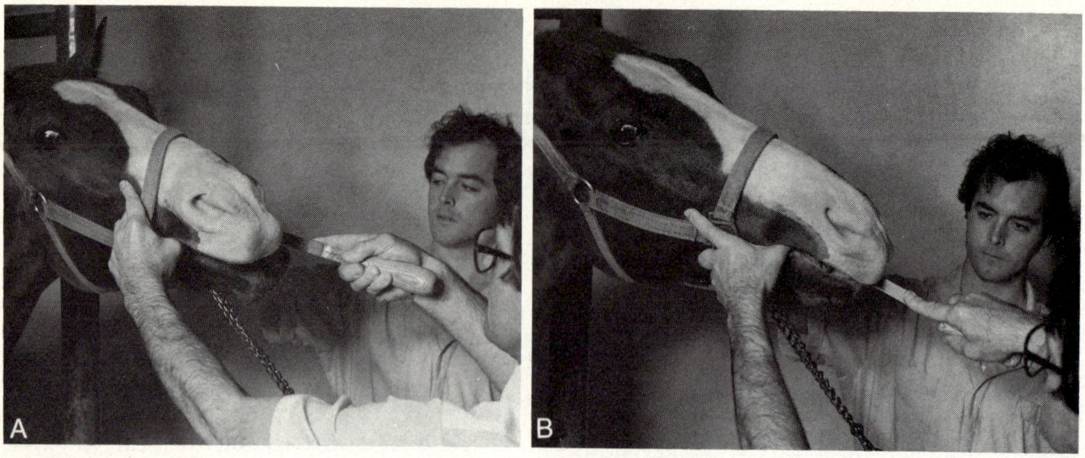

Figure 15–2. *A,* Floating the upper arcade using the angled float. *B,* Floating the lower arcade using the straight float.

When more extensive floating is necessary, as when grinding down a protruding tooth, a speculum should be used and the horse should be tranquilized, sedated, restrained, or given general anesthesia as needed. Usually, rasping is only necessary to remove any sharp enamel points that may abrade or cut the tongue and cheeks and to level any projections above the table surfaces. These projections are usually removed by five or six strokes with the rasp over the arcade. The rasp should not be placed flat on the arcade but should be held at an angle to the occlusal surface—lingually on the lower arcade and buccally on the upper arcade. A slightly angled rasp is used on the upper arcade and a straight rasp used on the lower arcade. When floating the upper arcade, neither the assistant's arm nor the nose band of the halter or speculum should press against the horse's cheek, since the back of the rasp may injure the buccal mucosa. If the horse shakes the head or moves it up and down, it is important to move with the horse so that the rasp does not injure the mouth. The assistant should hold the head firmly and steadily but should not hold the soft part of the nose so firmly that breathing is interfered with (Fig. 15–2).[2–4]

Removal of Wolf Teeth and Dental Caps

A dental elevator can be used to loosen the wolf tooth, which is then extracted with small animal straight canine tooth or incisor forceps. Dental caps may be removed with an elevator, using molar forceps or finger extraction.

Tooth Cutting

Cutting forceps with hardened jaws have been designed to remove projecting portions of molars. Forceps with a compound fulcrum supply sufficient force to the cutting edge to sever the tooth cleanly, though operators with strong arms can use the simple forceps satisfactorily. A speculum should be used in this operation. After cutting, the teeth should be floated to remove loose fragments or sharp corners. If special cutters are not available, large hooks and irregularities can be removed by striking carefully with a heavy hammer and a sharpened heavyweight cold chisel.

Tooth Extraction

Each case must be evaluated after a thorough clinical and radiological examination.[1] General anesthesia with a cuffed endotracheal tube to protect the airway from dental debris and hemorrhage is essential. If the tooth is grossly diseased or fractured, it can be manipulated and extracted through the mouth by hand with the use of dental forceps. For the majority of cheek teeth, however, extraction is best carried out by trephination and repulsion.

The site for trephination is selected from radiographs and anatomical landmarks. The skin site is closely clipped and is prepared for a sterile surgical incision. The skin incision is shaped to fit the anatomical site. A longitudinal, straight incision is used for the rostral lower teeth and a curved lateral flap is used for the caudal lower teeth. A circular disc gives satisfactory exposure of the rostral

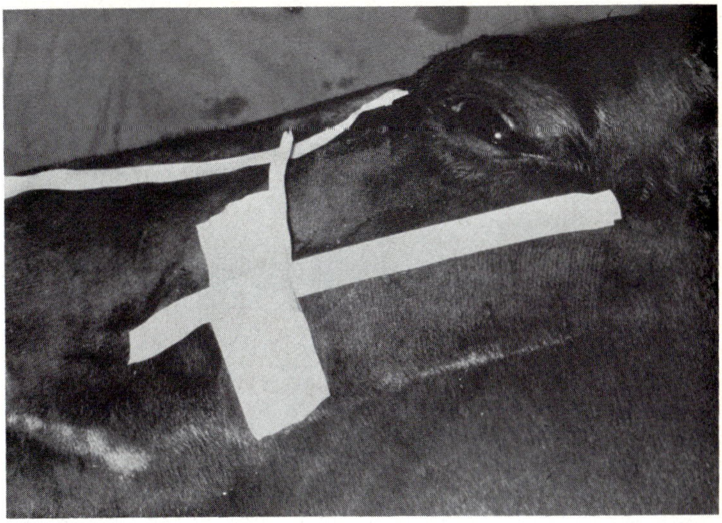

Figure 15–3. Lateral view of left maxilla. Tapes represent the limits of the maxillary paranasal sinus of the third cheek tooth.

upper teeth, though in some cases a skin and sinus flap technique may be preferred.

Care must be taken to avoid damaging the facial artery and vein, the parotid salivary duct, and the dorsal buccal branch of the facial nerve. Access to the caudal maxillary cheek is gained via the frontal and caudal maxillary sinuses.

After the skin has been incised, the periosteum is elevated and a trephine is used to expose the apex of the affected tooth. A stainless steel punch and a heavyweight steel orthopedic mallet are used to repel the tooth. It helps to have an assistant drive the punch while the operator ensures that the correct tooth is being extracted. Palpation of the exposed crown and the solid sound of good contact are the best guides. It is essential that the angle of repulsion be correct in both the caudorostral and the buccolingual planes. The correct caudorostral plane varies considerably with the age of the horse and the tooth involved. It is comparatively easy for the punch to slip from the exposed apex of the diseased tooth. If this happens, it may damage the root of an adjacent tooth. More seriously, it may continue along the alveolar plane and into the mouth, causing large fragmentary fractures of alveolar bone or of the entire thickness of the mandible. If the punch slips medially from the exposed root of upper teeth, there is a danger that the palatine artery may be sectioned. Such trauma will lead to severe hemorrhage and will require suture ligation. A common problem arising from teeth with primary impaction, or from movement of adjacent teeth secondary to the decay process in the diseased tooth, is that the tooth may be difficult to drive with the punch. It may then be necessary to use a chisel to divide the tooth along its vertical axis and remove it in fragments (Figs. 15–3 through 15–5).

Following extraction of the tooth, the alveolar socket should be thoroughly curetted, and any necrotic bone, remnants of apical granulomata, tooth fragments, or nodules of cementum should be removed. Infection within the paranasal sinuses must be washed

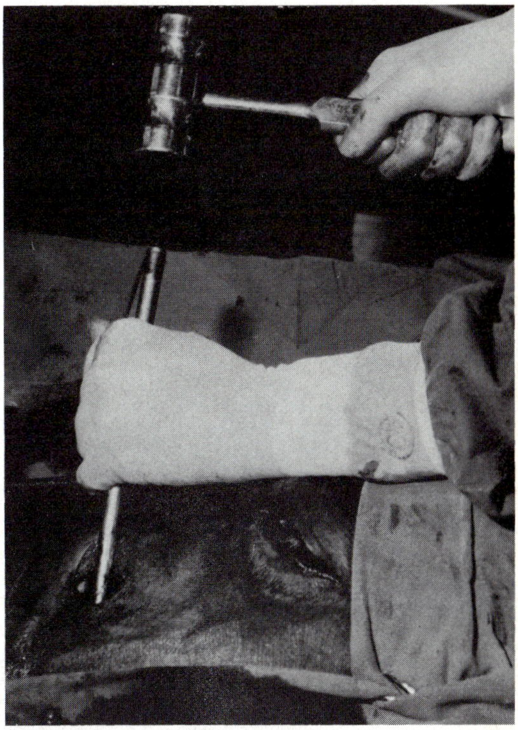

Figure 15–4. Punch used through a maxillary trephine to repel the third cheek tooth.

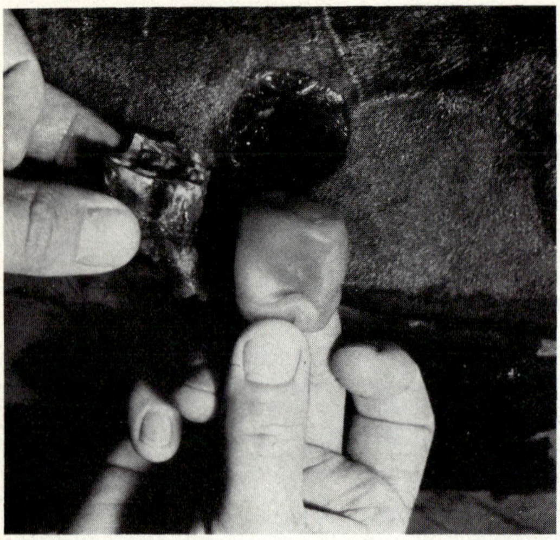

Figure 15–5. Extracted tooth and alveolar plug (dental wax).

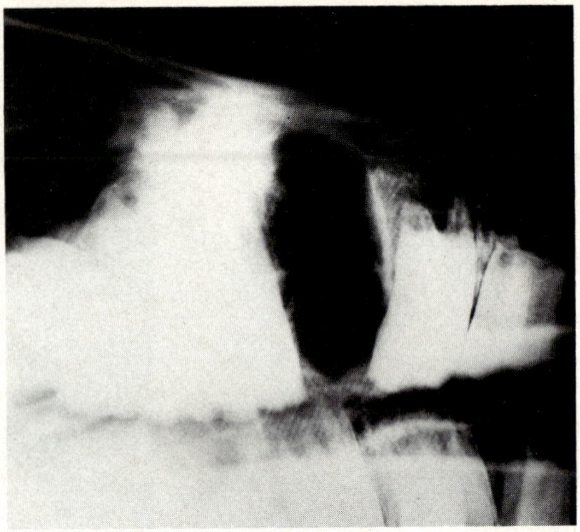

Figure 15–6. Postoperative radiograph after extraction and effective curettage.

out, and a frontal sinus irrigation trephine incision must be made. Postoperative radiographs should always be examined to ensure that all sequestrae have been removed (Figs. 15–6 and 15–7).

Special care is needed to gain access to the caudal upper teeth (the fifth and sixth teeth), and special punches are available to make contact through the frontal and caudal maxillary paranasal sinuses (see Fig. 15–1). In some cases, it may be easier to expose the caudal teeth via a lateral buccostomy. Using a dental elevator, periosteal elevator, or orthopedic chisel, the lateral alveolar plate can be removed and the tooth can be extracted.[4] If this approach is used, the surgeon must ensure that vital structures (facial nerve, facial artery, and parotid salivary duct) are identified and preserved.

Primary postextraction treatment of the alveolar socket is aimed at achieving an oral seal to prevent food and saliva from contaminating the socket. The external trephine and socket are cleansed by daily irrigation via either the paranasal sinus or the external trephine hole. An oral seal can be achieved using a variety of materials (e.g., dental wax [Fig. 15–8], soft acrylic cement, or gutta percha) to form a dental plug. This plug prevents contamination of the socket by food and saliva, and the socket fills with healthy granulation tissue that matures into fibrous tissue and bone. The plug should be removed after 1 month if it has not been shed spontaneously.

In a series of 142 dental extractions in the horse, it was found that 32 required reexploration and general anesthesia.[5] The

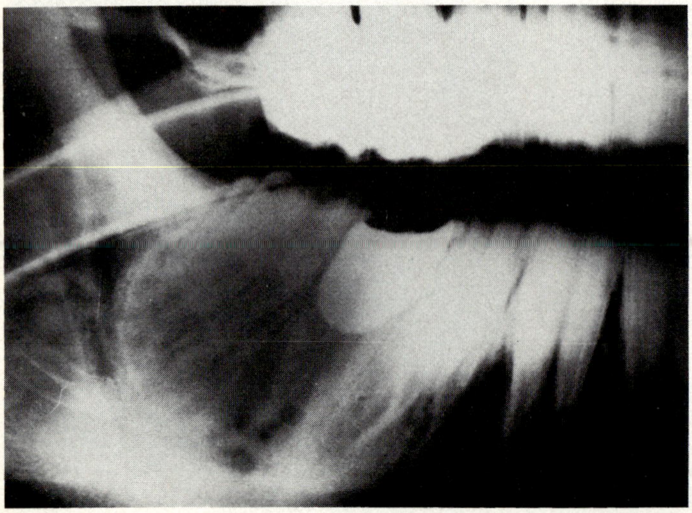

Figure 15–7. Gutta percha plug after extraction of the fifth lower cheek tooth.

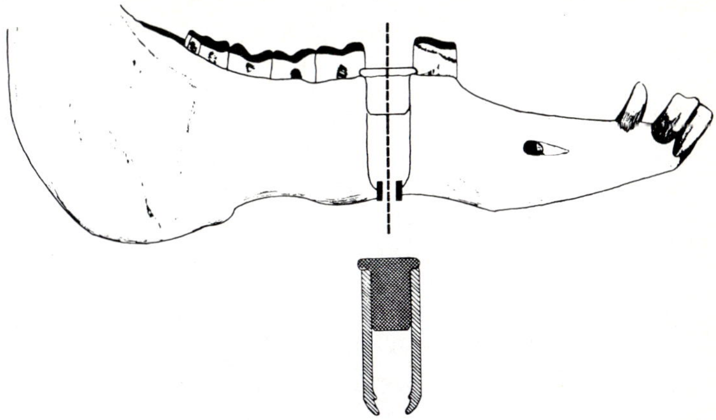

Figure 15–8. Diagram illustrating the ideal position of alveolar socket plug. (From Mansmann RA, McAllister ES: Equine Medicine and Surgery, 3rd ed. Santa Barbara, American Veterinary Publications Inc., 1982.)

main problems were persistent socket infection, sequestration, or the reappearance of dental sinuses or fistulae. In many cases, remnants of periodontal membrane proliferated, and nodules of cementum were produced. Some of these nodules were 5 mm to 10 mm and were not visible on the immediate postextraction radiographs. Overenthusiastic curettage of the alveolar socket during surgery can expose the reserve crown of adjacent teeth and may be the source of the subsequent reappearance of dental disease symptoms, such as fistula formation and sinus empyema.

CORRECTIVE DENTISTRY

Oral trauma can result in dental maleruption and malalignment. In some cases, it is necessary to extract malaligned or displaced teeth. Gap closure can then be encouraged using monofilament wire loops. It has been noted that some forms of malalignment have a genetic base (e.g., parrot mouth), and discretion is advised in advocating corrective surgery.

An upper incisor wire brace that is secured to the first cheek tooth on each side can afford some correction. Such a brace retards the extension of the upper diastema and incisive bone, thereby arresting the development of the overbite.

DENTAL, MANDIBULAR, AND MAXILLARY FRACTURES

Fractured teeth may occur from two main causes. The first, extension of the dental decay process, has been described. The second cause is acute trauma from kicks, falls, or gunshot wounds, or trauma in association with mandibular and maxillary fractures. In many cases there is exposure of the pulp, and pulpitis results. In general, treatment is aimed at stabilizing the crowns, and the arcade may still function even though the teeth are no longer vital. In other cases, fractured teeth will need to be extracted.

The mandibular and incisive bones are the most frequently fractured in the head of the horse.[6–8] Such fractures follow acute trauma—some may be iatrogenic and many involve incidents in which the horse's jaw becomes entangled. The flight reaction then results in the fracture of the mandibular or maxillary symphysis or incisive bone by gate latches, automatic waterers, hay racks, and so on.

Each fracture must be thoroughly evaluated, considering soft tissue, nerve, vascular, and salivary wounds. Many are open fractures, and antibiotic therapy (procaine penicillin G 22,000 IU/kg twice daily) is advisable, in addition to routine antitetanus prophylaxis. Early management, wound debridement (Fig. 15–9 A–C), and repair are necessary. Any delay will result in dehydration and debility of the horse, together with local contamination and infection that will hinder osteosynthesis.

Wire fixation, pins and wires, lag screw fixation, and V-bar techniques, together with bone plating and Kirschner devices, have all been described with successes reported.[6] Combination techniques using pins, bars, and acrylics may be developed to enable the horse to continue feeding during the healing period.

In severe trauma, the successful outcome of the case will depend upon the successful alimentation of the horse and preservation of the airway. The latter can be achieved using a tracheostomy tube, and the horse can be fed through either a nasogastric tube or a cervical esophagostomy.[9]

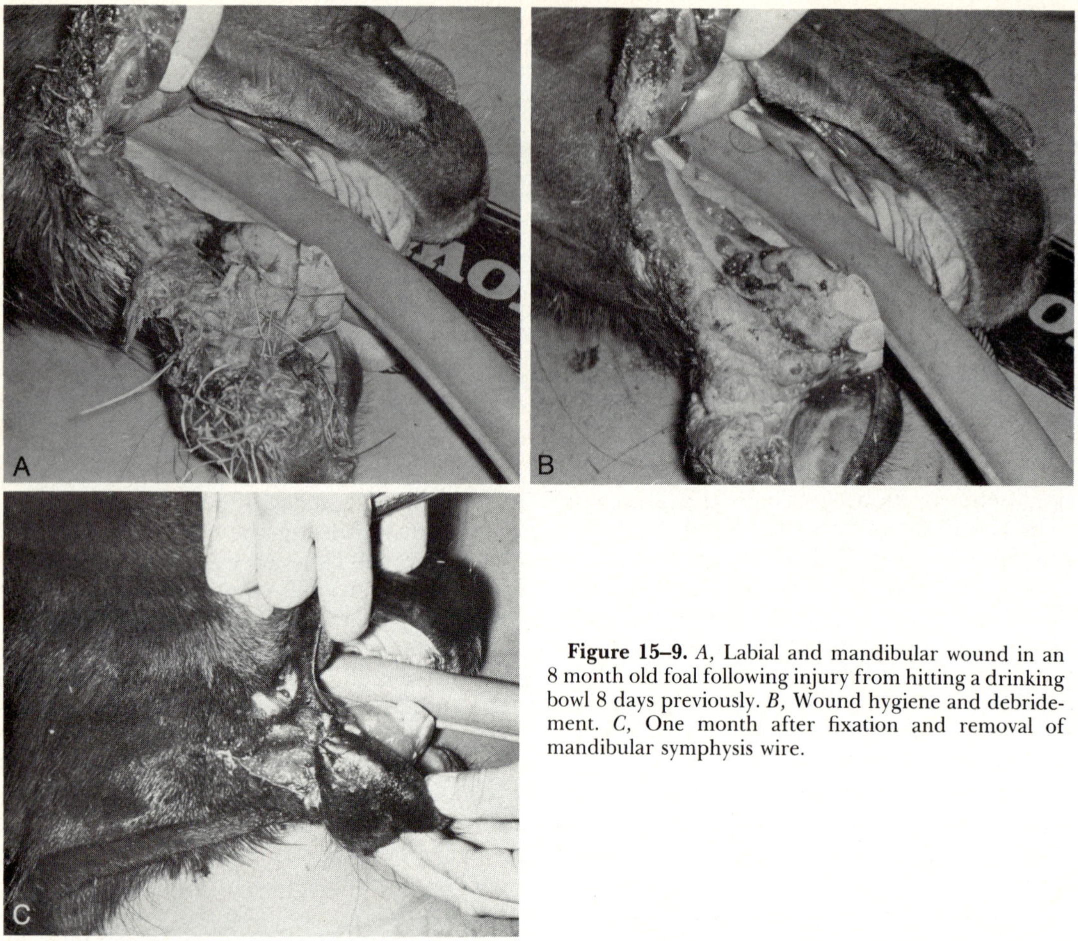

Figure 15–9. *A,* Labial and mandibular wound in an 8 month old foal following injury from hitting a drinking bowl 8 days previously. *B,* Wound hygiene and debridement. *C,* One month after fixation and removal of mandibular symphysis wire.

CLEFT PALATE SURGERY

In recent years, a number of publications have described the surgical repair of cleft palate in foals and weanlings.[10] Emphasis is correctly placed on early surgery and on the value of mandibular symphysiotomy in affording sugical exposure.[11] However, limited discussion has been given to the results, and though closure may be effective in reducing the nasal regurgitation, it is not possible to achieve a normal palatopharyngeal arch. Hence, normal laryngopalatine function is not achieved; thus the value of these procedures must be questioned.

References

1. Baker GJ: Some aspects of dental disease in the horse. *Equine Vet J* 2:105–110, 1970.
2. Hofmeyr CFB: Comparative dental pathology (with particular response to caries and paradontal disease in the horse and the dog). *J South Afr Vet Med Assoc* 29:471–481, 1960.
3. Cook WR: Dental surgery in the horse. *Proc Br Equine Vet Assoc* 34–44, 1965.
4. Evans LH, Tate LP, LaDow CS: Extraction of the equine 4th upper premolar and 1st and 2nd upper molars through a lateral buccotomy. Proceedings of the Twenty-seventh Meeting of the American Association of Equine Practitioners, 1981, pp. 249–252.
5. Baker GJ: Diseases of the teeth and paranasal sinuses. *In* Mansmann RA, McCallister ES (eds.): Equine Medicine and Surgery, 3rd ed. Santa Barbara, California, American Veterinary Pub. Inc., 1982, pp. 437–458.
6. Turner AS: Mandible and maxilla fractures. *In* Mansmann RA, McCallister ES (eds.): Equine Medicine and Surgery, 3rd ed. Santa Barbara, California, American Veterinary Pub. Inc., 1982, pp. 997–1000.
7. Sullins KE, Turner AS: Management of fractures of the equine mandible and premaxilla (incisive bone). *Comp Contin Ed* 4:S480–S490, 1982.
8. Pascoe J: Specific aspects of dental surgery. Fractures of the mandible and maxilla. Proceedings of the Symposium on Surgery and Diseases of the Oral Cavity. *Aust Equine Vet Assoc* 21–39, 1981.
9. Freeman DE, Naylor JM: Cervical esophagostomy to permit extraoral feeding of the horse. *J Am Vet Med Assoc* 172:314–320, 1978.
10. Nelson AW, Stashak TS: Cleft palate. *In* Robinson NE: Current Therapy in Equine Medicine. Philadelphia, WB Saunders Co., pp. 177–181, 1983.
11. Jones RS, Maisels DO, DeGeus JJ, Lovius BBJ: Surgical repair of cleft palate in the horse. *Equine Vet J* 7:86–91, 1975.

Section Three

Oral Diseases in Other Species

Chapter Sixteen

Anatomy of the Oral Cavity, Eruption, and Developmental Abnormalities in Ruminants

AH Andrews

ANATOMY

Cattle, sheep, and goats are members of the suborder Ruminantia, order Artiodactyla. A large gap or diastema conveniently separates the teeth of these animals into two groups, rostral (formerly anterior) and caudal (formerly posterior). The ruminants have both a temporary and a permanent dentition; incisor teeth are not present in the upper jaw in either set of these teeth. Instead, a substantial layer of fibrous tissue is found over the body of the premaxilla at which point the dental alveoli would be placed; this is covered by a thick, horny epithelium, which forms the dental pad.

Deciduous Dentition

There are 20 deciduous teeth, of which 8 are rostral. All the rostral teeth have a similar spatulate shape (Figs. 16–1 and 16–2). Because of their resemblance to each other conventional veterinary and agricultural terminology referred to them as incisors[1] and the dental formula was written thus:

$$2\left(i\frac{0}{4}\ c\frac{0}{0}\ p\frac{3}{3}\ m\frac{0}{0}\right) = 20$$

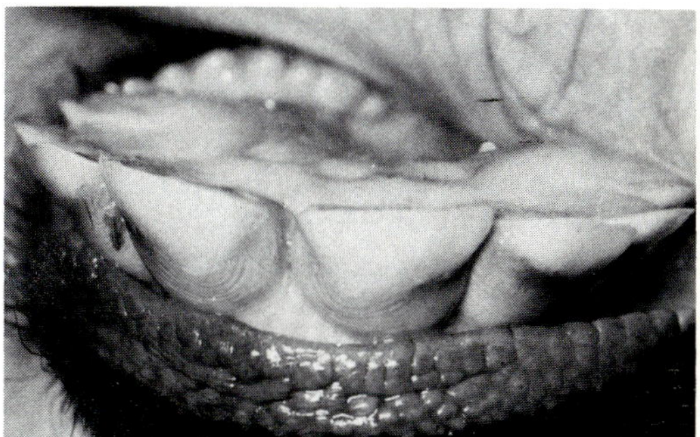

Figure 16–1. Rostral teeth in a 1 day old calf.

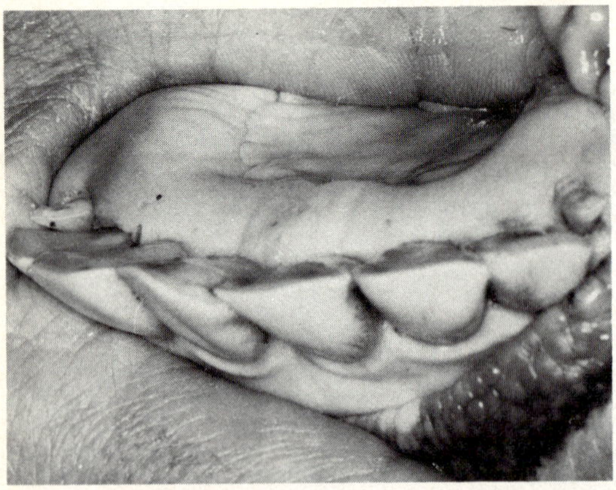

Figure 16–2. Rostral teeth of a 3 year old cow. There are three pairs of permanent incisors and one pair of temporary teeth.

Ruminants are, however, placental (eutherian) animals, which, by definition, have a maximum of three pairs of incisors and one pair of canine teeth per jaw.[2] Thus, the corner rostral tooth is a modified canine tooth. The work of dental anatomists supports such an assumption,[3–5] though the term was only accepted "under protest" by Tomes.[3] The corner rostral tooth does take on a caniniform shape in some deer, for example, the muntjac *(Muntiacus reevesi)*, and the duration of eruption is often longer in this last pair of teeth. The dental formula is therefore more correctly written thus:

$$2\left(i\frac{0}{3}\ c\frac{0}{1}\ p\frac{3}{3}\ m\frac{0}{0}\right) = 20$$

The cheek teeth form the remainder of the temporary dentition. There are 12 of these teeth, and they consist of 3 premolars in each caudal part of the maxilla and mandible.

Permanent Dentition

There are 32 permanent teeth, 8 of which are rostral in the lower jaw. The considerations that apply to the anatomical status of the corner teeth in the deciduous dentition also apply to the permanent dentition. The three pairs of premolars in each jaw are supplemented by three pairs of upper and lower molars. These latter teeth have no temporary precursors.

The dental formula of the permanent dentition[1] can be written thus:

$$2\left(I\frac{0}{4}\ C\frac{0}{0}\ P\frac{3}{3}\ M\frac{3}{3}\right) = 32$$

or more correctly:

$$2\left(I\frac{0}{3}\ C\frac{0}{1}\ P\frac{3}{3}\ M\frac{3}{3}\right) = 32$$

Incisors and Canines

These rostral teeth can be named from the center outward as the first pair, second pair, third pair, and fourth pair. They can also be described as central, medial, or first intermediate; lateral or second intermediate; and corners or canines, respectively. The construction (haplodontal) of these rostral teeth in both the temporary and permanent dentitions is simple (Fig. 16–3).

Cattle. In cattle, the rostral teeth have a short crown of spatulate shape and are arranged in a broad arch. The labial surfaces of the teeth are almost straight and are directed rostrally and dorsally to contact the dental pad, the angle of contact being acute. The occlusal surface of the tooth is white and is covered with enamel that is soon removed with mastication to reveal a central area of yellow primary dentin. The crowns of the central incisors are the largest, and the size of each succeeding pair decreases so that the canines are smallest. The root is rounded and is separated from the crown by a distinct neck. The fixation of the rostral tooth roots in the mandibular alveoli allows a small amount of dorsoventral movement. The bone in the surrounding alveoli is cancellous in nature.

The rostral tooth roots are usually positioned close together so that their crowns radiate outward, and initially there is often a small amount of overlap between each crown and the tooth medial to it. Initially, the dental

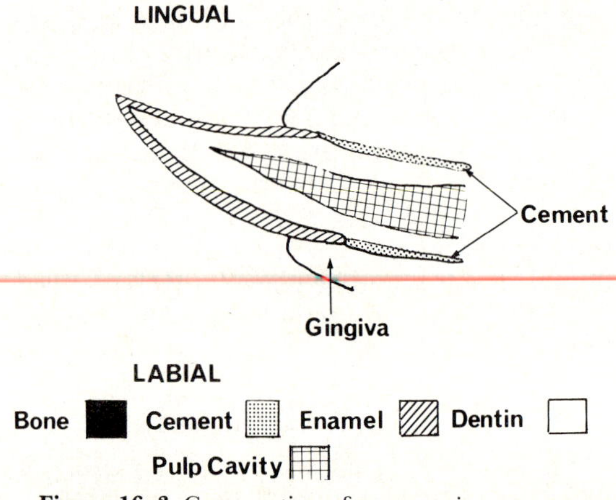

Figure 16–3. Cross section of an emerging permanent central incisor tooth.

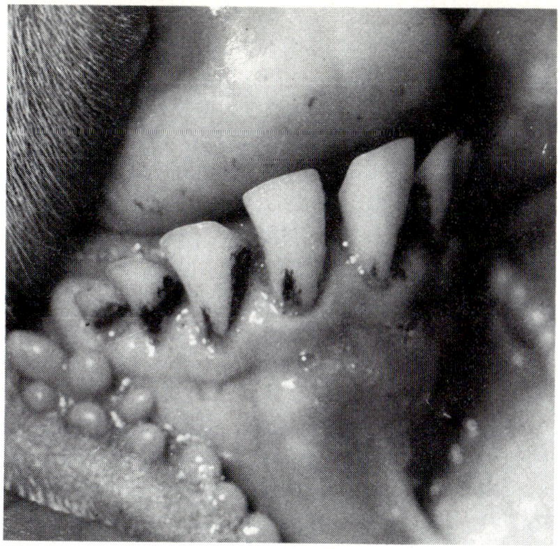

Figure 16–4. Rostral temporary teeth in a 3 to 4 month old goat kid.

arch exhibits a pronounced arc. In cattle, the tooth crown is formed prior to emergence; once it is fully erupted, the gingival margin is at the crown-root junction.

Sheep and Goats. The rostral teeth in sheep and goats (Fig. 16–4) have long, narrow crowns with no distinct neck, and they are arranged in a very curved arch. The labial surfaces of the teeth are very convex, and the dorsal edge is sharp for cropping forage. The roots of the rostral teeth tend to be firmly embedded in their alveoli.

The deciduous teeth are replaced by their permanent successors (Figs. 16–5 and 16–6).

Posteruption Changes. Increased age results in the retraction of the gingivae, thereby exposing the root. Enamel covers the occlusal

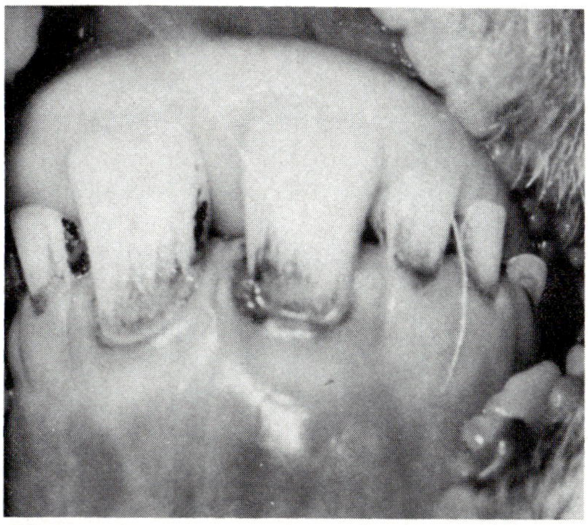

Figure 16–5. A 1 year, 4 month old sheep with permanent central incisors and three pairs of temporary rostral teeth.

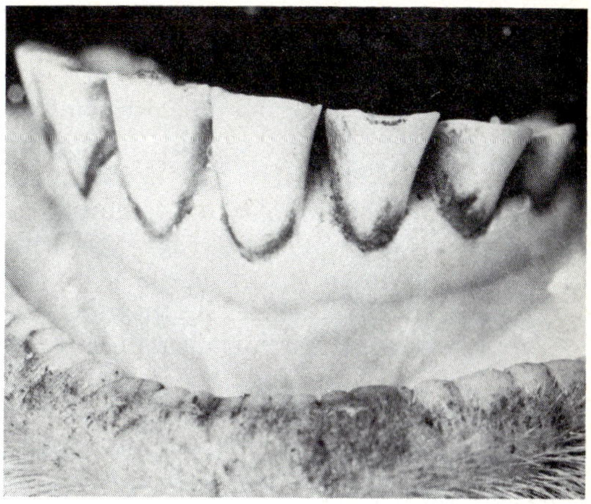

Figure 16–6. This 4 year old male goat has all permanent rostral teeth.

surface of the tooth, and as wear proceeds a thin layer of dentin is exposed, which assumes an oval shape and later encloses an area of darker secondary dentin. As attrition occurs, the dentinal layers become rectangular and then square. The rostral border of the outward surface is at first higher than the caudal border, producing a curved dental arcade for all eight rostral teeth. As attrition advances, the occlusal surface becomes hollow, and the rostral and caudal tooth borders are about the same height. The gradual erosion of the teeth results in a change in the dental arch from curved to almost straight, and later there is a separation between each of the crowns. Further attrition results in the teeth becoming little more than stumps. The lingual surface of the tooth is pitted by ridges. When these ridges have been removed and the crown enamel is lost, the tooth is said to be leveled.

Lower Cheek Teeth

There is a large gap, or diastema, separating the rostral teeth from the caudal, or cheek, teeth. Three premolar and three molar teeth are found in each half of the mandible. Only the premolar teeth are represented in the temporary dentition. There is a progressive increase in size from the rostral to the caudal cheek teeth in both the mandible and the maxilla.[1] The occlusal surface of the teeth is described as selenodont; that is, the cusps in cross section are crescent-shaped.[6] When compared with those in other groups of animals, the molar teeth in ruminants possess very high crowns and are referred to as hypselodont. The lingual surface of the crown is higher than the buccal surface; the former has longitudinal ridges on its surface and the latter is convex.

Some anatomists consider it correct to number the premolar teeth from the diastema caudally as the second, third, and fourth teeth.[7] This takes into consideration the fact that the number of premolars in mammals is four per quadrant.[8] However, there is neither an upper nor a lower first premolar, and in practice the premolars are enumerated from the rostral tooth backward as the first, second, and third premolar or cheek teeth. The molars are likewise considered as the first, second, and third molars or the fourth, fifth, and sixth cheek teeth.

Cattle. The deciduous first lower premolar in cattle is a small, low-crowned tooth consisting of a single cusp. It usually possesses two roots, but they may be fused. Only the caudal part of the occlusal surface is in contact with the upper teeth. The deciduous second premolar is irregular, and the occlusal surface is roughly triangular. The tooth has both a rostral and a caudal root. The deciduous third premolar has three complete cusp units, which are supported by three roots. The extra root arises from the lateral cusp of the middle unit and is between the rostral and caudal roots.

The first permanent premolar (Fig. 16–7) is similar to the temporary tooth but is larger. Both the second and third permanent premolars tend to be similar to the second temporary premolar. Their shape on the occlusal surface is irregular, and two deep grooves are usually present on the lingual surface. In some animals, the caudal groove of the second premolar is absent and is replaced by a small infundibulum. The teeth have two roots—one rostral root that tends to be vertical and one caudal root that is inclined caudally. An accessory third root is sometimes present in the third permanent premolar.

The lower molars are narrower than the upper ones. The first and second molar teeth display four cusps, which are arranged in rostral and caudal pairs or units. An infundibulum separates the cusps of each unit, and tubercles are found labially between the two units. There is a root arising from each unit—the rostral one being vertical and the caudal one tending to be directed caudally. The height of the crown is greater on the lingual edge than on the buccal edge of the tooth. The third molar is unusual in that besides the four cusps found in the other two molars there is a fifth cusp that is attached caudally. A tubercle is present labially between the rostral and caudal units. The roots are still two, but the caudal one tends to be enlarged, triangular, directed caudally, and grooved on its lingual and buccal surfaces.

Upper Cheek Teeth

The convex lingual surface of the upper teeth crowns is shorter than the labial surface, and the latter has three longitudinal ridges. The cheek teeth increase in size from the first premolar to the third molar.

Cattle. The temporary first premolar in cattle is a small tooth of irregular shape (Fig. 16–8). The medial border of the tooth is somewhat rounded, and with wear the occlusal surface tends to become straight but inclines dorsally and reaches a point rostrally. One or more infundibula are found toward the lingual surface of the tooth. There are two main roots, but a small third root is often found just rostral and lingual to the caudal root. The temporary second premolar has

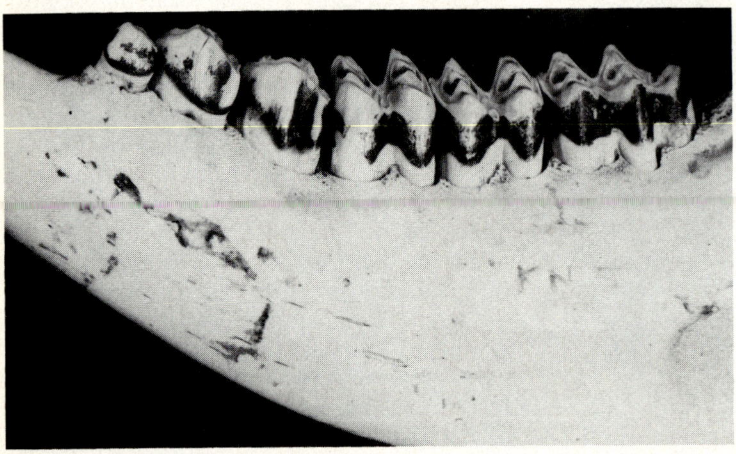

Figure 16–7. Bovine mandible showing permanent teeth.

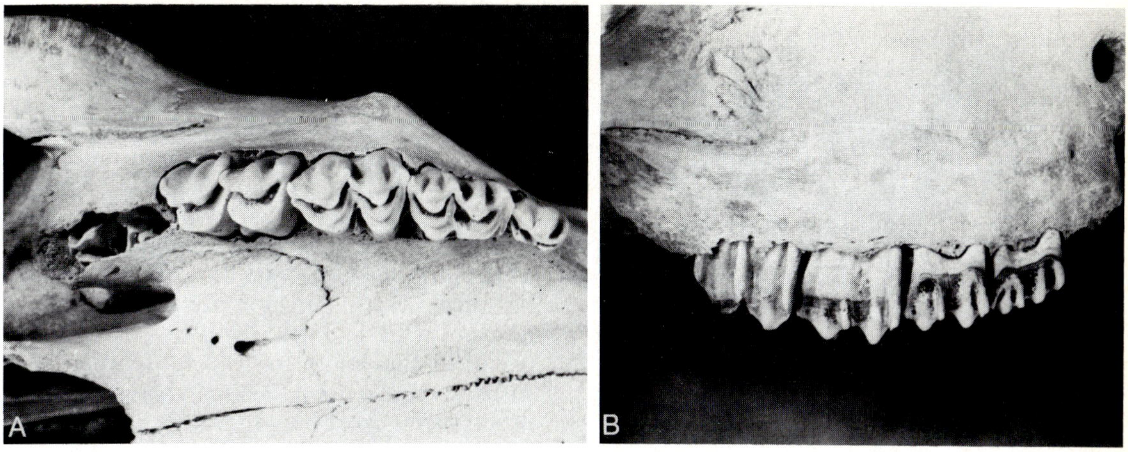

Figure 16–8. *A* and *B*, Temporary upper premolar teeth with first molar starting to erupt in an approximately 8 month old cow.

four major cusps arranged in rostral and caudal units. An irregular infundibulum is present between the cusps of each unit. It is crescent-shaped, with its concave border placed lingually. The buccal border is higher than the lingual border in this tooth and in the other cheek teeth. A single root is placed rostrally and two roots are placed caudally. The third temporary premolar has a shape that is similar to that of the second deciduous premolar, except there is a small tubercle placed lingually between the rostral and caudal units. There are a broad root placed lingually and smaller rostral and caudal roots placed labially.

The permanent first premolar (Fig. 16–9) is a single unit consisting of two cusps separated by a crescent-shaped infundibulum. The tooth has a rounded rostral border. There are two roots—rostral and caudal. The second and the third permanent premolars are similar and consist of a single large unit with a long infundibulum between the cusps. There are a broad root lingually and two roots buccally. The caudal roots of the second premolar consist of a broad rostral one and a smaller caudal one. There is a tendency for the rostral root of the third premolar to be less broad than the rostral root of the second premolar, but it is still larger than the distal root.

The crowns of all three upper molar teeth are similar, consisting of four cusps that are combined in pairs to form rostral and caudal units. The cusps in each unit are separated by a crescent-shaped infundibulum, which is concave buccally. Each tooth has three roots; one is beneath each buccal cusp and a wider one is present lingually. Vertical grooves are found on the side of the root facing the other

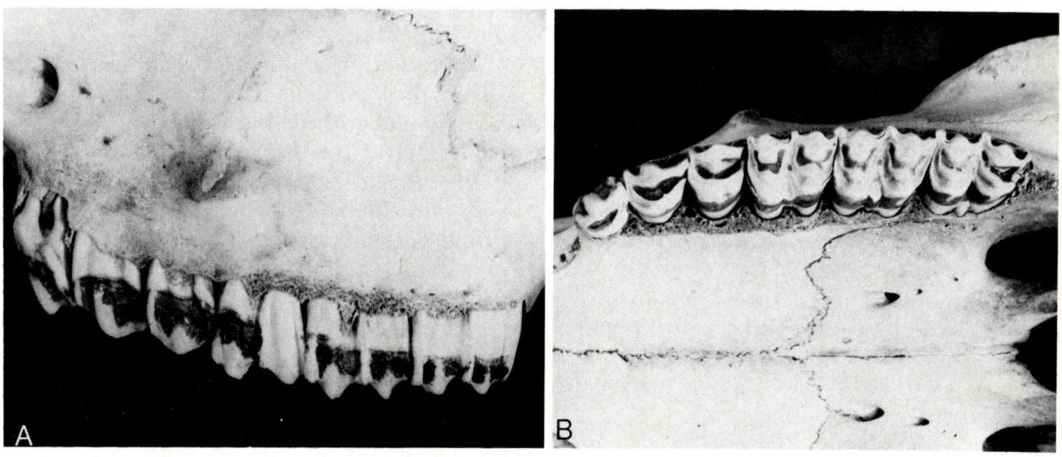

Figure 16–9. *A* and *B*, Upper permanent teeth of an approximately 4 year old cow.

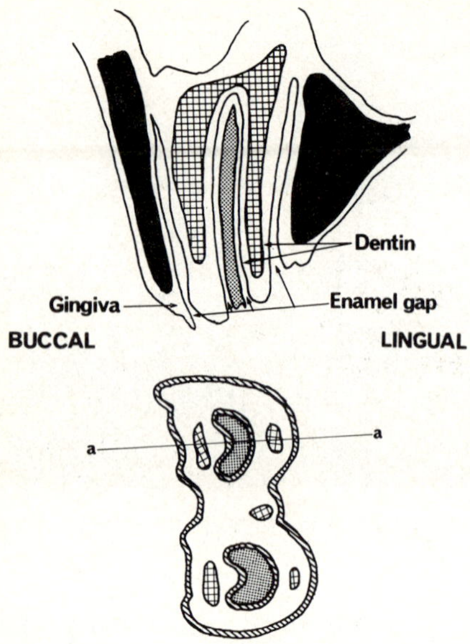

Figure 16–10. Vertical and transverse sections of an erupting upper second molar tooth. (See Fig. 16–3 for shading key.)

roots. There is a second groove on the lingual surface of the lingual root.

The molars of cattle have long crowns (hypselodontal), which continue to grow for some time after occlusal contact is made.[9] Constant use of the molars results in wear, which tends to be greater in soft cementum than in the harder enamel. As a result, sharp edges and cup-like erosions are produced, which provide a suitable surface for the shredding of herbage. This forms a very effective grinding mechanism when the lower teeth are swung upward against their counterparts. As attrition of the tooth crown occurs, the tooth erupts further to compensate. Although this resembles a continuously erupting tooth, roots are formed.

The anatomy of the vertical and transverse sections of an erupting second upper molar are seen in Figure 16–10. The tooth consists of an outer layer of enamel, which also borders the deep infundibula. Cementum may be present on the outside of the enamel and is particularly noticeable on the teeth of older animals, in which more of the crown is exposed following wear. An unusual form of less dense tissue resembling cementum fills the infundibulum and is often cellular in the newly formed tooth. Dentin forms the major part of each cusp and with wear, secondary dentin is exposed in the areas in which the pulp cavity previously existed.

Sheep and Goats. Morphologically, the cheek teeth of sheep and goats resemble those of cattle. They are covered with a thinner layer of cement, which often becomes discolored by food and takes on a black or silver-gray color. The occlusal surfaces of the teeth tend to be more sloped than those in cattle, because the difference in width between the upper and the lower jaws is greater in sheep and goats than it is in cattle.[10] Consequently, the lingual border of the lower tooth's occlusal surface and the buccal border of the upper tooth's occlusal surface tend to be very sharp. Attrition tends to become uneven with age so that two depressions occur in the lower teeth, one between the third premolar and the first molar and the other at the third molar level.[11]

Examination of the Cheek Teeth

In the living cow, examination of the cheek teeth is limited by their location and proximity to the buccal mucosa and the tongue.[12] Consequently, less information is available for these teeth than for the rostral teeth. Examination requires a good source of light, preferably positioned so that few shadows are produced.

The Drinkwater gag (Fig. 16–11) is useful for separating the cheek teeth, thereby allowing examination of the other half of the mouth. Practice will often allow satisfactory inspection of the molar teeth without a gag, provided that the animal is satisfactorily restrained (usually in a crush) so that no side to side, backward, or forward movement is possible. The ability to open the mouth in sheep is very restricted, so examination of the cheek teeth is difficult; however, it can be undertaken with a suitable gag (Fig. 16–12), light source (Fig. 16–13), and angled dental mirror. Room for examination is also restricted in goats; the cheek teeth are forced apart by a gag, and then an angled mirror and light source can be used.

Examination should reveal any hemorrhage, ulcer, vesicle, papule, pustule, or other lesion involving the labia, hard palate, gingivae, tongue, or buccal area. However, in many cases digital examination is also necessary and can be extremely helpful when defining and removing foreign material as well as when defining dental anomalies and soft tissue lesions. However, any such examination must be performed with a gloved hand because of the possibility of zoonotic infection such as rabies, bovine papular stomatitis, contagious pustular stomatitis, and foot and mouth disease, among others. The protected hand is also less likely to be traumatized by the teeth or jaws.

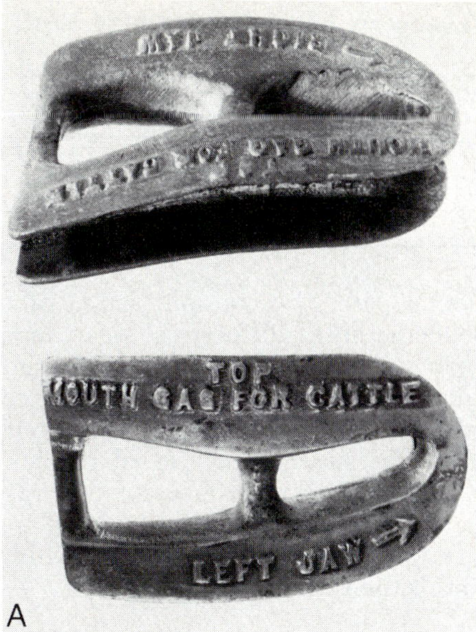

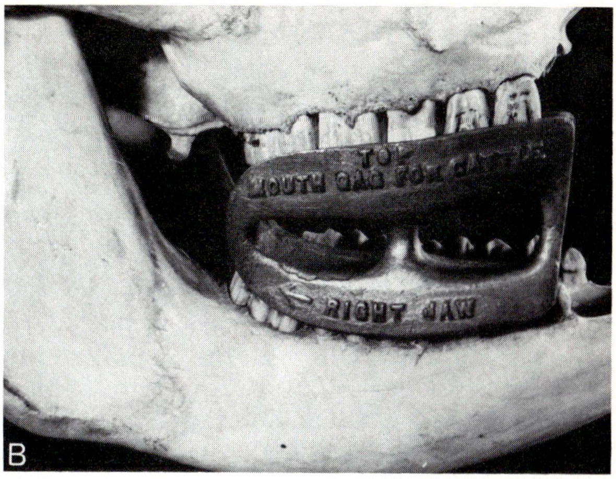

Figure 16–11. *A,* Drinkwater gag. *B,* The gag in position.

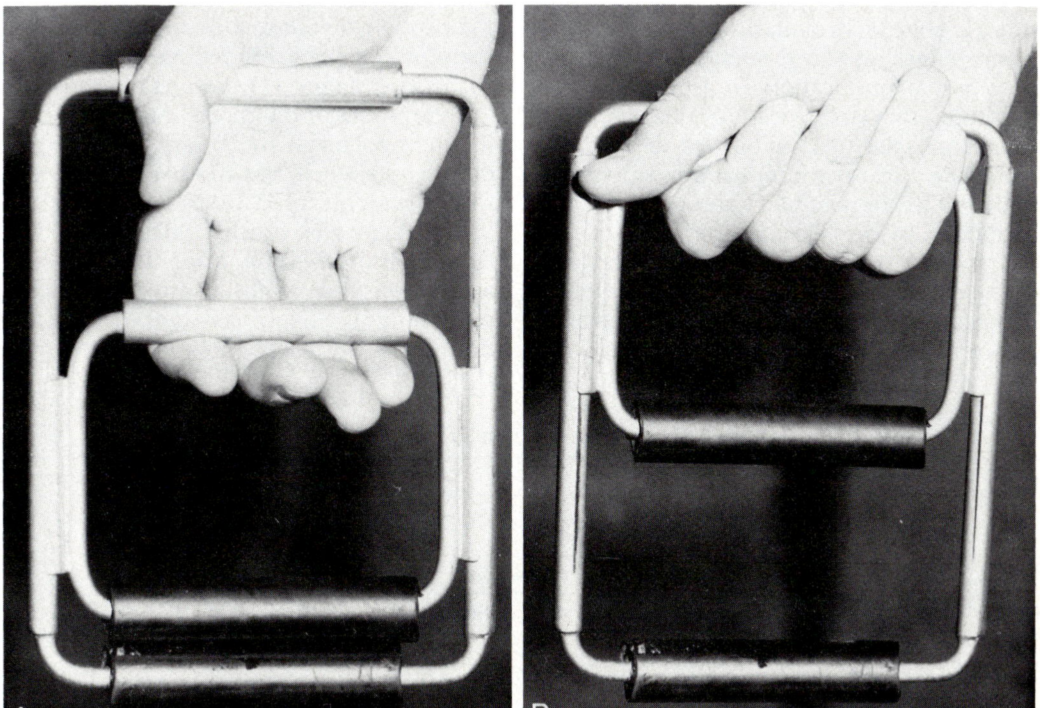

Figure 16–12. Gag for sheep and goats. *A,* In closed position for insertion. *B,* In open position for oral examination.

Figure 16–13. Pencil torch for oral examination.

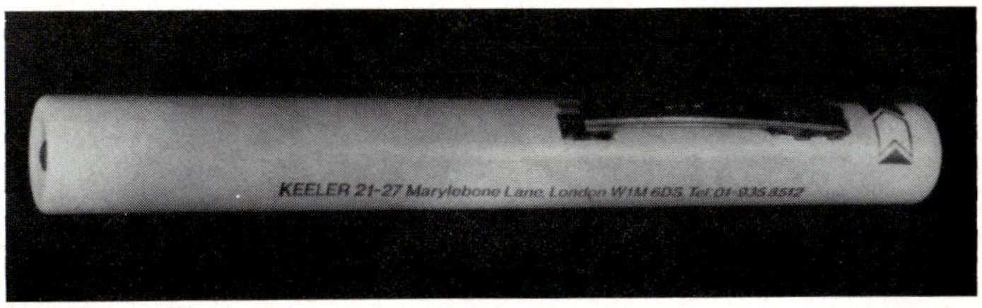

PREHENSION AND MASTICATION

Seizing and passing food into the mouth (prehension) in cattle is performed mainly by the tongue, which is muscular and long and can be protruded from the mouth. The tongue can be curled around a tuft of grass, which is then drawn into the mouth and is incised between the rostral teeth and the dental pad. The lips, though muscular, have a limited range of movement. In sheep, the tongue does not protrude from the mouth, but it does assist the rostral teeth in introducing food into the mouth, and the food is then nipped off. A philtrum or a cleft upper lip facilitates close grazing by sheep. Goats, which do not have a philtrum, do not graze as closely as sheep and use their teeth to strip bark and obtain twigs or tree branches. All ruminants drink by creating a negative pressure that sucks up liquid.

To ensure initial digestion of food in the rumen, it must be broken down into particles of short length and large surface area, either during initial mastication or during the remastication that follows regurgitation. The masseter muscles tend to be well developed. Side to side and up and down movements of the mandible are possible. Lateral movement is facilitated by the fact that the width of the lower jaw is less than that of the upper jaw. Excessive rostral tooth attrition, which would otherwise occur, is prevented by the replacement of the upper incisors and canines with the dental pad. The constant action of the cheek teeth causes differential wear among the enamel, dental, and cement components, helping to maintain a rough surface for continued grinding. Consequently, sharp edges occur on the lingual surfaces of the lower teeth and the buccal surfaces of the upper teeth. During mastication the bolus of food is thoroughly mixed and moistened with saliva and is then swallowed.

Table 16–1. Interval from First Emergence to Full Emergence of Permanent Rostral Teeth in Cattle

Rostral Tooth	Reference 23	Reference 24	Reference 25 (Zebu)
1st	5.9 wk	7.4 wk	12 wk
2nd	4.4 wk	7.8 wk	16 wk
3rd	5.3 wk	9.4 wk	16 wk
4th	9.8 wk	14.4 wk	24 wk

TOOTH ERUPTION

Eruption of the teeth can be divided into various stages. Prefunctional eruption involves two stages, (1) the intraosseous phase (development of the tooth in the bone crypt), which is followed by (2) an intraoral phase that ceases when the tooth is in apposition with the dental pad or the apposing tooth (the tooth against which it will occlude). Functional eruption occurs after the teeth are in apposition and results in the tooth height's remaining relatively constant despite attrition.

Table 16–2. Rostral Tooth Eruption in Cattle

Tooth	Germany[28]			Britain[29]	France[30]	Germany[31]
	Early Maturing	Mid-maturing	Late Maturing			
	Deciduous Teeth					
i1	Before birth	Before birth	Before birth	Before birth	Before or some days after birth	
i2	Before birth	Before birth	Before birth	Before birth	Before or some days after birth	
i3	Before birth	Before birth	2–6 d	Before birth–1–2 wk	14 d	
c	Before birth	2–6 d	6–14 d	Before birth–1–2 wk	2–3 wk	
	Permanent Teeth					
I1	1 yr 5 mo	1 yr 9 mo	2 yr 1 mo	1 yr 2 mo–2 yr 1 mo	1 yr 6 mo	1 yr 10 mo–2 yr
I2	1 yr 10 mo	2 yr 3 mo	2 yr 8 mo	1 yr 5 mo–3 yr	2 yr 6 mo	2 yr 4 mo–2 yr 7 mo
I3	2 yr 8 mo	3 yr	3 yr 4 mo	1 yr 10 mo–3 yr 4 mo	3 yr 6 mo	3 yr–3 yr 4 mo
C	3 yr	3 yr 9 mo	4 yr 4 mo	2 yr 8 mo–4 yr	4 yr 6 mo	3 yr 6 mo–4 yr 1 mo

Table 16–3. Rostral Permanent Tooth Eruption in Zebu Cattle (Months)

Tooth	Pakistan[32]		Cameroon[33]	Brazil[34]	Brazil[35]
	Sahiwal	Dajal			
I1	31.7	30.2	26	28.2	27.6
I2	40.0	39.2	32	35.4	34.8
I3	48.1	49.2	39	41.9	43.2
C	51.5	61.4	54	50.8	51.2

Table 16–4. Rostral Permanent Tooth Eruption in Buffalo (Pakistan[32])

Tooth	Months
I1	32.5
I2	39.8
I3	47.7
C	54.6

Factors Influencing Tooth Eruption

The eruption of teeth depends on various factors. Eruption of permanent teeth in the zebu type of cattle *(Bos indicus)* is slower than that in the European type of cattle *(Bos taurus)*.[13] Breed also seems to have an influence. The permanent teeth of Shorthorn cattle erupt before those of contemporary Aberdeen Angus, Hereford, Friesian, and Jersey cattle.[14, 15] Herefords have been shown to be slower in tooth eruption than other breeds, including Friesian, Aberdeen Angus, and dairy shorthorn.[16, 17] Calves from Jersey and Ayrshire parents had delayed emergence of some incisor pairs when compared with Friesians.[18] Similar breed differences occur in sheep, with the Wiltshire crosses replacing their first incisor pair before other crosses.[19] Other investigators, however, have not found differences in the age of eruption among breeds.[20–22]

Severe malnutrition with low body weight will delay eruption and, in some cases, the formation of teeth. A low plane of nutrition reduces incisor tooth eruption in cattle[14] and sheep.[19]

The time of year at birth can affect eruption; teeth in animals born between October and December emerged earlier, whereas the teeth of those born from January to March emerged later.[18]

Eruption of the bovine incisors in females occurred later than those in males in one report,[16] but other studies have not found consistent differences.[20]

Individual variation occurs in the eruption of teeth in cattle; teeth in some individuals may erupt as much as 5 months earlier or later than the mean eruption time.

Eruption of Rostral Teeth

Eruption of the permanent rostral teeth has been used for many years to estimate the age of ruminants for agricultural, veterinary, and archaeological purposes. Such knowledge has been considered important because it provides a quick check on the certified age of an animal, or it acts as a guide when no information is available. This is useful for the farmer in the market as well as for the research worker who is confronted with an animal of unknown age. Eruption status is also used as a criterion governing the entry of animals to various classes at agricultural and fatstock shows, and also as a guide when animals younger or older than certain ages receive subsidies from government departments wishing to promote certain trends in agriculture. When a national scheme is

Table 16–5. Rostral Tooth Eruption in Sheep

Deciduous Teeth

Tooth	*Britain*[29]	*Germany*[10]	*United States*[1]	*Britain*[36]
i1	Birth–1 wk	Before birth–up to 8 d	Birth–1 wk	Birth–1 mo
i2	Birth–1 wk	Before birth	1–2 wk	Birth–1 mo
i3	Birth–2 wk	Before birth	2–3 wk	Birth–1 mo
c	Birth–3 wk	Birth–up to 8 d	3–4 wk	Birth–1 mo

Permanent Teeth

Tooth	*Britain*[36]	*Britain*[29]	*Germany*[10]		*United States*[1]	*France*[38]	*France*[37]	*France*[39]
			Early Maturing	Late Maturing				
I1	12–15 mo	12–18 mo	12 mo	18 mo	12–18 mo	15–16 mo	15–18 mo	15–17 mo
I2	21 mo	18–24 mo	21 mo	24 mo	18–24 mo	24 mo	27 mo	21–27 mo
I3	27 mo	27–36 mo	27 mo	36 mo	30–36 mo	20–36 mo	42 mo	27–32 mo
C	31–36 mo	33–48 mo	36 mo	48 mo	42–48 mo	36–42 mo	48–54 mo	40–46 mo

Table 16–6. Eruption of Rostral Teeth in Goats

Deciduous Teeth

Tooth	*Britain*[29]	*Germany*[10]
i1	Birth	Birth
i2	Birth	Birth
i3	Birth	Birth
c	1–3 wk	1–3 wk

Permanent Teeth

Tooth	*Turkey*[40]	*Britain*[29]	*Britain*[29]	*Germany*[10]	*India*[41]	*Britain*[36]
		IMPROVED BREEDS	ROUGH BREEDS			
I1	15 ± ½–1 mo	15 mo	15 mo	15 mo	15–16 mo	14 mo
I2	24 ± 1–2 mo	21 mo	27 mo	21 mo	19–23 mo	24–36 mo
I3	31 ± 3½–4½ mo	27 mo	36 mo	27 mo	22–25 mo	36–48 mo
C	40 ± 6 mo	36 mo	40 mo	36 mo	26–30 mo	48–60 mo

Table 16–7. Classification of First and Second Molar Tooth Development

Molar Code Number	Stage of Development
0	First molar absent
1	Rostral part erupting, caudal part not visible
2	Rostral part one-fourth up, caudal part not visible
3	Rostral part one-fourth up or more, caudal part erupting
4	Rostral part one-half up, caudal part well erupted
5	Rostral part three-fourths up, caudal part one-half up or less
6	Rostral part three-fourths up or more, caudal part more than one-half up
7	Rostral part fully up, caudal part three-fourths up
8	Rostral and caudal parts fully up

Table 16–8. Cheek Teeth Eruption in Cattle

Temporary Teeth

Tooth	*?Mandibular 1834 France*[44]	*Mandibular 1855 England*[45]	*?Mandibular 1891 United States*[46]		*?Mandibular 19th Century France*[30]	*?Mandibular 1909 England*[47]	*?Mandibular 1943 Germany*[28]		
			PRECOCIOUS ANIMALS	COMMON ANIMALS			EARLY	MEDIUM	LATE
Premolar 1	6–12 d	After birth by 1 mo	6–12 d	18–30 d	Before or some days after birth	By 1 mo	Before birth	Soon after birth	14–21 d
Premolar 2	Soon after birth	After birth by 1 mo	Birth	After birth	Before or some days after birth	By 1 mo	Before birth	Soon after birth	14–21 d
Premolar 3	Soon after birth	After birth by 1 mo	Birth	After birth	Before or some days after birth	By 1 mo	Before birth	Soon after birth	14–21 d

Permanent Teeth

Tooth		*?Mandibular 1834 France*[44]	*?Mandibular 1839 France*[50]	*?Mandibular 1855 England*[45]	*?Mandibular 1891 United States*[46]	*?Mandibular 1894 France*[37]	*?Mandibular 19th Century France*[30]	*?Mandibular 1909 England*[47]	*?Mandibular 1943 Germany*[28]		
									EARLY	MEDIUM	LATE
Premolar	1		22 mo	30 mo	30 mo	29–31 mo	18 mo	30 mo	24 mo	26 mo	28 mo
	2		28–32 mo	30 mo	18 mo	29–31 mo	30 mo	30 mo	24 mo	26 mo	28 mo
	3		38–48 mo	30–36 mo	36 mo	34–35 mo	42 mo	36 mo	28 mo	31 mo	34 mo
Molar	1	6–12 mo	4–6 mo	6 mo	18 mo	6–7 mo	6–9 mo	6 mo	5 mo	5 mo	6 mo
	2	18 mo	16–22 mo	15 mo	24 mo	15–18 mo	30 mo	12 mo	15 mo	16 mo	18 mo
	3	24–30 mo	44–52 mo	24 mo	30 mo	25–28 mo	48–60 mo	24 mo	24 mo	26 mo	28 mo

adopted for controlling or eradicating certain diseases, age determination can form a guide if a group must be exempted from testing or injection because of age.

Most reports giving values for eruption of the rostral teeth do not state whether the figures are based on one stage of tooth eruption, such as the first appearance through the gingivae (emergence), or whether they include all stages of intraoral eruption. The time from the first appearance of the tooth to its being fully emerged (occluding with the dental pad) has been studied very little; available figures are given in Table 16–1.

Tables 16–2 through 16–6 give the eruption times of the deciduous and permanent rostral teeth for cattle of European, zebu, and buffalo types as well as for sheep and goats. The intraosseous development of bovine teeth can be established by radiography,[26] and has been studied.[20, 27]

Eruption of Cheek Teeth

Eruption of the cheek teeth has been studied much less than the eruption of rostral teeth. The lower cheek teeth erupt before their upper counterparts, and in the molar teeth the rostral unit emerges prior to the caudal one, so it has been possible to divide the intraoral eruption process in cattle into several stages (Table 16–7).

Table 16–9. Cheek Tooth Eruption in Buffalos[51]

Tooth		Temporary	Permanent
Premolar	1	4–7 d	34 mo
	2	5–8 d	47 mo
	3	4–7 d	48 mo
Molar	1		15 mo
	2		17 mo
	3		32 mo

It is not usually clear from published reports if values given are for lower or upper tooth eruption nor is it clear which stage is referred to. Most reported studies are based on the lower teeth of cadavers. In the live animal, it is extremely difficult to assess lower cheek teeth because they are hidden by the tongue and cheek. However, with practice and with the animal restrained, the upper molar teeth can be examined relatively easily (page 240). Values for deciduous and permanent cheek tooth eruption in cattle, buffalo, sheep, and goats are given in Tables 16–8 through 16–14.

The eruption of the cheek teeth can provide information about the age of an animal before rostral tooth emergence has occurred. Because the various stages of the intraoral eruption of each tooth can be studied (Tables 16–13 and 16–14), the age of an animal can be defined more exactly. Cheek teeth normally remain *in situ* in archaeological speci-

Table 16–8. Cheek Teeth Eruption in Cattle (*Continued*)

Temporary Teeth

Mandibular 1949 England[48]	*?Mandibular 1959 United States*[36]	*Mandibular 1960 United States*[20]	*?Mandibular 1961 United States*[1]	*?Mandibular 1969 England*[29]	*?Mandibular 1971 Holland*[49]
Around birth	Birth to 1 mo	2 wk	Birth to 2 wk	Birth to 3 wk	Birth to 1 wk
Around birth	Birth to 1 mo	2 wk	Birth to few d	Birth to 3 wk	Birth to 1 wk
Around birth	Birth to 1 mo	Birth	Birth to few d	Birth to 3 wk	Birth to 1 wk

Permanent Teeth

Mandibular 1949 England[48]	*?Mandibular 1959 England*[37]		*Mandibular 1960 United States*[20]	*?Mandibular 1961 United States*[1]	*?Mandibular 1969 England*[29]	*?Mandibular 1971 Holland*[49]
	HIGHLY BRED	COMMON				
26–27 mo	24 mo	30 mo	30–36 mo	24–30 mo	24–30 mo	24–30 mo
26–27 mo	24 mo	30 mo	24–30 mo	18–30 mo	18–30 mo	18–30 mo
33 mo	33 mo	36 mo	30–36 mo	30–36 mo	28–36 mo	20–36 mo
6 mo	6 mo	6 mo	5–6 mo	5–6 mo	5–6 mo	6 mo
12 mo	12–15 mo	15–18 mo	12 mo	12–18 mo	15–18 mo	12–18 mo
24 mo	21 mo	24 mo	24–30 mo	24–30 mo	24–30 mo	24–30 mo

Table 16–10. Cheek Tooth Eruption in Zebu Cattle[52]

Tooth		Temporary	Permanent
Premolar	1	Birth–1 mo	24 mo
	2	Birth–1 mo	24 mo
	3	Birth–1 mo	36 mo
Molar	1		6 mo
	2		18 mo
	3		24 mo

mens, whereas the rostral teeth are lost. Although it is not possible to undertake radiography in the conscious animal, some work has been undertaken on the development of the lower[20,42] and upper[43] cheek teeth. Development of the cheek teeth in sheep has also been studied.[11]

Gingivitis Resulting from Eruption

Eruption can result in a severe gingival reaction. In some sheep and cattle, the gum is carried with the erupting tooth, forming an "eruptive collar" of very vascular tissue that is part of the dental sac or follicle.[54] Occasionally the tooth can be nearly fully erupted before the gum is pierced and starts to recede; marked generalized inflammation with connective tissue proliferation may result. Bacterial infection also is often present, with a varying amount of purulent exudate. The gingivitis can persist for many months and may result in the formation of scar tissue. Although this gingival reaction is very common in cattle, it is unusual in sheep and goats. The resulting inflammation can cause

Table 16–12. Cheek Tooth Eruption in Goats

Temporary Teeth			
Tooth		*Britain*[29]	*Germany*[11]
Premolar	1	3 mo	3 mo
	2	3 mo	3 mo
	3	3 mo	3 mo

Permanent Teeth					
Tooth		*Britain*[29]		*Germany*[11]	*Turkey*[40]
		Improved Breeds	Rough Breeds		
Premolar	1	17 mo	20 mo	17–20 mo	Approximately 22 mo
	2	17 mo	20 mo	17–20 mo	Approximately 22 mo
	3	17 mo	20 mo	17–20 mo	Approximately 22 mo
Molar	1	5–6 mo	5–6 mo	5–6 mo	3 mo
	2	8–10 mo	12 mo	8–10 mo	11 mo
	3	18–24 mo	30 mo	18–24 mo	20 mo

inappetence and loss of condition in otherwise healthy animals. This is particularly the case in 1½ to 3 year old cattle who are forced to self-feed silage from an impacted clamp or when the grass is of a particularly fibrous nature.

Posteruption Changes. As the permanent cheek teeth are used, attrition occurs. However, the height of the exposed crown remains almost constant. This is because of the continued eruption of the tooth following apposition with its counterpart in the other dental arcade. If the apposing tooth is lost, progression of the tooth continues, producing a crown that is distorted and taller than that of its neighbors. The continued eruption of the cheek teeth is due to the deposition of secondary cement and dentin to the roots, thereby slowly raising the crown from its alveolus. This deposition of cementum can

Table 16–11. Cheek Tooth Eruption in Sheep

Deciduous Teeth				
Tooth		*Britain*[29]	*Germany*[11]	*United States*[1]
Premolar	1	Birth–6 wk	Before birth up to 4 wk	2–6 wk
	2	Birth–6 wk	Before birth up to 4 wk	2–6 wk
	3	Birth–6 wk	Before birth up to 4 wk	2–6 wk

Permanent Teeth					
Tooth		*England*[29]	*Germany*[11]		*United States*[1]
			Early Maturing	Late Maturing	
Premolar	1	21–24 mo	3 mo	3 mo	18–24 mo
	2	21–24 mo	9 mo	9 mo	18–24 mo
	3	21–24 mo	18 mo	18 mo	18–24 mo
Molar	1	Upper: 5 mo Lower: 3 mo	21 mo	24 mo	Upper: 5 mo Lower: 3 mo
	2	9–12 mo	21 mo	24 mo	9–12 mo
	3	18–24 mo	21 mo	24 mo	18–24 mo

Table 16–13. Age in Days at Each Stage of First Upper Molar Development[53]

Molar Code Number*	Minimum Age	Maximum Age	Median Age
0	—	237	—
1	162	258	208
2	191	282	227
3	201	310	259.5
4	224	359	292
5	245	380	340
6	286	405	370
7	305	448	373.5
8	311	512	429

*See Table 16–7.

also occur on the crown, producing a ridged effect. As crown attrition occurs, the relationship among enamel, dentin, and cementum changes. Following eruption, the tooth is covered by enamel, but wear exposes the dentin rostrally and then caudally. These areas of exposed dentin can be diagrammatically represented,[40] and they gradually unite, forming a double square shape in the first and second lower molars (□□), which is the main pattern for cheek teeth.

DEVELOPMENTAL ABNORMALITIES OF TEETH

Gross Abnormalities

Absence of Rostral Teeth. Rostral anodontia (complete absence of all deciduous or permanent teeth) and oligodontia (many teeth missing and those present of reduced size) are both extremely rare. However, hypodontia, or partial anodontia, in which a few teeth are absent, is quite common and results from the absence of or failure of development of one or more tooth buds.

Table 16–14. Age in Days at Each Stage of Second Upper Molar Development[53]

Molar Code Number*	Minimum Age	Maximum Age	Median Age
0	—	514	—
1	400	542	497
2	417	562	532.5
3	444	602	540
4	502	697	560
5	481	771	621.5
6	569	728	631
7	520	782	658
8	539	879	694.5

*See Table 16–7.

More cases occur in the permanent dentition than in the temporary dentition. If the permanent tooth is lacking, the temporary tooth may be retained.[55] Partial anodontia usually is not associated with other developmental abnormalities. Complete absence of temporary and permanent rostral teeth on one side of the mandible can occur. The most common rostral pair deficiency is that of the temporary[55] or permanent canines; this condition is usually bilateral in cattle, sheep, and goats. Diagnosis can be confirmed by radiography.

Absence of Cheek Teeth. From my experience, the absence of one or more cheek teeth is more common than the absence of rostral teeth, though detailed surveys are lacking. The tooth most commonly absent in cattle, sheep, and goats is the first permanent lower premolar. This tooth may be absent on one or both sides, and the temporary predecessor may also be absent. The condition has also been seen in archaeological specimens dating from Neolithic times.[56] In the primitive British Chillingham breed, the first premolar was considered to be absent.[57] Loss of teeth can be inherited in some species,[58] though other factors can be involved, including those that interfere with the formation of the tooth bud during fetal growth, such as nutritional deficiencies in pregnancy, endocrine dysfunction in the mother, and the severe effects of pyrexia and ectodermal toxins.[59] Other teeth fail to develop rarely; absence of the first upper molar in cattle has been reported.[60] Radiography is necessary to confirm the diagnosis. Breeding studies to establish a pattern of inheritance in cattle or sheep have not been conducted.

Absence of Cusps. The third mandibular molar consists of five cusps, four of which are arranged into rostral and caudal pairs or units. An infundibulum separates the cusps of each unit, and the fifth cusp is attached to the caudal unit. However, the fifth cusp commonly is absent in modern and archaeological specimens of cattle, sheep, and goats.[54] Other animals may have only rudimentary fifth cusps.[61] Such abnormalities are easily seen only on *postmortem* examination.

Supernumerary Rostral Teeth. Additional teeth occur much less frequently than does partial anodontia. Specimens with 24 rostral teeth,[62] double dentition,[63] and an extra permanent incisor[55] have been described. Occasionally rudimentary canine teeth are found in the maxilla in cattle,[64] goats,[64] and sheep.[65]

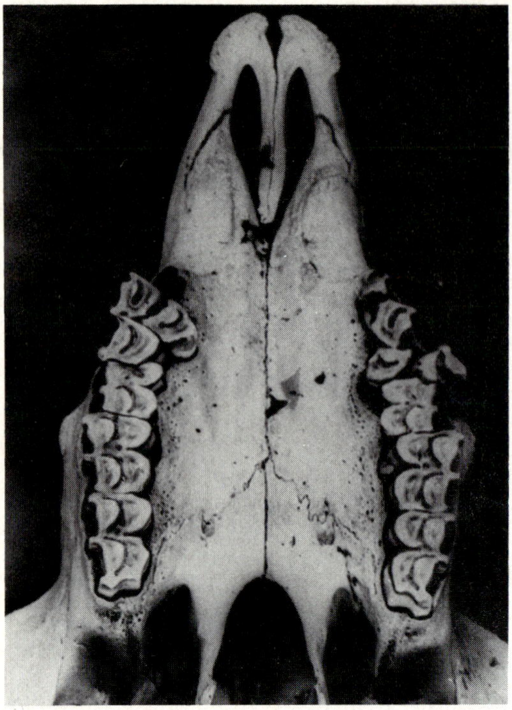

Figure 16–14. Mouflon with additional premolar teeth of the second premolar type with consequent irregular alignment and rotation of some teeth. (Courtesy of B. Noddle.)

Supernumerary Caudal Teeth. This is very rare. When it occurs, the premolar teeth are usually involved (Fig. 16–14).

Increased Root Formation. This is not uncommon in cheek teeth. There is often a tendency in the first premolar for a third root to develop from the caudal one.[66]

Retention of Temporary Teeth with Permanent Tooth Eruption. In some animals, the deciduous rostral teeth are retained for some time after the eruption of the permanent successors. In sheep, the commonly persisting temporary teeth are caudal to the permanent teeth.[54] Persistence also occurs with maleruption of the permanent successors.[67]

Accessory Cusps on Rostral Teeth. The labial surface of bovine rostral teeth may show a secondary cusp. The cusp is of varying size, but it may be quite considerable. The teeth most commonly affected are the permanent incisors. Following use, the cusp is normally lost by natural attrition.

Macrodontia of Rostral Teeth. Occasionally, exceptionally large pairs of rostral teeth are produced in cattle and sheep. The teeth often develop a three- or four-sided appearance rather than a two-sided one with concave and convex surfaces. The roots of such teeth are also enlarged.

Macrodontia of Cheek Teeth. This appears to be rarer than the rostral form of macrodontia and may just be a relative increase in size.

Parts of Cheek Teeth Developing Independently. Two individual teeth have been observed to develop from the rostral and caudal parts of the second lower molar. The anomaly was bilateral.[55] The two individual units were smaller than the normal tooth. In the lower third molar three different parts were produced.

Failure of Tooth Eruption. This may be due to teeth being abnormally positioned or the normal eruptive process failing to occur. It is very unusual for the condition to occur in ruminants, since the jaws are not overcrowded with teeth. It is most likely to occur in the cheek teeth. Confirmation of the diagnosis is by radiography.

Partial Eruption. This is due to cessation of root growth, thereby allowing only partial eruption of the crown, because of an injury to the developing tooth. The condition is extremely rare.

Impeded Eruption. Normally, this results from the premature loss of a tooth, which allows the neighboring teeth to partially migrate into the vacated space, preventing the eruption of the successor. Other cases can occur as a result of brachygnathia. The tooth is absent grossly but can be seen on radiographs. It is an extremely rare abnormality.

Prolonged Temporary Dentition. The temporary teeth may be retained if the premature successors are absent. Any systemic illness that occurs during the process of permanent tooth development may also delay eruption in cattle,[55] sheep,[54] and goats. Other problems, such as malnutrition, deficiency diseases, or lack of thriftiness resulting from parasitic gastroenteritis, can also lead to retarded eruption.

Alignment Irregularities

Crowded Rostral Teeth. Slight alignment irregularities occur, especially in the permanent central incisors; such irregularities may only indicate that the 90° rotation that occurs in normal eruption is not complete. In many instances in sheep[54] and cattle,[55] these conditions are self-correcting with subsequent jaw development. However, they may persist.[62]

Crowded Cheek Teeth. Occasionally there are irregularities in the position of the cheek

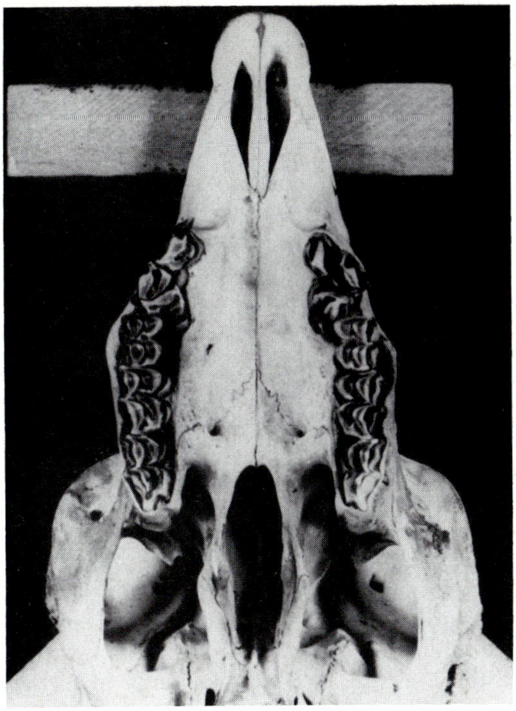

Figure 16–15. Maxilla of mouflon showing overcrowding of the cheek teeth with displacement and rotation of the third permanent premolar. (Courtesy of B. Noddle.)

teeth. This can particularly affect the premolar teeth; a goat with the third right premolar and the second left premolar displaced inward has been reported;[62] it has also been seen in the mouflon[67] (Fig. 16–15).

Displaced Cheek Teeth. Affected calves show the six lower premolars impacted or erupted in an abnormal position. The condition does not affect the upper premolars or rostral teeth and leads to the death of the calf during the first week of life. The abnormality is inherited as a single recessive gene.[69] It has also been reported in the goat.[62]

Rotation of Rostral Teeth. The permanent teeth are sometimes rotated 90° or 180° in their alveoli.[62] The problem appears to be a developmental anomaly in that there is usually no overcrowding, and it affects both members of the pair.

Rotation of Cheek Teeth. This condition has not been reported in the temporary dentition. Rotation of the cheek teeth occasionally occurs, and is most common in the first permanent mandibular premolar.[55] Rotation is usually about 90°.

Malposed Rostral Teeth. The permanent rostral teeth may erupt outside the normal dental arch and appears to occur particularly in Hereford cattle. Often, these teeth do not serve a useful purpose and may cause trauma during prehension and mastication.

Malposed Cheek Teeth. Occasionally, the cheek teeth erupt outside the dental arch or at unusual angles. These conditions affect mainly the permanent premolars. This lack of contact may result in an abnormally long crown for the teeth in the apposing jaw.

Crowded Cheek Teeth. This condition is unusual because of the long diastema. When crowding occurs, it will normally result in partial rotation of a tooth.

Enlarged Interdental Space. Spaces often develop between the cheek teeth, which allows the introduction and impaction of feed material, thereby causing gingivitis and, in some cases, resulting in a breakdown of the periodontal membrane. Space between the second and third lower premolar teeth is common. The caudal part of the temporary second premolar tends to impinge on this area during the eruption of its permanent successor and ultimately becomes wedged in the gap.

Compositional Abnormalities

Dental Hypoplasia. This condition is often associated with fluorosis, but dental hypoplasia, discoloration, and enamel erosion can occur in the deciduous rostral teeth of calves following the dam's exposure to radiation,[70] though the cheek teeth are relatively normal. The differentiating odontoblasts and ameloblasts are sensitive to radiation, resulting in the temporary or permanent cessation of dentin and enamel matrix formation.

Hypoplasia of the Temporary Dentition. This condition is relatively uncommon, particularly when compared with hypoplasia of the permanent successors. However, the labial surfaces of the third incisor teeth in calves often contain a hypoplastic pit near the mesial border.[55] The pit is of no detriment to the animal and does not extend completely through the enamel layer.

Hypoplasia of the Permanent Teeth. Disturbances occurring during permanent tooth development may cause abnormalities in the erupted tooth. Causes include prolonged pyrexia, malnutrition, deficiency diseases, and toxicity (such as fluorosis). The ameloblasts that are active at the time of the disturbance tend to reduce or cease enamel formation, and they are not reactivated after the insult has ended, so enamel defects in that area are not repaired. However, the ameloblasts that are not activated at the time of the disturbance are unaffected, and they assume their predetermined function. In minor disruptions, the enamel becomes pitted; in more severe cases, the outer layers of enamel may be minimal or nonexistent and the tooth is small.

Hypocalcification and Abnormal Calcium Salt Formation. Calcium salts of reduced quantity may be produced and may involve all the tooth constituents or just the enamel layer. The amount of calcium present in this condition may be normal, but the inorganic salts of the teeth are not of constant composition, so the salts produced may be of reduced hardness. It is seen in cattle[55] and sheep[54] and can be the result of imbalances in calcium, phosphorus, and vitamin D, of parathyroid and other endocrine disturbances, of drought conditions, or of exposure to excessive fluoride.

Teeth of Poor Quality. This condition has been described as affecting the permanent teeth more frequently than the temporary teeth,[55] but it involves all the teeth. Although the teeth look normal, there is an increased rate of wear, and they may be slightly more translucent.

Brown Teeth. This condition can occur in the temporary and permanent teeth and may involve all the dental layers. The distribution of the pigmentation may be patchy and may be of genetic origin.[71]

Incomplete Enamel Maturation. This condition is more common in the permanent teeth than in the temporary teeth, and it may involve all or part of the enamel, which is soft, opaque, and yellow-brown. The dentin is also affected, allowing bacterial penetration. Usually both teeth in a pair are affected. It is thought to be the result of a defective tooth germ. The putrefaction will often involve the alveolus and gingivae, resulting in pus formation that produces a foul smell.

Chalky Teeth. A chalky appearance of the tooth (dull, nontranslucent surface) can result from systemic and dietary disturbances. The systemic disturbance form affects all or part of the enamel in both teeth in a pair; the condition involves the whole enamel layer and is caused by a fault in production of the interprismatic substance. A second form, caused by dietary deficiency and imbalance, can cause the enamel of all the permanent teeth to be soft, chalky, and opaque. The teeth often become brown-yellow because of pigment absorption. Not all animals in a group will be affected to the same extent, and the condition can be corrected in those teeth that are still forming by adjusting the diet.

Enamel Flecks. These small opaque spots in the enamel on the labial surface in both the temporary and the permanent dentition occur in one or more rostral teeth in 65 percent of all mature cattle.[55] Both teeth in a pair are usually affected, and there may be multiple flecks on a tooth. It is common in certain cattle families. The spots are white to yellow-brown or black, and they darken with age. It has been suggested that the cause is a lack of the interprismatic layer or hypocalcification.[71] When these flecks reach the occluded surface they are rapidly worn away, resulting in the formation of a notch. The eroded underlying areas are prone to caries formation.

Irregular Enamel. The deposition of enamel in the incisor teeth can be abnormal, resulting in an irregular surface on either the permanent rostral or the permanent cheek teeth. The prism structure is also laid abnormally in affected animals. The durability of the enamel is normal.

Vertical Folds on Rostral Tooth Surface. Folding of the dentin and enamel junction before tissue formation causes a deep vertical pit on the labial surface of the rostral teeth. The tooth is still functional.

Odontoma. This condition affects the lower or upper cheek teeth, mainly in cattle. The tumors can be divided into two types.[72] Those that are derived from the whole dental germ and contain enamel, cement, and dentin are known as ameloblastic odontomas. The other type is ameloblastoma derived from enamel epithelium. The lesion may be calcified or uncalcified and may be connected with the dental alveoli. It may either interfere with tooth eruption or cause a bulge in the maxillary or mandibular bone.

Cementoma. These are regions of cemental hyperplasia on the roots of teeth. This condition is quite common in sheep and usually affects the cheek teeth.

Hamartoma. An occasional mass attached to the erupting bovine cheek teeth[73] (particularly the molar teeth) has been found. The mass is often adherent to a cusp or cusps and is raised above the level of the surrounding tissue. Histological examination (Fig. 16–16) shows a trabeculate structure; some of the intertrabeculate areas are empty or contain

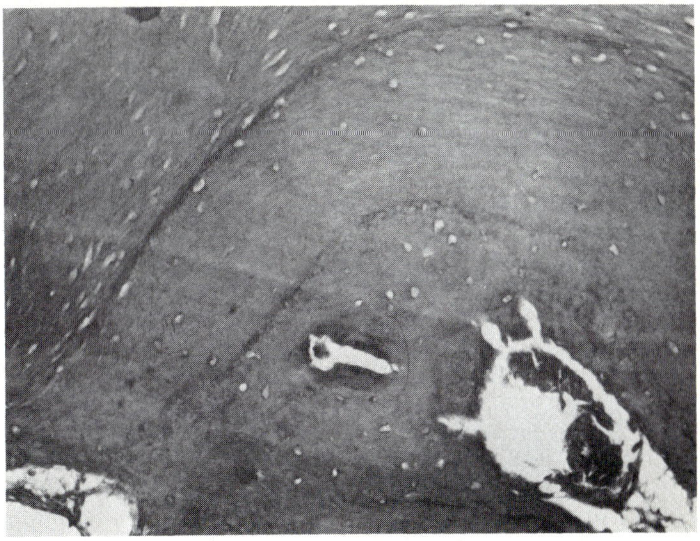

Figure 16–16. Longitudinal section of a hamartoma on the second molar of a steer. (Delafield's hematoxylin, magnification × 40.)

the remnants of vascular tissue. The structure appears to consist of cement rather than bone, and no dentin or enamel is found.

Clinical Significance of Congenital Abnormalities

Most abnormalities are isolated incidents and rarely affect the animal significantly. If several similar cases occur, the etiology should be investigated; abnormalities caused by poor nutrition can be prevented or corrected.

DEVELOPMENTAL ABNORMALITIES OF THE MANDIBLE, MAXILLA, AND MOUTH

Mandibular Prognathism (Brachycephalism, Overshot Jaw). "Prognathism" is the term used when the lower jaw protrudes beyond the upper jaw. Mandibular length is usually normal, and the condition is more correctly referred to as brachycephalism. There is a minor degree of prognathism in almost all calves (Fig. 16–17) and in many sheep and goats at birth, but it disappears following weaning. The condition is considered a serious defect in all ruminants, because it may affect the apposition of the upper and lower cheek teeth or the contact of the rostral teeth with the dental pad, impairing the ability to graze and masticate. At one time, pedigree bulls received a British reproductive license only if the two central pairs of incisors were in contact with the rostral half of the dental pad. A survey in Britain showed that 3.3 percent of dairy breeds and their crosses, 13 percent of Shorthorns and their crosses, and 14 percent of beef breeds and their crosses had some extent of prognathism;[74] the distribution among animals with temporary or permanent teeth was similar, suggesting there was little change with maturation. In my experience, prognathism often improves with age. A similar finding occurred in the offspring of one bull. In these calves, prognathism was present at birth; this was hard to detect at 3 months of age and was nonexistent by 1 year of age. It

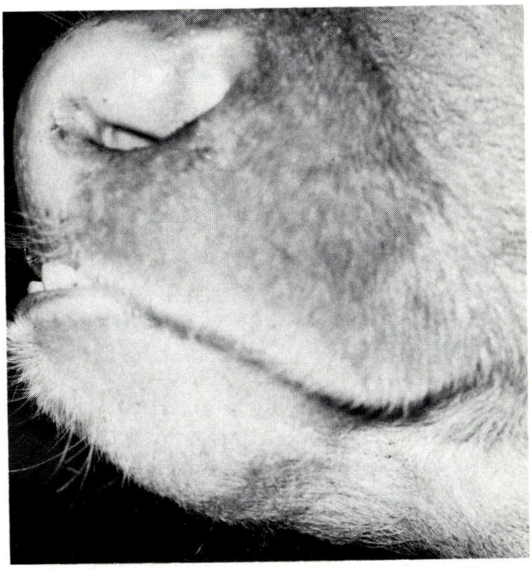

Figure 16–17. Mandibular prognathism (overshot jaw) in a young calf. This is normal during the first few weeks of life.

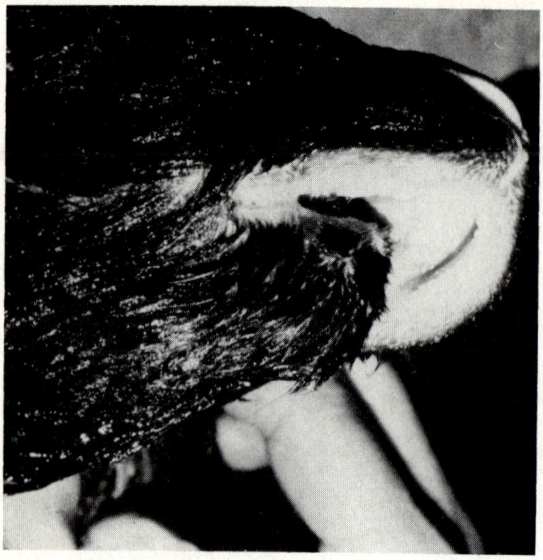

Figure 16–18. Severe brachygnathia in a calf. (Courtesy of A. Ash.)

was suggested in this case that the inheritance had an autosomal dominant pattern with incomplete penetrance.[75]

Mandibular Brachygnathia (Parrot Mouth, Parrot Beak, Undershot Jaw). A short mandible may be difficult to distinguish from dolichocephaly ("superior prognathism"). This defect may occur in an otherwise normal animal. The degree of the defect varies considerably, but if it is severe (Fig. 16–18), impaction of the cheek teeth may occur.[76] The condition can occur with other congenital defects, such as autosomal trisomies and chromosomal abnormalities. Brachygnathia is one of the characteristics of osteopetrosis in Aberdeen Angus cattle.[77] It is also present in the severe congenital skeletal abnormality known as acroteriasis congenita.[78]

Other Jaw Abnormalities. Lateral deviation of the face with normal mandibular development is occasionally seen.

The absence of the mandible is extremely rare and is usually fatal.[79] The jaw may be absent in animals born with other rare and lethal facial syndromes, such as facelessness.[80] Extreme reduction in the size of the mandible has been reported.[81]

Epignathus (the presence of a second, smaller part of the jaw bone attached to the mandible or maxilla) and otognathia (a rudimentary accessory mandible containing teeth, lips, and buccal mucous membranes that is found at the base of the pinna) occur rarely. Otognathic lesions may be continuous with the pharyngeal mucous membrane through the branchial fistula, and may contain a rudimentary tongue connected to the normal organ. Others form a pocket. Otognathia has been recorded in sheep.

Rotation of the rostral mandible has been observed in cattle.[55] The result is a lack of effective apposition of the teeth with the dental pad; thus, the teeth can take little part in prehension. The rotation may be due to a congenital defect or to trauma.

Slow or reduced development of the mandible may result in crowding of the rostral teeth. In normal eruption, the teeth undergo rotation as well as rostral movement; crowding prevents normal rotation.

The presence of a second jaw bone or a partial one that is the same size as the original jaw bone (dignathus) is a rare congenital condition.

Achondroplasia (Dwarfism, Bulldog Calf). This condition includes many congenital defects. The animals have short legs, wide and short-domed heads, and protruding mandibles. The head is excessively large, with a protruding forehead, bulging eyes, and obstructed respiratory passages. The tip of the tongue protrudes from the mouth, and the maxillae are distorted. Following birth, growth is reduced owing to abdominal distention and persistent bloat. There are two genetic forms of the condition—one is an autosomal dominant trait that is found in the Dexter breed, and the other is a simple recessive trait that is most common in Hereford and Aberdeen Angus cattle but also occurs in Shorthorns and Holsteins.

Cleft Chin. In some cattle, particularly Herefords, there is an obvious notch at the mandibular symphysis, which can result in the central incisors being directed slightly toward each other, causing a loss of enamel and dentin from their medial borders.

Cleft Palate. This is the most commonly reported congenital midline defect of the face, and it occurs in cattle (Fig. 16–19), sheep, and goats. Some cases are associated with other congenital defects, such as arthrogryposis,[82] and it is occasionally seen in animals with the "crooked calf disease" syndrome caused by feeding lupins *(Lupinus sericeus* and *L. caudatus)* to pregnant cattle in the second and third months of gestation.[83] It has been seen in acroteriasis congenita (a severe congenital condition), which involves absence of limbs and facial skeleton defects.[78] Ingesta escapes from the nostrils during feeding. Treatment has not been attempted in ruminants.

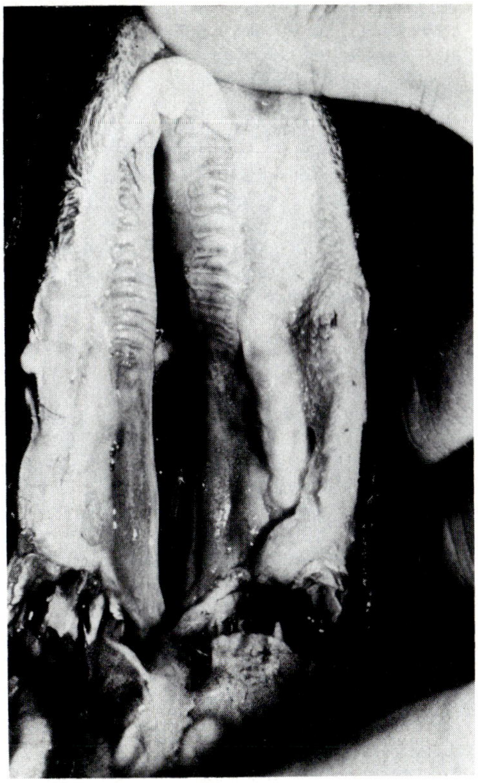

Figure 16–19. Cleft palate in a calf. (Courtesy of A. Ash.)

Harelip (Cheilognathoschisis). This condition is seen occasionally in cattle and goats. It usually occupies a median position, but it may be lateral in all species, including sheep. A bilateral condition also affecting the maxilla has been reported in Texel sheep.[84] A familial tendency for harelip has been reported in Shorthorn cattle.[85] The lip edges may be incised, provided that there is sufficient tissue, and the skin edges may be sutured with nonabsorbable material.

Tongue Abnormalities. "Smooth tongue" (epitheliogenesis imperfecta) has been recorded in Holstein, Friesian, and Brown Swiss cattle. The lingual filiform papillae are small, resulting in the smooth tongue effect. The calves tend to be unthrifty, produce excessive salivation, and have a poor, stary coat. The condition is inherited through an autosomal recessive gene.

The absence of the tongue (aglossia) in ruminants is exceptionally rare. The presence of a small tongue (hypoglossia) is unusual and usually accompanies agnathia or micrognathia. An excessively large tongue (macroglossia) that protrudes between the rostral teeth and the dental pad is unusual. It has been tentatively recognized in the belted Galloway, but the relative size of the tongue tended to decrease with increasing age.

Glossoschisis (forked tongue, snake tongue) is recognized very occasionally.

References

1. Sisson S, Grossman JD: The Anatomy of the Domestic Animals, 4th ed. Philadelphia, WB Saunders Co., 1953, pp. 451–454.
2. Young JZ: The Life of Vertebrates, 2nd ed. Oxford, Oxford University Press, 1962, p. 575.
3. Tomes CS: A Manual of Dental Anatomy: Human and Comparative, 3rd ed. London, J & A Churchill, 1889, pp. 387–415.
4. Tims HWM, and Henry CB (eds): Tomes' Manual of Dental Anatomy: Human and Comparative, 8th ed. London, J & A Churchill, 1923, p. 462.
5. Loomis FR: Dentition of artiodactyls. *Bull Geogr Soc Am* 36:583–604, 1925.
6. Scott JM, Symons NBB: The dentition of ungulates. *In* Dental Anatomy, 7th ed. London, Churchill Livingstone, 1974, pp. 429–435, 445.
7. St. Clair LE: Teeth. *In* Getty R (ed): Sisson and Grossman's The Anatomy of the Domestic Animals, 5th ed, Vol. 1. Philadelphia, WB Saunders Co., 1975, pp. 866–872.
8. Jones ND, St. Clair LE: The cheek teeth of cattle. *Am J Vet Res* 18:536–542, 1957.
9. Listgarten MA: A light and electron microscopic study of coronal cementogenesis. *Arch Oral Biol 13*:93–114, 1968.
10. Nickel R, Shummer A, Seiferle E: Teeth, general and comparative. *In* The Viscera of the Domestic Animals. Translated and revised by Sack WO. First English ed, Berlin, Verlag Paul Parey, 1973, pp. 75–99.
11. Weinreb MM, Sharav Y: Tooth development in sheep. *Am J Vet Res* 25:891–908, 1964.
12. Garlick NL: The teeth of the ox in clinical diagnosis. II. Gross anatomy and physiology. *Am J Vet Res* 15:385–394, 1954.
13. Kikule SE: Age changes in the teeth of Zebu cattle. *E Afr Agric J* 19:86–88, 1953.
14. Joubert DM: On the effect of breed and nutritional plane on dentition in the cow. *Proc Br Soc Anim Prod,* 111–116, 1956.
15. Tulloh NM: A study of the incisor teeth of beef cattle. *Aust J Agric Res* 13:350–361, 1962.
16. Andrews AH, Wedderburn RWM: Breed and sex differences in the age of appearance of the bovine central incisor teeth. *Br Vet J* 133:543–547, 1977.
17. Brookes AJ, Hodges J: Breed, nutritional and heterotic effects on age of teeth emergence in cattle. *J Agric Sci Camb* 93:681–685, 1979.
18. Wiener G, Forster J: Variation in the age of emergence of incisor teeth in cattle of different breeds. *Anim Prod* 35:367–373, 1982.
19. Wiener G, Purser AF: The influence of four levels of feeding on the position and eruption of incisor teeth in sheep. *J Agric Sci Camb* 49:51–55, 1957.
20. Brown WAB, Christofferson PV, Massler M, Weiss MB: Postnatal tooth development in cattle. *Am J Vet Res* 21:7–34, 1960.
21. Bonsma JC, Neser FWC: Practical application of growth studies on cattle. The relationship between chest girth and weight. *Farm S Afr* 26:365–374, 1951.

22. Graham WC, Price MA: Dentition as a measure of physiological age in cows of different breed types. *Can J Anim Sci* 62:745–750, 1982.
23. Wiener G, Donald HP: A study of variation in twin cattle. IV. Emergence of permanent, incisor teeth. *J Dairy Res* 22:127–137, 1955.
24. Andrews AH, Green DA, Harrop AE: Observations on the age of shedding of the deciduous and the eruption of the permanent anterior teeth in a herd of Friesian cattle. *J Agric Sci Camb* 82:139–146, 1974.
25. Dumas R, Lhoste P: Les signes de l'age chez le zebu. Etude des incisives de replacement. *Rev Elev Med Vet Pays Trop* 19:357–363, 1966.
26. Christofferson PV, Weiss MB: Technique for dental radiography in cattle. *J Am Vet Med Assoc* 133: 496–498, 1958.
27. Andrews AH: The relationship of bovine rostral tooth development to age determined by post-mortem radiographic examination of cattle aged between 12 and 24 months. *J Agric Sci Camb* 97:97–102, 1981.
28. Ellenberger-Baum: Handbuch der Vergleichenden Anatomie der Haustiere, 18th ed. Revised by Zietzschmann HCO, Ackernecht E, Grau H. Berlin, Springer, 1943, pp. 356–357.
29. Silver IA: The ageing of domestic animals. *In* Bothwell D, Higgs F (eds): Science in Archaeology: A Survey of Progress and Research, 2nd ed. London, Thames and Hudson, 1969, pp. 283–302.
30. Chauveau A: Traité d'anatomie comparée des animaux domestiques, 4th ed. Paris, 1888 (quoted by ref. 29).
31. Habermehl KH: Die Altersbertimmung bei Haust—und Laboriteren. Berlin, Paul Parey, 1975.
32. Ishaque SM, Khan AW, Khan MA: Studies on the eruption of teeth in buffaloes, Sahiwal and Dajal cattle of Pakistan. Proceedings of the 18th–19th Pakistan Scientific Conference, Part III, 1967, pp. G 34–35.
33. Dumas R, Lhoste P: Les signes de l'age chez le Zebu. Etude des incisives de replacement. *Rev Elev Med Vet Pays Trop* 19:357–363, 1966.
34. Chieffi A, Paiva OM, Veiga JS: Contribuicão para o estudo da cronologia dentaria no zebu. *Revua Facultida Medicin.* Brazil, Veterinary University at Sao Paulo 3:251–269, 1948.
35. Prata H: Cronometria dentária no zebú. Institute de Zootechnia, Rio de Janeiro, Brazil. Publication No. 26, 1951, pp. 1–12.
36. Miller WC, Robertson EDC: Practical Animal Husbandry, 7th ed. Edinburgh and London, Oliver and Boyd, 1959, pp. 407–413.
37. Cornevin C, Lesbre X: Traité de l'âge des animaux domestiques d'après les dents et les productions épidermiques. Paris, B. Ballière et fils, 1894, pp. 270–299.
38. Girard NF: Traité de l'âge du cheval, 3rd ed. Publiée avec des changements et augmentée de l'âge du boeuf, du mouton, du chien et du cochon. Revised by Girard J. Paris, Béchet jeune, 1834, pp. 94–133.
39. Velu H: Chronologie de la calcification et de l'éruption des dents d'adulte chez le mouton marocain. *Bull Acad Vet France* 11:167–170, 1938.
40. Deniz E, Payne S: Eruption and wear in the mandibular dentition as a guide to ageing Turkish Angora goats. *In* Wilson B, Grigson C, Payne S (eds): Ageing and Sexing Animal Bones from Archaeological Sites. British Archaeological Reports, series 109, 1982, pp. 155–205.
41. Reddi BS: Eruption of incisor teeth in Jamunapari goats. *Ind Farm* 31:27–29, 1982.
42. Andrews AH: The relationship of bovine mandibular cheek tooth development to age determined by post-mortem radiographic examination of cattle aged between 12 and 24 months. *J Agric Sci Camb* 98:109–117, 1982.
43. Andrews AH: The relationship of maxillary cheek tooth development to age determined by post-mortem radiographic examination of cattle aged between 12 and 24 months. *J Agric Sci Camb* 99:105–114, 1982.
44. Girard NF: Traité de l'âge du cheval, 3rd ed. Publiée avec des changements et augmentée de l'âge du boeuf, du mouton, du chien et du cochon. Revised by Girard J. Paris, Béchet jeune, 1834, pp. 94–133.
45. Simonds JB: On the teeth of the ox, sheep and pig as indicative of the age of the animal, being the substance of two lectures delivered before the Royal Agricultural Society of England. *J Roy Agric Soc* 15:276–362, 1855.
46. Huidekoper RS: Age of the Domestic Animals. Philadelphia, FA Davis, 1891, pp. 158–174.
47. Barton FT: The Stock Owner's Manual. London, Everett and Co., 1909, pp. 112–113.
48. Brown GT: Dentition as Indicative of the Age of the Animals of the Farm, 9th ed. London, John Murray, 1949, pp. 5–6, 35–46.
49. Dyce KM, Wensing CJG: Essentials of Bovine Anatomy. Utrecht, A Oosthoek's Uitgeversmatchappij NV, 1971, pp. 11–14.
50. Rousseau LFE: Anatomie Comparée du Système Dentaire chez L'homme et Chez les Principaux Animaux. Paris, JB Ballière, 1839, pp. 227–236.
51. Macgregor R: The domestic buffalo. Fellowship thesis. Royal College of Veterinary Surgeons, 2nd series. No. 111, 1939, pp. 1–76.
52. Lall HK: Dentition in Indian Cattle. *Ind J Vet Sci* 18:37–39, 1948.
53. Andrews AH: Eruption of the maxillary first and second molar teeth in cattle as a method of estimating age. *Br Vet J* 139:355–360, 1983.
54. Suckling G: The normal development of incisor teeth in sheep and some anomalies. Sheep and Beef Cattle Society of the New Zealand Veterinary Association. Proceedings of the Society's 9th Seminar. Lincoln College, July 6th and 7th, 1979, pp. 1–3.
55. Garlick NL: The teeth of the ox in clinical diagnosis III. Developmental anomalies and general pathology. *Am J Vet Res* 15:500–508, 1954.
56. Andrews AH, Noddle BA: Absence of premolar teeth from ruminant mandibles at archaeological sites. *J Arch Sci* 2:137–144, 1975.
57. Meek A, Gray RAH: Animal remains. *In* Forster RH, Knowles WH: Corstopitum—Report on the excavations in 1910. *Archaeol Aeliana,* 3rd series. 7:220–267, 1911.
58. Stones HH, Farmer EP, Lawton F: Abnormalities in number, size and form of the teeth. *In* Oral and Dental Diseases, 4th ed. London, ES Livingstone, 1962, pp. 138–152.
59. Thoma KH, Goldman HM: Developmental abnormalities of the dentition. *In* Oral Pathology, 5th ed. St. Louis, The CV Mosby Co., 1960, pp. 23–72.
60. Garlick NL: The teeth of the ox in clinical diagnosis I. Developmental anatomy. *J Vet Res* 15:226–231, 1954.
61. Jackson, JW: Animal remains. *In* Bersu G: The Roman Villa, Huccleaote. *Trans Br Glouc Arch Soc* 55:370–375, 1933.
62. Colyer F: Variations and Diseases of the Teeth of Animals. London, John Bale, Sons and Danielsson, Ltd., 1936, pp. 1–750.

63. Baldi B: Anomalia dentaria in un bovino. *Nuova Vet* 24:19–21, 1948.
64. Dekeyser PL, Derivot J: Sur la présence de canines supérieures chez les bovidés. *Bull de L'I Fan* 18:série A 1272–1281, 1956.
65. Benson SB: Occurrences of upper canines in mountain sheep *(Ovis canadensis)*. *Am Midland Nature Notre Dame* 30:786–789, 1943.
66. Tucker R: Teratomorphic dentition in cattle. *Aust Vet J* 29:31, 1953.
67. Bruère AN, West DM, Orr MB, O'Callaghan MW: A syndrome of dental abnormalities in sheep. 1. Clinical aspects on a commercial sheep farm in the Wairarapa. *New Zealand Vet J* 27:152–158, 1979.
68. Noddle BE: Personal communication, 1983.
69. Heizer EE, Hervey MC: Impacted molars—a new lethal in cattle. *J Hered* 28:123–128, 1937.
70. West JL: Enamel hypoplasia of the deciduous incisor teeth of a calf. *Am J Vet Res* 34:839–840, 1973.
71. Thoma KH: Oral Pathology, 3rd ed. St. Louis, The CV Mosby Co., 1950, pp. 267–271, 286.
72. Jubb KVF, Kennedy PC: The upper alimentary system. *In* Pathology of the Domestic Animals, 2nd ed., Vol. 2. New York, Academic Press, 1970, pp. 1–44.
73. Andrews AH: A cemental abnormality in the bovine molar tooth. *Vet Rec* 92:318, 1973.
74. Donald HP, Wiener G: Observations on mandibular prognathism. *Vet Rec* 66:479–482, 1954.
75. Meyer VH, Becker H: Eine erbliche Kieferanomalie beim Rind. *Dent Tierarzl Wschr* 74:309–310, 1967.
76. Grant HT: Underdeveloped mandible in a herd of dairy Shorthorn cattle. *J Hered* 47:165–170, 1956.
77. Leipold HW, Doige CE, Kaye MM, Cribb PH: Congenital osteopetrosis in Aberdeen-Angus calves. *Can Vet J* 11:181–185, 1970.
78. Rieck GW, Baehr H: Akroteriasis congenita beim deutschen schwarzbunten Rind. *Dent Tierarzl Wschr* 74:356–364, 1967.
79. Ely F, Hull FW, Morrison HB: Agnathia, a new bovine lethal. *J Hered* 30:105–108, 1939.
80. Leipold HW, Dennis SM, Huston K: Congenital defects of cattle: Nature, cause and effect. *Adv Vet Sci Comp Med* 16:103–150, 1972.
81. Deniz E: A rare malformation: Extreme agnathia in a male calf. *Ankara University Fakulty Dergisi* 13:281–291, 1966.
82. Leipold HW, Crates WF, Radostits OM, Howell WD: Arthrogryposis and associated defects in newborn calves. *Am J Vet Res* 31:367–374, 1970.
83. Shupe JL, Binns W, James LF, Keeler RF: Lupine, a cause of crooked calf disease. *J Am Vet Med Assoc* 151:198–203, 1967.
84. Hoekstra P, Wensvoort P: Cheilognathoschisis in Texel sheep. *Tijschr Diorgeneesk* 101:71–76, 1976.
85. Wheat JD: Harelip in Shorthorn cattle. *J Hered* 51:99–101, 1960.

Chapter Seventeen

Acquired Diseases of the Teeth and Mouth in Ruminants

AH Andrews

ACQUIRED CONDITIONS OF THE TEETH

Dental Caries

In my experience in Britain, true dental caries appears to be rare; this is contrary to the findings in American cattle.[1] Most cases occur in older animals, though cavities can be found in both the temporary and the permanent dentition. In most animals there appears to be little pain, and there is no inhibition of the normal prehensive and masticatory processes. Dental caries is less common in the teeth of animals with fluorosis.

Although caries can involve primary dentin, it commonly affects the exposed secondary dentin, and the tissue appears black. As the process continues, the diseased tissue is lost, producing a hollowed-out pattern. Deposition of secondary dentin is accelerated more ventrally in the tooth; the dentin is of poor quality, so the disease process continues. The neck of incisor teeth may be affected in sheep.[2] In some cases, the apex of the root becomes infected, which can lead to periodontal abscess formation.

Caries in enamal usually affects defective areas, such as enamel flecks, rather than the normal tissue.[1] The condition is self-limiting; the infected enamel fleck tends to be lost, leaving an uninfected enamel pit. The pits produced may contain black pigment.

Excessive Attrition of Rostral Teeth

The excessive attrition of rostral teeth in cattle, sheep, and goats is a common problem in Africa, Australia, and New Zealand, and to a lesser extent elsewhere. They undergo rapid wear, which leads to difficulties in prehension and mastication. This severe attrition is most often seen in breeding ewes 5 years or older.[3] It causes unthriftiness and loss of condition, and can be of considerable economic importance. Mouth examination reveals excessively worn teeth; often they are only short stumps. The teeth may also be loose, missing or fractured. This condition can be confused with periodontal disease that causes tooth loss ("broken mouth") in sheep (page 266). In some cases, excessive attrition occurs in cattle and sheep on the same farm. Attrition in sheep has been reported in conjunction with other conditions, such as osteopathy of the mandibular bone, maleruption of the permanent rostral teeth, and the formation of dentigerous cysts.[4]

In Rhodesia, the rostral teeth of Herefords had an increased rate of wear, because of a decrease in tooth enamel hardness, when compared with indigenous native cattle.[5] Affected animals tended to possess a brachygnathic occlusion.[6] In New Zealand sheep, increased attrition and early tooth loss was thought to be partially due to some of the constituents (such as acids and enzymes) in the herbage consumed.[7] These substances acted on the tooth dentin, and increased attrition resulted from the rough constituents (such as fiber, silica) in the grass. This is now thought to be of less importance in sheep than is the amount of soil ingested. In certain areas of New Zealand where soil structure is "poorly developed" and badly drained, much soil tends to be ingested when pasture growth is low and when heavy stocking rates occur.[8] Supplementing the feed at times when little grass is available, as well as decreasing the stocking rate, can considerably reduce the rate of wear,[9] but the supplemental feed must replace a large amount of the animal's daily feed intake. If there is limited supplementation, it may encourage further grass and soil ingestion.[10] Nutrition also will influence tooth hardness; in growing sheep in Australia, a calcium:phosphorus imbalance or a calcium-deficient diet predisposes to tooth wear[11] and appears to depress the development of enamel and dentin.[12] The inclusion of 1 percent ground limestone in the diet of growing sheep should provide an adequate amount of calcium for normal enamel and dentin formation. Cattle and sheep should be examined prior to the period when attrition will occur (usually winter), and those with badly worn teeth should be culled or provided with adequate supplementary feed. The use of caps or crowns for incisors has been tried as a means of reducing attrition.[13] In one particularly severe syndrome in New Zealand, the provision of copper by injection and addition to the feed helped reduce attrition in temporary teeth.[4]

Fluorosis (Fluoride Poisoning)

Fluorosis is caused by the ingestion of small amounts of fluorine in the feed or drinking water of cattle, sheep, and goats. In nature, fluorine is present, in differing amounts, as fluoride (the combined form), and exists in the atmosphere, vegetation, water, and soil. Usually its presence in one or a combination of these elements, causes the fluorosis. Ingestion in small amounts produces no obvious abnormalities. However, levels of more than 100 parts per million (ppm) in the dry ration are likely to cause fluorosis. Although high levels of fluoride can be present in soil and surface water, plants do not generally absorb much of it. Most cases are due to the contamination of pasture or water with smoke, vapor, or dust from aluminum foundries or brickworks. Supplementary feeding of phosphates or the use of superphosphate fertilizers can cause fluorosis. Acute fluorosis results in ruminal stasis, with diarrhea or constipation, excitability, convulsions, anorexia and, in most cases, death.

In chronic fluorosis, the bones or teeth are involved. More work has been undertaken in cattle than in sheep. Experimental fluorosis has been studied recently.[14] The deciduous dentition is not affected, but the permanent successors are, and the severity of abnormality will depend upon when exposure occurs relative to the permanent tooth development. Thus, it is not seen in animals who are brought into affected areas after the permanent teeth have formed. There is mottling (seen as areas of pigmentation varying from yellow to brown to black), hypoplasia, hypocalcification, and excessive attrition (Fig. 17–1). Although the rostral teeth are affected, the cheek teeth are also abnormal. Both enamel and dentin are involved. A method of grading rostral tooth fluorosis is available.[15] 0 = normal; 1 = questionable effect, slight enamel change; 2 = slight effect, slight mottling; 3 = moderate effect, obvious mottling; 4 = marked effect, definite mottling, hypoplasia, and hypocalcification; and 5 = severe effect, definite mottling,

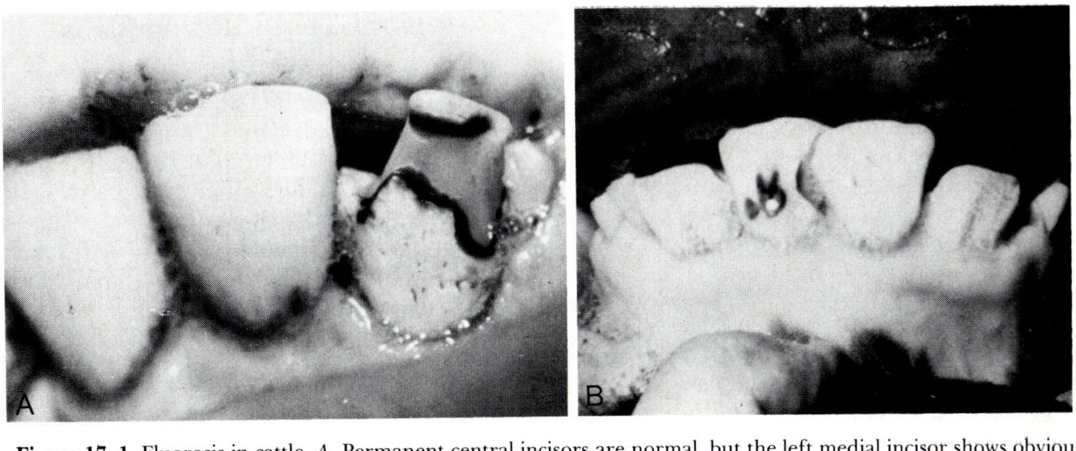

Figure 17–1. Fluorosis in cattle. *A*, Permanent central incisors are normal, but the left medial incisor shows obvious mottling of the enamel, along with hypoplasia and hypocalcaemia, with exposure of the underlying dentin. *B*, The central and medial permanent incisors show enamel mottling and the right central incisor has discoloration and pitting. The central incisors also overlap at their medial surfaces. (Courtesy of J Allcock.)

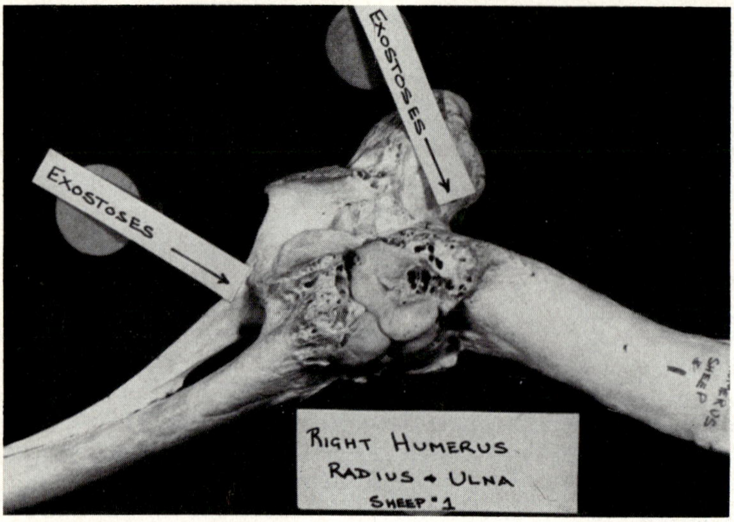

Figure 17–2. Fluorosis. Humerus of a sheep with multiple exostoses around the elbow joint. (Courtesy of J Allcock.)

discoloration, hypoplasia, and hypocalcification.

There is rapid and uneven wear in the cheek teeth. In some cases infection of the alveoli occurs, making prehension and mastication painful and causing loss of teeth. The bones tend to be enlarged (Fig. 17–2), and lameness and unthriftiness may be seen. The mandible is often palpable and sometimes is visibly enlarged. Diagnosis is usually made from the knowledge that the animal has access to environmental contamination plus the analysis of feed and water samples. The normal blood concentration of fluorine is 0.2 mg/dl; it may be raised, though not always, in fluorosis. The fluorine in urine is usually 2 to 6 ppm, but it may be quite elevated in fluorosis. Postmortem analysis of fluorine in teeth and bones is very useful. The main method of treatment for chronic fluorosis is to remove the animal from the source of fluoride. Adequate concentrates, calcium, and phosphorus should be given. The use of aluminum salts, such as aluminum chloride, aluminum sulfate, and calcium aluminate, reduces the storage of fluorine in bone, but only by about 30 per cent.

Fractured Teeth

The rostral teeth are capable of a certain amount of movement in their alveoli; thus, fracture of these teeth in ruminants is unusual. However, fractures can occur in both temporary and permanent dentition and tend to be transverse.

Fractures of the cheek teeth occur much more frequently than do fractures of the rostral teeth. This is partly true in cattle because of their indiscriminate eating habits. The fracture may involve the separation of the margins or the cusps of the lower cheek teeth. Fractures of the occlusal surface may subsequently become smooth from attrition. Other fractures run ventrally and labially and do not involve the root. The majority of these problems will be found incidentally, without signs of discomfort to the animal.

When teeth become split along their length, including the root, mastication is painful, resulting in reduced feed intake and loss of condition. The problem may be indicated by the frequent drooling of bubbling saliva. Examination under xylazine will normally reveal the fractured tooth. Removal may require the use of local anesthesia, but usually the fractured parts are loose and can be removed with molar forceps.

Rostral Tooth Retropulsion

Trauma can occasionally cause a rostral tooth to be driven caudally into its alveolus.[1] This force may also be ventral, causing the root to penetrate the alveolar bone and allowing the tooth to lie under the gingivae in contact with the labia. The tooth usually is not lost, and any alveolar damage or fracture heals, though the tooth tends to remain in its abnormal position.

ACQUIRED CONDITIONS OF THE MOUTH

Stomatitis

Stomatitis involves inflammation of the gum mucosa (gingivitis) (Fig. 17–3), the lin-

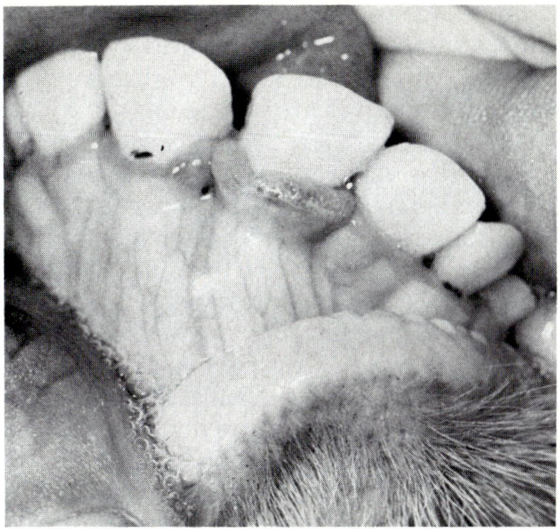

Figure 17–3. Localized gingivitis of unknown origin in a calf.

gual mucosa (glossitis), and the palate (palatitis). Such processes can be diffuse or localized and can involve many types of inflammation, including ulcerative, purulent, vesicular, catarrhal, and diphtheritic. Etiologically, viral conditions probably predominate, but bacteria and fungi can cause similar lesions. Trauma may also result from injuries, accidents, or careless dentistry or administration of medications. Foreign bodies may produce a catarrhal stomatitis, and similar lesions can occur with frozen feeds, grass, cereal awns, or prickles and spines on plants. Many chemical agents, such as acids, alkalis, mercury compounds, and chloral hydrate, are caustic and can cause catarrhal inflammation. Ingestion of some plants may also induce the condition (Fig. 17–4).

The signs vary according to the severity and cause of the condition. Often there is a considerable amount of drooling and a reluctance to eat and swallow. When necrosis or pus is present, the animal may become toxemic. Manipulation and examination of the lip and mouth is usually resented. Treatment often requires forced feeding, often by stomach tube, until the lesions begin to heal. Local treatment may include mouthwashes of antibiotics, antiseptics, or mild astringents.

Foreign Bodies

Sharp foreign bodies can cause laceration and the introduction of bacteria causing infection. Grass awns and seeds may penetrate soft tissues, resulting in abscess formation or allowing the entry of specific organisms, such as *Actinomyces bovis.* In addition, they can enter the alveolar space between the teeth and the gingivae and produce a marked gingivitis. Cattle in phosphorus-deficient areas may develop a pica, involving osteophagia that can result in foreign bodies being lodged in the mouth or pharynx.

Yellow bristle grass *(Setaria lutescens)* has grass seeds with spiny awns that cause a mechanical stomatitis in cattle. Most cases involve the tongue, but the buccal mucosa may also be affected.

INFECTIONS OF THE ORAL CAVITY

Viral Diseases

Many major viral diseases cause oral lesions. The following section includes a brief summary of the epizootiology of each disease, and a description of the oral lesions. Many of these diseases are of major epizootological (economic) and public health importance. Further information on these aspects, and laboratory diagnosis of these diseases, is available elsewhere.[16]

Ulcerative Dermatosis of Sheep. In America, it has been reported that ulcerative dermatosis of sheep is caused by a virus that is very similar to the one that causes contagious pustular dermatitis, though the former is less contagious than the latter. The lesions are much more erosive and destructive, and there is no pus. They occur on the feet, legs, genitalia, nares, and lips. Often, the dermatosis between the lips and the nares is in-

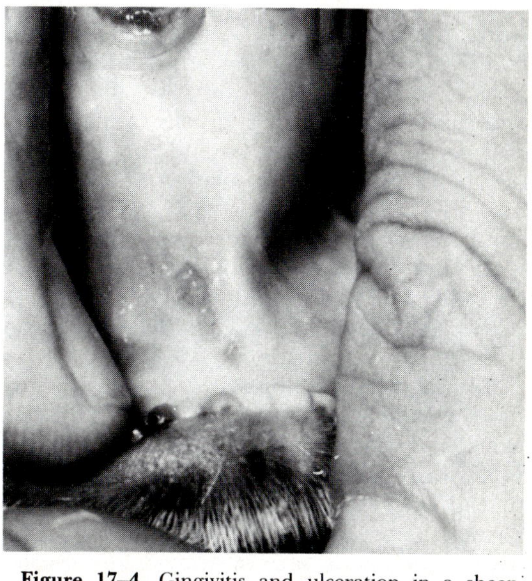

Figure 17–4. Gingivitis and ulceration in a sheep following contact with giant hogweed *(Heracleum mantegazzianum).*

fected, and in severe cases the oral mucosa is involved. Isolation of the virus and distribution of the lesions assist in the diagnosis.

Sheep-pox and Goatpox. Although the sheep-pox virus causes a high mortality in sheep of all ages, it is most severe in lambs. Most cases occur in Europe and the Middle East. Young animals show depression, pyrexia, and profuse oculonasal discharge; those that survive develop skin lesions. In severe cases there are lesions of the buccal mucosa. Usually, treatment is not undertaken, since the disease is highly contagious. Diagnosis is by examination of the characteristic lesions that start as areas of erythema, which is followed by firm raised papules with hyperemia at their bases. A yellow vesicle is then formed, which ruptures and produces a scab, and this is the stage usually seen. Control is achieved through slaughter and vaccination.

The goatpox virus is distinct from the virus that causes sheep-pox. The condition is usually severe in sheep as well as in goats. The main lesions are on the lips and oral mucosa as well as on the udder and teats. Diagnosis is by recognition of the characteristic lesions, which are similar to the lesions of sheep-pox.

Contagious Pustular Stomatitis (Contagious Ecthyma, Orf). The paravaccinia virus is part of the pox virus group and can infect both sheep and goats. The lesions occur on lambs and kids and are seen mainly on the oral mucocutaneous junction and on the skin of the muzzle and nostrils, though the buccal mucosa is also involved. There is usually a proliferative lesion of papules, with inflammation, ulceration, and granulation. The lesions interfere with sucking, causing the lambs to lose condition and transmitting disease to the teats and udder of the dams. Diagnosis is confirmed by the appearance and distribution of the lesions, the histological characteristics, and isolation of the virus. The use of oxytetracycline or gentian violet spray helps in reducing infection. Prevention is through the use of a live intradermal vaccine given to dams and the lambs or kids before the period of risk. The disease can be transmitted to humans.

Bovine Papular Stomatitis. This very common infection of cattle in most parts of the world is caused by a paravaccinia virus of the pox group. The virus appears to be identical to the one that causes the teat lesions of pseudocowpox. Infection can occur in humans. The disease can be seen in animals 10 days of age or older, and it is particularly common in animals less than 2 years old. Immunity appears to be short-lived, and individual animals may be infected more than once. Most animals are infected at some time in their lives. There are few generalized signs. Occasionally, there is a transient pyrexia and inappetence. When signs are severe, concurrent bacterial infection is present. The lesions start as red papules and then develop a more characteristic form that is partly or completely circular or oval. There are three zones in this outer layer of hyperemia, inside of which is a narrow, raised, pale area of hyperplasia; the major central part of the lesion is depressed, is gray or brown, and becomes necrotic. In some cases, the lesions coalesce, but at no stage are vesicles present. The main areas affected are the nares, muzzle, and buccal mucosa, particularly around any erupting teeth. Although lesions may heal in 1 to 2 weeks, successive crops tend to arise before the earlier lesions disappear. Diagnosis is confirmed by observation of the characteristic lesions, the histopathological characteristics, and isolation of the virus. Treatment is not usually required.

Ulcerative Stomatitis. The virus causing this disease affects only cattle and was first recorded in America. The lesions occur mainly on the dorsal surface of the tongue, but they may be present elsewhere in the buccal cavity—on the muzzle, the nostrils, and the rostral turbinates. Although no pyrexia is seen, there may be some inappetence and loss of body weight. Histologically, the lesions are distinct from those of papular stomatitis, because in the former there are no inclusion bodies, and both erosions and ulcerations are apparent.

Mucosal Disease–Bovine Viral Diarrhea. The pestivirus concerned appears to be similar in both forms of this disease, and differs only in the epidemiology. Bovine viral diarrhea usually occurs when infection first enters a herd, with low mortality but high morbidity. Mucosal disease is seen subsequently with few animals showing clinical signs, but those that do have a high mortality. The incubation period is usually 1 to 3 weeks, and the signs include a diphasic temperature rise in experimental infection. In acute cases, animals tend to be dull, with inappetence, profuse watery diarrhea, loss of condition, and reduced milk production. Abortion and congenital abnormalities may occur. There are keratitis and conjunctivitis and, often, pedal lesions. Erosions occur on the nares and muzzle. The most noticeable erosions in the mouth are on the hard palate, though others are often present on the gingivae, the buccal papillae, and the dorsal and lateral lingual surfaces. The lesions may coalesce to form large, necrotic membranes. Saliva tends to be held in the mouth. Lesions usually heal in about 2 weeks. However, in chronic cases, several cycles of lesions may develop, particularly on the labial commissures, and the animals may show intermittent diarrhea and loss of condition. Diagnosis is confirmed by the clinical signs, isolation of the virus, or rising serological titers. The only treatment available is supportive.

Proliferative Stomatitis. This viral disease infects mainly calves between 2 and 8 weeks old. Cases occur in animals of other ages who have previously been exposed to chlorinated naphthalenes. The incubation period is about a week. Initially a congested and erosive lesion that becomes proliferative is seen. Lesions tend to be localized, yellow-brown, crusty plaques, and they remain a few weeks before healing. They usually start near the rostral teeth, but later they may involve the hard palate, lips, tongue, and buccal mucosa. Usually, there is little sign of systemic illness, though inappetence may be seen. Diagnosis is usually based on the age of the animal, the history, and the apearance of the lesions.

Foot and Mouth Disease. This highly contagious disease is caused by one of seven strains of enterovirus. The disease is present in most parts of the world, except Australia, New Zealand, and North America. It affects cloven-hoofed animals, including cattle, sheep, goats, pigs, and deer. The severity of disease depends on the subtype and the species involved. Morbidity approaches 100 percent, but mortality tends to be less than 10 percent, except in young animals. Human infection is infrequent. The incubation period in natural infection is usually 4 to 10 days. The infected animals show pyrexia, dullness, stomatitis, and lameness resulting from vesicular lesions in the coronary region. Vesicles that are 1 cm or larger in diameter appear on the buccal mucosa, the tongue, and the hard palate. The vesicles rupture easily, releasing a yellow fluid. In the initial stages, there is severe pain, which is exhibited by lip smacking, reluctance to eat, and the drooling of strings of saliva. As the lesions heal, the pain is relieved, but there is often a long period of convalescence with reduced productivity, and considerable economic impact. Death is often the result of myocardial involvement. Signs in pigs, sheep, and goats are normally milder, with fewer mouth lesions than there are in cattle. Diagnosis depends on the signs and identification of the virus by morphological characteristics and fluorescent antibody or complement fixation tests. A rise in antibody titer can be detected in chronic cases. Most countries without the disease have policies to prevent its introduction or its eradication if inadvertent entry should occur. In countries where disease is a constant threat or where the condition is enzootic, vaccination programs are usually undertaken.

Vesicular Stomatitis. This condition is highly contagious and is caused by a rhabdovirus. The virus infects mainly horses, but cattle, pigs, and, occasionally, humans may also be infected. Calves are quite resistant to disease and sheep are usually naturally infected. The disease occurs in both North America and South America. Infection can spread by direct contact between animals, but it normally gains entry through some form of wound. Mosquitoes and biting flies can spread infection. The incubation period is 2 days or more and in cattle is followed by a mild pyrexia and vesicular lesions, which are similar to those of foot and mouth disease, on the buccal mucosa, the dental pad, the dorsum of the tongue, and the labia. The vesicles rupture rapidly and are often missed, resulting in a painful mouth typified by drooling and inappetence. Foot lesions are uncommon except in pigs. Recovery is usually rapid. Diagnosis depends on virus isolation and fluorescent antibody testing. Treatment is mainly symptomatic and includes the use of mouthwashes. Prevention is mainly by hygiene and quarantine.

Rinderpest (Cattle Plague). This is a highly contagious disease of cattle caused by a myxovirus that can also infect other ruminants and pigs. Infection is common in parts of Africa and Asia. Morbidity rates in cattle approach 100 percent, with a mortality rate of about 50 percent. The incubation period is 3 to 9 days. Affected animals show systemic signs, including pyrexia, dullness, a drop in milk yield, and ocular and nasal lesions that are serous and then purulent. Oral lesions develop about 2 to 3 days after the temperature rises and consist of focal ulcers that are first present on the lower lip, the adjacent gum, the cheek mucosa, and the ventral surface of the tongue. There is no vesiculation. Lesions spread all over the buccal cavity and often tend to coalesce. Lesions also occur on other mucosal surfaces. Other signs develop, including diarrhea, tachypnea, abdominal pain, dehydration, recumbency and, in many cases, death. In sheep, oral cavity lesions are less frequent and involve mainly soft palate erosion and abscessation of the tonsils. Salivation tends to occur less frequently than in cattle. Diagnosis depends on the signs, evidence of high morbidity and mortality, virus isolation, and fluorescent antibody tests. There is no treatment. Attenuated vaccines are used for prevention.

Malignant Catarrhal Fever (Bovine Malignant Catarrh). This disease, found mainly in African cattle and buffalo, is caused by a herpesvirus. Cases have been recorded in other parts of the world, including North America, Europe, and Australia. Lesions in sheep and goats are minimal, though these animals have been incriminated in spread of the disease. The incubation period is 18 to 38 days. Spread is not by contact. Usually, individual cases occur, but in some instances morbidity is high. Most affected animals die. The disease takes several forms, including peracute, intestinal, head and eye, and mild forms. Signs of the head and eye syndrome include pyrexia, depression, anorexia, enlarged lymph nodes, mucopurulent nasal discharge with necrosis of nasal mucosa, ocular discharge, blepharospasm, corneal edema, and congested scleral vessels, diarrhea, and neurological signs. In the mouth, there is hyperemia, initially with small erosions at the mucocutaneous junctions followed by extensive erosion of the oral mucosa, including the tips of the labial papillae, the tongue, the cheeks, and the hard and soft palates. Following death, histological examination shows a necrotizing vasculitis. Signs are helpful in arriving at a diagnosis, but suitable techniques for viral isolation are not available. There is no effective therapy. Control is achieved through isolation of infected animals.

Blue-Tongue. The virus concerned in this disease has several strains, is transmitted by insects, and affects mainly sheep, though cattle, goats, and wild ruminants can be infected. The condition occurs in Africa and has been reported from parts of Europe, North America, Asia, and Australia. The incubation period is less than a week, and the virus may persist for long periods after recovery. Usually blue-tongue infects individual animals or small groups; epizootic situations are rare. The condition tends to be more severe in sheep in good condition or in those given excess exercise or exposed to strong sunlight. Following an initial temperature rise, there is hyperemia of the buccal and nasal mucosae, with copious, frothy salivation and nasal discharge, which later becomes mucopurulent and bloody. The face, ears, lips, gingivae, and tongue become swollen and edematous, and later the epithelium is shed with ulceration and often secondary infection. The lateral surfaces of the tongue tend to ulcerate and become swollen and bluish-purple. There are involuntary labial movements, and swallowing often is painful. Diarrhea may be present, and respirations tend to become rapid and noisy from obstruction. Some animals develop lameness and recumbency from laminitis and coronitis, which may include the presence of a purple band above the coronet. Death occurs in about 6 days; other animals enter a long convalescence with a loss of condition and wool and often cracking of the skin and hooves. Infection in most cattle and goats goes unnoticed, though a few develop a milder form of the sheep syndrome. Serological diagnosis is possible in sheep, but in cattle it depends on injecting blood into susceptible sheep. Control primarily involves keeping the disease out of uninfected countries. In enzootic areas vaccination is practiced.

Infectious Bovine Rhinotracheitis (Rednose). This condition is the result of bovine herpesvirus 1 infection and is primarily an upper respiratory and reproductive disease. However, a separate intestinal syndrome can occur in newborn calves following the introduction of a carrier to an uninfected herd. Infectious bovine rhinotracheitis (IBR) is present in most parts of the world. Affected calves show conjunctivitis, rhinotracheitis, and pyrexia. In the oral cavity, there is inflammation of the soft palate, with the production of small gray pustules followed by necrosis. About 90 percent of affected calves die. Diagnosis depends on virus isolation from nasal or fecal swabs or postmortem findings. Treatment is directed mainly at counteracting dehydration and secondary infection. Control of this type of IBR is by vaccination of the dams.

Papillomatosis. The common wart in cattle is caused by a species-specific virus. Although most warts occur on the skin, they are sometimes present in the nose, muzzle, or labia. Older suckler cows in bracken areas often have oral papillomata, and in such cases other papillomata that are found in other parts of

Table 17–1. Therapy for Animals with Necrobacillosis

Drug	Initial Dose (per kg/Bodyweight)	Maintenance Doses	Duration
Sulfadimidine	0.2 g	Half of initial dose twice daily	Up to 5 d
Sulfamerazine	0.2 g	Half of initial dose twice daily	Up to 5 d
Sulfanilamide	0.2 g	One third of initial dose three times daily or half of initial dose twice daily	Up to 5 d
Sulfamethoxypyridazine	22 mg	One dose sometimes, otherwise dose interval variable	Usually up to 3 doses
Penicillin	10,000 U	Same as above	3–5 d
Oxytetracycline	10 mg	Same as above	3–5 d
Streptomycin	10–15 mg	Same as above	3–5 d

the gut may give rise to alimentary squamous cell carcinoma.

Bacterial Diseases

Necrobacillosis. This disease is caused by the introduction of *Fusobacterium necrophorum (Fusiformis necrophorus, Sphaerophorus necrophorus)* into wounds in the oral cavity or pharynx. The oral form occurs mainly in calves up to 3 months old. The less common laryngeal form can be found in animals up to 2 years old. Most cases are sporadic, but outbreaks of the oral form can occur if hygiene is poor. The oral form is often seen in the region of the cheek teeth. In early cases, the main sign is a swelling of the cheek in an otherwise bright animal. If the disease is untreated, anorexia, pyrexia, and depression follow. The lesion is painful to external or internal palpation, and often the deep ulcerative area on the cheek is packed with feed. Some cases will also involve an area of the tongue apposing the cheek lesions, and in neglected cases the breath is foul-smelling. Bacterial culture helps confirm the diagnosis. Treatment is with sulfonamides or antibiotics, such as penicillin, streptomycin, or oxytetracycline (Table 17–1). No supportive treatment is required provided that therapy starts early. Fluids and multivitamin injections may be indicated in severely affected animals. Control involves isolation of the infected animal and keeping feeding buckets separate. Improvements in hygiene are helpful in preventing the disease.

Actinobacillosis (Wooden Tongue). *Actinobacillus lignierisii* infection occurs in cattle, sheep, and goats. The ingestion of contaminated feed or pasture is usually involved, and infection enters through a wound. The disease is worldwide, and in cattle it leads to the production of a hard, swollen, and painful tongue. The animal is reluctant to eat and salivates excessively, though the animal's temperature is usually normal. The tongue shows nodules and ulcers laterally, and if the condition is untreated it becomes shrunken, hard, and immobile. The local lymph nodes, including the submaxillary and parotid nodes, may become infected. In sheep and goats, deep or superficial lesions (which may discharge thick, yellow pus) occur on the face, nose, lower lip, lower jaw, or elsewhere. Local lymph nodes may become infected.

Diagnosis is by identification and culture of the organism. Therapy involves sulfonamides or antibiotics (Table 17–1) or erythromycin, 2.5 mg/kg bodyweight for 3 to 5 days. Sodium iodide intravenously (8 g/100 kg bodyweight at 10-day intervals if necessary. Potassium iodide administration for a week at a dose (for cattle) of 6 g to 10 g daily is helpful. There is always the possibility that infection may recur; following treatment, the animal should be fattened and slaughtered.

Necrotic Stomatitis. Besides *Fusobacterium necrophorum* infection, necrosis of the mucosa can result from chemicals (acids, alkalis, chloral hydrate, lime) or excessive local heat or cold. Secondary bacterial infection can also develop.

Purulent Stomatitis. Following injury or abrasions from feed or foreign bodies, *Corynebacterium pyogenes* infection may occur with varying degrees of pus formation.

Anthrax. Infection with *Bacillus anthracis* results in peracute death or an acute syndrome in cattle, sheep, and goats, with anorexia, pyrexia, ruminal stasis, rapid respirations, dyspnea, and collapse. The mucosae, including those of the oral cavity, tend to become congested and hemorrhagic. In some cases, phlegmonous stomatitis or occasionally local edema of the tongue occurs.

Periodontitis. This condition is described

in the section on Infections of the Mandible, Maxilla, and Mouth.

Fungal Infections

Bovine Nocardiosis (Bovine Farcy, Mycotic Lymphangitis). The main infection is a mycotic dermatitis caused by *Nocardia farcinicus* or *Nocardia dermatonomus.* The main lesions tend to be in lymphatic vessels and lymph nodes that occur in the cheeks, in the parotid area, or on the mandibular bone;[17] however, they can occur in many other sites. Typically, the lesions consist of localized, thickened swellings that may develop sinuses or ulcerate, discharging a thick, odorless, yellow or gray pus. The organism can usually be detected in the pus. Treatment is by intravenous sodium iodide injections (20 percent solution at a dose of 1 g/12.5 kg), repeated at 10-day intervals until the lesions have resolved.

Inflammatory Reactions

Phlegmonous Stomatitis. This condition is a deep-seated stomatitis that produces a serous or purulent discharge after filling a wound or infection.[18] Malignant catarrhal fever, rinderpest, and occasionally anthrax and mucosal disease can produce phlegmonous stomatitis. The wound can result from injury to incisor teeth or deep penetration by foreign bodies. Deep ulceration or vesiculation can occur following burns, which are either electrical or from caustic drugs such as ammonia or chloral hydrate crystals. There is usually a sudden onset of anorexia, with salivation and pain if eating is attempted. There may be submandibular edema. If the tongue is involved, it will be swollen and will protrude. In the mouth the mucosa has a deep purple color and is swollen; there is usually a serous or purulent discharge that may produce a foul smell. Treatment is local with the possible use of parenteral antibiotics (Table 17–1); in superficial cases healing takes only a few days, but with deeper lesions, recovery may take several weeks.

Allergic Stomatitis (Clover Disease). This disease has been reported in the southern part of the United States in cattle who graze on red clover, ladino clover, or Dutch white clover. Most cases are recorded in early spring or autumn, and lesions are similar to those produced by photosensitization. Most cases are mild. Affected animals show skin lesions, reddened nostrils, and crusty foci on the muzzle. There is hyperemia of the buccal mucosa, with discrete, superficial erosions and salivation. In a more severe form, there are dermatitis and stomatitis, with numerous ulcers on the labia, hard palate, and caudal part of the tongue. Treatment consists of taking the animals off the offending pasture and keeping them out of sunlight. Antihistamine or corticosteroid injections may be required in some animals.

Conditions Caused by Poisoning

Photosensitization. This condition is the result of the sensitization of the outer body layers to light. There are many causes, including the presence of aberrant pigments such as porphyrins, exogenous photosensitizing agents such as St. John's wort *(Hypericum perforatum),* or hepatogenous photosensitization caused by the accumulation of phylloerythrin, as well as unknown causes. Unpigmented parts of the body, usually including the face, muzzle, ears, eyelids, and teats, are involved. In the oral cavity, the lips and ventral third of the tongue are involved, causing a diffuse superficial mucosal slough. Diagnosis of the condition is normally made on the type and distribution of the lesions. It is often difficult to determine the etiological agent. Treatment is often of limited value. Removing the animal from direct sunlight and preventing further intake of any photosensitizing substances are helpful.

Chronic Mercury Poisoning. A catarrhal stomatitis is produced from chronic mercury poisoning in cattle, with gingivitis and tooth loss ensuing. Systemic signs include chronic diarrhea, depression, inappetence, alopecia, incoordination, convulsions, and other neurological signs. Diagnosis is often difficult without estimating the mercury concentration in kidney tissue; feces and urine mercury concentrations may be high, as may urinary levels of alkaline phosphatase and gamma-glutamyltranspeptidase. Intravenous injection of sodium thiosulfate may be helpful—for cattle, 15 g to 30 g in 100 ml to 200 ml water, followed by 30 g to 60 g orally four times daily until recovery occurs.

Chronic Arsenic Poisoning. This condition can result in erythema of the buccal mucosa and ulceration. Lesions may also be present on the muzzle, and there is often reddening of the conjunctival mucosa and, in some cases, there are skin lesions. Other, more general signs include poor growth and a dry staring coat. Diagnosis is made by testing arsenic levels in hair or in the liver. Therapy with sodium thiosulfate (see section on Chronic Mercury Poisoning) or dimercaprol (British Anti-Lewisite) may be helpful.

ACQUIRED CONDITIONS OF THE MANDIBLE, MAXILLA, AND MOUTH

Mandibular Fractures

Fractures of the mandible occur from trauma and typically occur during attempts at restraint. Many mandibular fractures heal well with conservative treatment. Plates, wires, and methylmethylacrylate splints can be used.[19] The introduction of an intramedullary pin, ventral to the first incisor and directed caudally, can also be helpful.[20] In bilateral fractures, a pin can be used in each mandible and stabilized with a Kirschner apparatus. Feed should be in the form of concentrates and grain, with hay being introduced later. It is prudent to give broad-spectrum antibiotics for 7 to 10 days, and saline mouthwashes may be necessary.

Infections

Actinomycosis (Lumpy Jaw). Actinomycosis is an infection of cattle, occurring worldwide, that is caused by *Actinomyces bovis.* It is less commonly diagnosed in Britain at present than it was formerly. The organism is a frequent inhabitant of the mouth and respiratory tract of cattle, and infection usually enters via a wound or dental alveolus, particularly during the eruption of teeth. The disease is commonly seen in animals 1 to 3 years old. The mandible is more often affected than is the maxilla, and the cheek tooth region is usually involved. Initial signs are few until the hard, initially painless swelling is noticed. The swelling may be diffuse or localized, or may involve the ventral edge of the ramus, and may progress slowly or rapidly. Other signs may include difficulty in eating and loosening of some of the cheek teeth. As the lesion progresses, the mass may protrude into the oral cavity or cheek skin and may rupture, producing a sinus that discharges thick, yellow-green pus containing small, hard, yellow "sulfur granules." The sinuses tend to heal and others break out. Local spread of infection to surrounding muscle and connective tissue can occur, but the local lymph nodes are not involved. Lesions can occur in other soft tissues. The main bony lesion shows necrosis with subsequent osteomyelitis. Diagnosis is made by demonstrating the organism in the pus, particularly in the granules, and by cultures. Treatment is with sulfonamides or antibiotics (erythromycin, 2.5 mg/kg/bodyweight for 4 to 5 days; see also Table 17–1). Sodium or potassium iodide can be used as for actinobacillosis (page 263). Oral doses of isoniazid (10 mg to 20 mg/kg) for a month can be useful but cannot be used in animals that produce milk for human consumption because it is excreted in the milk. The infected animal should be isolated because it is a focus of infection. It is advisable to fatten and slaughter the animal after recovery.

Rostral Mandibular Abscess. Particularly in sheep, grass seeds or other feed may penetrate the alveolus, or a rostral tooth may be retropulsed by trauma. The resulting damage may allow the introduction of bacteria, with development of osteomyelitis and swelling of the bone in the rostral mandible. Teeth may become loose and are lost. In other cases, a sinus that may open to the outside develops, discharging a fluid, foul-smelling pus. Following drainage, the wound may heal, but the thickened mandible remains. In some animals, antibiotic therapy is helpful; in others it is necessary to remove the causative agent, such as the grass seed. If the discharge persists, it is often best to extract the involved rostral tooth.

Caudal Mandibular or Maxillary Abscesses. These abscesses often develop in the region of the third premolar and the first and second molar teeth. Most cases involve the mandible. Food is trapped between the succeeding teeth or between the tooth and the gingival margin, resulting in penetration of the alveolus and entry of infection. Swelling of the mandible or maxilla caused by osteomyelitis may be palpable. The tooth becomes loose, and mastication with lateral movement of the mandible is painful. The tooth may ultimately be lost. In other cases, a sinus develops, which may discharge into the mouth or to the outside. Antibiotics may assist in the treatment of some animals. In others, extraction of the affected cheek teeth may be necessary. A molar extraction forceps, with the jaws at right angles to the handles, is best for this procedure (see Fig. 17–11 *C*, page 270).[21]

Both rostral and caudal mandibular or maxillary abscesses may result from periodontal disease.

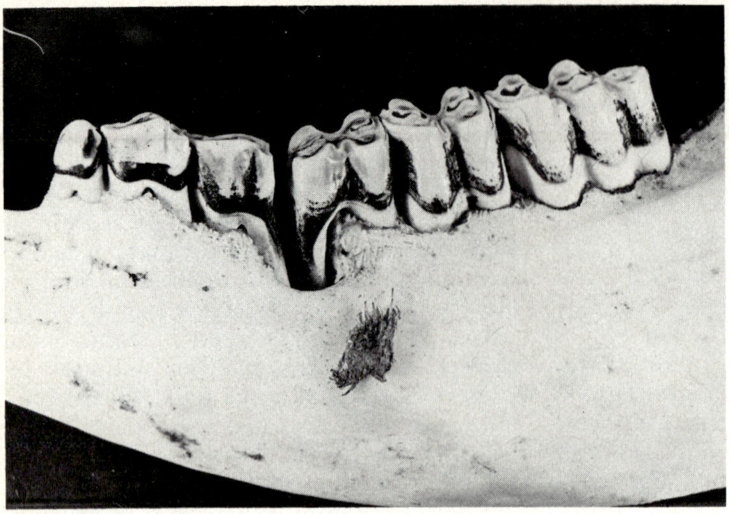

Figure 17–5. Periodontitis of the mandible in a 9 year old Friesian cow that developed alveolitis, allowing the space between the third premolar and the first molar to be packed with feed material, which, in turn, resulted in bone erosion, swelling, and sinus formation. The impacted feed can be seen in the center of the mandible. (Courtesy of B Noddle.)

Periodontitis

Cattle. Periodontitis is much less common in cattle than in sheep. It has been recorded mainly in Brazil, where it is known as "cara inchada" or swollen face.[22] It is a periodontitis of calves and older zebu cattle and is associated with a chronic ossifying periostitis of the maxilla that influences the eruption of both the temporary and the permanent cheek teeth. The mandible is affected less frequently.[23] There is usually an obvious hard, bony swelling; examination of the mouth reveals loss of teeth or loose cheek teeth, with deep periodontal pockets around the teeth.

Affected cattle usually also have diarrhea and loss of condition, and they eventually die. The syndrome is seen only in specific areas, and transferring cattle to non-affected areas results in improvement. There appears to be an association of disease with low-fertility pastures in which Guinea grass *(Panicum maximum)* predominates. The type of lesions found have been considered to be consistent with bacterial infection[24] that might be present, particularly in the Guinea grass areas. It is not uncommon to find cases of alveolitis at postmortem examination (Fig. 17–5).

Sheep (Paradontal Disease, Alveolar Periostitis, "Broken Mouth"). The term "broken mouth" refers to the loss of some rostral teeth in the adult sheep (Fig. 17–6). It is considered to be of economic importance in Britain, New Zealand, and Pakistan. Periodontal disease is by no means new, being found in many archaeological specimens from neolithic times onward.[25] Broken mouth was commonly present (73 percent of the time) in sheep slaughtered when they were 5 to 6 years old,[26] and 69 percent of hill-bred sheep had some tooth loss.[27] It is an important cause for culling hill-bred sheep because farmers contend that the sheep lose condition,[28] though it is not so important on good grazing in lowland situations.[27] Prevalence varies among farms, breeds, and seasons, advancing more quickly in the summer and autumn.[29, 30]

Characteristics of the Rostral Teeth. The rostral teeth are in shallow sockets and are mobile. The periodontal ligament that anchors the roots in their sockets is wide and loosely organized.[31, 32] Lingually, large bundles of collagen fibers attach the tooth to the alveolar bone running roughly at right angles to the tooth axis, and they can accept the forces to which the rostral teeth are sub-

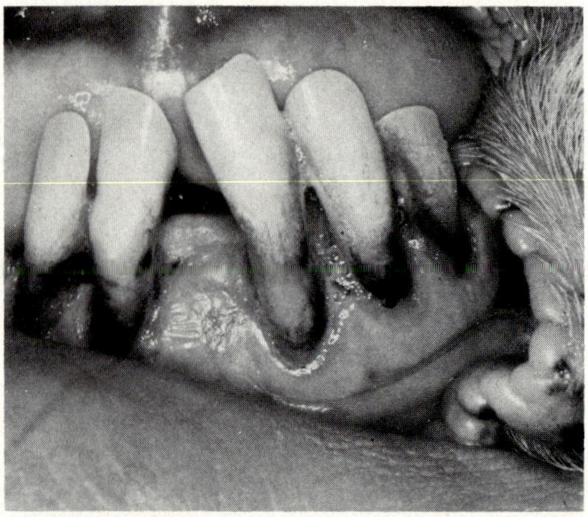

Figure 17–6. Broken mouth (periodontitis) in a ewe.

jected. The caudal teeth are initially without root formation and are kept in their alveoli by the unerupted crown plus the coronal cement.

Classification of Periodontitis in Sheep. Two types of periodontitis are generally recognized. One affects mainly the rostral teeth and results in the premature loss of teeth, and is referred to as "broken mouth."[33] The other affects both rostral and caudal teeth, but primarily the latter, and is an acute periodontitis beginning as gingivitis and resulting in the development of deep periodontal pockets and loosening of the teeth.

In the first type, the rostral teeth appear normal, but there is a marked migration rostrally from their sockets, which is soon accompanied by a degradation of the peripheral alveolar bone, together with a rapid increase in the depth of the periodontal pockets between the tooth and periodontal tissue. The depth of the pocket is often closely related to the severity of plaque formation. The result of this progressive periodontitis is that the rostral teeth have limited bone support, and they are held in position mainly by collagen fibers of the apical periodontium. This process may occur without much overt gingivitis,[34] though in some cases inflamed gingivae may be present underneath fecal-like debris and calculus. In other cases, a purulent gingivitis is seen.[30] Most work has involved the rostral teeth, since they are easier to examine and measure, but similar changes occur in the caudal region[30] and affect both the lingual and buccal sides of the teeth. The cheek teeth are not lost as frequently, because more of the tooth is surrounded by alveolar bone, and the stresses on the teeth differ from those acting on the rostral ones. Extensive work undertaken on mandibles after death has shown abnormalities, including loss of alveolar bone, swelling of alveolar bone often with increased porosity, uneven tooth line, discoloration of the mandible, and sinus formation (Fig. 17–7).[25] Of 217 adult mandibles examined, 59 (27 per cent) had advanced disease and 15 (7 percent) had slight periodontal disease. Loss of alveolar bone with some swelling occurred more frequently between the third premolar and the first molar teeth. Cheek teeth normally are loose rather than missing.[35] The lower teeth are more likely to be lost than are the upper teeth.

The second form of periodontitis has been described mainly in New Zealand and is acute in nature.[36] It affects mainly the molar teeth

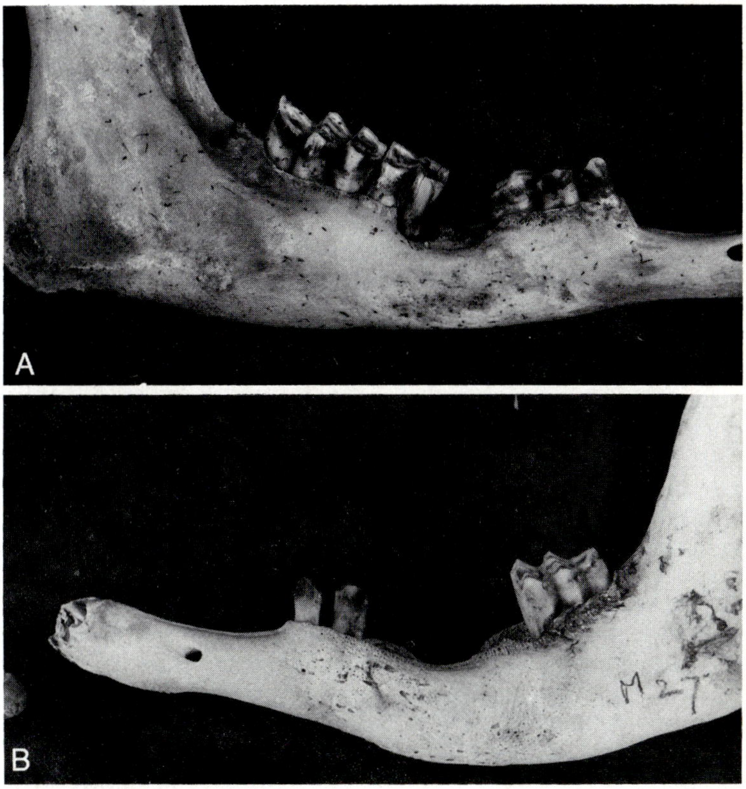

Figure 17–7. Periodontitis. *A,* Right mandible of a goat showing bone erosion and loss of first molar tooth. *B,* Left mandible of a mouflon showing loss of all but the first and second premolar and third molar teeth. The mandibular bone is slightly swollen with increased porosity. (Courtesy of B Noddle.)

and occurs in late winter or early spring, producing an ulcerative and necrotic gingivitis. It may involve all periodontal tissues and produces a fetid smell. Erosion of the periodontium around the molar roots can occur and can lead to chronic abscess formation.[37] The classic descriptions given, however, do not completely embrace the observations of a possible acute inflammatory condition superimposed on a chronic periodontitis.[38, 39]

Etiology, Symptoms, and Treatment. Various factors have been considered important in "broken mouth," and of these, genetic traits, environmental influences, and infection with a particular type of plaque-forming bacteria are probably most important.[24] The factors influencing the synthesis of collagen, which is a major component of the periodontal ligament, may also be important; they include manganese ions, oxygen, vitamin C, ferrous ions, the copper enzyme lysyl oxidase, and an adequate supply of protein.[40] Mechanical trauma, such as eating frozen turnips, may also be of importance.[41]

The clinical signs vary considerably; often no signs are noticeable if rostral teeth are involved. However, on examining the mouth there may be calculus formation and gingival recession, and in some cases pus can be expressed from the alveoli. There may be some discomfort on mastication, but this is much more noticeable if the cheek teeth are involved. Mastication may occur on one side only, with the mouth being held open between each jaw movement. In some cases, drooling and pressure on the teeth may produce discomfort.[21] If there is bone involvement, the swelling of the maxilla or mandible will be palpable. Most cases of cheek tooth involvement are first indicated by a loss of condition.[21] Although it is not always the case, the presence of "broken mouth" often suggests loose cheek teeth.

Little can be offered in terms of therapy, since the etiology is still doubtful. If the rostral teeth are very loose and much gingival retraction is present, it is probable that pain occurs with prehension and mastication. In such cases, it is best to extract the tooth following the use of a sedative, such as xylazine, and local anesthesia. Tooth clipping has also been practiced. Sheep can survive adequately without rostral teeth provided that they do not have to graze too closely on pasture or remove silage from tightly packed clamps (Fig. 17–8). The use of a daily dose of streptomycin sulfate (1 g) for 5 to 7 days has been of value in the early stages of the disease.[3] The observation that the presence of loose cheek teeth must be extremely painful to the sheep during mastication led to the suggestion that any loose cheek teeth should be removed under sedation and local anesthesia.[21] The procedure is performed with the aid of a gag and using dental forceps having jaws that are at right angles to the handle (see Fig. 17–11 *C*, page 270). The technique has increased the productive life of affected animals. A steel brace, fitted around permanent incisors and held in position with dental plastic, can be used in an attempt to overcome "broken mouth." Few critical, long-term evaluations have been undertaken of this commercially available product. However, results in trials on hill sheep have not been encouraging. In Australia, a method of filing teeth with a special gag has also been used. However, since the present state of knowledge about periodontitis in sheep suggests that inflammation of the gingivae and subsequent loss of tissue are major factors, the apparatus would seem to be of little benefit.

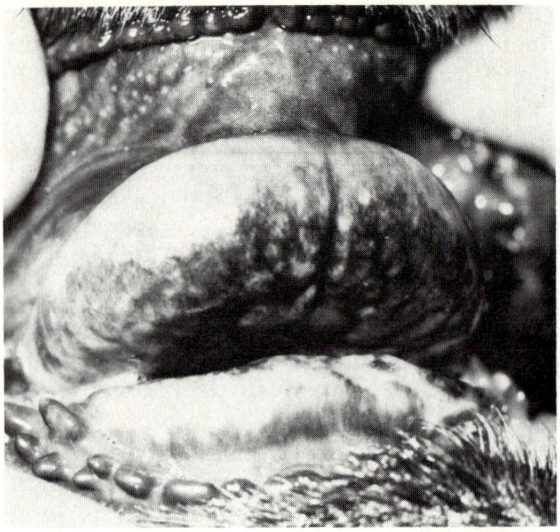

Figure 17–8. Broken mouth in a lowland ewe that was surviving with no teeth.

Dentigerous Cysts

Dentigerous cysts have been reported in ruminants, particularly sheep,[2] and may be associated with excessive rostral tooth attrition, maleruption of the permanent rostral teeth, and osteopathy of the mandibular bone.[4] There is a swelling of the mandible that is often obvious, both visibly and on palpation. Radiographs demonstrate the cystic nature of the swelling.

Oral Neoplasms

Neoplasms of the oral structures in ruminants are rare. Most are squamous cell carcinomata. There is usually a marked invasion of tissue. The gums or hard palate are involved in cattle. There is usually a considerable amount of bone erosion, resulting in loosening or displacement of the cheek teeth. On examination, a large, grayish, ulcerated mass is present, often with a fetid smell. The tumors usually invade the adjacent sinuses, which can result in bulging of the face. They can also invade local or regional lymph nodes, the nasal cavity, the orbital cavity, or the cranial cavity.[42]

Osteodystrophia Fibrosa

Osteodystrophia fibrosa is caused by resorption of calcium from bone and its replacement by fibrous connective tissue. It can result from calcium, phosphorus, or vitamin D deficiencies or from primary or secondary hyperparathyroidism. Hypocalcemia can result in increased parathyroid activity; secondary parathyroidism in animals can occur when there is nutritional deficiency and chronic renal disease. It is seen most commonly in the goat,[43] it is seen occasionally in cattle, and it is rarely seen in sheep. The condition occurs in the growing animal and consists of a bilateral swelling of the mandible (Fig. 17–9), maxilla, or both. The swelling is soft and painless. Often the animal drools and cannot eat properly. Radiographs reveal poorly mineralized bone, and there is rotation of the cheek teeth so that the crowns are directed lingually and the roots buccally. It may be possible to cut the bone with a knife, and there are often fractures of long bones. Blood calcium levels may be reduced and alkaline phosphatase levels may be raised. Treatment is to ensure a ratio of calcium:phosphorus of at least 2:1 in the diet, and this can perhaps be accomplished by adding ground limestone.

Tooth Extraction

Tooth extraction in cattle and sheep should involve general anesthesia (thiopental and halothane-oxygen) or deep narcosis (xylazine) and local anesthesia. Local anesthesia is obtained by infiltrating the involved tissues rather than by using a nerve block. No attempt should be made to remove teeth in the fully conscious animal because the roots are often deceptively well imbedded, and severe damage to the alveolar bone and mucosa may result. The gingivae are incised ventrally in a vertical direction over the tooth until the bone is reached (Fig. 17–10 *A* and *B*). The surrounding periodontal tissue is broken down by means of appropriate-sized dental elevators (Figs. 17–10 *C* and 17–11 *A*). The tooth is grasped and traction is applied only when the tissue has been broken down on all sides (Fig. 17–10 *D*).

If the tooth does not show signs of movement, it must be further separated from its alveolus using the elevators. Traction should follow alignment with the tooth. The roots tend to curve vertically and caudally. The tooth should be raised dorsally and vertically or caudally.

Molar teeth can be extracted in cattle by means of elevators and molar forceps (Fig.

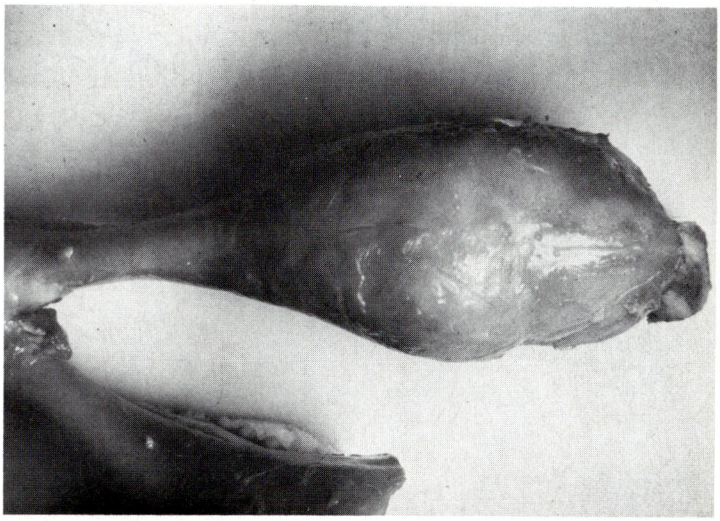

Figure 17–9. Osteodystrophia fibrosa of the mandible in a goat.

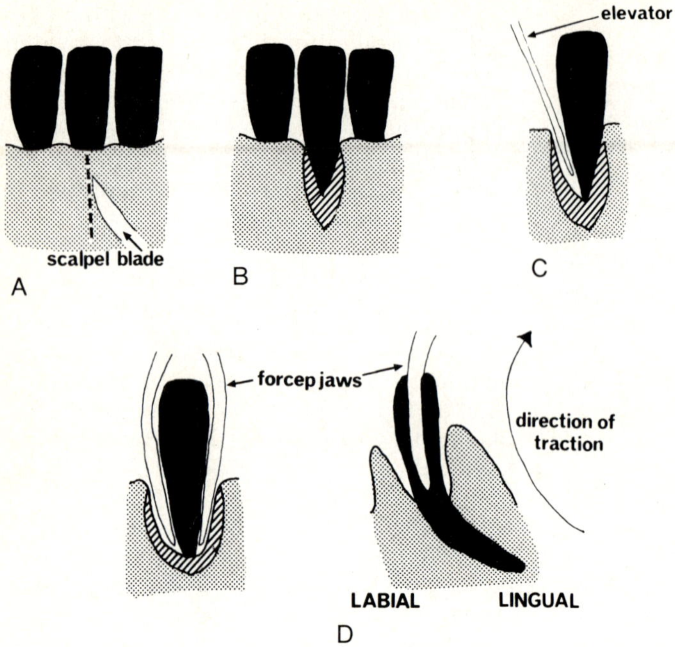

Figure 17–10. Rostral tooth extraction. *A,* A scalpel is used to incise gingiva. *B,* A cut is made down to the level of the bone. *C,* Periodontal tissue is broken down with a tooth elevator. *D,* The tooth is grasped with dental forceps and removed.

17–11 *B*). Again, much attention must be paid to ensure an adequate breakdown of the periodontal ligament. The degree to which the mouth can be opened is limited in sheep and goats; in most cases there is very little room to work. Generally, if molar teeth or adjacent bone is diseased, they are very mobile and are easily extracted. A pair of molar forceps with the jaws at right angles to the handle (Fig. 17–11 *C*) is best for this work. There is no need to occlude the opened alveoli. Prophylactic antibiotic therapy (see Table 17–1) should be provided at the time of extraction to prevent the possibility of hematogenous spread of bacteria and septicemia.

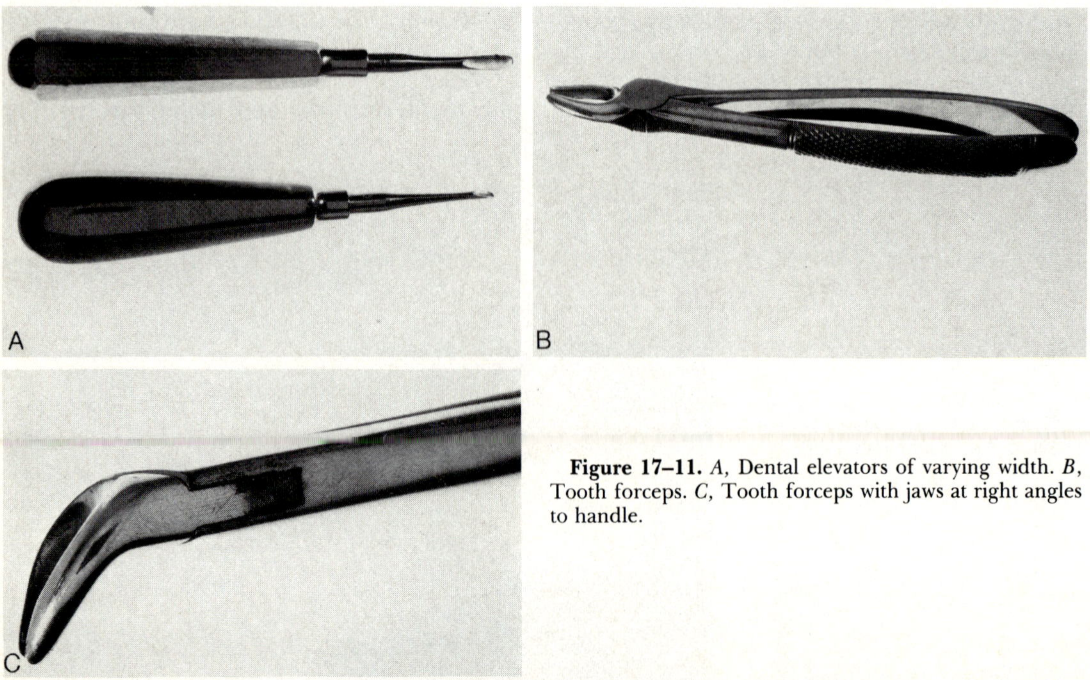

Figure 17–11. *A,* Dental elevators of varying width. *B,* Tooth forceps. *C,* Tooth forceps with jaws at right angles to handle.

References

1. Garlick NL: The teeth of the ox in clinical diagnosis. III. Developmental anomalies and general pathology. *Am J Vet Res* 15:500–508, 1954.
2. Colyer F: Variations and Diseases of the Teeth of Animals. London, John Bale, Sons and Danielsson Ltd., 1936, pp. 1–750.
3. Jensen R: Diseases of the digestive system. *In* Jensen R (ed.): Diseases of Sheep. Philadelphia, Lea & Febiger, 1974, pp. 209–213.
4. Bruère AN, West DM, Orr MB, O'Callaghan MW: A syndrome of dental abnormalities in sheep. 1. Clinical aspects on a commercial sheep farm in the Wairarapa. *New Zeal Vet J* 27:152–158, 1979.
5. Steenkamp JDG: Effect of the brittle hardness and abrasive hardness of enamel on degree of attrition of deciduous teeth of representative breeds of *Bos indicus* and *Bos taurus* origin. *Agroanimalia* 1:23–34, 1969.
6. Steenkamp JDG: Differences in manner of occlusion of representative indigenous and exotic breeds of cattle and effect on wear of deciduous incisor teeth. *Agroanimalia* 2:85–92, 1970.
7. Barnicoat CR, Hall DM: Attrition of incisors of grazing sheep. Nature 185 (No. 4707):179, 1960.
8. Healy WB, Ludwig TG: Ingestion of soil by sheep in New Zealand in relation to wear of teeth. *Nature* 208 (No. 5012):806–807, 1965.
9. Healy WB, Cutress TW, Michie C: Wear of sheep's teeth. IV. Reduction of soil ingestion and teeth wear by supplementary feeding. *New Zealand J Agric Res* 10:201–209, 1967.
10. Steenkamp JDG: Wear in bovine teeth. Paper presented to 2nd Symposium on Animal Production. South Africa Society of Animal Production (Rhodesia Branch), Salisbury. pp. 11–23, 1969.
11. Franklin MC: Influence of diet on dental development in sheep. *Australian C.S.I.R.O. Bulletin* 252, 1950.
12. McRoberts MR, Hill R, Dalgarno AC: Effects of deficient diets on teeth of growing sheep. *J Agric Sci Camb* 65:1–27, 1965.
13. Boley LT. Bovine tooth capping. *Mod Vet Pract* 43(8):47–49, 1962.
14. Suckling GW, Purdell-Lewis D: Macroscopic appearance, microhardness and microradiographic characteristics of experimentally produced fluorotic lesions in sheep enamel. *Caries Res* 16:227–234, 1982.
15. Shupe JL, Olson AE: Fluoride toxicosis. *In* Amstutz HE (ed): Bovine Medicine and Surgery, 2nd ed., Vol. 1. Santa Barbara, American Veterinary Publications Ltd., 1980, pp. 475–488.
16. Mostafa IE: Studies of bovine farcy in the Sudan. II. Mycology of the disease. J Comp Pathol 77:231–236, 1967.
17. Blood DC, Radostitis OM, Henderson JA: Veterinary Medicine. 6th ed., London, Balliere Tindall, 1983.
18. Amstutz HE: Diseases of the mouth. *In* Amstutz HE (ed): Bovine Medicine and Surgery, 2nd ed, Vol. 2. Santa Barbara, American Veterinary Publications Ltd., 1980, pp. 650–656.
19. Colahan PT, Pascoe JR: Stabilization of equine and bovine mandibular and maxillary fractures, using an acrylic splint. *J Am Vet Med Assoc* 182:1117–1119, 1983.
20. Johnson JH, Hull BL, Dorn AS: The mouth. *In* Anderson, NV (ed): Veterinary Gastroenterology. Philadelphia, Lea & Febiger, 1980, pp. 337–371.
21. Andrews AH: Clinical signs and treatment of aged sheep with loose mandibular and maxillary cheek teeth. *Vet Rec* 108:331–333, 1981.
22. Camargo WV de A, Fernandes NS, Santiago AMH: Contribuição ao estudo de "Cara inchada" em bovinos. *Biologico* 47:183–185, 1981.
23. Döbereiner J, Tokamia CH, Rosa IV: Cara inchada, a periodontal disease of cattle in Brazil. Proceedings of 9th International Congress on Diseases of Cattle, Vol. 2. Paris, 1976, pp. 1133–1139.
24. Page RC, Schroeder HE: Periodontitis in other mammalian animals. *In* Periodontitis in Man and Other Animals. A Comparative Review. Basel, S Karger, pp. 58–221, 1982.
25. Noddle B: Personal communication, 1983.
26. Herrtage ME, Saunders RW, Terlecki S: Physical examination of cull ewes at point of slaughter. *Vet Rec* 95:257–260, 1974.
27. Spence, JA: Studies into the pathogenesis of early tooth loss (broken mouth) in sheep. FRCVS Thesis, Vol. I, pp. 1–124; Vol. II, pp. 1–95, 1982.
28. Miller WC, West GP: Black's Veterinary Dictionary, 6th ed. London, Adam and Charles Black, 1962, p. 126.
29. Quarterman J, Dalgarno AC: Observations on the development of periodontal disease in hill sheep and the effect of selenium injections. *Res Vet Sci* 9:41–47, 1968.
30. Spence JA, Aitchinson GV, Sykes AR, Atkinson PJ: Broken mouth (premature incisor loss) in sheep: the pathogenesis of periodontal disease. *J Comp Pathol* 90:275–292, 1980.
31. Cutress TW: Incisive apparatus of the sheep. *Res Vet Sci* 13:74–76, 1972.
32. Spence JA: Functional morphology of the periodontal ligament in the incisor region of the sheep. *Res Vet Sci* 25:144–151, 1978.
33. Hitchin AD, Walker-Lane J: Broken mouth in hill sheep. *Agric* 66:5–8, 1959.
34. Lyle-Stewart W, Hatt SD, Cresswell E: Dental conservation in sheep, preliminary report of a clinical trial. *Vet Rec* 78:40–44, 1966.
35. Richardson C, Richards M, Terlecki S, Miller WM: Jaws of adult culled ewes. *J Agric Sci Camb* 93:521–529, 1979.
36. Salisbury RM, Armstrong MC, Gray KG: Ulceromembranous gingivitis in sheep. *New Zeal Vet J* 1:51–52, 1953.
37. Cutress TW, Ludwig TG: Periodontal disease in sheep. 1. Review of the literature. *J Periodontol* 40:529–534, 1969.
38. Mackinnon MM: A pathological study of an enzootic paradontal disease of mature sheep. *New Zeal Vet J* 7:18–26, 1959.
39. Hart KE, Mackinnon MM: Enzootic paradontal disease of adult sheep in the Bulls-Santoft area. *New Zeal Vet J* 6:118–123, 1958.
40. Millar KR: Factors that can influence the supported tissue of teeth. Sheep and Beef Society of the New Zealand Veterinary Association. Proceedings of the Society's 9th Seminar, Lincoln College. July 6–7, 1979, pp. 4–10.
41. Benzie D, Kay RNB, Gill JC: Effects of frozen turnips and mineral supplements on incisor tooth loss in sheep. *Proc Nutr Soc* 40:115A, 1981.
42. Jubb KVF, Kennedy PC: The upper alimentary system. *In* Pathology of Domestic Animals, 2nd ed, Vol. 2. Academic Press, New York, 1970, pp. 1–44.
43. Andrews AH, Ingram PL, Longstaffe AJ: Osteodystrophia fibrosa in young goats. *Vet Rec* 112:404–406, 1983.

Chapter Eighteen

Oral and Dental Disease in Pigs

CE Harvey and RHC Penny

ANATOMY[1]

Unlike the other major species of veterinary interest, the domestic pig *(Sus scrofa domesticus)* is omnivorous. Its teeth and other important oral structures reflect a combination of carnivorous (large canine teeth for grasping and tearing) and herbivorous (grinding molar teeth) functions. The shape of the skull has been modified to be effective when rooting for food, though the primitive dolichocephalic shape has been changed by selection to a more mesocephalic shape in some modern breeds.

Premaxilla, Maxilla, and Mandible

The bones carrying the teeth are massive when compared with the rest of the skull. They form a long snout with a large surface area for masticatory muscle attachment on the dorsally extended temporal fossa, which peaks at the parietal crest and on the wide zygomatic arch (Fig. 18–1). The thickness of the dental ridge and the thickness of the maxilla itself combine to contain the roots of the premolar and molar teeth. There is no need for the roots of the teeth to penetrate into the nasal passageways. Thus, nasal discharge is an unlikely consequence of dental disease in pigs when compared with some other species. The general shape of the oral surface of the maxilla and the palate is a rectangle (Fig. 18–2 *A*); thus, the cheek teeth form two parallel rows rather than an arch.

The mandible is particularly thick, the vertical ramus being very broad. The roots of the teeth (even those of the canine teeth) extend only about halfway into the dorsoventral depth of the horizontal ramus (see Fig. 18–1). The mandible is a single bone, which is formed from two halves that unite rostrally soon after birth. The general shape of the mandible is in the form of a V. The lower cheek teeth form two parallel lines to match the upper cheek teeth; thus, the long axis of a line through the cheek teeth is offset at an angle to the long axis of the horizontal ramus of the mandible (Fig. 18–2 *B*). There is a medial bony projection at the caudal end of the horizontal ramus to accommodate this divergence. The temporomandibular joint has a broad articular surface on its temporal side, permitting considerable rostrocaudal movement, but only limited transverse movement, in addition to hinge movement.

Oral Cavity

The commissures of the lips are set well back on the cheek, allowing the mouth to be opened rather widely in a cooperative animal; the lips themselves are thick and are not capable of much movement or stretching. The snout is a very strong but exceedingly mobile structure. The jaws form a long oral cavity, the space of which is filled mostly by the fleshy tongue, which is long but is not capable of extending very far out of the mouth. The tongue has taste-sensing papillae on its dorsal aspect and a distinct fold for the epiglottis on its dorsocaudal aspect. The dorsal surface of the mouth is formed by the hard palate, with a mucosal surface thrown into mediolateral ridges separated by a midline furrow. The incisive papilla is obvious at the rostal end of the palate.

Teeth

The dental formulae of the deciduous and permanent dentitions of the pig are

$$D: 2(i\,\tfrac{3}{3}\,c\,\tfrac{1}{1}\,p\,\tfrac{3}{3}) = 28$$
$$P: 2(I\,\tfrac{3}{3}\,C\,\tfrac{1}{1}\,P\,\tfrac{4}{4}\,M\,\tfrac{3}{3}) = 44$$

Eruption times are in Table 18–1.

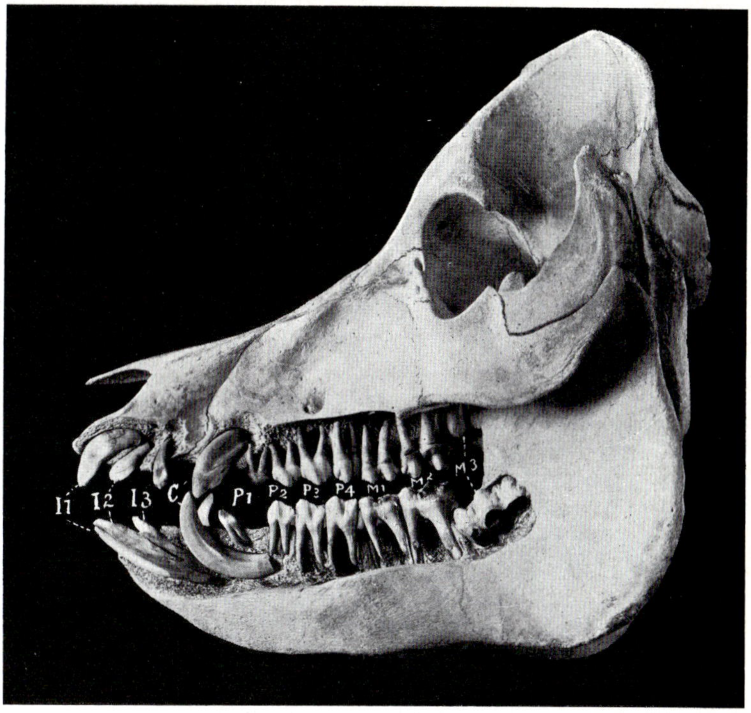

Figure 18–1. Lateral view of the skull of an 18 month old pig. Bone covering the roots of the teeth has been removed. C = canine; I = incisor; M = molar; P = premolar. (From Getty R: Sisson and Grossman's Anatomy of the Domestic Animals, 5th ed. Philadelphia, WB Saunders Co., 1975.)

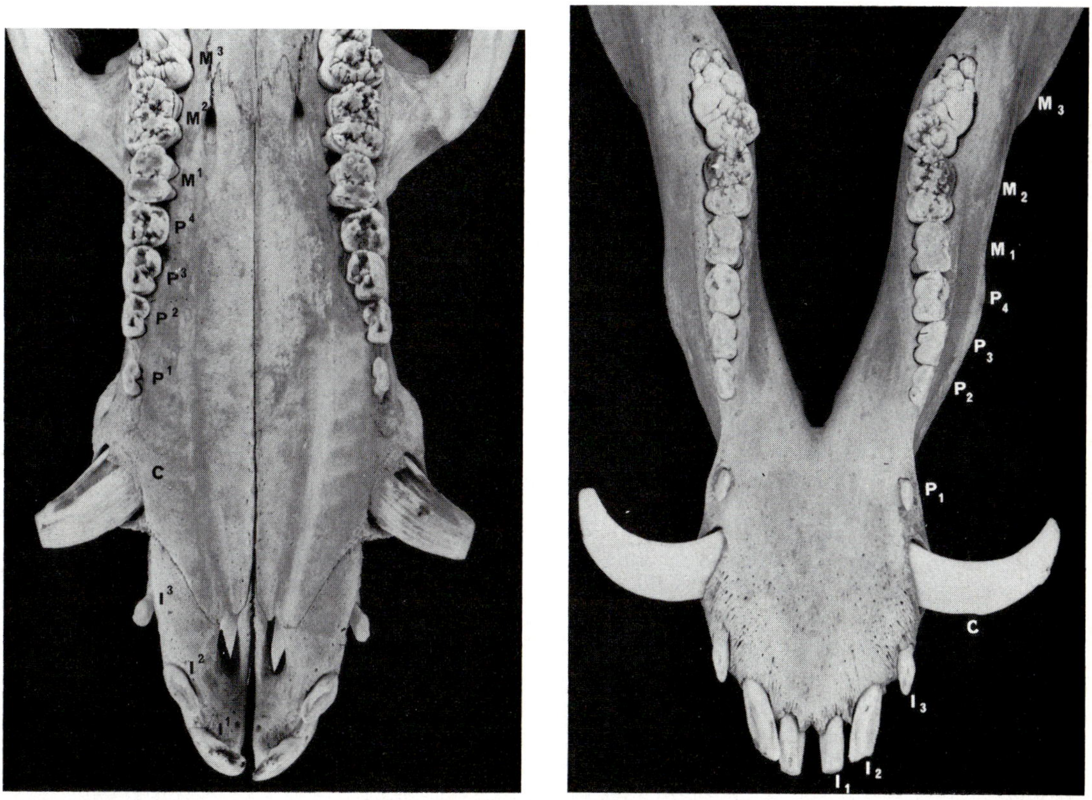

Figure 18–2. *A,* Ventral view of the maxilla and palatine bones of a mature pig with the teeth in place. *B,* Dorsal view of the mandible and lower teeth of a mature pig. (From Getty R: Sisson and Grossman's Anatomy of the Domestic Animals, 5th ed. Philadelphia, WB Saunders Co., 1975.)

Table 18–1. Dental Eruption Times in the Pig

Tooth	Deciduous	Permanent
I1	2–4 wk	12 mo
I2 upper	2–3 mo	16–20 mo
lower	1–2 mo	16–20 mo
I3	Before birth	8–10 mo
C	Before birth	9–10 mo
P1	5 mo	12–15 mo
P2	5–7 wk	
P3 upper	4–8 d	
lower	2–4 wk	
P4 upper	4–8 d	
lower	2–4 wk	
M1		4–6 mo
M2		8–12 mo
M3		18–20 mo

The shape of the deciduous teeth is very similar to that of the permanent teeth.

The four medial incisor teeth (I1, I2) are larger than the lateral incisor tooth and lie rostral to it, with a diastema of 2 cm to 3 cm separating them. The central and middle incisor teeth are also usually separated, but by a smaller interdental space; these teeth on the upper and lower jaws form an occluding set for grasping. The upper incisors are curved, with the crowns pointing ventrally. The lower incisors are almost straight and point rostrodorsally. The crowns of the incisor teeth are incompletely covered by enamel, and the lingual or occlusal surface is covered by cementum.

The canine teeth are separated from the lateral incisor tooth by a diastema of 3 cm to 4 cm. The canine teeth in adult male pigs are well developed (see Fig. 18–2) and may project between the lips to be visible as external tusks. The crowns are triangular in cross section and are covered by enamel only on the lateral (convex) surface. The roots remain open so that the tooth continuously erupts as it is worn by occlusion. The rostral surfaces of the upper canine teeth occlude against the caudal surfaces of the lower canine teeth.

There is space between the canine teeth and the main line of cheek teeth; in the upper jaw, it is between the canine and the first premolar teeth, and in the lower jaw it is between the first and second premolar teeth. The cheek teeth are progressively larger from a rostral to a caudal direction (see Fig. 18–2). The crowns of all the cheek teeth are relatively short and are covered by enamel; those of the premolar teeth are ridged, which allows the shearing of ingesta. The molar teeth crowns have an occlusal table thrown into folds or mounds, which permits crushing or grinding of ingesta. The number of roots varies: the lower first premolar has one; the upper first and second premolars and the lower second and third premolars have two; the upper third premolar and the lower fourth premolar have three; the lower first and second molars have four; the upper fourth premolar and the lower third molar have five; and the upper first, second, and third molars have six.

Pharynx

The soft palate is long and thick and often has a midline caudal projection—the uvula. The tonsils are less distinct than in other veterinary species, but other scattered areas of lymphatic tissue are visible in the oropharynx and on the root of the tongue. The tonsils are a major entry point for disease-producing organisms, and they have a rich surface flora that often includes pathogenic organisms, including *Erysipelothrix rhusiopathiae.*[2]

Glands Supplying the Oral Cavity

The serous parotid glands are large triangular structures lying on the side of the face and neck caudal to the masseter muscle; the duct runs over the surface of the masseter muscle to enter the mouth on the mucosal surface of the cheek at the level of the upper fouth premolar or first molar tooth.

The seromucinous mandibular gland is a small oval structure with a rostral projection. It lies between the parotid gland laterally and the muscles of the neck and pharynx; the duct runs rostrally, opening on the lateral surface of the frenulum of the tongue with the sublingual gland. The sublingual gland, which is also seromucinous, consists of two parts—a small caudal part that feeds into a distinct duct that runs with the mandibular duct and a larger rostral part that opens through a series of small ducts into the sublingual furrow.

There are several other areas of saliva-secreting glandular tissue that are less well defined, including the palatine, the ventral and dorsal buccal, and the labial glands. There is no anatomically distinct gland in the position of the zygomatic (orbital) gland of carnivores.

ORAL EXAMINATION

The oral cavity of pigs is not very accessible. Although the mouth opens rather widely when compared with other large veterinary species, lack of patient cooperation often prevents inspection of the cheeks, palate, and cheek teeth. In a suckling piglet or a cooperative animal, the incisor and canine teeth, the gingivae, and the tongue can be inspected. Fortunately, the area available for inspection is usually sufficient to observe the lesions caused by vesicular diseases, which are the most important infectious oral diseases of pigs. Full inspection of the oral cavity and pharynx requires sedation or anesthesia. Because of the expense and time involved, it is rarely done, with the result that there is little documented information on dental abnormalities in pigs.

Radiographic examination of oral structures is rarely performed, though radiographs are sometimes used for the diagnosis of atrophic rhinitis or when certification of the presence of normal turbinates is required.

ORAL DISEASES

It is rarely economical to treat oral diseases in pigs. Periodontal disease, the major oral disease of many other species, has not been reported to any great extent in pigs; a recent compilation of studies on periodontal disease in humans and in other animals does not contain reference to the pig.[3] The anatomy and diet of pigs are sufficiently similar to those of humans that a predisposition to peridontal disease seems likely; factors that affect the incidence of periodontal disease—such as the microbiology of the periodontal pocket, plaque formation, and salivary pH—have received little attention in pigs. Since periodontal disease is a slowly developing, but progressive, condition, the apparently low incidence is probably due to the relatively young age of most pigs at slaughter.

When clinical signs suggest the presence of oral disease, recognition of a cause is essential because of the potential economic loss and epizootiological considerations associated with the common oral diseases of pigs.

Vesicular and Ulcerative Oral Lesions

The diseases that cause vesicles or erosions on the oral mucosa (most typically on the tongue, lips, and gingivae), and on the snout, are foot and mouth disease, vesicular exanthema, vesicular stomatitis, and swine vesicular disease. The vesicles are formed from a bleb of clear fluid that accumulates from acute necrosis of oral epithelium, particularly of the stratum spinosum. The vesicles usually rupture soon after formation, leaving a hemorrhagic, eroded surface that heals rapidly if secondary bacterial infection does not become established.

It is impossible to differentiate the diseases causing vesicles by clinical observations alone. Fever is also common with all four of the diseases just named, and the first indication of abnormality may be anorexia, which results when the oral lesions cause discomfort to the animal during eating. Lameness, or an unwillingness to rise or move around, may also be seen, because vesicular lesions occur frequently on the feet, typically on the coronary band and bulbs of the heel. Lesions occasionally arise at other sites, such as the teats of nursing sows. They are more common on the feet than in the mouth in swine vesicular disease. Drooling may be seen and is more common in vesicular stomatitis. Abortion may occur in pregnant females who have foot and mouth disease or vesicular exanthema. Diarrhea is sometimes seen in vesicular exanthema.

These four conditions are caused by highly communicable viruses, and foot and mouth disease and vesicular stomatitis can be transmitted to other species (see Chapters Fourteen and Seventeen). Swine vesicular disease has been seen in humans and causes a flulike syndrome with production of antibodies. Because of the contagious nature of these diseases, prompt laboratory differentiation[4] is essential, a description of which is beyond the scope of this text.

Occasionally, ulcerative lesions are seen on the tongues of suckling pigs as part of the exudative dermatitis syndrome.[5] The skin lesions in affected animals are widespread, making differentiation from the vesicular diseases already described easy. The cause is *Staphylococcus hyicus.* Ulcerative granulomata caused by *Borrelia suilla* may involve the lips and cheeks and may spread to the labial mucosa.

Occasionally, tongue ulcers without vesicles are seen in pigs living in close contact with cattle which have the glossitis-respiratory syndrome. Ulcers may also occur on the tip of the tongue from trauma caused by damaged or sharp-edged feeding troughs. Widespread acute necrosis and erosion of the oral mucosa may be seen in the acute stage of paraquat poisoning.

Excessive Salivation

Drooling is seen in some disease syndromes, though rarely as a single clinical sign. Toxicity is the most common cause. Agents that are known to cause salivation in pigs include lead, levamisole, organophosphate and carbamate insecticides, paraquat (acutely, presumed from the carrier solvent), and nitrates from poisonous plants. The pattern of other clinical signs, or environmental evidence, is usually sufficient to provide a tentative diagnosis. Drooling may be seen as foaming at the mouth if chewing movements are also stimulated by the toxic agent. Other causes include a burned mouth from food that is too hot or a foreign body that is caught around a tooth. Salivation can be seen in pigs with rabies and in adult pigs with Aujeszky's disease (pseudorabies).

Abnormal Jaw Movements

Another non-specific sign that is seen with some toxic agents, such as chlorinated hydrocarbons and levamisole, is chattering jaws or facial muscle fasciculations, and it can also be seen in pigs with rabies. The signs of neuromuscular dysfunction are generally not limited to the head and neck area.

Grinding of the teeth is common in pigs of any age. The cause is not known. It could be a habit, or it could result from eruption pain or irritation of the teeth or gingivae from foreign bodies, excessive tooth wear, or caries.

Facial and Neck Swelling

The most common cause of swelling in the head and neck is bacterial infection, particularly with *Streptococcus* spp.[4, 6] Beta-hemolytic streptococci are common in the tonsils of healthy pigs, and they are a common cause of acute septicemia or chronic localized infections in many places in the body. *Streptococcus suis,* type 2, may also be carried in the tonsils of apparently healthy pigs. Abscesses, most often caused by Lancefield group E streptococci, are found predominantly in the head and neck. The bacteria enter the body through the tonsillar epithelium. Clinical signs occur only when the abscess is large enough to interfere with respiration or swallowing.

The major importance of this condition is the economic loss associated with condemnation of part or all of a carcass during meat inspection. Treatment of an established abscess consists of administration of an appropriate antibiotic (penicillin, tetracycline), surgical drainage, or resection. When the incidence of bacterial abscesses is high, the environment should be examined for sources of skin or mucous membrane punctures (such as rough edges of pens or troughs or unclipped deciduous teeth), and hygiene practices should be reviewed. Autogenous vaccines or feeding of a ration that contains tetracycline at 50 g to 400 g/ton can be used to obtain an immediate reduction in the incidence of abscesses. A phlegmonous pharyngitis and cellulitis occurs from the same cause in young pigs and may cause death.[2]

Less common causes of neck swelling include *Clostridium novyi* infection (usually accompanied by sudden death), anthrax that is limited to the pharyngeal lymph nodes, tuberculosis, and lymphosarcoma. Some of these lesions may cause cervical edema, respiratory distress, or dysphagia, or they may not be noticed until slaughter. It is very rare for neoplasms other than lymphosarcoma to occur in the head and neck area of pigs.

Occasionally, *Candida albicans* is the cause of maxillary swelling from infection ("thrush") of the nose, gingivae, and lips of young pigs, and is precipitated by either antibiotic administration or vitamin A deficiency. Affected piglets are dull, they lose their appetite, and they vomit. Black-gray to yellow-green diarrhea is seen. The lesions in the oral cavity appear as yellow-white crusts, mainly on the tongue, palate, and pharynx. About 50 percent of affected piglets die.[7] Diagnosis is made by examining a smear of the oral crusts or by culture. Antifungal agents have been used for treatment.[8]

With the exception of experimental biotin deficiency, nutritional deficiencies very rarely cause oral signs or lesions. Severe protein deprivation results in the increased keratinization of the buccal mucosa; scrapings of the mucosa can be used to assess the severity of the malnutrition.[9]

Fusobacterium necrophorum (Fusiformis necrophorus, Sphaerophorus necrophorus) is a common cause of necrobacillosis of oral tissues. If this infection gains entrance as a result of damage to the gingivae during tooth clipping, severe necrosis of the lips and tongue may result. Care should be taken to avoid the gingivae during tooth clipping, and the instrument must be keep clean.[4] Other uncommon causes of upper or lower jaw swelling and infections include actinomycosis and actinobacillosis; the lesions are similar to those seen in cattle (pages 263, 265). "Actinomycotic" lesions may be caused by *Actinomyces* spp. or by staphylococci.[2]

CONGENITAL ABNORMALITIES

The most common congenital abnormality affecting the oral structures of pigs is a short upper jaw (brachygnathia superior, Fig. 18–3). It is seen as an "almost normal" breed-associated feature in some strains of English large white and the now uncommon middle white breeds. The defect is often mild, but in severe cases, it can cause spectacular malocclusion. A short or twisted upper jaw is also a sign of atrophic rhinitis in pigs. Mandibular malalignment is an acquired condition that is discussed further on.

Harelip, cleft palate, absence of the jaw, and other cranial abnormalities occur sporadically in pigs and are sometimes associated with tongue abnormalities.[10, 11] The cause may be an inherited defect or an insult occurring *in utero*.[12] Affected animals usually die within a few days after birth.

Congenital dental abnormalities have been observed infrequently in pigs. Overgrowth of the continuously erupting tusks of wild boars is common and may occasionally result in penetration through the maxilla or palate;[13] these large tusks are used as charms or talismans by some Pacific Island natives. Congenital porphyria occurs occasionally and may cause a pink discoloration of one or more teeth.[2]

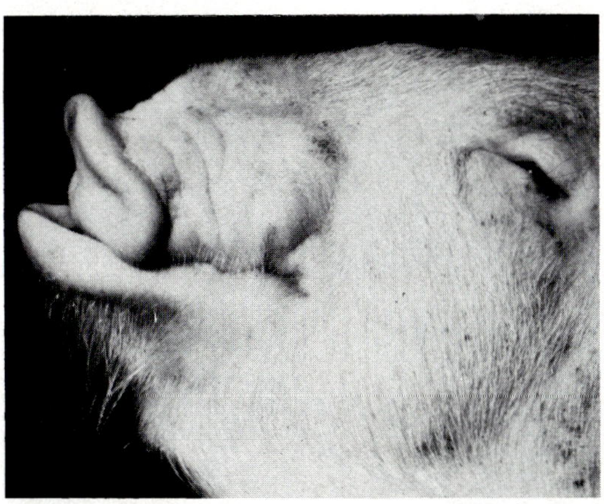

Figure 18–3. Deformed maxilla and snout in a pig. This abnormality could be due to a congenital defect or atrophic rhinitis.

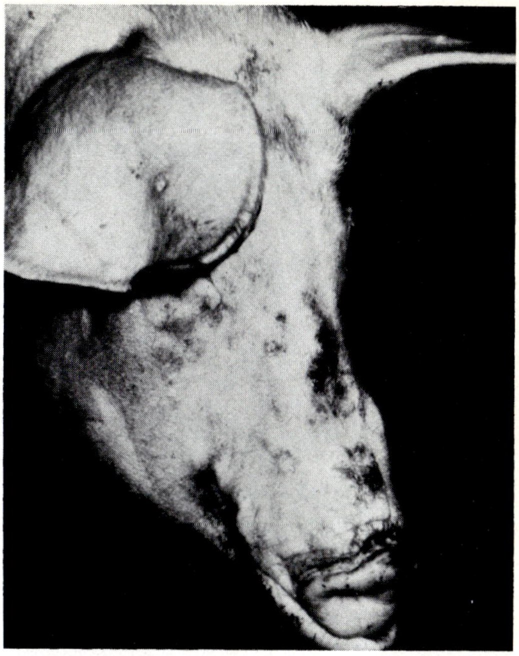

Figure 18–4. Deviated mandible of a pig.

ACQUIRED TOOTH AND JAW ABNORMALITIES

Mandibular Malalignment

Deviation of the lower jaw to the right or left in association with changes in the temporomandibular joint (Fig. 18–4) is common in many breeds of pigs in Britain.[14, 15] It is seen most commonly in pigs which are housed intensively in stalls or on tethers, and the deviation occurs toward the source of food and water in 90 percent of affected animals, suggesting that head movements and snout pressing are likely causes. Deviation has to be very severe to interfere with mastication.

The importance of this condition is that it can be confused with twisting of the snout caused by atrophic rhinitis.[16] To differentiate the two conditions, an imaginary line is drawn from a point in the middle of the skull between the eyes down the nasal peak to bisect the snout. If the line deviates to one side, the snout is twisted, and the cause is likely to be atrophic rhinitis. If the line passes through the center of the snout, the cause is mandibular malalignment.

Two types of deviation are recognized. In type A, the convexity of the articular surface is lost, with reduced curvature along both longitudinal and transverse axes and loss of height in the vertical ramus. In type B, the

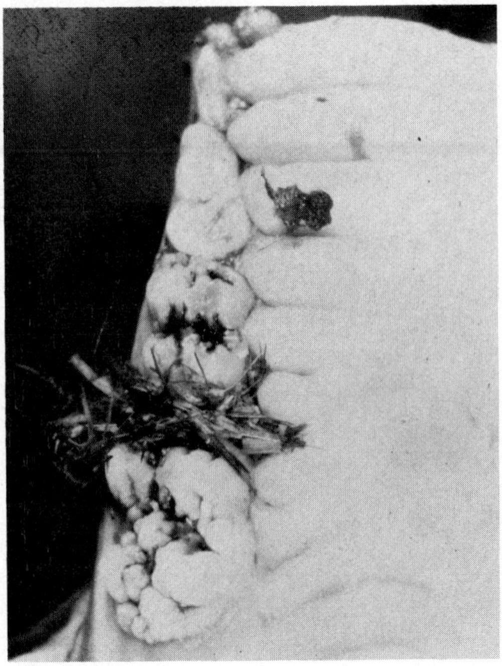

Figure 18–5. Straw wadded between upper cheek teeth of a pig.

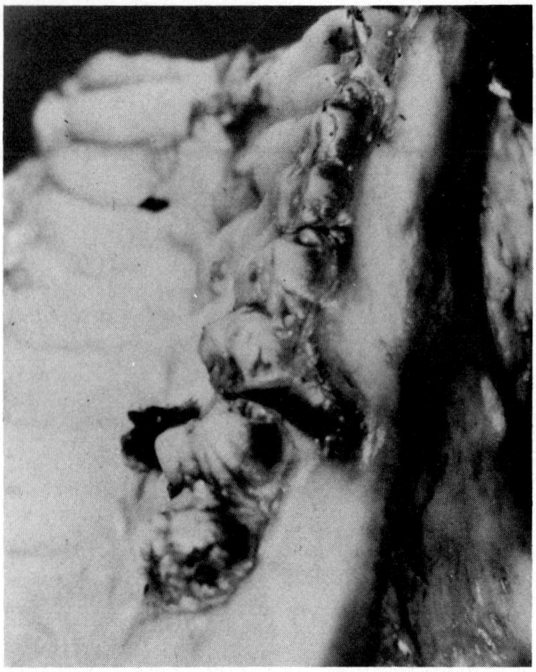

Figure 18–6. Gingivitis caused by impaction of foreign material between the upper cheek teeth of a pig.

condyle is relatively normal, but the height of the vertical ramus is reduced.

Osteoarthrosis and osteoarthritis have been observed in the temporomandibular joints of growing pigs. There are eburnation, cartilage lifting, and synovitis. The usual cause is *Erysipelothrix rhusiopathiae* infection.[17]

Dental Abnormalities

Pigs are notoriously inquisitive animals and will chew on and play with non-food objects, but they rarely swallow them. Foreign bodies lodged around, between, or in teeth were found in 5.3 percent of 2701 pigs examined at slaughter.[16] Wads of straw (Fig. 18–5) or pieces of wood wedged between teeth caused a localized gingivitis (Fig. 18–6). In pigs who were fed garbage, tinfoil was often wedged tightly between tooth cusps, resembling dental amalgam.

Abnormal wear of cheek teeth (Fig. 18–7) was observed in 37 percent of pigs.[16] It was present in both jaws and on both sides, was often bilaterally symmetrical, and was most obvious in the middle cheek teeth, in which a trench was formed. Chewing on the bars of pens or partitions, a common observation in modern pig units (Fig. 18–8), is a likely cause.

Caries has been found on the crowns of molar teeth (Fig. 18–9) in rare instances,[13, 18] and a severe form was found in 9 of 2701 pigs examined at the time of slaughter.[16] Pigs who are fed a carbohydrate-rich diet and are inoculated with a cariogenic oral flora will develop caries;[9] the size, difficulty of han-

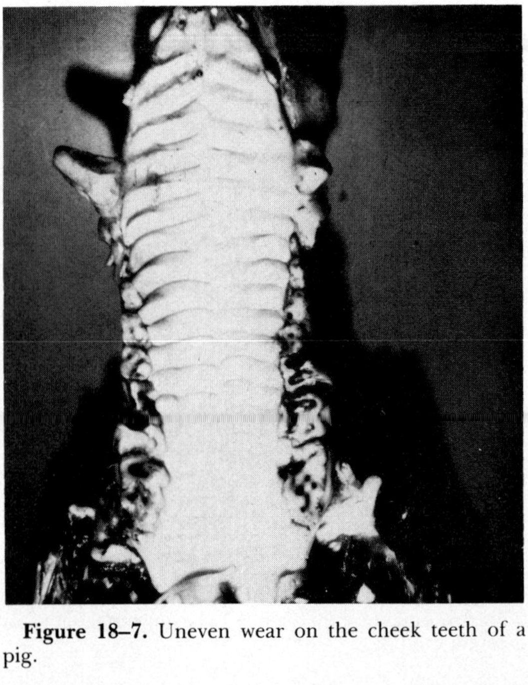

Figure 18–7. Uneven wear on the cheek teeth of a pig.

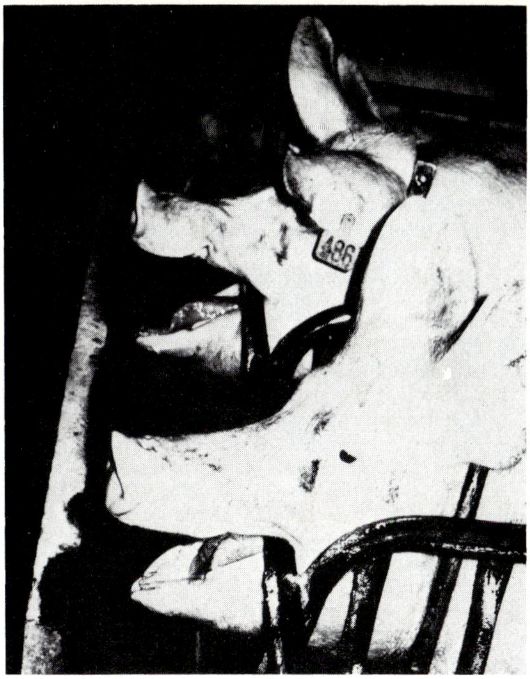

Figure 18–8. Pigs chewing the bars restraining them in stalls.

dling, and expense of pigs—even miniature pigs—has prevented the widespread adoption of this otherwise excellent animal model of human caries.

Calculus accumulates in large quantities in pigs, but differs in its mineral composition from that of humans.[9] For this reason, it has not been studied in any depth. A blackish discoloration that could be scraped off the teeth was observed in 29 percent of pigs examined at slaughter (Fig. 18–10).[16] The frequency apparently increased with age.

Clinically obvious periodontal disease is

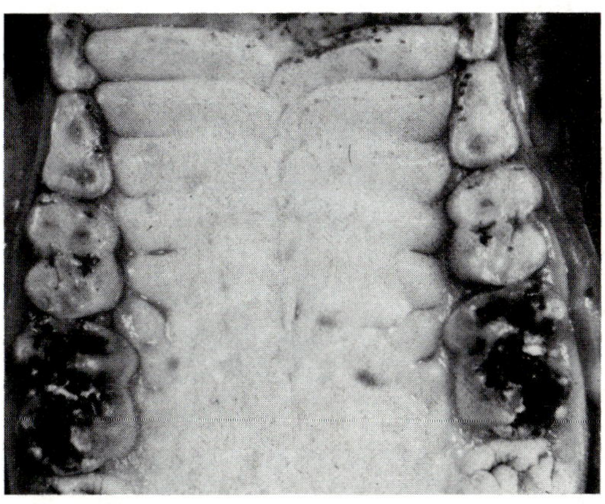

Figure 18–9. Bilateral caries lesions in the upper molar teeth of a pig.

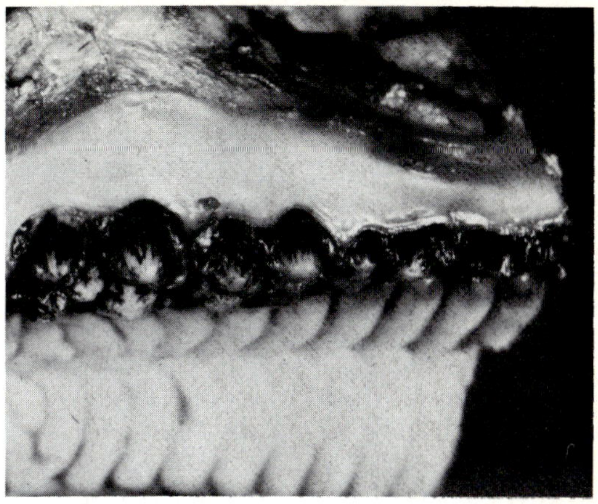

Figure 18–10. Darkly stained calculus on the surface of upper cheek teeth of a pig.

rare (page 275).[3] Maxillary or mandibular osteomyelitis occurs sporadically and secondary to strepococcal infection or endodontal or periodontal disease.

The potential uses of the pig as a model for human dental diseases have been described.[9, 19, 20]

ORAL SURGERY

Oral surgery in pigs is generally limited to clipping selected deciduous teeth, cutting the tusks of boars, and lancing abscesses.

The upper and lower canine and lateral incisor teeth of baby pigs ("needle teeth") are routinely clipped soon after birth to prevent damage to the dam. A pair of side-cutting pliers or dog-nail clippers is used to clip off the teeth just above the gingival margin. Shattering the root (a potential cause of gingival streptococcal or *Sphaerophorus* infection) or causing jagged edges that may traumatize the tongue and impede nursing should be avoided.

Adult canine teeth are often resected every 3 to 6 months in boars in order to reduce the risk of injury to handlers and sows. Sedation or anesthesia may be used, but in most cases a cord snare is applied to the snout behind the tusks, and the free end is passed around a strong bar to provide access to the tusks. A wooden rod is placed in the mouth to keep the jaws open, and the tusks are sawed off 2 mm to 3 mm above the gingival margin using a length of embryotomy wire equipped with handles. Hack-saws or bolt cutters should not be used in order to prevent fracture of the tooth's root and damage to adjacent soft tissues.

Surgical techniques for cannulation, transposition, and resection of the major salivary glands of pigs for experimental purposes have been described.[21]

References

1. Getty R: The Anatomy of the Domestic Animals, 5th ed. Vol. 2. Philadelphia, WB Saunders Co., 1975.
2. Jubb KVF, Kennedy PC: Pathology of Domestic Animals, Vol. 1. New York, Academic Press, 1963.
3. Page RC, Schroeder HE: Periodontitis in Man and Other Animals. Basel, S Karger, 1982.
4. Leman AD: Diseases of Swine, 5th ed. Ames, Iowa, Iowa State University Press, 1981.
5. Andrews JJ: Ulcerative glossitis and stomatitis associated with exudative epidermitis of suckling pigs. *Vet Pathol* 16:432–437, 1979.
6. Woods RD, Ross RF: Streptococcosis of swine. *Vet Bull* 46:397–400, 1976.
7. McCrea MR, Osborne AD: A case of "thrush" (candidiasis) in a piglet. *J Comp Pathol Ther* 67:342–344, 1957.
8. Osborne AD, McCrea MR, Manners MJ: Moniliasis in artificially reared pigs and its treatment with nystatin. *Vet Rec* 72:237–241, 1960.
9. Navia JM: Animal Models in Dental Research. University, Alabama, University of Alabama Press, 1977.
10. Huston R, Saperstein G, Schoneweis D, Leipold HW: Congenital defects in pigs. *Vet Bull* 48:465–675, 1978.
11. Bille N, Neilsen NC: Congenital malformations in pigs in *post mortem* material. *Nord Vet Med* 29:128–136, 1977.
12. Ollivier L, Sellier P: Pig genetics: a review. *Ann Genet Sel Anim* 14:481–544, 1982.
13. Colyer J: Variations and Diseases of the Teeth of Animals. London, J Bale, 1936.
14. Muirhead MR: Mandibular malalignment in the pig. *Br Vet J* 136:141–145, 1980.
15. Done JT: Facial deformity in pigs. *In* Grunsell CSG, Hill FWG (eds): Vet Ann 17th issue, Bristol, Wright Scientechnica, 1977, pp. 96–102.
16. Penny RHC, Mullen PA: Atrophic rhinitis of pigs: abatoir studies. *Vet Rec* 96:518–521, 1974.
17. Cross GWA: A study of some joint and skeletal abnormalities of pigs. MVSc Thesis, University of Sydney, Australia, 1974.
18. Andrews AH: Dental caries in an experimental domestic pig. *Vet Rec* 93:257–258, 1974.
19. Jump EB, Weaver ME: Miniature pig in dental research. *In* Bustad LK, McClellan RO (eds): Swine and Biomedical Research. Seattle, Frayn Pub Co., 1966, pp. 543–552.
20. Weaver ME: Miniature pig as an experimental animal in dental research. *Arch Oral Biol* 7:17–24, 1962.
21. Denny HR, Messervy A: Surgical techniques for the extirpation of the submandibular salivary glands and the collection of salivary secretions in the pig. *Vet Rec* 90:650–654, 1972.

Chapter Nineteen

Oral Disease in Laboratory Animals: Animal Models of Human Dental Disease

SL Yankell

The three oral diseases covered in this chapter—caries, calculus (tartar), and periodontitis, are the primary ones treated by both the dental and veterinary professions. Animal models that exhibit these diseases have yielded much information on both etiology and treatment. Since the 1950s, there have been four major reviews or presentations of data on dental diseases in rodents and primates,[1–4] which are the animals covered in this chapter and used most frequently in dental research. There is little data on the incidence and prevalence of naturally occurring dental diseases in these species.

When the dentition of laboratory animals is compared with that of humans, (Table 19–1), it is interesting to observe that only the Old World monkeys, exemplified by rhesus, have a permanent tooth dental formula and a growth mode similar to that of humans. New World monkeys, as exemplified by the marmoset, have a dental formula that is close to that of humans; however, they have an additional premolar and one additional last molar. In the rodent species, all incisor growth is continuous, that is, the teeth continue to erupt throughout the lifespan. The incisors and molars of guinea pigs and rabbits continuously erupt, whereas only the incisors in mice, rats, and hamsters show continuous eruption patterns. The molar teeth of mice, rats, and hamsters are the teeth that have

Table 19–1. Dentition of Laboratory Animals and Humans[1,3]

Species	Dental Formula of Permanent Teeth				Growth Mode of Teeth	
	Incisors	*Canines*	*Premolars*	*Molars*	*Incisors*	*Molars*
Mouse, rat, hamster	$\frac{1}{1}$	$\frac{0}{0}$	$\frac{0}{0}$	$\frac{3}{3}$	Continuous	Limited
Guinea pig	$\frac{1}{1}$	$\frac{0}{0}$	$\frac{0}{0}$	$\frac{4}{4}$	Continuous	Continuous
Rabbit	$\frac{2}{1}$	$\frac{0}{0}$	$\frac{3}{2}$	$\frac{3}{3}$	Continuous	Continuous
Ferret	$\frac{3}{3}$	$\frac{1}{1}$	$\frac{3}{3}$	$\frac{1}{2}$	Limited	Limited
Dog	$\frac{3}{3}$	$\frac{1}{1}$	$\frac{4}{4}$	$\frac{2}{3}$	Limited	Limited
Pig	$\frac{3}{3}$	$\frac{1}{1}$	$\frac{4}{4}$	$\frac{3}{3}$	Limited	Limited
Marmoset	$\frac{2}{2}$	$\frac{1}{1}$	$\frac{3}{3}$	$\frac{2}{2}$	Limited	Limited
Rhesus monkey	$\frac{2}{2}$	$\frac{1}{1}$	$\frac{2}{2}$	$\frac{3}{3}$	Limited	Limited
Human	$\frac{2}{2}$	$\frac{1}{1}$	$\frac{2}{2}$	$\frac{3}{3}$	Limited	Limited

Table 19–2. Advantages and Disadvantages of Laboratory Animals for Use in Dental Research

Species	Advantages	Disadvantages
Mouse, rat, hamster	Small Inexpensive to purchase, house and feed Available in pure-bred strains Available with defined gnotobiosis	Continuously erupting incisors Shallow pits, fissures (hamsters) Less susceptible to caries (mice) Diet and microbial flora must be carefully defined to induce disease
Guinea pig, rabbit	As stated under Mouse, rat, hamster Also docile	Continuously erupting incisors and molars Enamel composition and coverage different from humans
Dog	Docile Susceptible to calculus and periodontal disease	Not caries prone Purchase and housing costs
Pig	Susceptible to caries, calculus, periodontal disease	Cost (as stated under Dog). Size Difficult to handle
Monkey	As stated under Pig	Cost. Size Prone to systemic infections, diseases Ferocious

been studied most often in dental research projects.

The advantages and disadvantages of laboratory animals in dental research are presented in Table 19–2. All the rodent species have essentially the same advantages—that is, they are small; they are inexpensive to purchase, house, and feed; and they are available in purebred strains. Rats especially have the additional advantage of being commercially available with a defined microbial status (Table 19–3). How these factors relate to the onset and progress of dental disease will be discussed further on.

Although primates provide the extreme advantage that their dentition is similar to that of humans and they have a similar onset and progress of several dental diseases, their benefits are perhaps outweighed by their cost and size and the difficulty of maintaining them under standard laboratory conditions. In addition, the daily or topical treatment of these animals is extremely difficult.

Table 19–3. Microbiological Status of Commercially Available Rats[4]

Terminology	Definition
Conventional	No specific microbial flora
Gnotobiotic	Known microbial flora
Specific pathogen–free (SPF) or barrier maintained	No pathogenic or defined flora
Germ free	No viable microorganisms

THE RAT MODEL

Rats are the most frequently used animals in dental experiments. The primary similarity between the rat and humans is the shape of the molar teeth, though rat molars have thinner enamel on the occlusal surfaces.[5]

One of the major breakthroughs occurring in dental research was the demonstration that when infected with specific bacterial strains, germ-free rats developed carious lesions. Animals who were not inoculated with these strains, but were receiving a caries-prone diet, did not develop caries. This result indicated that dental caries was indeed a transmissible bacterial disease.[6] This research was further extended to animals who were not gnotobiotic (Table 19–3), but who had a known microbial flora (defined as those animals who were germ-free but were inoculated with one or more pure cultures of microorganisms).[7] The research was then further widened to include conventional animals who were deprived of their microflora through the use of antibiotics and were then superinoculated with an antibiotic-resistant microorganism.[8,9] Through the use of these procedures, and by housing animals that were thought to be "caries susceptible" with those defined as "caries-resistant," an increased development of disease was observed. Similar results were shown to occur in hamsters and are discussed later in this chapter. The primary finding to emerge from these experiments was the recognition of *Streptococcus mutans* as the organism used to superinfect conventional, gnotobiotic, or specific pathogen–free animals who then developed crevice (pit and fissure) caries. In describing carious lesions, three types are apparent. (1) Caries on smooth surfaces are influenced primarily by adherent plaque. (2) Root surface caries are smooth-surface carious lesions that occur below the cemento-enamel junction. They occur chiefly when the gingival tissue has lost its attachment, recession has occurred, and the dentinal root surface areas are exposed to the oral environment. Plaque is also the primary factor affecting the incidence of disease in this type of caries. (3) Crevice, or pit and fissure caries, result mainly from impaction and adherence of food particles and are dependent upon the eating patterns of the animal species.[10] Other modifying influences on all types of carious lesions include tooth form, occlusion, and the relationship of the contiguous soft tissues.[2]

With the establishment of *Streptococcus mutans* as a primary culprit in pit and fissure caries, several researchers attempted to combine inoculations to determine the synergism and antagonism of various bacterial strains in producing both plaque and caries in rats. By using a combination of *Streptococcus mutans* and *Actinomyces viscosus,* Swiss researchers routinely produced extensive plaque formation and smooth surface and fissure caries in short-term experiments.[11] The use of *Actinomyces viscosus* has been studied further in the production of calculus and periodontal disease factors in rats.[12] In our laboratories, inoculation with *Actinomyces viscosus* increased alveolar bone resorption (a sign of periodontal disease) in one commercially available rat strain but not in another.[13] Interestingly, rats in their natural habitat have been found to be infected with *Streptococcus mutans* and are considered to be a reservoir of this organism.[14]

Differences in the patterns of disease occurreance among various commercially available rat strains have also been related to eating patterns. Under similar experimental conditions, animals have been shown to develop different patterns of caries, plaque or calculus formation, or bone resorption. An apparatus has been developed that regulates the frequency and amount of food available.[15] The two primary purposes for this control are to eliminate the non-specific effects of dietary variables on food intake and to impose on the animals widely different eating patterns in order to investigate effects of caries activity. By programming the device for feeding 12, 18, 24, or 30 times daily, a highly significant positive correlation has been found between the frequency of eating and the incidence of caries. This apparatus has further been used to provide a single test food that could be taken orally; all other essential nutrients were administered to the animals through gastric intubation. In this way, the cariogenic potential of a defined food could be determined in a simple, unequivocal reproducible manner.[16] The specific cariogenicity of a food is based on its composition and its frequency of adminstration; an example of results obtained with this procedure is shown in Table 19–4. The cariogenic potential index (CPI) is expressed using a ratio of 1 for the cariogenicity of sucrose.

Table 19–4. Relative Cariogenicity of Foods in Rats[15]

Food	Cariogenic Potential Index
Sucrose	1
Chocolate cookie with soft filling	1.40
Presweetened cereal (60% sucrose)	0.94
Potato chips	0.84
Unsweetened cereal (2% sucrose)	0.45
No sugar orally	0

In evaluating the susceptibility of animals, it was observed that age is an important factor.[17] It is known that, because of increased mineralization, teeth become more

Table 19–5. Caries-Promoting Diets for Rats[3]

	Diet		
Component	*NIDR 2000* (%)	*MIT 200* (%)	*MIT 305* (%)
Sucrose	56	67	5
Cornstarch	—	—	62
Skim milk powder	28	—	—
Lactalbumin	—	20	20
Whole wheat flour	6	—	—
Alfalfa leaf meal	3	—	—
Brewers yeast	4	—	—
Whole liver	1	—	—
Sodium chloride, iodized	2	—	—
Cellulose	—	6	6
Cotton seed oil	—	3	3
MIT salt mixture	—	3	3
Vitamin mixture	—	1	1

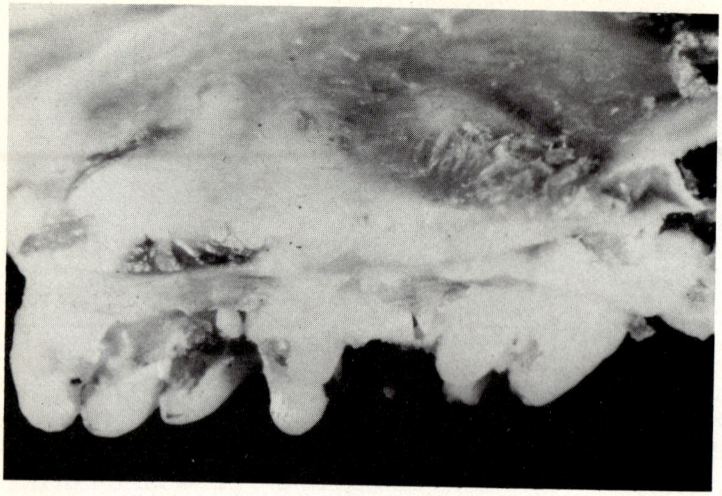

Figure 19–1. Extensive caries on upper first and second molar teeth of a rat.

resistant to caries as they are exposed to the oral environment. Rats are usually started on caries experiments at the age of 20 to 22 days, when they are first weaned from the mother. At this point, the third molars have not fully erupted and may be susceptible to both topical and systemic effects of agents used to prevent caries.

Many caries-promoting diets have been used for rodent species.[3] Three of the more frequently used diets are presented in Table 19–5. Two of these diets have a very high sucrose level (greater than 50 percent), whereas the MIT diet 305 has only a 5 per cent sucrose level, yet produces a similar caries incidence. Apparently the normal or superimposed inoculum in the oral cavity has the ability to metabolize both cornstarch and sucrose with similar cariogenic effects.

With the development of procedures to artificially induce caries, it became necessary to accurately assess the carious lesions. In rodent species, it is necessary to evaluate caries under magnification after the experiment has been completed. The first quantitative caries assessment was developed by Keyes.[18] He attempted to diagnose and evaluate caries development from early enamel lesions to rampant activity (Fig. 19–1). An attempt was made to estimate the linear spread of the carious lesions in units or areas, and each tooth surface was assigned a given surface number according to its size (Table 19–6). Each surface of each upper or lower molar has a maximum score; however, difficulty has been encountered when evaluating caries on smooth *versus* pit and fissure surfaces. A recent attempt to define this problem has been developed[19] (Table 19–7). By staining, differences between smooth and sulcal surfaces can be better demonstrated. The Keyes procedure calls for single sectioning of the molar teeth. The Zurich method of scoring caries has refined this procedure by sectioning the molar teeth into six to eight sections.[20] Using the Swiss procedure, the teeth are also stained, and smooth surface lesions are differentiated from moderate or advanced dentinal fissure lesions.

Although cariogenic diets are often high in sucrose content, diets potentiating calculus and periodontal disease contain higher levels of calcium and phosphate products. Attempts have been made to evaluate plaque formation both *in situ* and postmortem. Calculus deposits must be dried in order to be seen; therefore, deposits can only be evaluated postmortem in rats. With both plaque and calculus

Table 19–6. Keyes' Rat Caries Scoring Method[18]

Surface	Upper Molar No.			Lower Molar No.		
	1	*2*	*3*	*1*	*2*	*3*
	Maximum Score					
Buccal	6	4	3	6	4	4
Morsal	0	0	0	1	2	1
Lingual	6	4	2	6	4	4
Sulcal	5	3	2	7	5	2
Proximal	1	2	1	1	2	1

Table 19–7. Comparison of Carious Lesion Appearance on Smooth versus Sulcal Surfaces[19]

Lesion	Smooth	Sulcal
	Treatment Prior to Scoring	
	Intact, Not Stained	*Sliced, Stained*
Enamel (E)	White, opaque, no break in surface	Dye has not penetrated into dentin
Slight dentinal (Ds)	Dry, crumbly surface enamel appearance	Dye penetrates to one third of dentinal depth
Moderate dentinal (Dm)	Exposed dentin	Dye extends to two thirds of dentinal depth
Extensive dentinal (Dx)	Dentin is softer or missing, color may be dark	Dye penetrates through dentin, which may be soft or missing

Table 19–8. Rat Calculus Scoring Method[23]

Description of Calculus Deposits	Deposit Classification		
	Light	*Medium*	*Heavy*
	Assigned Score		
On mesial surface of first molar	0.75	1.00	1.25
Extending from mesial surface to either side of first molar	1.75	2.00	2.25
On first molar and extending to either side of second molar	2.75	3.00	3.25
On first and second molars and extending to either side of third molar	3.75	4.00	4.25

scoring methods, attempts are made to describe the deposit according to light, medium, and heavy classifications (Fig. 19–2). An attempt is made to define which tooth surface areas are covered by the deposits.[21,22] An example of a calculus scoring method used in our laboratory is presented in Table 19–8.[23] Recently, methods have been developed to quantitate root surface caries.[24]

With the development of sophisticated and reproducible test procedures,[25] the testing of agents to inhibit the disease process has also received much attention (Fig. 19–3).[26] Topically applied fluoride products have a similar efficacy in preventing caries in both rats and humans. The effects of topically applied stannous or sodium fluoride compounds are shown in Table 19–9. At similar concentrations, the use of stannous fluoride has been demonstrated to be significantly superior to sodium fluoride.[27] The fluoride levels used in this experiment are similar to those in commericially available fluoride toothpastes. The use of stannous chloride alone shows some inhibition of caries and is essentially comparable to sodium fluoride.

Toothbrushing with a modified toothbrush inhibits both plaque scores and caries severity.[28] When compared with control (unbrushed) scores, two brushing procedures and topically applied fluoride solution inhibit crevice or occlusal plaque. With increased brushing times, increased efficacy is observed

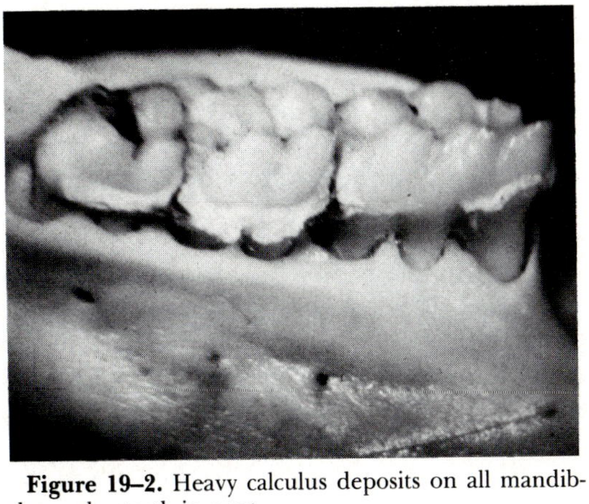

Figure 19–2. Heavy calculus deposits on all mandibular molar teeth in a rat.

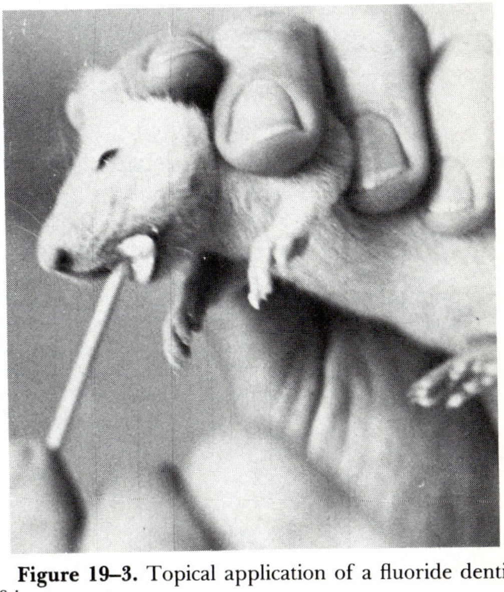

Figure 19–3. Topical application of a fluoride dentifrice to a rat.

Table 19–9. Effect of Topically Applied Tin or Fluoride Compounds on Caries in Rats[27]

Treatment	Concentration (ppm) Tin:Fluoride	% Reduction in Caries Compared with Control
SnF_2	3120:1000	37
NaF	—:1000	13
$SnCL_2$	3120:—	10

Table 19–11. Effects of Chlorhexidine or Sodium Fluoride on Plaque and Caries in Rats[29]

Treatment	Plaque Units	Smooth Surface Caries Units	Advanced Dentinal Fissure Lesions
Chlorhexidine	1.3	4.2	5.1
Sodium fluoride	3.6	2.6	5.6
Chlorhexidine and sodium fluoride	1.4	3.3	2.9
Control	3.6	10.6	9.8

(Table 19–10). All three treatment regimens are essentially similar in reducing caries severity when compared with control scores. Antibacterial agents are receiving increased attention in both experimental and clinical evaluations. As an example of activity in the rat plaque and caries model (Table 19–11), the effects of an antibacterial agent, chlorhexidine, is compared with that of sodium fluoride.[29] Chlorhexidine alone is excellent in reducing plaque scores; no enhancement of effect is seen with the combination of chlorhexidine and sodium fluoride. Sodium fluoride alone shows no activity on plaque when compared with controls. Sodium fluoride is the most effective of the agents tested in reducing smooth surface caries units, whereas the combination of chlorhexidine acetate and sodium fluoride is more effective on advanced dental fissure lesions than is either test agent by itself.

The use of the rat model will continue to be extremely important in the refinement and testing of individual test agents and of combinations as they are developed for clinical testing.

THE HAMSTER MODEL

Hamsters are another widely used species and have many of the advantages that rats have (low cost, ready availability, reproducible methods, easy handling). In addition, these animals can be examined *in situ* because the mouth can be opened more widely than is possible in rats.

Table 19–10. Effect of Brushing or Topical Fluoride on Plaque and Caries in Rats[28]

Treatment	Cervical Plaque Score	Occlusal Plaque Score	Caries Severity
15-sec brushing	2.12	1.94	12.52
60-sec brushing	1.42	1.02	12.63
250 ppm F from NaF	1.42	0.79	14.39
Control	2.21.	1.94	19.04

Much of the initial research on the transmissibility of periodontal disease and caries by specific organisms was performed on hamsters. Many of the factors evaluated in this species (age of the animal, dietary requirements, inoculation procedures, and caries scoring) are similar to those described for rats.[30–32]

The major disadvantage of the hamster is that the molar teeth do not have an extensive occlusal anatomy, and, therefore, they do not have the potential to develop pit and fissure caries.

THE PRIMATE MODEL

Primates are the third major species used in dental research. They are most similar to the clinical situation in regard to the arrangement and shape of the dentition. Caries are rarely found in younger wild or captive primates. More frequently, caries in older animals are attributed to enamel fractures that expose dentin at food impaction sites or to occlusal attrition.[14] In the laboratory, several primate species have been studied, including spider monkeys,[33, 34] macaques[35] and marmosets.[36]

Primates are the most expensive animal species to purchase and, because of import restrictions, are becoming increasingly difficult to obtain. Extreme care is necessary in their handling; these animals cannot be treated topically or examined *in situ* unless they are sedated or anesthetized. Old World monkeys harbor an oral flora that contains a wide range of species similar to those found in humans.[37] Biochemical reactions in plaque from monkeys are similar to those in plaque from humans. When young monkeys are fed high-sugar diets, they develop carious lesions that are clinically, radiologically, and histologically extremely similar to the clinical disease processes in humans. A review of dental caries in primates has been published recently.[38]

THE FERRET MODEL

The albino ferret has both a deciduous and a permanent set of teeth.[39] Interest in ferrets as a dental research animal has been based primarily on the works of King.[40, 41] A similarity to the human periodontal disease process was reported consistently. It was concluded that plaque and calculus were precursors of gingival changes, a fact that is now well-accepted in humans. Ferrets are routinely used for vaccine testing and production, influenza and other viral research, and immunological research procedures; however, I am not aware of research using the ferret as a gingivitis or periodontal disease model.

OTHER SPECIES MODELS

Significant dental disease findings have been published on several other rodent and lagomorph species, including the cotton rat,[42, 43] the rice rat,[44, 45] the gerbil,[46] and the rabbit.[47] Difficulties with using these species include the aggressiveness of both the cotton rat and the rice rat, and the continually erupting molars of gerbils and rabbits. For these reasons, these species are no longer in major use in dental research.

In earlier studies, many attempts were made to use gnotobiotic and conventional mice in caries research. The primary difficulty appears to have been that caries-producing organisms were not easily implantable in this species.[48, 49] Recently Kamp and associates[50] have reported a rapid and reproducible induction of caries in a specific strain of mice infected with *Streptococcus mutans* and fed a synthetic powder diet containing 30 per cent sucrose during the 10-week experiment. Since mice are valuable as an immunological assay model, the use of this species could prove to be valuable in further studies on experimental dental caries.

References

1. Johansen E, Keyes PH: Production and evaluation of experimental animal caries: A Review. *In* Sognnaes RF (ed): Advances in Experimental Caries Research. Washington, DC, Amer Assoc Adv Sci, 1955, pp. 1–46.
2. Keyes PH: Similarities and differences in dental caries in various species. *In* Harris RS (ed): Art and Science of Dental Caries Research. New York, Academic Press, 1968, pp. 185–199.
3. Navia JM: Animal Models in Dental Research. Birmingham, Alabama, The University of Alabama Press, 1977, pp. 1–466.
4. Briner WW: Rodent model systems in dental caries research: rats, mice, and gerbils. Tanzer JM (ed): Microbiology Abstracts (Suppl.), Washington, DC, 1981, pp. 111–119.
5. Muhlemann HR, König, KG: Ciba Symp, 1965; 13:65–71.
6. Fitzgerald RJ: Dental caries research in gnotobiotic animals. *Caries Res* 2:139–146, 1968.
7. Larson RH: Response of Harvard caries-susceptible and caries-resistant rats to a severe cariogenic challenge. *J Dent Res* 44(6):1402–1406, 1965.
8. Larson RH: Genetic and Environmental Factors in Experimental Dental Caries. Environmental Variables in Oral Disease. Washington, DC, Amer Assoc Adv Sci, 1966, pp. 89–101.
9. Guggenheim B, Regolati B: Interrelation of eating pattern, plaque formation and caries incidence in 5 stocks of rats. *Helv Odont Acta* 16:1–12, 1972.
10. König KG, Larson RH, Guggenheim B: A strain-specific eating pattern as a factor limiting the transmissibility of caries activity in rats. *Arch Oral Biol* 14:91–103, 1969.
11. Regolati B, Guggenheim B, Muhlemann HR: Synergisms and antagonisms of two bacterial strains superinfected in conventional Osborne-Mendel rats. *Helv Odont Acta* 16:84–88, 1972.
12. Baer PN: Use of laboratory animals for calculus studies. *Ann NY Acad Sci* 153:230–239, 1968.
13. Kavanagh BJ, Eby R, Leung FC, Yankell SL: Effect of inoculation on bone resorption scores in two rat strains, *J Dent Res* 51:1000–1004, 1972.
14. Shklair IL: Natural occurrence of caries in animals—animals as vectors and reservoirs of cariogenic flora. Tanzer JM (ed): Symposium on Animal Methods in Cariology. Microbiology Abstracts (Suppl.), Washington, DC, 1981, pp. 41–48.
15. König KG, Schmid P, Schmid R: An apparatus for frequency-controlled feeding of small rodents and its use in dental caries experiments. *Arch Oral Biol* 13:13–26, 1968.
16. Bowen WH, Amsbaugh SM, Monell-Torrens S, Brunelle J, Kuzmiak-Jones H, Cole MF: A method to assess cariogenic potential of foodstuffs. *J Am Dent Assoc* 100:677–681, 1980.
17. Larson RH, Fitzgerald RJ: Caries development in rats of different ages with controlled flora. *Arch Oral Biol* 9:705–712, 1964.
18. Keyes PH: Dental caries in the molar teeth of rats. II. A method for diagnosing and scoring several types of lesions simultaneously. *J Dent Res* 37:1088–1099, 1958.
19. Larson RH: Merits and modifications of scoring rat dental caries by Keyes' method. *In* Tanzer JM (ed): Symposium on Animal Models in Cariology. Microbiology Abstracts (Suppl.), Washington, DC, 1981, pp. 195–203.
20. Konig KC: Moglichkeiten der Kariesprophylaxe beim menschen and ihre unter suchungen in kurzfristigen rotten experiment. Bern and Stuttgart, Hans Huber, 1966.
21. Stookey GK: Plaque scoring—evaluation in living animals. *In* Tanzer JM (ed): Microbiology Abstracts (Suppl.), Washington, DC, 1981, pp. 205–213.

22. Shern RJ, Monell-Torrens E, Couet KM, Kingman A, Bowen WH: Post-mortem evaluation of dental plaque in rats. *In* Tanzer JM (ed): Symposium on Animal Models in Cariology. Microbiology Abstracts (Suppl.), Washington, DC, 1981, pp. 215–221.
23. DePalma PD, Loux JJ, Hutchman J, Dolan MM, Yankell SL: Anticalculus and antiplaque activity of 8-hydroxy quinoline sulfate. *J Dent Res* 55(2): 292–298, 1976.
24. Rosen S, Doff RS, App G, Rotilie J: A topographical scoring system for evaluating root surface caries. *In* Tanzer JM (ed): Symposium on Animal Models in Cariology. Microbiology Abstracts (Suppl.), Washington, DC, 1981, pp. 175–182.
25. Larson RH, Amsbaugh SM, Navia JM, Rosen S, Schuster GS, Shaw JH: Collaborative evaluation of a rat caries model in six laboratories. *J Dent Res* 56(8):1007–1012, 1977.
26. Yankell SL: Enhancing the usefulness of rats in dental caries studies. *Lab Anim* 5(4):24–27, 1976.
27. Francis MD: The effectiveness of anticaries agents in rats using an incipient carious lesion method. *Arch Oral Biol* 11(2):141–148, 1966.
28. Yankell SL, Emling R, Cancro LP, Moreno OM: Effects of toothbrushing or topical fluoride on plaque and caries. *J Dent Res* 62 (Abstr. No. 914), 1983.
29. Regolati B, Schmid R, Mühlemann HR: Combination of chlorhexidine and fluoride in caries prevention: An animal experiment. *Helv Odont Acta* 18(2):12–16, 1974.
30. Keyes PH, Fitzgerald RJ, Jordan HV, White CL: The effect of various drugs on caries and periodontal disease in albino hamsters. *Adv F Res Dent Caries Prev* 1:159–177, 1962.
31. Jordan HV, Keyes PH: Aerobic, gram-positive, filamentous bacteria as etiologic agents of experimental periodontal disease in hamsters. *Arch Oral Biol* 9:401–414, 1964.
32. Strålfors A, Thilander H, Bergenholtz A: Correlation between caries and periodontal disease in the hamster. *Arch Oral Biol* 12:1213–1216, 1967.
33. Goldman HM: Periodontosis in the spider monkey—a preliminary report. *J Periodontol* 18:34–40, 1947.
34. Ranney RR, Zander HA: Allergic periodontol disease in sensitized squirrel monkeys. *J Periodontol* 41:12–21, 1968.
35. Levy BM: The nonhuman primate as an analogue for the study of periodontal disease. *J Dent Res* 50:246–53, 1971.
36. Friedman LA, Levy BM, Ennever J: Epidemiology of gingivitis and calculus in a marmoset colony. *J Dent Res* 51(3):803–806, 1972.
37. Bowen WH: A bacteriological study of experimental dental caries in monkeys. *Int Dent J* 15:12–53, 1965.
38. Bowen WH: Dental caries in primates. *In* Tanzer JM (ed): Symposium on Animal Models in Cariology. Microbiology Abstracts (Suppl.), Washington, DC, 1981, pp. 131–135.
39. Berkovitz BKB: Tooth development in the albino ferret *(Mustela putorius)* with special reference to the permanent carnassial. *Arch Oral Biol* 18(4):465–471, 1973.
40. King JD, Rowles SL, Little K, Thewlis J: Chemical and x-ray examination of deposits removed from the teeth of golden hamsters and ferrets. *J Dent Res* 34(5):650–660, 1955.
41. King JD: Experimental production of gingival hyperplasia in ferrets given "epanutin" (sodium diphenylhydantoin). *J Exp Pathol* 33:491–489, 1952.
42. Thompson DT, Vogel JJ, Phillips PH: Certain organic substances and their effects upon the incidence of dental caries in the cotton rat. *J Dent Res* 44(3):596–599, 1965.
43. Vogel JJ, Phillips PH: A shortened dental caries assay with the cotton rat. *Proc Soc Exp Biol Med* 108:829–830, 1961.
44. Gupta OM, Shaw JH: Periodontia—periodontal disease in the rice rat. I. Anatomic and histopathologic findings. *Oral Surg Oral Med Oral Pathol* 9:592–603, 1956.
45. Mulvihill JE, Susi FR, Shaw JH, Goldhaber P: Histological studies of the periodontal syndrome in rice rats and the effects of penicillin. *Arch Oral Biol* 12(6):733–744, 1967.
46. Moskow BS, Wasserman BH, Rennert MC: Spontaneous periodontal disease in the mongolian gerbil. *J Periodont Res* 3(2):69–83, 1968.
47. Horodyski B, Slowik T: Radiograph of periodontal disease in humans and experimental periodontal disease in rabbits. *Czas Stomat* 19(11):1191–1195, 1966.
48. Gibbons RJ, Socransky SS: Enhancement of alveolar bone loss in gnotobiotic mice harboring human gingival bacteria. *Arch Oral Biol* 11(8):847–848, 1966.
49. Dick HM, Trott JR: Immunity and inflammation as synergistic mechanisms in the pathogenesis of periodontal disease. *J Periodont Res* 4(2):127–140, 1969.
50. Kamp EM, Huis in't Veld JHJ, Havenaar R, Dirks OB: Experimental dental caries in mice. *In* Tanzer JM (ed): Symposium on Animal Models in Cariology. Microbiology Abstracts (Suppl.), Washington, DC, 1981, pp. 121–130.

Chapter Twenty

Oral Disease in Captive Wild Animals

WB Amand and CL Tinkelman

INTRODUCTION

Oral disease in captive wild animals has not been documented in any comprehensive fashion. Only three papers that deal specifically with general dental pathology in zoo animals are available.[1–3]

Infections of the oral cavity may or may not be directly related to primary dental disease. Microbial infections or by-products of these microbes may directly affect oral tissue and dental supporting structures, as well as attack the dentition itself by producing caries. Alternatively, a primary dental defect, such as a fracture of a lower canine tooth, may result in an infected pulp cavity, producing an apical abscess with subsequent erosion to adjacent bone, which leads to osteomyelitis and a draining fistulous tract.

From the foregoing, it is clear that a comprehensive examination of the oral cavity should be carried out whenever a captive wild animal is restrained or sedated for other reasons.

DENTAL FORMULAE

The dental formulae of zoo animals often has been observed cursorily, but has rarely been studied in detail, except for historical value. Diet, feeding and chewing habits, social harmony, sexual dominance, and age determination are all affected by the number, shape, and position of the teeth (Table 20–1).[3] A young animal with erupting deciduous teeth should be fed a diet that is more abrasive than that fed to an adult to aid in exfoliation. When a mixed dentition exists, there is normally a change in occlusion and chewing ability, as well as a possible weight loss. Colyer[4] pointed out that improper eruption patterns can cause food and tooth impaction, periodontal disease, caries, and an eventual behavior problem.

ORAL DEVELOPMENT

Eruption

The eruption of deciduous teeth in exotic animals has not been well studied. The incisors, canines, and premolar teeth form the primary dentition, since there are no deciduous molar teeth. A knowledge of the eruption times of both deciduous and permanent teeth is helpful. These events have been studied best in primates, particularly in those species used in laboratories.

Primates. The order of tooth eruption in primates has been outlined.[5] The study sample included 2394 wild and 514 captive primate specimens. It was found that in the permanent dentition (1) the canine teeth of males erupt later and more slowly than those of females, (2) the teeth of the lower jaw erupt before the corresponding teeth of the upper jaw, and (3) attrition of the permanent teeth is rare before the dentition is complete. The deciduous dentition erupts earlier in small monkeys than in apes and earlier in apes than in humans. In all primates, eruption of the first molar teeth is followed by a comparatively long interval before additional teeth are added to the permanent dentition. In the gorilla, the earliest deciduous teeth to erupt are the incisors and the upper first premolars.

Variations in the order of permanent incisor tooth eruption are seen more often in the chimpanzee than in the gorilla. In the latter, the upper second incisors may appear before the lower teeth, but in the former, a fairly wide range of variation is seen (e.g., the second molars may precede the second

Table 20–1. Representative Formulae for Permanent Dentition

Species	Incisor	Canine	Premolar	Molar
Marsupials				
Opossum	5/4	1/1	3/3	4/4
Macropods	3/1	0,1/0	2/2	4/4
Insectivores				
Solenodon	3/3	1/1	3/3	3/3
Tenrecs	2/3	1/1	3/3	3,4/3
Moles	2 1/3,2	1/0,1	3,4/3,4	3/3
Chiroptera				
Fruit bat	2/2	1/1	3/3	2/3
Leaf-nosed bats	1/2	1/1	1,2/2	3/3
Vampire bat	1/2	1/1	2/3	0/0
Primates	2/2	1/1	3/3	3/3
Edentates				
Armadillo (nine-banded)	7 7/9,9	(primitive peglike teeth)		
Giant anteater	0/0	0/0	0/0	0/0
Two-toed sloth	0/0	1/1	4/3	0/0
Lagomorphs				
Pika	2/1	0/0	3/2	2/3
Rabbits and hares	2/1	0/0	3/2	3/3
Rodents				
Squirrels	1/1	0/0	1,2/1	3/3
Beaver	1/1	0/0	1/1	3/3
Porcupines	1/1	0/0	1/1	3/3
Capybara	1/1	0/0	1/1	3/3
Guinea pig	1/1	0/0	1/1	3/3
Carnivores				
Ursids	3/3	1/1	4/4	2/3

incisors). The appearance of the premolar teeth does not seem to follow any definite order in either the chimpanzee or the gorilla.[5, 6]

Infant primates often have "teething gingivitis" as a result of deciduous eruption. Tender, swollen jaws, diarrhea, and pyrexia may be observed. Pediatric aspirin, kaolin-pectin suspension, and teething toys are helpful in pacifying the infants.[7]

Large Cats. The eruption sequences of the deciduous teeth of the large exotic cats have been described in detail.[8] The incisor and canine teeth erupt at different times in cats, but the eruption time for the first "grinders" is strikingly uniform. The tiger exhibits the longest interval before the other permanent teeth erupt, and the lion has the shortest interval before eruption.

Elephant. The dental eruption of the elephant is unique among mammals. Elephants have six complete sets of molar teeth. The newborn elephant has the first and second molars in place at birth. The first set of molars are worn away, and the roots are resorbed as the second set comes forward. Each successive molar is pushed forward in the jaw by the replacement molar behind it. As the clinical crown is worn and its blood supply is compromised by the pressure from the new molar behind it, the crown fractures transversely in sections. These pieces of crown are either swallowed or spit out, and the remaining roots are resorbed. Each molar consists of complex ridges or lamellae of dentin covered with enamel, with cementum between the ridges. Each successive set of molars is composed of progressively larger

Table 20–1. Representative Formulae for Permanent Dentition *(Continued)*

Species	Incisor	Canine	Premolar	Molar
Carnivores *(Continued)*				
Procyonids	$\frac{3}{3}$	$\frac{1}{1}$	$\frac{3,4}{3,4}$	$\frac{2}{2}$
Mustilids	$\frac{3}{3}$	$\frac{1}{1}$	$\frac{2,4}{2,4}$	$\frac{1}{1,2}$
Canids	$\frac{3}{3}$	$\frac{1}{1}$	$\frac{4}{4}$	$\frac{2}{3}$
Felids	$\frac{3}{3}$	$\frac{1}{1}$	$\frac{3}{2}$	$\frac{1}{1}$
Sea lion	$\frac{3}{2}$	$\frac{1}{1}$	$\frac{4}{4}$	$\frac{1,3}{1}$
Hyaenids	$\frac{3}{3}$	$\frac{1}{1}$	$\frac{4}{3}$	$\frac{1}{1}$
Tubliodontae				
Aardvarks	$\frac{0}{0}$	$\frac{0}{0}$	$\frac{2}{2}$	$\frac{3}{3}$
Proboscidea				
Elephants	$\frac{1,1}{0,0}$	$\frac{0,0}{0,0}$	—	$\frac{6,6}{6,6}$
Hyrax	$\frac{1}{2}$	$\frac{1}{1}$	$\frac{4}{4}$	$\frac{3}{3}$
Sirenians				
Manatee	$\frac{0}{0}$	$\frac{0}{0}$	$\frac{0}{0}$	$\frac{6}{6}$
Perissodactyla				
Rhinoceros	$\frac{0,3}{0,3}$	$\frac{0,1}{0,1}$	$\frac{3,4}{3,4}$	$\frac{3}{3}$
Zebras	$\frac{3}{3}$	$\frac{1}{1}$	$\frac{3,4}{3,4}$	$\frac{3}{3}$
Tapirs	$\frac{3}{3}$	$\frac{1}{1}$	$\frac{3,4}{4}$	$\frac{3}{3}$
Atiodactyla				
Warthog	$\frac{1}{3}$	$\frac{1}{1}$	$\frac{3}{2}$	$\frac{3}{3}$
Collared Peccary	$\frac{2}{3}$	$\frac{1}{1}$	$\frac{3}{3}$	$\frac{3}{3}$
Hippopotamus	$\frac{2,3}{1}$	$\frac{1}{1}$	$\frac{4}{4}$	$\frac{2}{3}$
Camelidae	$\frac{1}{3}$	$\frac{1}{1}$	$\frac{3}{2}$	$\frac{3}{3}$
Llama	$\frac{1}{3}$	$\frac{1}{0,1}$	$\frac{2}{2,3}$	$\frac{3}{3}$
Chevrotain	$\frac{0}{3}$	$\frac{1}{1}$	$\frac{3}{3}$	$\frac{3}{3}$
Cervids (Deer)	$\frac{0}{3}$	$\frac{0}{1,1}$	$\frac{3}{3}$	$\frac{3}{3}$
Giraffe	$\frac{0}{3}$	$\frac{0}{1}$	$\frac{3}{3}$	$\frac{3}{3}$
Antelope	$\frac{0}{3}$	$\frac{0}{1}$	$\frac{3}{3}$	$\frac{3}{3}$

teeth. In the African elephant, the sixth molar begins to move forward at 26 to 30 years of age. After the sixth molar is worn, the accuracy of estimating age becomes less sound, since the only criterion is the degree of wear of the sixth molar teeth, which are the only molars left at 45 to 49 years of age.[9]

Elephant tusks are incisor teeth. Ivory is composed of dentin, cartilagenous material, and calcium salts. Deciduous tusks are present at birth and the tips are covered with enamel. They are replaced by permanent tusks at about 1 year of age.[11] Tusks are gently curved and are usually directed downward and forward, the tips tending to the midline. Variations are not uncommon. They may project horizontally with a slight curve upward and outward, one tusk may be horizontal and the other vertical, or they may cross one another, usually turning inward. The irregular eruption of elephant teeth occurs more frequently in captivity. A plaster cast of "Jumbo" made in 1822, showed that rostral and caudal teeth were malpositioned.[4]

Other Species. Aardvarks also have a nontraditional eruption pattern. The deciduous teeth do not break through the gums and are vestigal. The rostral teeth erupt first and are lost, being replaced by more caudal teeth that grow throughout the life of the animal. The teeth are columnar, lack roots, and are surrounded by a cementum-like layer instead of enamel. The typical tooth is made up of hexagonal prisms of dentin surrounded by tubular pulp cavities, hence, the name Tubulidontata.[12, 13]

Unlike primates, both the deciduous and permanent upper teeth in giraffes erupt slightly before the corresponding lower teeth.[14] The permanent teeth do not begin eruption until after 3 years of age, and then they begin progressively with the emergence of the molars and proceed rostrally, with the exception of the canines, which do not erupt until the giraffe is 6 years of age or older. The low-crowned molars are characteristically rugose, unlike any other mammal, and the enamel is always smooth.

Some marsupials have no deciduous teeth, and among the placental mammals, the deciduous dentition may be lost *in utero*.[15]

The teeth of the zebra and other exotic equine species, as well as the rhinoceros, are used for determining the age of these species.[10]

Dental Abnormalities

Anomalies of the dentition may result from abnormal tissue development, dysplasia, or environmental influences. Developmental abnormalities consist of irregularities in number, size, shape, structure, position, and eruption of teeth. Non-developmental anomalies generally result in discoloration or damage to the integrity of the tooth structure and can affect either the entire primary or secondary dentition or only specific teeth.

Failure of Eruption. The eruption of primary and permanent teeth takes place in a set sequence and time range. Failure of teeth to erupt may be a manifestation of another anomalous dental condition, or it may be mistaken for agenesis of teeth, as demonstrated by Marshall's work on martens *(Martes americana)*.[16] Mechanical factors, odontomata, and follicular cysts are generally responsible for the failure of eruption. Eruption is influenced by malpositioned buds, supernumerary teeth, and retained teeth. Pathological bone that prevents eruption has been reported in the mandrill, the bear, and the cat.[4]

Anatomical Defects in Teeth. In a study of 179 teeth in 78 primate skulls, many dental abnormalities comparable to those of humans were found.[17] The developmental microscopic defects were principally in the tooth enamel structure. The presence of interglobular dentin, which is suggestive of frank defects in the calcification process, was found in 12 percent of the teeth examined. Molars were affected more often. There were many grooves on the enamel surfaces of the incisors, which were probably due to temporary arrests in development. These defects were seen most often in chimpanzees, orangutans, and gibbons.

In their native environment in India the teeth of wild rhesus monkeys *(Macaca mulatta)* appear to be remarkably free from developmental defects, the enamel surface being extremely smooth and the internal structures being homogenously formed and calcified. In contrast, the teeth of anthropoids were much more prone to faulty development, with three types of dentin and various irregularities of the surface texture and internal surface of enamel. The teeth of the anthropoids were found to be more comparable to those of humans.[17]

In one study, free-ranging pongids showed less-frequent enamel hypoplasia than did zoo-reared animals. A sample of wild cercopithecoids was almost entirely free from developmental defects, whereas animals examined at primate centers and zoos had varying degrees of hypoplasia.[18]

Hypoplasia of teeth varies in its severity. It can range from simple pitting of the enamel to total loss of the enamel covering. In captive animals, the degree of hypoplasia is usually mild, but it is often closely related to bone disease and deficient calcification. Captive baboons seem to be affected more often, with only the upper central incisors being afflicted. The enamel organ of this tooth may be more unstable than other enamel organs and may be the first to show defects when mineralization is altered.[18]

Enamel hypoplasia is usually more rare and milder in animals in the wild than in those in captivity. In the wild state animals are seldom, if ever, exposed to an alteration in environment that is so drastic and permanent as the environment of captivity, though a period of food shortage can alter the animal's metabolism. The conditions of captivity are much different than the environment wild animals are adapted for, and any tissue abnormalities can often be attributed to these altered surroundings.

Hypoplasia of any of the calcified dental tissues changes the color of the teeth. Discoloration may cause the deposition of a film, pigment, or calculus on the surface of the enamel, exposed dentin, or cementum, resulting in color changes or stains. An example is the staining of teeth in raccoons *(Procyon lotor)* with aluminum.[15]

Attrition

Teeth that grow continuously are kept within normal limits by attrition. If the teeth are displaced from an injury or if the opposing tooth is displaced or lost, the teeth may

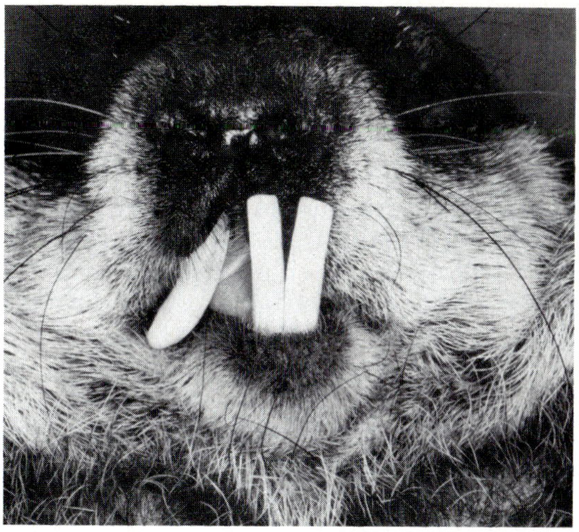

Figure 20–1. Woodchuck with displaced and overgrown incisors.

grow to an extreme size. Rabbits and rodents are affected most frequently. The upper incisors of these animals approach one another as they emerge from the bone until the medial borders come into contact, which provides the attrition necessary for normal size. If contact is lost, the teeth grow in an outward direction, piercing the skin and eventually causing death (Fig. 20–1).

Excessive overgrowth also occurs in the tusks of hippopotamuses, the incisors of beavers, and the beaks of many exotic birds.[4] In captivity, the animals that are prone to loss of normal attrition must be carefully monitored. When excessive overgrowth does occur, the teeth can be (1) extracted, (2) filed down on a periodic basis, or (3) treated endodontically to remove the pulp, thereby eliminating the source of growth.

A study of Weddell's seal showed a correlation between tooth wear and the mortality of adults. Abrasion to upper canine teeth from chewing on ice to maintain breathing holes resulted in pulp infections, fractures, and abscesses.[19]

Dental Sexual Dimorphism

The occurrence of sexual dimorphism in the size of canine teeth suggests that function is not wholly alimentary; variations are often used to study functional relationships among diet, predator defense, and threat display and aggression.

Apart from the Hominidae, all primate families' canine teeth show some degree of projection beyond the tooth row; projection is usually more pronounced in the upper jaw than in the lower jaw. The degree of projection and stoutness of the tooth varies considerably, particularly among the Cebidae. Callicebus, for instance, shows relatively little projection, whereas the canines in Chiroptes are long and extremely stout. The longest and sharpest canines are found among ground-living Cercopithecoidae, and the most massive are found among the Pongidae.[20]

For instance, there is no doubt judging from the massive form and the evidence of wear in the gorilla that the canines are not mere adornment; they are probably used for stripping bark. The skulls of adult females appear to have a human-like fragility when compared with the massive skulls of the adult males; their teeth are much smaller also. The females are far less susceptible to the occurrence of supernumerary teeth; as a result they suffer less frequently from alveolar absorption.[21] The slender, dagger-like canines of baboons have a non-alimentary function that is associated with the role of the male in the social organization of the troop; the dominant male controls mainly by the threat of aggression. Threat also operates in the defense against predators; an aggressive display by large male gibbons discourages attack by cheetahs or leopards. Macaques also exhibit a striking sexual dimorphism in the size of their canine teeth.[22]

Communication through facial expression increases the importance of the front teeth; the "grin" of most primates and the "snarl" of the baboon and mandrill are displays of profound significance for primate communication.[20]

Canine tooth size in females of different species varies with social structure. In general, females of monogamous species have larger canines than females of polygamous species. In monogamous species, it is presumed that the female is more often involved in territorial disputes and heterosexual aggression.[23]

Of the larger land mammals, elephants show the most striking example of sexual dimorphism involving dentition, with the male elephant exhibiting greater development of the incisors (tusks).

Dental Adaptations to Diet

Many wild animals have teeth that are adapted for an abrasive diet. If the diet is too soft in captivity, abrasion will be absent and excessive tooth growth may occur. Many ungulates suffer from irregular tooth wear in captivity. A maned wolf, *Chrysocyon jubatus,* has canine teeth that will continue to grow if the floor of their living area is too hard, since it digs with its teeth, which causes wear in nature.[24] In primates, dental adaptations to diet are not very noticeable. The most extreme behavioral adaptation is that of Daubentonia, which adopts a rodent-like gnawing action for excavating wood-boring insects. Other adaptations that can be correlated to diet are the large size of the molars in the gorilla, who is a bulk vegetarian; the sharply pointed molar cusps of Tarsius, Aotus, and Galago, which are related to their largely insectivorous habits; and the unique form of the upper and lower molars in the leaf-eating howler monkeys.[20]

In carnivores, a pair of cheek teeth (upper last premolar and lower first molar) are often developed as specialized shearing teeth and are called carnassials. They are most developed in cats and are least developed in those carnivores that have omnivorous diets (Ursidae-Procyonidae). The giraffe has molars that are characteristically rugose to aid in the lateral grinding of food. Vegetarian hippopotamuses have heavy front teeth and lips that help crop the huge amount of vegetation that they eat. The edentates (anteaters, sloths, armadillos) are, as the name signifies, without teeth. Anteaters are the only living mammal totally without teeth; other edentates lack incisors and canines, but some have continuously growing cheek teeth. The Hyaenidae have exceptionally strong premolars that help in their scavenging on the kill of other species.

The dentition of all pinnipeds is designed for catching and holding prey. The teeth of the walrus are the most specialized of this group; they are formed for gathering mollusks and crushing the shells. The canine teeth (tusk) bear enamel briefly after eruption, and only at the tip, the adult crown being entirely dentin.[7]

OCCLUSAL ABNORMALITIES

Variation in the Number and Shape of Teeth

Anomalies of tooth shape and size frequently coexist, and they are usually associated with anomalies of tooth number. An increase in size may actually be a step toward hyperdontia.[15] Seemingly unrelated characteristics, such as the time and the order of eruption of certain teeth, have a statistically demonstrable relationship to tooth number and size.[25]

There is evidence that animals from the same district may exhibit similar variations—for example, the upper second premolars were absent in three species of *Colobus badius rufomitratus* from the Tana River. The distribution of this subspecies is very local, being restricted to the lower part of the river near the coast.[4]

Accessory or abnormally formed cusps on the teeth of wild animals are not uncommon. Incisors and canines often show an increased size of the lingual tubercle. The lower premolars have a greater change in crown shape than do the upper premolars; dasyurid marsupials often show fused or divided premolar crowns.[26]

Supernumerary teeth probably originate from local influences. Disturbances affecting the cells of odontogenesis, such as inflammation or excess pressure, are likely causes.[27] They may imitate the shape of a normal tooth or may be formed atypically. Supernumerary teeth are found twice as frequently in the maxilla as in the mandible and seldom occupy a functional position. The number of supernumerary teeth rarely exceeds one in each of the archs of the dentition. In a study of almost 30,000 skulls, the percentage of supernumerary teeth was found to vary among species: in carnivores it was 2.3 percent, in

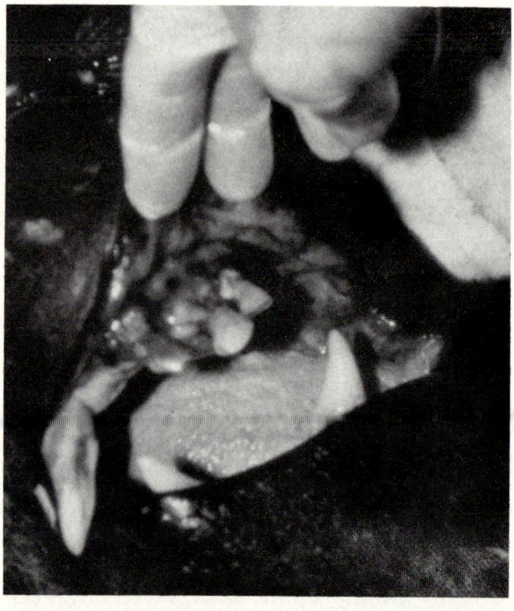

Figure 20–2. Upper left canine of Massa, a 53 year old male lowland gorilla, showing a rostral shift and a lateral rotation of position.

primates it was 1.3 percent, in marsupials, it was 1 percent and in artiodactyls, conies, and rodents it was less than 1 percent.[4]

Position of Teeth. Colyer gives a most thorough report of the variable positions of teeth in most orders and subspecies.[4] In Figure 20–2, the upper canine teeth of Massa, the oldest gorilla in captivity, showed a rostral shift and a slight rotation laterally; this movement was probably due to the loss of so many teeth from periodontal disease.

There is evidence that certain animals tend to develop particular types of abnormalities—for example, a characteristic variation in the Colobus monkeys and in the leaf monkeys is an irregular arrangement of one or both upper first incisors, and in the gorilla, the lower canine tooth erupts toward the midline. In primates, carnivores, artiodactyls, and marsupials, the premolars are usually malpositioned, whereas in perissodactyls, proboscids, and conies it is the incisors that are malpositioned. Among lagomorphs, the incisors are more commonly maloccluded than are either the premolars or the molars.[28]

The types of abnormalities seen in the captive animal are similar to those seen in the animal in the wild state, but as a rule they are more marked. The prevalence of malpositioned teeth in many groups of mammals averages between 5 and 12 percent of the species examined, and among primates, prevalence rates of up to 40 percent are common. In animals raised in captivity, the prevalence may double or triple. For example, in the wild state Papio and Macaques show a common but slight abnormality in the premolar teeth; in the captive animal these abnormalities are generally more marked and may take the form of extreme displacement of the teeth.

In the captive animal, bone diseases affect the position of the teeth. If the teeth are to develop normally, bone growth must proceed normally. Insufficient bone growth results in the teeth assuming positions that are somewhat similar to those in which they developed; excess growth tends to displace the teeth and in some cases produces extreme irregularities.

In rickets, there is a displacement rather than a crowding of the teeth. The degree of displacement depends on the position of the developing teeth and the duration of the disease. The teeth that have erupted are the least affected, and the upper teeth are usually more affected.[4]

Dental Injuries

Injuries to the teeth are common in zoo animals, and occur either from the aggressive activity of other animals or from contact with their environment, such as bars and concrete slabs.

Deciduous Teeth. A traumatic injury to one of these teeth can cause a plethora of problems for the animal. Pulp exposure can lead to pulp death and necrosis, which, if unattended, will cause abscess formation and damage to the permanent successor. Displacement of a deciduous tooth can cause soft tissue damage and occlusal disharmony, as well as injury to the permanent tooth. The result of such an injury could be arrested growth, ankylosis, abnormal calcification, or lateral displacement.

Permanent Teeth. The pathology of injury to the permanent teeth is similar to the events in domesticated species (Chapter Six). The most remarkable example is the elephant; a traumatic blow to an immature tusk can lead it to grow into one or more bends or into a spiral. The pulp of the tusk also has strong recuperative powers. An abscess from an injury can be walled off by secondary dentin and can maintain its ability to generate normal dentin. Longitudinal fractures of a tusk are common and are usually followed by functional dentinal repair. A split tusk can be healed by the application of a tight metal ring that is held in place by lag screws until secondary dentin forms. It is also possible that if a tusk is split into pieces, each segment will grow separately and be covered by ivory. It is usual, however, for the pulp to abscess when injured.[9] The canine is most often the traumatized tooth. There are numerous reports of this tooth being fractured or displaced in ursids, felids, and large primates in a zoo population. Abnormal occlusion and possibly starvation can result (Fig. 20–3).[29–30]

DIAGNOSTIC TECHNIQUES

Pain is a significant sign of dental disease and injury. Loss of appetite and subsequent weight loss, excessive salivation, and constant rubbing of a particular area can be signs of oral pain.

Small captive animals can often be examined in their cages or normal habitat without being anesthetized. However, definitive di-

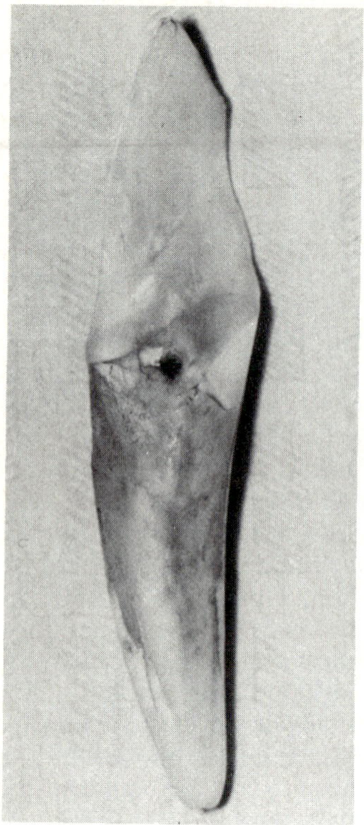

Figure 20–3. Fractured upper incisor of an Asiatic lion, showing root canal exposure.

agnosis and treatment require chemical restraint.

Radiology. Portable x-ray machines can be used *in situ*, though a developing tank must also be nearby for times when a rapid diagnosis is needed. A periapical film can be taken using human dental film and a small dental cone on the x-ray machine; however, it is difficult or impossible to use these films in very small mouths. Lateral jaw and oblique films are often advantageous if the beam is positioned to minimize overlapping.

Equipment

Veterinary dental equipment has to be mobile, portable, and comprehensive.[31] Treatment may have to be rendered in a cage, laboratory, or in an outdoor habitat. The equipment should be kept simple, avoiding elaborate, costly, and difficult to maintain gadgets. The following are the major items needed:

1. An air-operated handpiece unit. We use a large suitcase with a motor that drives a slow-speed handpiece, air syringe, suction, and a focused light source (Fig. 20–4).
2. An electrosurgical unit.
3. An ultrasonic scaling device.
4. A portable x-ray unit with a portable developer.
5. Surgical, restorative, endodontic, and periodontal instruments and supplies.

Clinical Examination

An oral examination should be done with rubber gloves, a dental mirror and explorer, tongue depressors, a periodontal probe, and a good light. Hard tissue (teeth and bone) should be examined for calculus, caries, fractures, and mobility. Soft tissue (lips, tongue, cheeks, palate, pharynx, and gingivae) should

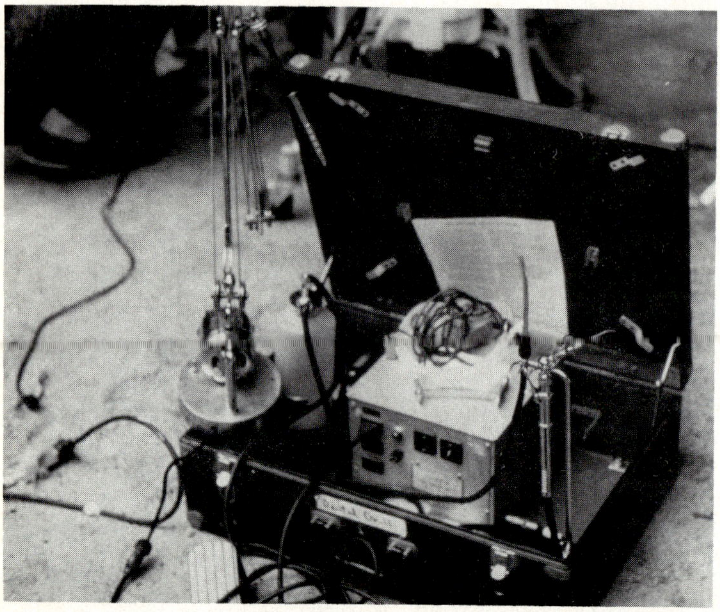

Figure 20–4. Portable dental unit used at the Philadelphia Zoo.

be examined for swelling, bleeding, ulceration, and color change. The gingival sulcus around the teeth, especially the canines and molars, should be probed for pocket depth. A measurement of more than 3 mm indicates a need for further examination.

If the animal is not intubated, the jaws should be closed to inspect the occlusion. The relationship of the upper and lower canine and molar teeth should be noted. Wear facets, malalignment, fractured cusps, and interference with movement should be investigated and corrected.

DENTAL THERAPEUTIC TECHNIQUES

The treatment of oral disease in captive wild animals requires a working knowledge of head and neck anatomy, oral pathology, dental radiology, periodontal and endodontic therapy, and oral surgery.

The literature contains many case reports of varied diagnoses, techniques, and materials. They vary from extraction of an elephant tusk[32] to making a set of dentures for a donkey.[33] Root canal therapy dominates the case histories, probably because of the frequency of canine fracture and the ease of detection. The animals most affected are lions, tigers, bears, and primates.[34, 35] Mandibular fractures occur in a varied range of exotic animals, from the large cats[36, 37] to the snapping turtle.[38]

The most difficult part of dental care is in preparing for the unexpected. Often, a simple root canal treatment becomes a complicated case because of size, curvature, and occlusion. Endodontic instruments for humans are too small and too short for a Siberian tiger's 6-in (15-cm) canine. A periodontal scaler will barely scrape the plaque off a zebra's molars and will not remove any of the large amounts of accumulated calculus. Repairing the beak of a toucan is very dissimilar to extracting a molar from a primate. Anesthetic risk is also a factor in the preparation for treatment. The multiple visits and adjustments that permit perfection in human dentistry are not available or practical in veterinary dental care. The dentist has "to get in, get it done right the first time, and get out."[39]

Endodontics

Endodontics is the most commonly used procedure for oral pathology in exotic animals. Considering the diversity in length, diameter, and accessibility of the pulp chamber of the teeth, it is one of the most difficult procedures encountered. The three basic steps in endodontics are (1) access, (2) instrumentation and debridement, and (3) obturation (Chapter Six). There are very distinct differences in equipment and materials when treating large exotic animals. Forier used modified saw blades to debride the canals of polar bears;[29] others used spoon curettes,[40] multiple barbed broaches wrapped together, large drill bits,[41, 42] and hydrogen peroxide.[30] We found that soldering the working end of a normal endodontic instrument to 0.036 orthodontic wire gave us an instrument with sufficient length, flexibility without breakage, and varying size. Root canals can be filled or obturated with zinc oxide and eugenol paste or gutta percha, depending on the size and length of the canal. A rubber dam or some method of isolating the tooth should be used in order to prevent debris or irrigating solutions from falling into the mouth and blocking the airway.

Elephant tusks present a challenging case for endodontics.[43] An exposed root canal can lead to the loss of the tusk by infection. Large hand drills, lots of irrigation, and zinc oxide–eugenol paste have been used successfully. A rule of thumb for estimating the length of the canal is that the distance between the elephant's eye and the distal portion of the sulcus is equal to the distance from the sulcus to the end of the pulp tissue in the tusk. Younger elephants have longer tusks. If just the end of the canal is exposed, conservative measures can be used, since the recuperative powers are excellent; the end is bathed with antibiotics and is covered with either a sterile medical-grade silicone plug or sterile epoxy molded around the tusk. A broad-spectrum antibiotic given systemically is necessary. The plug should be left on for a few months while the tusk heals by forming secondary dentin.[9]

Restorative Techniques

The clinical crown must be restored after treating a fracture or caries or after endodontic therapy to give it a functional contour. Composite filling materials are useful because they are strong, esthetic, and easy to use. It is not always possible to restore the tooth to its original form. There are occasions when only a little tooth structure remains, and a cast non-precious metal crown has to be fabricated (Chapter Six), which requires a second treatment episode.

Periodontal Techniques

A Cavitron and hand instruments, including large ronguers, are needed to remove the calculus build-up, especially in carnivores. We have often used diamond burs and regular pliers to remove the large pieces of calculus. Regular scalers and curettes are good for subgingival cleaning, which should be done whenever possible. If left, subgingival calculus will remain as a constant irritant and will cause gum breakdown and periodontal disease (Chapter Five).

Exodontia

Instruments used for tooth extraction in humans (forceps, elevators, and root picks) can almost always be used satisfactorily for tooth extraction in exotic animals. However, bone density, shape, and size will often alter the best-prepared plans.[37] Tooth removal, especially the canines of carnivores, is usually done surgically. There are times when conventional instruments are useless, as in extracting an elephant's tusks. A 20-in (50-cm) pipe wrench was used to remove the tusk from an 11-year-old African elephant, because 48 days of antibiotics and irrigation had failed to heal the infected canal.[32]

ORAL INFECTIONS

Normal Oral Flora

The normal microbial flora of the healthy oropharynx has been described in comparatively few wild species of mammals and even more rarely in birds and reptiles. Thus, interpretation of culture results is frequently difficult and may require multiple samples from numerous specimens of the same species in order to make accurate interpretations.

The major work on normal oral flora has been in primate species that are used for dental research. For example, when the normal oral flora of *Macacca sp.* was studied, a variety of aerobic and anaerobic bacteria were isolated.[44] Herpesvirus simiae was recovered from the saliva of clinically normal *Macaccas*,[45] as were protozoa such as *Trichomonas buccalis* and *Entamoaeba gingivalis*.[46]

There is little information on the normal oral flora of birds. As in other species, the results of such cultures will undoubtedly be influenced by the nature of the environment as well as by the usual food eaten. Most data on oral flora in birds have been obtained during attempts to diagnose palatine and sublingual abscesses, which are usually the sequellae of hypovitaminosis A or rhinitis-sinusitis infection that may drain into the oropharynx via the choanal slit in the roof of the mouth. The results of such "oral" cultures are usually very unsatisfactory and misleading because they often represent contamination from the upper respiratory tract. Only with extreme care and patience using swabs of suitable size is one able to obtain clean cultures from the oral cavity of a bird.

Like birds, the normal oral flora of reptiles has been only rarely investigated. *Pseudomonas, Proteus, Klebsiella, Escherichia, Micrococcus,* and *Corynebacterium* spp. have been found to be normal bacterial inhabitants of the oral cavity of healthy King snakes; gram-negative organisms far outnumber gram-positive organisms in this cavity.[47] Similar findings have been reported in garter snakes.[48] Many snake mouths are seemingly devoid of readily recoverable bacteria.[49] *Aeromonas hydrophilia* was isolated from the oral cavity in 85 percent of normal American alligators *(Alligator mississipiensis)* studied.[50] No studies reporting the oral flora of healthy turtles could be found.

Caries

The different orders and genera of animals show a varying degree of susceptibility to caries, and the disease is much more common in captive animals than in those in the wild. Major factors in the etiology of caries in exotic animals have been proposed, such as: (1) action of micro-organisms; (2) structural tooth defects; (3) tooth fractures; (4) malpositioned teeth, which create areas of food impaction; and (5) improper diet, particularly one that is high in carbohydrates.[3]

The type of caries in the captive animal usually differs from that found in the animal in the wild state. Zoo animal caries invariably begins at locations in which food can lodge. Molars are more affected in captivity, whereas incisors are more frequently affected in the wild. Caries often starts in exposed dentin in those animals that are prone to excessive attrition of the enamel, such as the baboon. With the increase of attrition, enamel is worn at the point of contact, increasing the possibility of food impaction and subsequent cavity formation. The upper incisors show the earliest signs of decay; monkeys have a habit of pulling at food with their front teeth, which leads to abnormal attrition. This can lead to caries, soft tissue damage, and supporting bone loss.[4]

Exotic cats often develop caries because of their propensity to fracture enamel by biting bars or large objects, thereby exposing the more-susceptible dentin to caries. Simple caries is sometimes difficult to differentiate from penetrating fractures into the pulp, especially when the fault is at the rostral or caudal surface of the tooth. Caries is extremely rare in the deciduous teeth of monkeys and apes. In the permanent dentition, caries is more frequent in the adult than in the young. Gorillas have very few cavities, chimpanzees and orangutans have more. Caries is very rare in Colobinae and is common in Lasiopyginae; it is extremely rare in howlers but is comparatively frequent in other platyrrhines. Wide differences in the frequency of caries exist in other groups of primates. In more than half of teeth with caries, the cavities occur in the same teeth on the right and the left sides of the jaw. Caries is found more commonly in the upper jaw than in the lower jaw.[5]

In 85 captive lemurs examined, only two cases of caries were found. In wild rodents, no cavities were found, but there were many in the captive rodents. Only 4 cases of caries were found in more than 2000 ungulates. Carnivores in the wild state are practically caries-free, as are ursidae and marsupials.[4] Dental caries is reported to be common in the opossum *(Didelphis virginiana)*.[51] In 180 skulls examined from free-ranging nutria *(Myocastor)*, 11 percent had carious teeth.[52] Caries has also been reported in the hyrax and the hippopotamus. Labial and lingual caries was reported in the fifth molar teeth of a 27 year old African elephant in captivity. Examination of several hundred elephant jaws from East Africa failed to reveal similar lesions in wild animals. It was suggested that the caries may have resulted from an abnormal diet, namely, the feeding of this elephant by the public.[53]

It is generally accepted that caries is initiated by acid-producing bacteria that adhere to the teeth from food and dental plaque. In the wild, purely flesh-eating carnivora are free from caries, and caries is also extremely rare in these species in captivity. In captive exotic animals, caries of the enamel is frequent and occurs in those animals receiving a fermentable carbohydrate in their diet, such as buns, breads, and biscuits. Animals with a diet of grass are almost immune to caries. In captivity, however, other foodstuffs are added, making equine species more susceptible to decay.

The captive wild animal not receiving a "natural diet" becomes more prone to decay from an alteration in the character of the diet; an effort must be made to reduce the feeding of soft, carbohydrate-filled foodstuffs.[54]

Dentoalveolar Abscess

Dentoalveolar abscesses are also found more often in captive animals than in those in the wild. Abscessation of the pulp and apical tissues of the root arise from infection through the pulp, and are initiated as a result of tooth crown fracture, attrition, or carious extension into the pulp, or they are secondary to periodontitis.[2]

The clinical signs of abscessed teeth may range from a unilateral swelling on the affected side to draining facial fistulae or sinus tracts. Elevated rectal temperature, anorexia, depression, tenderness of the affected area, and fetid breath may be observed. Fistulous tracts opening from the maxillary or malar area just ventral to the medial canthus of the eye occur with abscessation of the root of the upper canine or carnassial teeth. Abscesses of the lower teeth drain ventrally through the submandibular area.

Dentoalveolar abscesses have been reported in the California sea lion and walrus. Walruses consistently have problems with their tusks from trauma during capture or confinement. Extraction is extremely difficult, and correction is accomplished by establishing drainage and by antibiotic therapy.[7]

The long incisors of certain marsupials are liable to fracture and exposure of the pulp. The canines of polar bears *(Thalarctos maritimus)* may become abraded on the cages, exposing the pulps. Bone destruction, resulting from apical abscesses of these teeth, produces drainage into the nasal fossa and above and through the ventrum of the mandibular rami.[4]

The formation of draining sinus tracts on the face and chin areas of primates is a relatively common occurrence. The upper canines are affected more often than the lower ones. These dental problems are often overlooked in animals until facial swelling or drainage occurs. Even after producing open drainage through the skin, the condition is often mistaken for a superficial dermatological lesion.[55]

In some cases of dentoalveolar abscesses of canine teeth in squirrel monkeys *(Saimiri sciureus),* maxillary sinus fistulation is produced because of erosion of the maxillary bone.[56] Endodontic and antibiotic therapy provide satisfactory results.

Other zoo animals in whom tooth abscesses have been reported include gazelles, tapirs, and elephants. In some cases, osteitis of the mandible and even death can be a consequence of such infections.[57, 58]

Periodontal Disease

Gingivitis is a common occurrence in exotic animals, especially in captive cats. The major causes of gingivitis, other than dental plaque and calculus, include secondary infection following injury, malnutrition, viral infections, and kidney disease. The clinical signs are halitosis, anorexia, careful chewing motions, and excessive salivation.

Dietary differences from the wild state to a captive state are often substantial. The consistency of food has an effect upon the composition and rate of dental plaque formation. Softer diets produce more bacterial plaque than do harder diets. In short, diet consistency and texture more than likely play a role in the etiology of oral disease.

Periodontal disease causes a transient bacteremia during daily routines such as mastication or teeth cleaning. Diet influences the diversity of the bacterial content and the composition of dental plaque. Consequently, there is a relationship among diet, oral pathology, and systemic health.[59]

Four timber wolves *(Canis lupus)* were used to test a soft diet *versus* a hard, dry, extruded dog food. It was found that the hard diet caused much less accumulation of plaque on the upper fourth premolar, the lower first molar, and the upper and lower canine teeth than did a soft, moist, meat-based diet. This was probably due to the mechanical action of the food that acted as a dietary toothbrush.[60]

Diets also have a reported effect on gorillas.[21] In zoos, the principal foods of fruit and primate cake are of relatively soft consistency, whereas the plant foods of wild gorillas often possess a fibrous quality that takes a greater toll on the teeth. We can, therefore, expect less wear in the teeth of aged apes in captivity and more decay and disease from the sweet, sticky foods in their diets. In 1969, Massa, an

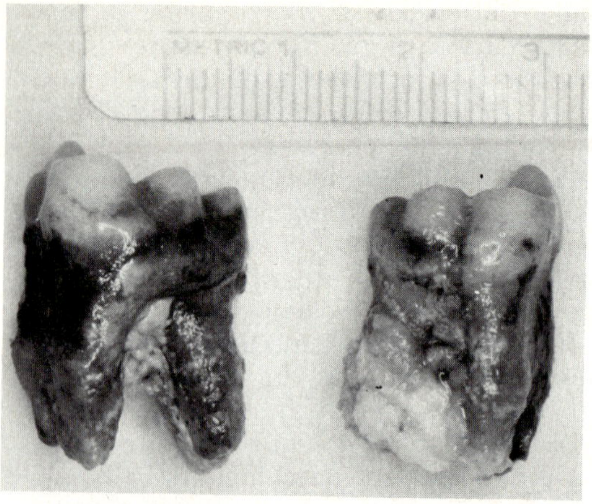

Figure 20–5. Severe periodontal disease of Massa's molars (see also Fig. 20–2), showing a huge accumulation of calculus.

aged western lowland gorilla in the Philadelphia Zoo, required extraction of 17 teeth; in 1983, 6 more teeth were taken out. Advanced periodontal disease, with suppuration, mobility, and excessive calculus, was present (Fig. 20–5).

In addition to diet, the stress of capture, confinement, and transportation of exotic animals is manifested by excessive chewing, biting, and clenching, all of which lead to increased periodontal disease.

The veterinary staff of zoos must examine the diets of exotic animals from a variety of viewpoints: (1) food preferences in the wild; (2) occupational value of food items not necessarily related to nutritional value; and (3) practical considerations relating to the availability, perishability, or economy of foodstuffs.[54] In addition to the nutritional value, exotic animals need food that will use their dentition and masticatory apparatus to prevent loss of teeth and possible systemic disease. Veterinarians at the National Zoo have added oxtails to the diet of their carnivores, drastically reducing tartar build-up and periodontal disease.[61] Whole ox femurs are fed once a week to the tigers at the Detroit Zoo, with similar beneficial results.[62]

Lumpy Jaw in Macropods

Lumpy jaw is a condition seen whenever Macropodidae species (kangaroos and wallabies) congregate in large numbers, though the prevalence is much lower in free-ranging animals than in captive ones. The condition is also referred to as "jaw disease," "necrobacillosis," nocardiosis, streptothricosis, and actinomycosis.

Since the last century, infectious lesions of the jaws and adjacent tissues have been recognized as a major cause of death of macropods in captivity.[63] The early investigators attributed the lesions to the "necrosis bacillus." Although poor management is now well recognized as predisposing macropods to jaw infections, the etiological agents incriminated are numerous despite the fact that disease descriptions are similar. A strictly aerobic actinomycete named *Nocardia macropodidarum* was considered to be the causative agent at one time.[57]

Recent studies would suggest that *Fusobacterium necrophorum* plays a major role in the etiology of lumpy jaw.[64] However, a variety of other organisms, such as *Staphylococcus, Streptococcus,* coliforms, *Bacteroides sp., Corynebacterium pyogenes, Actinomyces,* and *Nocardia spp.,* have also been incriminated as primary or secondary etiological agents.[65]

Molar progression or the accumulation of calicified deposits on the teeth of macropods, or both, may permit the entry of an opportunist organism, which is frequently already present as a normal part of the oral flora,[66–68] a key event in the initiation of lumpy jaw.[69] Many infections have been found around erupting molars. Further, trauma to periodontal tissue induced by the feeding of coarse, dry hay may be an important factor in the establishment of the etiological agent in the jaw.[70] The soft tissue and skeletal lesions are typical and have been extensively described elsewhere.[63, 65, 71–77]

Medical and surgical treatment of lumpy jaw gives variable results; successful treatment invariably depends on early diagnosis and intensive therapy. Radiological examination is helpful in confirming a diagnosis and assessing prognosis (Fig. 20–6). Radical debridement of affected tissue, extraction of involved teeth, and a 6 wk to 8 wk course of an appropriate antibiotic, such as ampicillin, chloramphenicol, or oxytetracycline, is recommended.[64] Unless appropriate attention is given to an aggressive control program, recurrence is not uncommon.

The most effective control measure lies in proper management. A high-density population and its associated stress must be avoided. Reduction in environmental fecal contamination, especially around feeding stations, will significantly reduce the incidence of the disease.[70]

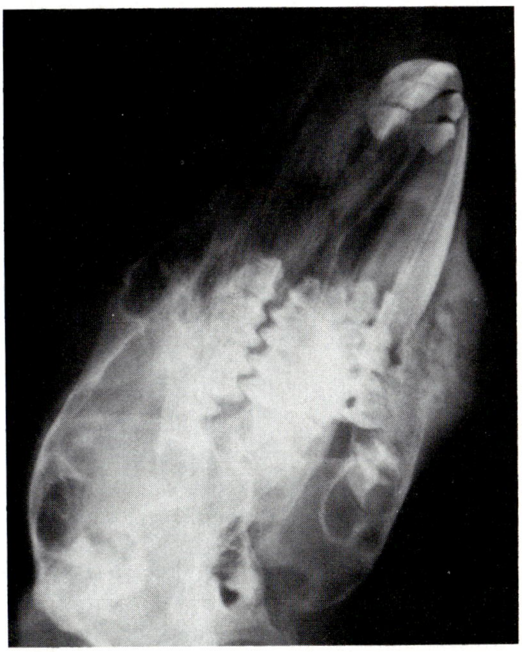

Figure 20–6. Oblique radiograph of the jaw in a kangaroo, illustrating the soft tissue swelling seen in lumpy jaw.

Fluorosis

Chronic fluorosis occurs in animals receiving more than a minute amount of fluorine in the diet over long periods of time. Such poisoning occurs in animals who eat pasturage or forage contaminated by airborne residues from aluminum factories, phosphate refineries, and similar industrial installations, or in animals who drink well water that contains soluble fluorides to the extent of 10 parts per million (ppm) or more.[78]

The clinical signs of chronic fluorine poisoning as described in cattle include (1) mottling and abrasions of teeth, (2) intermittent lameness, (3) periosteal hyperostosis, and (4) demonstration of more than 6 ppm of fluorine in the urine.[79] (See Chapter Seventeen.)

The pathognomonic lesions of chronic fluorosis involve the teeth, the bones, and possibly the kidneys. The significant dental changes include (1) chalky areas, (2) mottling, (3) excessive attrition, and (4) hypoplastic pitting of the enamel.[78]

Chronic fluorisis has been reported in white-tailed deer.[80] The condition was especially prominent in the teeth, resulting in a brown to black discoloration of the premolars and molars, with spontaneous pitting and cracking of the teeth. The mandibles from deer exposed to excessive levels of fluoride had levels of 880 ppm to 7125 ppm, as compared with levels of 167 ppm to 560 ppm in normal animals.

Although it has not been reported among captive wild animals, chronic fluorosis could occur as a result of feeding contaminated food or water. "Slobbers," a syndrome seen in the guinea pig, may actually be chronic fluorosis.[81] A possible source of fluorine in guinea pig feed may be rock phosphate of high fluorine content, which is used as a component of pelleted feed. With this experience in mind, it is possible that other animals could be chronically poisoned by contaminated foods.

Stomatitis

The most essential structure of the oral cavity is the mucosal integument.[82] Homeostasis exists between the oral and the internal environment across the interface, which forms a protective barrier between the internal environment and an array of physical, chemical, and biological factors.

The protective properties of saliva supplement the mechanical barrier effect of the mucosa.[82] The immunosecretory products of the salivary glands, along with the immunological activity of the oral mucosa, constitute a first line of defense against a multitude of agents in the oral environment that have the potential of inducing disease.

Infectious Stomatitis

Mycotic Infections. Numerous mycotic agents have the potential to produce stomatitis. The mycotic organism most frequently isolated from the oral cavity is *Candida albicans.*[82] However, isolation of the organism is not necessarily synonymous with diagnosis of candidiasis (Moniliasis, thrush). *Candida* may be found (as a budded yeast) as part of the normal, commensal oral flora in a wide range of host species. However, when disease occurs, there is a change from the yeast phase to a mycelial or pseudohyphal form. Such pathogenic overgrowth is a reflection of the degree of host resistance resulting from genetic, nutritional, immunological, hormonal, or systemic disease, or in association with prolonged antimicrobial therapy.

The lesions typically consist of either localized or generalized white, curd-like membranous plaques that are loosely adherent to the mucosa. Upon removal of the membrane, a raw, bleeding surface remains. The surrounding mucosa is usually erythematous. Confirmation of the disease includes demonstration of the organism by direct smear and culture and possibly by histopathology.

The disease has been described in mammals (cetaceans, pinnipeds, marsupials, swine, primates, ursides, canidae, and primates), birds (pheasants, jungle fowl, ruffed grouse, quail, herring gulls, raptors, and a variety of companion bird species) and reptiles; however, in the latter the disease is more poorly documented.[7, 83, 84]

Treatment has included nystatin suspension (100,000 IU), chlorhexidine (Nolvasan) 0.2 percent solution, and ketoconazole (Nizoral-Jensen) used for a period of 7 to 10 days.

Other mycotic diseases that have the potential to infect the oral cavity include histoplasmosis, blastomycosis, cryptococcosis, coccidioidomycosis, and actinomycosis.

Vincent's Disease. Vincent's disease, or trenchmouth, has been reported sporadically in the veterinary literature. Among captive wild animals, the disease has been reported in primates.[85, 86] It appears to be caused by the association of at least two organisms—a fusiform bacillus *(Bacteroides)* and a spirochete *(Treponema spp).* This "fusospirochetal complex" characteristically causes localized granular ulceration of the gingivae.

Finding characteristic spiral organisms on stained smears of the lesions assists in making a diagnosis, and darkfield illumination may be helpful.

Treatment consists of topical gentian violet or a 1 percent hydrogen peroxide flush and parenteral penicillin.

Trichomoniasis. Known also as canker and frounce, trichomoniasis is a disease of the upper alimentary tract of pigeons and doves,[87–89] raptors,[90–92] canaries, sparrows, and other finches, as well as psittacines.[93–95] The causative organism is *Trichomonas gallinae.*

Affected birds may exhibit excessive salivation, awkward swallowing motions, erythema of the oral mucous membranes, and cankers, or caseous diphtheritic membranes of the mouth, caudal pharynx, and crop, or both.

A diagnosis of trichomoniasis is made by demonstrating the protozoan parasite in wet mounts of the exudate. The organism has a characteristic jerky circular motion. The shape of *T. gallinae* varies from round to pear-shaped, and its size is 6μ to $19\mu \times 2\mu$ to 9μ. Characteristically, there are four flagella. The differential diagnosis should include *Candida* infections, avian pox, vitamin A deficiency, and capillariasis.

Treatment consists of the oral administration of 2-amino-5-nitrothiazole (Enheptin-American Cyanamid) or metronidazole (Flagyl, Schering Corp.). Copper sulfate may be used in the drinking water.[7]

Viral Stomatitis. Viral diseases that cause oral lesions are best exemplified in the Felidae and the Artiodactyla.

Feline viral rhinotracheitis (FVRT) is widespread in exotic felids.[7] An outbreak in the Cincinnati Zoo in 1968 severely affected at least ten species of the genus Felis.[96] FVRT can cause severe lesions, including ulcers on the oral mucosa and the tongue.

Work done at both the St. Louis and the Brookfield Zoological Gardens suggests that all species of exotic cats will develop good levels of antibody within 14 days of vaccination with a modified live-virus FVRT vaccine.[7]

Feline calicivirus, a picorna virus, is most often associated with ulcerative stomatitis. FCV infection has been described in cheetahs.[97] The disease may be quite severe, with the more virulent strains producing pneumonia. Carrier states are quite common, thus survivors may pose a threat to other felids in the collection. Vaccination is reported to prevent the disease.[7]

Other feline viral diseases, such as feline panleukopenia, may be associated with stomatitis, though other tissues and organs are more typically affected.

A large number of exotic ruminants appear to be susceptible to a great variety of viral diseases.[7] Many of these viral infections affect the tissues of the oral cavity. Examples of such viral disorders in exotic Artiodactyla include malignant catarrhal fever, vesicular stomatitis, blue-tongue, rinderpest, and foot and mouth disease. They are described in Chapter Seventeen.

Avian "diphtheria" or pox is a viral disease that produces proliferative lesions on the epithelial surfaces of the skin and oral cavity. Poxes occur in both free-living and captive birds. The oral lesions usually take the form of diphtheritic membranes and must be differentiated from trichomoniasis, candidiasis, and hypovitaminosis A.

Since there is no specific treatment for most viral diseases, therapy must be directed toward supportive care, which includes both intensive fluid therapy and attention to nutritional requirements. The prophylactic use of parenteral antibiotics may help avoid secondary bacterial stomatitis.

Infectious Stomatitis of Reptiles. Infectious stomatitis of reptiles, also referred to as necrotic stomatitis, ulcerative stomatitis, ulcerative gingivitis, mouthrot, and oral canker, is perhaps the most common disease recognized in captive reptiles.[47, 49, 98–105]

Clinical signs are variable. Early signs may consist of anorexia, a cloudy, thick oral mucus, and petechial hemorrhages of the oral mucosa. In more advanced disease, the petechial hemorrhages on the gingivae may be associated with ulceration of the oral mucosae. In the more severe state, there is gingival edema, and the cloudy oral mucus contains clumps of caseous material (Fig. 20–7). Frequently, this caseous material adheres to the dental arches. Open-mouthed breathing often accompanies this condition. If left untreated, the infection may cause pneumonia, gastritis, and infection of the spectaculoconjunctival space.[103]

A number of factors may be responsible for initiating this disease. Oral trauma, malnutrition, and poor husbandry are considered important factors in precipitating infectious stomatitis in reptiles. Gram-negative bacteria are the predominant microbial organisms recovered in cases of mouthrot,

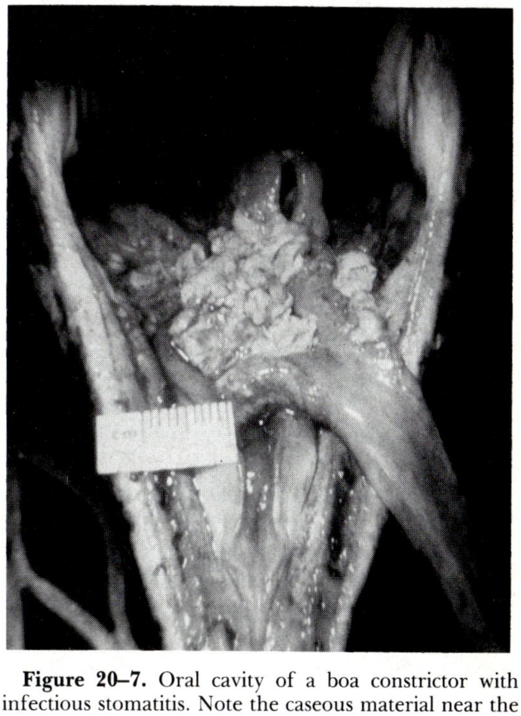

Figure 20–7. Oral cavity of a boa constrictor with infectious stomatitis. Note the caseous material near the glottis and the hemorrhage along the dental arcade.

with *Aeromonas, Proteus, Klebsiella,* and *Pseudomonas* spp. being the most frequent isolates.[103] Fungi, such as *Aspergillus* sp., and yeasts are occasionally seen in impression smears or are recovered on culture; however, these latter organisms are not considered primary causes of the infection.

Diagnosis is based on clinical signs and upon finding characteristic lesions in the mouth.

Treatment consists of (1) specific systemic antimicrobial therapy and oral antiseptics; (2) proper diet, including parenteral fluids, force feeding, and supplementation with ascorbic acid; and (3) husbandry improvements, especially temperature and moisture.[7, 105–107]

Non-Infectious Stomatitis. A number of non-infectious conditions may potentially cause stomatitis in captive wild animals, including physical agents, such as foreign bodies, trauma, thermal and electrical burns, and chemical agents, such as strong alkalis, acids, petroleum distillates, and heavy metals. Other non-infectious causes include metabolic disorders, such as diabetes mellitus and uremia; nutritional deficiencies, such as thiamine, riboflavin, niacin, pyridoxine, cyanocobalamine, folic acid, biotin, ascorbic acid, vitamin A, vitamin D, iron, and zinc; blood dyscrasias and reticuloendothelial diseases; allergic and toxic drug reactions; autoimmune disease; and imunosuppressive or immunodeficiency disorders.[82]

Clearly not all these non-infectious causes of stomatitis have been described in captive wild animals. However, all may possibly occur in wild animals, since they have been described in humans and domestic animals (see Chapters Four, Fourteen, Seventeen, and Eighteen).

Local Gingival Disease

Focal Epithelial Hyperplasia. A single case of focal epithelial hyperplasia has been reported in the oral cavity of a chimpanzee.[108] The lesions were plaque-like and were the same color as the normal oral tissue. No other clinical signs were recognized. The lesions regressed in size and number over a 10 month period without treatment.

Epulis, a non-neoplastic lesion that appears as a non-ulcerated, cauliflower-like growth at the gingival margin in many breeds of dog (Chapter Eight) has not been described to date in wild animals, though it is likely to occur in wild Canidae.

Gingival Hyperplasia Associated with Diphenylhydantoin Therapy. This condition occurs in humans. A similar lesion has been described in the gorilla undergoing therapy for idiopathic epilepsy.[109] Any animal undergoing prolonged diphenylhydantoin therapy should receive a periodic oral examination in order to detect the initial phases of gingival hypertrophy. Adjusting the dose of diphenylhydantoin may prevent worsening of the condition. In advanced stages, gingivectomy may be needed in addition to dosage adjustments.

LIPS, CHEEKS, AND BEAK

Specific disorders of the lips and cheeks are not commonly described in the veterinary literature on wild animals. It would be safe to assume, however, that the conditions affecting the lips and cheeks of domestic animals could also be seen in wild animals.

Of special interest are the cheek pouches that are seen in hamsters. These pouches are oral-cavity evaginations traveling alongside the head and neck to the scapula.[110] The pouches are lined with stratified squamous epithelium, are thin-walled, and are highly distensible. The cheek pouches serve the hamster as a food transportation mechanism. Occasionally, these pouches will become infected from the introduction of bacteria, from the retention of food, or from trauma associated with a foreign body. Under general anesthesia, the cheek pouches can be everted, cleaned, and treated locally. In extreme situations, an impaction of the pouch may occur with abscessation and associated oral pathology.

The beak or bill of birds and turtles is a very specialized oral structure that includes the upper and lower jaws and their keratinized covering. The beak combines the functions of prehension and mastication.[111] The size and shape of the beak varies greatly among species and to a great extent is correlated with feeding habits. The cutting edges may be serrated, ridged, or smooth. Beak growth is constant and the beak is worn down by the feeding and other oral habits of the species.

A number of beak abnormalities may be seen in birds, including overgrowth, splits, fractures, necrosis, and neoplasms.[112]

The most common deformity in birds is simple overgrowth resulting from malocclusion and insufficient normal wear (Fig. 20–8).[113] Problems of malocclusion seem to occur most frequently in psittacine species.

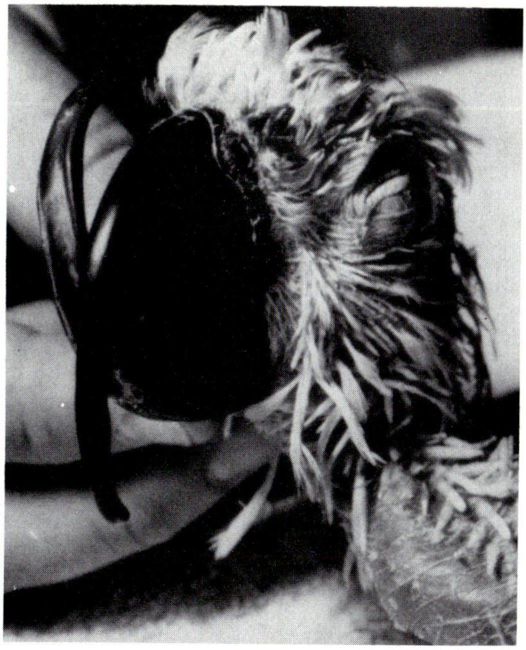

Figure 20–8. Malocclusion and beak overgrowth in a sulfur-crested cockatoo.

One of the most frequent causes of overgrown beaks in small psittacines (e.g., budgerigars) is a parasitic infection with the *Knemidocoptes pilae* mite (Fig. 20–9). This mite invades the matrix of the beak and burrows deep into it, destroying areas of the germinal tissue. The resulting difference in growth pattern leads to an overgrowth of both upper and lower beaks on non-occluding surfaces. Although elimination of the mite with a suitable parasiticide will prevent further damage, the existing deformity may be irreversible. In psittacines of advancing age, overgrowth of the upper beak may occur from loss of contour and straightening.[113]

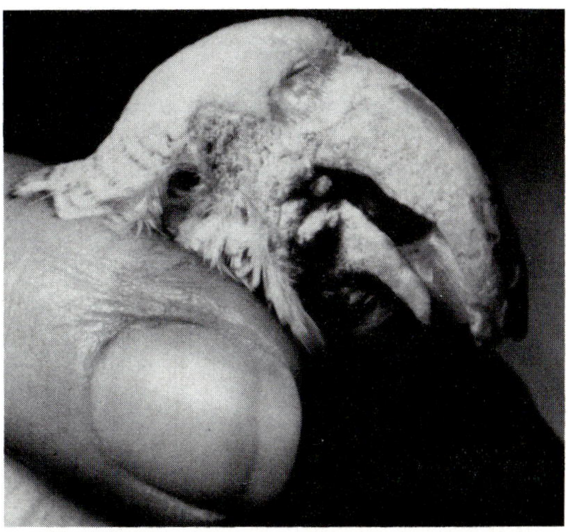

Figure 20–9. Beak deformity and overgrowth in a budgerigar infested with mites of the genus *Knemidocoptes.*

Other causes of beak deformity in both psittacine (hard-billed) and passerine (soft-billed) birds are mycosis, liver disease, malnutrition, specific nutritional deficiencies, rickets, and osteodystrophy. Hereditary and congenital deformities are seen infrequently.

Beak trauma as a consequence of falling or flying into a solid object may result in simple hemorrhage, a split in the beak, or complete avulsion. Simple hemorrhage into the substance of the beak frequently results in little more than some discoloration. Extensive hemorrhage between the laminae as a consequence of more severe beak trauma may result in some deformity. As the extravasated blood clots and dries, and as the beak grows, flaking and fractures may occur.[113]

Splits, fractures, and avulsions of the beak are cause for more concern and frequently require some degree of surgical intervention as well as intensive nursing care. Loss of beak tissue can be treated by constructing a wire and acrylic prosthesis.[114–116]

Beak neoplasms may result in significant deformity and complete or partial loss of the beak.

Conditions affecting the beaks in turtles are not well documented. The most frequently encountered condition in turtles appears to be simple overgrowth due to age or a soft diet, or both. As in birds, the treatment is simple trimming with an appropriate instrument, such as a toenail or cuticle nipper, or filing with a dental engine or Dremmel tool and bur.

TONGUE

The tongues of wild animals, birds, and reptiles are highly variable organs morphologically and for the most part are examples of adaptation to a particular diet.

The giraffe has a long, prehensile tongue that is used to reach, grasp, and remove the fine, leafy foliage while avoiding the long, sharp thorns of the acacia trees and shrubs that make up the bulk of the diet. Other mammals, such as the anteater, pangolin, and aardvark, also have long, dextrous tongues, but they are much more slender than the giraffe's and are used to probe for ants and termites.

Adaptations of the tongue in birds are also associated with the type of food eaten and the method of obtaining it.[117] For example, woodpeckers have long tongues with barbed tips that can protrude beyond the tip of the bill to extract grubs from burrows in and under the bark of trees. Hummingbirds, sunbirds, and honey-eaters have tubular tongues that are brushy at the tips to aid in sucking nectar out of flowers. Ducks and flamingos have tongues that are shaped so that water is forced out of the mouth through strainers on the edge of the bill.

The shape of the tongue among reptiles varies widely. Some lizards have fleshy tongues with expanded tips that can protrude a distance equal to more than half the length of the body to catch their prey. The wide, fleshy tongue of the croccodile occupies the entire floor of the mouth but cannot be protruded, and it is used to push food into the esophagus.

Diseases of the tongue that have been described in captive wild animals fall into two general catetgories: those resulting from trauma, and glossitis. Common sources of trauma are foreign bodies, such as thorns, plant awns, wood, and metal splinters, string, rubber bands, nails, staples, and so on, that become embedded in or encircle the tongue. External trauma from fighting or hitting fences, and from cage enclosures or chewing sharp objects, frequently produces tongue trauma. The trauma from malocclusion is a common cause of irritation to the tongue. Removal of foreign bodies and eliminating evident sources of trauma will usually bring about a rapid and complete recovery.

Glossitis caused by infectious agents is commonly seen in wild ruminants and exotic cats. The most frequently encountered microbe producing infectious glossitis in wild ruminants is *Actinobacillus*. A number of viral diseases, such as malignant catarrhal fever, vesicular stomatitis and blue-tongue also can cause glossitis (Chapter Seventeen).[7] Infectious glossitis is characterized by constant licking, chewing, and salivation. Necrotic stomatitis in marsupials frequently involves the tongue.[2] The infectious agents most often associated with glossitis in wild felids are the FVRV and the calicivirus. These diseases often cause tongue ulceration. Management and control are described on page 303.

Two unique conditions of the tongue have been observed.[118] The first occurred in an adult female reticulated giraffe who was born in captivity and had always exhibited a tongue-lolling behavior. At 10 years of age, the animal exhibited a sudden acute "paralysis" of the tongue and was unable to withdraw it back into her mouth (Fig. 20–10). No atrophy was noted. Nerve stimulation studies under general anesthesia failed to reveal any neuromuscular abnormalities. A complete physical examination, skull radiographs, and blood studies also failed to establish any abnormality. Approximately 80 percent of the tongue was amputated, and the animal experienced immediate postanesthetic complications and died. The necropsy was unremarkable. Histologically, the tongue had a marked diffuse fibrosis with chronic myodegeneration. There were diffuse foci of eosinophils. The hypoglossal nerves appeared normal. No etiological agent was seen to explain the condition.

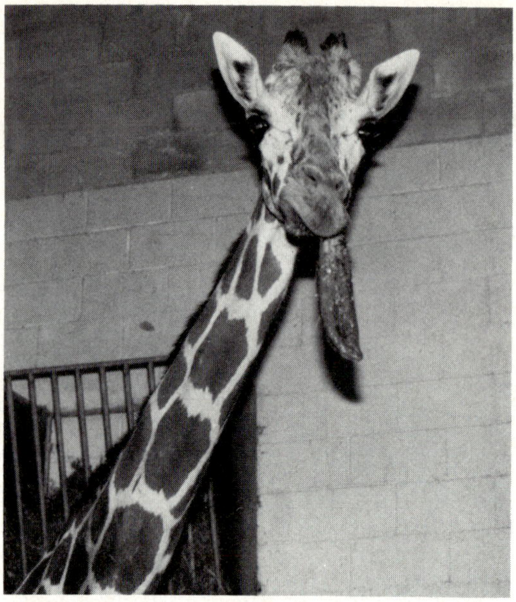

Figure 20–10. Paralysis of the tongue in a female reticulated giraffe.

A mature female giant anteater was noted at the time of necropsy to have a band of fibrous tissue within and encircling the tongue near its base, compromising the circulation and causing necrosis of the distal portion of the tongue. Again no causal agent could be identified.

The usual conditions affecting the tongue in birds are trauma and foreign bodies. Para- and sublingual abscesses associated with hypovitaminosis A are seen commonly in psittacine birds. These abscesses heal quickly following curettage and cautery.[119, 120] Supplemental vitamin A and dietary adjustments will usually prevent recurrences.

In reptiles, disorders of the tongue are most likely to be a result of trauma or foreign bodies. Generalized malnutrition will commonly result in glossitis.

OROPHARYNX, TONSILS AND SALIVARY GLANDS

There are very few references to conditions affecting the oropharynx in wild animals. Trauma has been associated with a foreign body granuloma in a rhesus monkey,[121] and ingestion of caustic chemicals with subsequent pharyngeal disease has been described in a woolly monkey.[122] Infections, abscesses, and neoplasms are all possible sources of oropharyngeal disorders.

Except for neoplasms, diseases of the salivary glands in captive wild animals have not been described.

No case of tonsillar disease in wild animals has been reported, though gross and histological studies are rarely performed on this tissue.

OROPHARYNGEAL NEOPLASIA

Based on the available literature, oral neoplasms of wild mammals appear to occur infrequently.

No tumors of the teeth or adnexa were

Table 20–2. Oropharyngeal Neoplasms—Philadelphia Zoological Garden 1908–1983

	Mammals	
Marsupialia		
Opossum	*(Didelphis virginiana)*	Fibro-osteoma of both maxillae
Opossum	*(Didelphis virginiana)*	Osteosarcoma of jaw
Opossum	*(Didelphis virginiana)*	Osteosarcoma of jaw
Primates		
White-handed gibbon	*(Hylobates lar)*	Squamous papilloma of pharynx
Orangutan	*(Pongo pygmaeus)*	Squamous cell carcinoma of esophagus
Rodentia		
Woodchuck	*(Marmota monax)*	Adenocarcinoma of salivary gland (or pharyngeal mucous glands)
Minnie Downs mouse	*(Pseudomys australis minnie)*	Adenocarcinoma of the parotid salivary gland
Carnivora		
Dingo	*(Canis familiaris dingo)*	Carcinoma of the parotid salivary gland
Arctic fox	*(Alopex lagopus)*	Glandular carcinoma of the nasal mucosa
Black bear	*(Ursus americanus)*	Epithelioma of the root of the tongue
Ring-tailed coati	*(Nasua nasua)*	Neuroepithelioma
Ring-tailed coati	*(Nasua nasua)*	Neuroepithelioma
Ring-tailed coati	*(Nasua nasua)*	Neuroepithelioma
Ring-tailed coati	*(Nasua nasua)*	Neuroepithelioma
Crab-eating raccoon	*(Euprocyon cancrivorus)*	Neuroepithelioma
Crab-eating raccoon	*(Euprocyon cancrivorus)*	Neuroepithelioma
Kinkajou	*(Potos flavus)*	Neuroepithelioma
Ring-tailed "cat"	*(Bassariscus astutus)*	Neuroepithelioma
American badger	*(Taxidea taxus)*	Oral squamous cell carcinoma
Mongoose	*(Mungos mungo)*	Neuroepithelioma
Genet	*(Genetta genetta)*	Oral carcinoma
Genet	*(Genetta genetta)*	Neuroepithelioma
Caracal	*(Lynx caracal)*	Osteochondroma in nasal area
Jungle cat	*(Felis chaus)*	Oral papilloma
African lion	*(Panthera leo)*	Adamantinoma of mandible
Siberian tiger	*(Panthera tigris)*	Oral fibrosarcoma
California sea lion	*(Zalophus californianus)*	Squamous cell carcinoma of the cheek
Artiodactyla		
Reticulated giraffe	*(Giraffa reticulata)*	Fibroma on wall of pharynx
Gazelle	*(Gazella isabella)*	Osteofibroma of maxilla
Nilgae	*(Boselaphus tragocamelus)*	Adamantinoma of the mandible
Blue duiker	*(Cephalopus monticola bicolor)*	Oral squamous cell carcinoma
	Birds	
American white pelican	*(Pelecanus erythronhynchos)*	Squamous cell carcinoma of the beak
	Reptiles	
Galapagos tortoise	*(Testudo vicinia)*	Squamous cell carcinoma of the jaw

found in a survey of 3127 zoo mammals necropsied over a 12 year period at the San Diego Zoo.[123] The only neoplasm reported in the oral cavity was an adenocarcinoma in a Syrian golden jackal, *Chrysocyon brachyurus.* A more recent report from the San Diego Zoo lists four additional cases of neoplasia affecting the oral cavity.[2] These recent cases include a papilloma of the gingiva in a white-tailed gnu, a non-malignant hemangioma of the tongue in a cheetah, a squamous cell carcinoma of the face that involved the maxillary sinus in a pronghorn antelope, and a pedunculated papilloma of the tongue in a Tasmanian devil.

The oral neoplasms seen at the Philadelphia Zoological Garden over a 75 year period are listed in Table 20–2.[124] Thirty-three individual specimens have been recorded. Thirty-one of them have occurred in mammals, with one each occurring in birds and reptiles.

Other sporadic cases of oral neoplasia have been recorded (Figs. 20–11 and 20–12).[7, 106, 125–129]

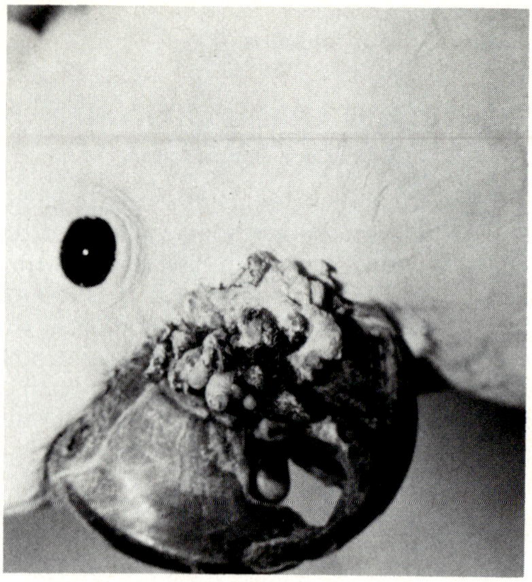

Figure 20–12. Multiple papillomae at the left commissure of the beak in a Moluccan cockatoo.

ORAL PARASITES

Oral parasites are rare in captive wild animals. The most often encountered oral parasites in mammals are external forms, such as ticks and leeches, that attach to the lips and cheeks and at the commissures of the mouth.

The two most common parasites of the oral cavity in birds are the trichomonad, *Trichomonas gallinae,* and the knemidocoptic mite, *Knemidocoptes pilae. T. gallinae,* the cause of canker-frounce, is discussed on page 302. *K. pilae* is responsible for severe beak deformity. This latter condition is discussed on page 305.

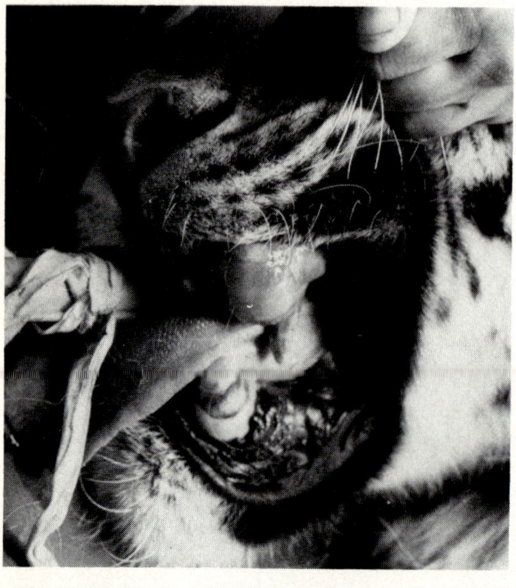

Figure 20–11. Oral fibrosarcoma in the region of the upper left canine in a male Siberian tiger.

Flukes are commonly observed in the mouth as well as in the esophagus, lung, intestine, and kidney of reptiles and amphibians.[7, 105, 130] Although these flukes are considered to be non-pathogenic, they may result in mouth gaping. Flukes are rarely transmitted in captivity because the molluscan or invertebrate intermediate host is usually absent.

Clinical signs are usually limited to the mouth gaping already noted and variable periods of anorexia. Diagnosis is made by finding adult flukes in the oral cavity or ova in the feces of infected animals. There is no specific, safe, or effective treatment of trematodes in reptiles. If indicated, the oral trematodes can be physically removed from the oral cavity by using a cotton-tipped applicator or blunt forceps.

References

1. Kazimiroff T: A report on the dental pathology found in animals that died in the New York Zoological Park in 1938. *Zoologica NY Zool Soc* 24(14):297–304, 1938.
2. Robinson PT: Oral pathology in mammals at the San Diego Zoo and Wild Animal Park. *Proc Am Assoc Zoo Vet* 96–98, 1979.
3. Robinson PT: A literature review of dental pa-

thology and aging by dental means in non-domestic animals. *Zoo Anim Med* 10:57–65(Pt. I); 81–91(Pt. II), 1979.
4. Colyer F: Variations and Diseases of the Teeth of Animals. London, John Bales and Sons and Danielsson Ltd., 1936.
5. Schultz AH: Eruption and decay of the permanent teeth in primates. *Am J Phys Anthrop* 19:489–588, 1935.
6. Willoughby DP: All About Gorillas. Cranbury, NJ, AB Barnes Co., 1978.
7. Wallach JD, Boever BJ: Diseases of Exotic Animals. Philadelphia, WB Saunders Co., 1983.
8. Schneider KM: The development of the teeth of the lion *(Panthera leo)*, with some observations about the teething of several other great cats and of the domestic cat. *Der Zoologische Garten* 22:240–361, 1959.
9. Schmidt M: Elephants. *In* Fowler, ME (ed): Zoo and Wild Animal Medicine. Philadelphia, WB Saunders Co., 1978.
10. Laws RM: Age criteria for the African elephant, *Loxodonta africana. East Afr Wildlife J* 4:1–37, 1966.
11. Altevogt R: Elephants. *In* Grzimek B (ed): Grzimek's Animal Life Encyclopedia. Mammals, Vol. 12, No. 3. New York,Von Nostrand Reinhold Co., 1975.
12. Rahm U: Aardvarks. *In* Grzimek B (ed): Grzimek's Animal Life Encyclopedia, Mammals, Vol. 12, No. 3. New York, Von Nostrand Reinhold Co., 1975.
13. Walker EP: Mammals of the World, 3rd ed., (2 Vols.). Baltimore, Johns Hopkins University Press, 1975.
14. Dagg AI, Foster JB: The Giraffe–Its Biology, Behavior and Ecology. New York, Van Nostrand Reinhold Co., 1976.
15. Hoff GL, Hoff DM: Dental anomalies in mammals. *In* Hoff GL, Davis, JW (eds): Noninfectious Diseases of Wildlife. Ames, Iowa, Iowa State University Press, 1982, pp. 100–108.
16. Marshall WH: Note on missing teeth in *Martes americana. J Mammal* 33:116–117, 1952.
17. Schuman EL, Sognnaes RF: Developmental microscopic defects in the teeth of subhuman primates. *Am J Phys Anthrop* 14:193–214, 1956.
18. Molnar S, Ward SC: Mineral metabolism and microstructural defects in primate teeth. *Am J Phys Anthrop* 43:3–17, 1975.
19. Stirling I: Tooth wear as a mortality factor in the Weddell seal, *Leptonychotes waddelli. J Mamm* 50:559–565, 1969.
20. Napier JR, Napier PH: A Handbook of Living Primates. London, Academic Press, 1967.
21. Cousins D: Dental disease in the Gorilla with special reference to alveolar regression. *Int Zoo News* 175:10–18, 1982.
22. Bramblett CA: Pathology in the Darajani baboon. *Am J Phys Anthrop* 26:331–340, 1967.
23. Harvey PH, Kavanagh M, Clutton-Brock TH: Canine tooth size in female primates. *Nature* 276:817–818, 1978.
24. Hediker H: Wild Animals in Captivity. New York, Dover Publications, 1964.
25. Schulze C: Development abnormalities of the teeth and jaws. *In* Gorlin RJ, Goldman HM: Thoma's Oral Pathology. St. Louis, The CV Mosby Co., 1970.
26. Archer M: Abnormal dental development and its significance in dasyurid and other marsupials. *Mem Queensland Mus* 17:251–265, 1975.
27. Bernier JL: The Management of Oral Disease. St. Louis, The CV Mosby Co., 1959.
28. Zeman WV, Fielder FG: Dental malocclussion and overgrowth in rabbits. *J Am Vet Med Assoc* 155:115–1119, 1969.
29. Forier RC, Miller T, Swigert J: Case report–root canal therapy on two polar bears. *Proc Am Assoc Zoo Vet* 213–214, 1975.
30. Brinkman RJ, Williams RV: Root canal and capping on a whitehanded gibbon. *J Zoo Anim Med* 6:26, 1975.
31. Fagan DA: Equipment and instrumentation and its relationship to veterinary dental care. *Proc Am Assoc Zoo Vet* 92–94, 1979.
32. Stringer BG: The removal of a tusk in an African elephant. *Proc Am Assoc Zoo Vet* 271–272, 1972–1973.
33. Nakagawa S: False teeth for a donkey. *Int Zoo Yr Bk* 5:196, 1965.
34. Tinkelman CL: Endodontic treatment of a Siberian tiger at the Philadelphia Zoological Garden. *Proc Am Assoc Zoo Vet* 99, 1979.
35. Sedwick CJ, Cooper RW: Dental fistula in the squirrel monkey *(Saimiri sciureus). J Zoo Anim Med* 3:26–27, 1972.
36. Kemp WB, Barton RA, Hyatt FD: Surgical correction of orofacial trauma in a lion cub. *J Zoo Anim Med* 7:9–11, 1976.
37. Milton JL, Silberman MS, Hankes GH: Compound comminuted fractures of the rami of the mandible in a tiger *(Panthera tigris):* A case report. *J Zoo Anim Med* 11:108–112, 1980.
38. Kuehn G: Case report—bilateral transverse mandibular fractures in a turtle. *Proc Am Assoc Zoo Vet* 243, 1972.
39. Fagan D: A discussion of endodontic techniques in carnivores. *Proc Am Assoc Zoo Vet* 94–96, 1979.
40. Wutzke G, Frye FL, Sorrokin G: Endodontic therapy and upper canine restoration utilizing dental techniques. *J Zoo Anim Med* 8:24–25, 1977.
41. Ross D: Root canal on an elephant. *Animal Kingdom*, December 1977.
42. Van De Grift ER: Root canal therapy on a Siberian tiger *(Panthera tigris Altaica). J Zoo Anim Med* 6:24, 1975.
43. Bush M, Heise DW, Gray CW, James AE: Surgical repair of tusk injury (pulpectomy) in an adult male forest elephant. *J Am Dent Assoc* 93:372–375, 1976.
44. Kelly FC: Bacteriology of artificially produced necrotic lesions in the oropharynx of the monkey. *J Infect Dis* 74:93–108, 1944.
45. Ruch TC: Diseases of Laboratory Primates. Philadelphia, WB Saunders Co., 1959.
46. Hegner R, Chu HJ: A comparative study of the intestinal protozoa of wild monkeys and man. *Am J Hyg* 12:62–108, 1930.
47. Page LA: Experimental ulcerative stomatitis in king snakes. *Cornell Vet* 51:258–266, 1961.
48. Mergenhagan SE: The bacterial flora of the common garter snake, *Thamnophis sirtalis sirtalis. J. Bacteriol* 71:739, 1956.
49. Burke TJ, Rosenberg D, Smith AR: Infectious stomatitis—a perspective. *Proc Am Assoc Zoo Vet* 190–196, 1978.
50. Gordon RW, Hazen TC, Esch GW, Fliermans CB: Isolation of *Aeromonas hydrophila* from the American alligator, *Alligator mississippiensis. J Wildlife Dis* 15:239–243, 1979.
51. Farris EJ: *In* Care and Feeding of Laboratory Animals. New York, John Wiley & Sons, 1950.
52. Schnitoskey F: Anomalies and pathological condi-

tions in the skulls of nutria from southern Louisiana. *Extrait de mammalia* 33:311–314, 1971.
53. Short RV: Notes on the teeth and ovaries of an African elephant, *Loxodonta africana,* of known age. *J Zool* (London) 158:421–425, 1969.
54. Fagan D: Diet consistency and periodontal disease in exotic carnivores. *Proc. Am Assoc Zoo Vet* 34–37, 1980.
55. Robinson PT: Multiple canine teeth fistulae in a red uakari monkey. *Vet Med Sm An Clin* 69:699, 1974.
56. Greenstein ET, Hirth RS: Maxillary sinus fistula in a squirrel monkey with a diseased canine tooth. *J Am Vet Med Assoc* 167:655, 1975.
57. Fox H: Diseases in Wild Animals and Birds. Philadelphia, JB Lippincott Co., 1923.
58. McGavin MD, Walker RD, Schroeder EC, Patton CS, McCracken MD: Death of an African elephant from probable toxemia attributed to chronic pulpitis. *J Am Vet Med Assoc* 183:1269–1273, 1983.
59. Cohen DW, Goldman HM: Oral disease in primates. *Ann NY Acad Sci* 85:889–909, 1960.
60. Vosburgh KM, Barbiers RB, Sikarskie JG, Ullrey DE: A soft versus hard diet and oral health in captive timber wolves *(Canis lupus). J Zoo Anim Med* 13:104–107, 1982.
61. Bush M, Gray C: Dental prophylaxis in carnivores. *Int Zoo Yr Bk* 15:223, 1975.
62. Colmery BH: Personal communication, 1984.
63. Bang B: Om Aarsagen til lakal Nekrose. Maanedskr. f. Abt. Dyrlaeger. 2:235, 1981–1. Cited by Beveridge WIB: *J Pathol Bacteriol* 38:467–491, 1934.
64. Butler R, Burton JD: Necrobacillosis of macropods—control and therapy. *Proc Am Assoc Zoo Vet* 137–140, 1980.
65. Finnie EP: Marsupials and monotremes. *In* Fowler ME (ed): Zoo and Wild Animal Medicine. Philadelphia, WB Saunders Co., 1978, pp. 399–426.
66. Beighton D, Miller WA: A microbial study of normal macropod dental plaque. *J Dent Res* 56:995–1000, 1977.
67. Samuel JL: Bacterial flora of the mouth and of lesions of the jaw in macropods. *In* Fowler ME (ed): Wildlife Disease of the Pacific Basin and Other Countries. California, Fruitridge Printing, 1982, pp. 56–58.
68. Samuel JL: The normal flora of the mouths of macropods (Marsupialia:Macropodidae). *Arch Oral Biol* 27:141–146, 1982.
69. Miller WA, Beighton D, Butler R: Histologic and osteological observations on the early stages of lumpy jaw. *In* Montali RJ, Magaki G (eds): The Comparative Pathology of Zoo Animals, Washington, DC, Smithsonian Institution Press, 1980, pp. 231–239.
70. Butler R: Epidemiology and management of "lumpy jaw" in macropods. *In* Fowler ME (ed): Wildlife Diseases of the Pacific Basin and Other Countries. California, Fruitridge Printing, 1982, pp. 58–61.
71. Tucker R, Millar R: Outbreak of nocardiosis in marsupials in the Brisbane Botanical Gardens. *J Comp Pathol* 63:143, 1953.
72. Watts PS, McLean SJ: *Bacteroides* infection in kangaroos. *J Comp Pathol* 66:159–162, 1953.
73. Wallach JD: Lumpy jaw in captive kangaroos. *Int Zoo Yr Bk* 11:13, 1971.
74. Boever WJ, Leathers C: Pulmonary and encephalic infection secondary to lumpy jaw in kangaroos. *J Zoo Anim Med* 4:13–16, 1973.
75. Finnie EP: Necrobacillosis in kangaroos. *In* Page LA (ed): Wildlife Disease. New York, Plenum Pub. Corp., 1976, pp. 511–518.
76. Potkay S: Diseases of marsupials. *In* Hunsaker D (ed): The Biology of Marsupials. New York, Academic Press, 1977, pp. 415–506.
77. Arundel JH, Barker IK, Beveridge I: Disease of marsupials. *In* Stonehouse B, Gilmore G (eds): The Biology of Marsupials. Baltimore, University Park Press, 1977, pp. 141–154.
78. Smith HA, Jones TC, Hunt RD: Veterinary Pathology, 4th ed. Philadelphia, Lea & Febiger, 1972, pp. 928–935.
79. Shupe L, Miner ML, Greenwood DA: Clinical and pathological aspects of fluorine toxicosis in cattle. *Ann NY Acad Sci* 111:618–637, 1964.
80. Karstad L: Fluorosis in deer, *Odocoileus virginionus. Bull Wildife Dis Assoc* 3:42–46, 1967.
81. Hard GC, Atkinson FFV: "Slobbers." *In* Laboratory guinea pigs as a form of chronic fluorosis. *J Pathol Bacteriol* 94:95–102, 1967.
82. MacDonald JM: Stomatitis. *Vet Clin North Am: Sm Anim Pract* 13:415–436, 1983.
83. Keymer IF: Mycoses. *In* Petrak ML (ed): Diseases of Cage and Aviary Birds, 2nd ed. Philadelphia, Lea & Febiger, 1982, pp. 599–605.
84. Cooper JE, Jackson OJ (eds): Diseases of the Reptiles. Vols. I and II. New York, Academic Press, 1981.
85. Migaki G, Seibold HR, Wolf RH, Garner FM: Pathologic conditions in the patas monkey. *J Am Vet Med Assoc* 159:549–556, 1971.
86. Van Riper DC, Fineg J, Day PW: Vincent's disease in the chimpanzee. *J Am Vet Med Assoc* 151:905–906, 1967.
87. Bullock BC: Trichomoniasis in pigeons. *Lab Anim Dig* 2:12–13, 1966.
88. Lund EE, Farr MM: Protozoa. *In* Hofstad M et al (eds): Infectious Diseases of Poultry, 5th ed., Ames, Iowa, Iowa State University Press, 1965, pp. 1056–1148.
89. Sileo L, Jr, Fitzhugh EL: Incidence of trichomoniosis in the band-tailed pigeons of southern Arizona. *Bull Wildlife Dis Assoc* 5:146, 1969.
90. Kocan RM, Herman CM: Trichomoniasis. *In* David JW, et al: Infectious and Parasitic Diseases of Wild Birds. Ames, Iowa, Iowa State University Press, 1971, pp. 282–290.
91. Rettig T: Trichomoniasis in a bald eagle *(Haliaeetus leucocephalus):* diagnosis and successful treatment with dimetridazole. *J Zoo Anim Med* 9:98–100, 1978.
92. Stone WB, Jones DE: Trichomoniasis in captive sparrow hawks. *Bull Wild Dis Assoc* 5:147, 1969.
93. Altman RB: Parasitic diseases of cage birds. *In* Kirk RW (ed): Current Veterinary Therapy VI. Small Animal Practice. Philadelphia, WB Saunders Co., 1977, pp. 682–687.
94. Greve JH: Parasitic diseases. *In* Fowler ME (ed): Zoo and Wild Animal Medicine. Philadelphia, WB Saunders Co., 1978, pp. 371–381.
95. Keymer IF: Parasitic diseases. *In* Petrak ML (ed): Diseases of Cage and Aviary Birds, 2nd ed. Philadelphia, Lea & Febiger, 1982, pp. 535–598.
96. Theobald J: Felidae. *In* Fowler ME (ed): Zoo and Wild Animal Medicine. Philadelphia, WB Saunders Co., 1978, pp. 650–667.
97. Sabine M, Hyne RHJ: Isolation of a feline picornavirus from cheetahs with conjunctivitis and glossitis. *Vet Rec* 87:794, 1970.
98. Heywood R: *Aeromonas* infections in snakes. *Cornell Vet* 58:236–241, 1968.

99. Burke TJ: Infectious stomatitis of snakes. *Proc Am Assoc Zoo Vet* 267–270, 1973.
100. Cowan DF: Diseases of captive reptiles. *J Am Vet Assoc* 153:848–859, 1968.
101. Kiel JL: A synopsis of some common bacterial diseases in snakes. *Southwest Vet* 27:33–36, 1974.
102. Richenback-Klinke H, Elkan E: The Principal Diseases of Lower Vertebrates. New York, Academic Press, 1965.
103. Wallach JD: Diseases of reptiles and their clinical management. *In* Kirk RW (ed): Current Veterinary Therapy IV. Philadelphia, WB Saunders Co., 1971, pp. 433–439.
104. Cooper JE: Bacteria. *In* Cooper JE, Jackson OF (eds): Diseases of the Reptiles, Vol. 1. New York, Academic Press, 1981, pp. 175–177.
105. Frye FL: Biomedical and Surgical Aspects of Captive Reptile Husbandry. Edwardsville, Kansas, Veterinary Medical Publishing Co., 1981.
106. Burke TJ: Infectious diseases of reptiles. *In* Fowler ME (ed): Zoo and Wild Animal Medicine. Philadelphia, WB Saunders Co., 1978, pp. 134–137.
107. Wallach JD: Mechanics of nutrition of exotic pets. *Vet Clin North Am* 9:405–414, 1979.
108. Tate CL, Conti PA, Nero EP: Focal epithelial hyperplasia in the oral mucosa of a chimpanzee. *J Am Vet Med Assoc* 163:619–621, 1973.
109. Fagan D, Oosterhuis J: Gingival hyperplasia induced by diphenylhydantoin in a gorilla. *J Am Vet Med Assoc* 175:960–961, 1979.
110. Harkness JE, Wagner JE: The Biology and Medicine of Rabbits and Rodents, 2nd ed. Philadelphia, Lea & Febiger, 1983, pp. 25–26.
111. Fagan DA: Oral disease in avian species. *Proc Am Assoc Zoo Vet* 30–32, 1981.
112. Arnall L: Conditions of the beak and claw in the budgerigar. *J Small Anim Pract* 6:135–144, 1965.
113. Altman RB: Conditions involving the integumentary system. *In* Petrak ML: Diseases of Cage and Aviary Birds, 2nd ed. Philadelphia, Lea & Febiger, 1982, pp. 368–371.
114. Sleamaker TF, Foster WR: Prosthetic beak for a salmon-crested cockatoo. *J Am Vet Med Assoc* 183:1300–1301.
115. Zenoble RD: Selected diseases of the head and face in caged birds. *Comp Cont Ed* 4:995–1004, 1982.
116. Woerpel RW, Rosskopf WJ, Jr, Holechek JD: Surgical repair of beak trauma in caged birds. *Vet Med Sm An Clin* 78:1068–1072, 1983.
117. Tollefson CI: Nutrition. *In* Petrak ML: Diseases of Caged and Aviary Birds, 2nd ed. Philadelphia, Lea & Febiger, 1982, pp. 220–249.
118. Amand WB: Personal communication, 1984.
119. Altman RB: Palatine and lingual abscesses in large psittacine birds. *Proc Am Assoc Zoo Vet* 127–130, 1967.
120. McCluggage D: Hypovitaminosis A associated with a sublingual abscess and dyphagia. *Proc Am Assoc Zoo Vet* 247–250, 1983.
121. Lord GH, Willson JE: Foreign body granuloma in a rhesus monkey. *J Am Vet Med Assoc* 153:910–913, 1968.
122. Amand WB, O'Brien JA, Tucker JA: Dysphagia in a woolly monkey *(Lagothrix lagothrica)* following a caustic esophageal burn. *J Am Vet Med Assoc* 157:706–711, 1970.
123. Effron M, Griner L, Benirschke K: Nature and rate of neoplasia found in captive wild animals, birds and reptiles at necropsy. *J Natl Cancer Inst* 5:185–198, 1977.
124. Snyder RL: Personnel communication, 1984.
125. Petrak ML, Gilmore CE: Neoplasms. *In* Petrak ML (ed): Diseases of Cage and Aviary Birds, 2nd ed., Philadelphia, Lea & Febiger, 1982, pp. 606–637.
126. Kollias GVJ: Tumors in zoo animals and wildlife. *In* Theilen GH, Madewell BR (eds): Veterinary Cancer Medicine. Philadelphia, Lea & Febiger, 1979, pp. 407–424.
127. Jacobson ER: Neoplastic diseases. *In* Cooper JE, Jackson OF (eds): Diseases of the Reptiles, Vol. 2. New York, Academic Press, 1981, pp. 429–468.
128. Perry RA, Bramhall A, Pass DA: Osteogenic sarcoma in the beak of a budgerigar *(Melopsittocus undulatus). Aust Vet Pract* 13:127, 1983.
129. Kast A: Malignes adenoameloblastom des gaumens bei einer tiger-python. *Frankfort Z Pathol* 7:135–140, 1967.
130. Marcus LC: Veterinary Biology and Medicine of Captive Amphibians and Reptiles. Philadelphia, Lea & Febiger, 1981.

Index

Note: Numbers in *italics* refer to illustrations; numbers followed by *t* indicate tables.